With contributions by

HAROLD ARLEN, M.D.
ARNOLD BERRETT, M.D.
ANDREW CANNISTRACI, D.D.S.
COSMO V. De STENO, D.M.D., Ph.D.
GEORGE EVERSAUL, Ph.D.
GEORGE FRITZ, Ed.D.
LAWRENCE A. FUNT, D.D.S., M.S.
SALLY GELB, B.A.
CLYDE A. HELMS, M.D.
RICHARD W. KATZBERG, M.D.
HANS KRAUS, M.D.
EDNA M. LAY, D.O.
MYRON LIEB, D.D.S.

PETER V. MADILL, M.D.
SIMON E. MARKOVICH, M.D.
EDWARD W. MARSH, D.M.D.
STEVEN G. MESSING, D.M.D.
HAROLD H. MOSAK, Ph.D.
HAROLD T. PERRY, D.D.S., Ph.D.
PAUL SCHEMAN, D.D.S.
ERIC P. SHABER, D.D.S.
LAWRENCE S. SONKIN, M.D., Ph.D.
BRENDAN STACK, D.D.S., M.S.
JEFFREY S. TARTE, D.D.S.
JOHN W. WITZIG, D.D.S.
IRA M. YERKES, D.M.D., M.S.

Clinical Management of
HEAD, NECK and TMJ PAIN and DYSFUNCTION

A MULTI-DISCIPLINARY APPROACH TO DIAGNOSIS AND TREATMENT

SECOND EDITION

Edited by
HAROLD GELB

Clinical Professor, University of Medicine and
 Dentistry of New Jersey,
Former Director, Temporomandibular Joint Clinic,
Department of Otolaryngology, New York Eye and
 Ear Infirmary, New York, New York

W. B. SAUNDERS COMPANY_____**1985**
PHILADELPHIA   LONDON   TORONTO   MEXICO CITY   RIO DEJANEIRO   SYDNEY   TOKYO

W. B. Saunders Company: West Washington Square
Philadelphia, PA   19105

1 St. Anne's Road
Eastbourne, East Sussex BN21 3UN, England

1 Goldthorne Avenue
Toronto, Ontario M8Z 5T9, Canada

Apartado 26370—Cedro 512
Mexico 4, D.F., Mexico

Rua Coronel Cabrita, 8
Sao Cristovao Caixa Postal 21176
Rio de Janeiro, Brazil

9 Waltham Street
Artarmon, N.S.W. 2064, Australia

Ichibancho, Central Bldg., 22-1 Ichibancho
Chiyoda-Ku, Tokyo 102, Japan

Library of Congress Cataloging in Publication Data
Main entry under title:

Clinical management of head, neck, and TMJ pain and dysfunction.

    Includes bibliographical references and index.
1. Head—Diseases. 2. Neck—Diseases. 3. Temporomandibular joint—Diseases. I. Gelb, Harold, 1925–   . II. Arlen,
Harold, 1932–   . III. Title: Head, neck, and TMJ pain and
dysfunction. IV. Title: Head, neck, and T.M.J. pain and
dysfunction. [DNLM: 1. Head. 2. Neck. 3. Pain. 4. Temporomandibular Joint Diseases. WU 140 C641]

RC936.C58   1985   617'.51   84–5600

ISBN 0–7216–4073–7

Clinical Management of Head, Neck and TMJ Pain and Dysfunction   ISBN   0–7216–4073–7

Last digit is the print number: 9   8   7   6   5   4   3   2   1

To
Sally, Michael, Lisa, and Cathy
whose patience and understanding simplified the task

CONTRIBUTORS

HAROLD ARLEN, M.D., F.A.C.S.
Associate Clinical Professor, University of Medicine and Dentistry of New Jersey, Rutgers Medical School, Newark, New Jersey; President, Medical/Dental Staff, John F. Kennedy Medical Center, Edison, New Jersey; Attending Physician, New York Eye and Ear Infirmary, New York, New York; Director of Otolaryngology, Muhlenberg Hospital, Plainfield, New Jersey
The Otomandibular Syndrome

ARNOLD BERRETT, M.D.
Associate Clinical Professor of Radiology, New York Medical College, New York, New York; Director of Radiology, Calvary Hospital, and Director of Radiology, Midtown Hospital, New York, New York
Radiology of the Temporomandibular Joint

ANDREW J. CANNISTRACI, D.D.S., F.A.C.D.
President, Biofeedback Society of New York, New York; Attending Dentist, Misericordia Hospital Medical Center, Bronx, New York
Biofeedback—The Treatment of Stress-Induced Muscle Activity

COSMO V. De STENO, D.M.D., Ph.D., F.A.C.D., F.A.C.P.
Clinical Professor of Prosthodontics, University of Medicine and Dentistry, School of Dentistry, Newark, New Jersey; Chief of Prosthodontics, Bergen Pines County Hospital, Paramus, New Jersey
The Pathophysiology of TMJ Dysfunction and Related Pain

GEORGE A. EVERSAUL, Ph.D.
Applied Kinesiology and the Treatment of TMJ Dysfunction

GEORGE FRITZ, Ed.D.
Director of Biofeedback Services, St. Luke's Hospital, Bethlehem, Pennsylvania
Biofeedback—The Treatment of Stress-Induced Muscle Activity

LAWRENCE A. FUNT, D.D.S., M.S.D.
Director, the Craniofacial Pain Center of Washington, Washington, D.C.; Lecturer, U.S. Naval Hospital, Bethesda, Maryland and Walter Reed Army Hospital, Washington, D.C.; Consultant, Monsaud Clinic, Baltimore, Maryland
Myofunctional Therapy in the Treatment of the Craniomandibular Syndrome

HAROLD GELB, D.M.D.
Clinical Professor, University of Medicine and Dentistry of New Jersey, Newark, New Jersey; Former Director, TMJ Clinic, New York Eye and Ear Infirmary, New York, New York
Patient Evaluation; Effective Management and Treatment of the Craniomandibular Syndrome; Conclusion

SALLY GELB, B.A.
Assistant Professor, University of Medicine and Dentistry of New Jersey, Newark, New Jersey
Myofunctional Therapy in the Treatment of the Craniomandibular Syndrome

CLYDE A. HELMS, M.D.
Associate Professor, Department of Radiology, University of California, San Francisco, California; Consultant, Department of Radiology, Veterans Administration Medical Center, San Francisco, California; Consultant, Department of Radiology, San Francisco General Hospital, San Francisco, California; Consultant, Department of Radiology, United States Air Force, Travis Air Force Base, Fairfield, California
Arthrography of the Temporomandibular Joint; The Significance of CT Scanning of the Temporomandibular Joint.

RICHARD W. KATZBERG, M.D.
Assistant Professor of Radiology, University of Rochester, School of Medicine and Dentistry, Rochester, New York; Clinical and Research Associate, Eastman Dental Center, Rochester, New York
Arthrography of the Temporomandibular Joint

HANS KRAUS, M.D.
Formerly Associate Professor of Physical Medicine, New York University, New York, New York
Muscular Aspects of Oral Dysfunction

EDNA M. LAY, D.O., F.A.A.O.
Associate Professor of Osteopathic Theory and Methods, Kirksville College of Osteopathic Medicine, Kirksville, Missouri; Consultant, Department of Osteopathic Manipulative Medicine, Kirksville Osteopathic Hospital, Kirksville, Missouri
The Osteopathic Management of Temporomandibular Joint Dysfunction

MYRON M. LIEB, D.D.S., F.A.G.D., F.I.C.D.
Director, Institute for Graduate Dentists, New York, New York
Oral Orthopedics

PETER V. MADILL, M.D.
Attending Physician, Palm Drive Hospital, Sebastopol, California
Traditional and Modern Acupuncture Modalities in the Diagnosis and Treatment of the Temporomandibular Joint Syndrome

SIMON E. MARKOVICH, M.D.
Clinical Associate Professor of Neurology, University of Miami School of Medicine, Miami, Florida; Senior Attending Neurologist, Cedars Medical Center, Miami, Florida; Consultant Neurologist, Mercy Hospital, Miami, Florida; Consultant Neurologist, Mt Sinai Medical Center, Miami Beach, Florida
Pain in the Head: A Neurological Appraisal

E. W. MARSH, D.M.D., M.S.
Private practice
Functional Considerations in Early Limited Orthodontic Procedures

STEVEN G. MESSING, D.M.D.
Private practice limited to periodontics and TMJ disorders, Albany, New York; Attending and Co-director of TMJ Clinic, St. Peter's Hospital, Albany, New York; Consultant, Sunnyview Hospital, Schenectady, New York
Arthrography of the Temporomandibular Joint

HAROLD H. MOSAK, Ph.D.
Professor, Alfred Adler Institute, Chicago, Illinois; Consultant, VA Hospital, Hines, Illinois; Consultant, VA Hospital, North Chicago, Illinois; Consultant, West Side VA Hospital, Chicago, Illinois
Does a "TMJ Personality" Exist?

H. T. PERRY, D.D.S., Ph.D.
Professor and Chairman, Department of Orthodontics, Northwestern University Dental School, Chicago, Illinois; Staff, Northwestern University Hospitals, Chicago, Illinois
Functional Considerations in Early Limited Orthodontic Procedures

MARIANO ROCABADO, P.T.
Professor and Physical Therapist, School of Dentistry, University of Chile, Santiago, Chile; Physical Therapist, Department of Maxillofacial Prosthesis and Traumatology, José Joaquin Aguirre University of Chile Hospital, Santiago, Chile
Arthrokinematics of the Temporomandibular Joint

PAUL SCHEMAN, D.D.S.
Director of Medical/Dental Affairs, Kingsbrook Jewish Medical Center, Brooklyn, New York
Radiography of the Temporomandibular Joint; Surgery of the Temporomandibular Articulation

ERIC PAUL SHABER, D.D.S.
Associate Professor, Oral and Maxillofacial Surgery, University of the
Pacific, San Francisco, California; Attending Maxillofacial Surgeon, Pacific
Medical Center, San Francisco, California; Attending Surgeon, Mt. Zion
Medical Center, San Francisco, California; Attending Surgeon, Veterans
Administration Medical Center, San Francisco, California; Consultant in
Oral and Maxillofacial Surgery, University of California, Irvine, California;
Consultant in Oral and Maxillofacial Surgery, Veterans Administration
Medical Center, Long Beach, California
The Significance of CT Scanning of the Temporomandibular Joint

LAWRENCE S. SONKIN, M.D., Ph.D.
Associate Attending Physician and Clinical Associate Professor of Medicine,
Division of Endocrinology, The New York Hospital, Cornell Medical Center,
New York, New York
Endocrine Disorders and Muscle Dysfunction

BRENDAN STACK, D.D.S., M.S.
Director, National Capital Center for Craniofacial Pain, Vienna, Virginia
Myofunctional Therapy in the Treatment of the Craniomandibular Syndrome

JEFFREY S. TARTE, D.D.S.
Attending Dentist, Department of Otolaryngology, New York Eye and Ear
Infirmary, New York, New York
The Role of Hypnosis in the Treatment of Craniomandibular Dysfunction

JOHN W. WITZIG, D.D.S.
Visiting Lecturer, Tufts University College of Dental Medicine, Boston,
Massachusetts and University of South Carolina College of Dental Medicine,
Charleston, South Carolina
Functional Jaw Orthopedics

IRA M. YERKES, D.M.D., M.S.
Clinical Instructor, Department of Orthodontics, Tufts University School of
Dental Medicine, Boston, Massachusetts
Functional Jaw Orthopedics

PREFACE

Some 10 years ago, I perceived the need for a book that would bring to the attention of all health professionals the most current clinical knowledge about the diagnosis and treatment of head, neck, and jaw disorders. All of us who have been involved in its preparation hope that this book will meet that need and that the concepts, diagnostic procedures, and therapeutic approaches presented herein will help health professionals provide total care of acutely and chronically ill patients.

We have attempted to overcome certain shortcomings of the traditional health care orientation by crossing specialty and professional boundaries, so that practitioners and students in all the fields covered in this book may benefit from the expertise of those in separate but related specialties. We have also attempted to impress upon the reader the need to train as many health specialists as possible in the care of patients with chronic illness.

Good fortune has blessed me with as fine a group of contributors as could be assembled at one time, and I am deeply grateful to them. All of us are indebted to the many people who, through team work, made significant contributions that were responsible for development of the concepts on which this book is based and the procedures described in it. Space does not permit listing of all of them, but I would like to mention certain individuals and groups whose influence over the last 25 years has been important to me. They are Willie B. May, D.D.S.; George Goodheart, D.C., the founder of the International College of Applied Kinesiology; the American Equilibration Society; the American Academy of Craniomandibular Disorders; Victor Stoll and the group for Orthopedic Research in Dentistry; Janet G. Travell, M.D.; Bernard Jankelson, D.D.S.; and the Sutherland Cranial Academy.

I owe special thanks to Joshua Johnson for his help with photography and to Carole Ping Thompson for her illustrations.

I am grateful to my wonderful office staff and to my personal secretary, Cathy Ward.

I am thankful to Carroll Cann, Sandy Reinhardt, and the many others at the W. B. Saunders Company who made all this possible.

And I thank my wife, Sally, my best friend and confidante, whose encouragement, patience, and devotion enabled me to complete this endeavor.

HAROLD GELB

It is not the critic who counts; not the man who points out how the strong man stumbled or where the doer of deeds could have done them better. The credit belongs to the man who is actually in the arena; whose face is marred by dust and sweat and blood; who strives valiantly; who errs and comes short again and again; who knows the great enthusiasms, the great devotions, and spends himself in a worthy cause; who, at the best, knows the triumph of high achievement; and who, at the worst, if he fails, at least fails while daring greatly so that his place shall never be with those cold and timid souls who knew neither victory nor defeat.

Theodore Roosevelt

CONTENTS

INTRODUCTION

Sound knowledge of neuromuscular function and dysfunction, and of psychosomatic influences, is necessary in order to treat syndromes of the craniomandibular complex successfully. In keeping with the theme of this book, namely, to develop the link between the various specialty areas of dentistry and medicine using the neuromuscular mechanism, the chapters that follow will address themselves to these relationships primarily on a clinical basis.

At present, a patient with facial or head pain first consults his family physician or internist, and a patient with ear, head, or neck symptoms consults an otolaryngologist, neurologist, or orthopedist. These practitioners, well aware of the complexity of symptomatology, try to rule out the etiological factors one by one. If the cause is found, it is treated immediately, and the symptoms subside. There are many cases that do not respond to treatment, however, and it is in these that the craniomandibular factors are often overlooked. This situation is encountered not only by medical specialists to whom the patient may be referred but also by family dentists.

Knowledge, experience, and proper training are most necessary in order to recognize the symptoms produced in the head and neck area by various conditions such as dental malocclusion with or without malposition of the jaw, loss of teeth, decrease in vertical distance between the jaws, poorly fitting dental prostheses, erratic eruption patterns, pipe clenching, abnormal swallowing, other injurious oral habits, unilateral mastication, and disease of the temporomandibular joints. One of the chief causes of head and neck pain is muscle spasm caused by such factors as mandibular malposition, muscle incoordination, and stress-induced bruxism and clenching.

It will readily be seen that much of what we know today of the etiology, diagnosis, and treatment of the temporomandibular joint syndrome is not new. Many major texts on this subject have been written by competent investigators, such as Sarnat and Laskin; Schwartz; Bell; Shore; Freese and Scheman; Grieder and Cinotti; Solberg and Clark; Morgan, Vamras, and Hall, and Zarb and Carlsson.

Recommended procedures for diagnosing and treating temporomandibular joint disorders, as described in the literature, most often reflect an approach influenced by the background and specialty practice area of the investigator. Not only must the maxillomandibular relations be checked, along with radiographic examination of the joints, but a complete history and physical examination are necessary. It is my belief that if the clinician permits the patient to tell his or her story, even before a detailed examination is made, the patient will tell you not only what is wrong, but also exactly how it should be treated. The need is only to listen.

A multiprofessional approach is necessary for the successful resolution of the craniomandibular syndrome. There is no place for intellectual isolationism in the holistic approach to the diagnosis and treatment of this clinical entity.

In essence, a new specialty area is appearing, that of the "pain doctors," the physicians, dentists, osteopaths, and other health professionals who are devoting their careers to the examination, study, and treatment of pain.

Dr. Arthur Freese, in his book entitled *Pain,* states, "When you consider that the practice of medicine is essentially the treatment of pain—the painful head, the painful appendix, the painful gall bladder or leg—then the doctor-patient relationship can be understood as a pain relationship. And the doctor is at his weakest dealing with chronic pain."

Dr. John J. Bonica, who heads the Pain Clinic at the University of Washington School of Medicine, states that "hundreds of thousands of suffering patients are not getting the relief they deserve. Others are subjected to a very high risk of accidental complications from improper therapy—like narcotic addiction, multiple, often useless, at times mutilating operations. Some of course give up medical care and go to quacks and spend an awful lot of money, and some even commit suicide." Dr. Bonica believes the reasons for this are that we have great gaps in our knowledge and that what we already know is being poorly utilized. The professional schools in this country have few courses, if any, devoted to the treatment and management of chronic pain states.

It will be the endeavor of this book to fill some of the voids that exist in the clinical management of the patient with chronic pain.

No attempt will be made to go into extensive discussions of the anatomic, physiologic, or histologic aspects of the subject matter, since that has been done many times before in the literature.

HAROLD GELB

The Pathophysiology of TMJ Dysfunction and Related Pain

COSMO V. De STENO, D.M.D., Ph.D.

In order to treat a diseased state effectively we must first arrive at a diagnosis which has been determined by careful scrutiny of those signs and symptoms presented by the patient. The ability to assimilate data compiled through clinical examination, medical and dental histories, and radiographic analysis is fundamental. More critical, however, is the ability to correlate this information to specific pathological alterations of the involved tissues. With specific reference to temporomandibular joint (TMJ) dysfunction, it is of paramount importance to have a working knowledge of the anatomy, physiology and biochemistry of the occlusion, musculature of the head and neck, and related TM joint structures before an adequate determination of pathological changes can be made.

Once the pathological alterations are determined, treatment should follow to return the affected tissues to a normal physiological state. Treatment procedures should be specific and not of a random nature.

This chapter will develop a concept designed to account for the three conditions necessary for TM joint dysfunction: predisposition, tissue alteration, and psychological dependence. These conditions will be referred to collectively as "the TMJ triad."

THE TMJ TRIAD

To understand the etiology and management of TMJ dysfunction we must understand those components that, when present in certain relation to each other, cause the precipitation of pain and dysfunction. These compo-

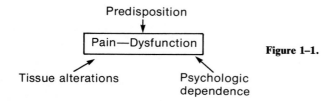

Figure 1–1.

nents can be categorized into the following three groups: (1) predisposition, (2) tissue alterations, and (3) psychological dependence (Fig. 1–1).

For TMJ dysfunction to be diagnosed all three components of the triad must be present. That is, the patient must be predisposed to TMJ dysfunction, the tissues (neuromuscular, skeletal, and dental) must be in some degree of pathological alteration, and lastly, there must exist a degree of stress sufficient to cause excessive muscle tension, clenching and/or bruxing of the teeth. The triad is potentially present in all individuals (Fig. 1–2). Not until all three components become involved do we see any clinical manifestation of TMJ syndrome. Once the triad develops, the syndrome precipitates and we observe the symptoms of TMJ dysfunction (Fig. 1–3). For example, an individual may be genetically predisposed to acquiring TMJ dysfunction. During his early life the occlusal relationship of the teeth changed, causing an altered maxillo-mandibular relationship.

We now have two of the three components necessary for the completion of the triad—predisposition and tissue alteration (Fig. 1–4). However, the level of stress necessary to complete the triad does not exist, and precipitation of the syndrome will not occur. When the level of psychological stress increases so that the degree of bruxing and clenching abnormally works and stresses the musculature, the triad is complete (Fig. 1–5).

Furthermore, we must consider not only existence but also degree. An intense individual may exhibit numerous wear facets (indicative of moderate to severe bruxing) and radiographic evidence of an altered condyle-fossa relationship, but may present no clinical symptoms of pain or dysfunction. In this case, predisposition may be absent (Fig. 1–6A) or not of a sufficient degree (Fig. 1–6B).

The degree of predisposition, tissue alterations, or psychological de-

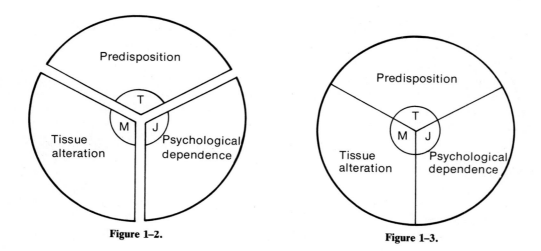

Figure 1–2.

Figure 1–3.

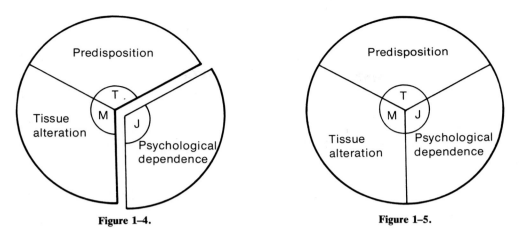

Figure 1–4.　　　　　　　　Figure 1–5.

pendence necessary for precipitation of the syndrome is unique to the individual (Fig. 1–6C, D). Similarly, we may find an individual exhibiting minimal levels of the triad or its individual components but suffering from a severe case of TMJ dysfunction (Fig. 1–7A, B, C). This example further illustrates the levels necessary for precipitation of dysfunction. Pain varies

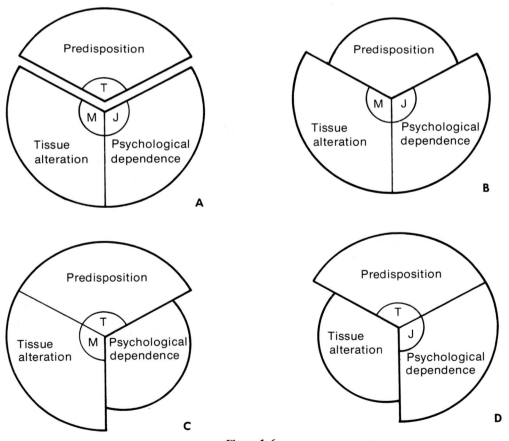

Figure 1–6.

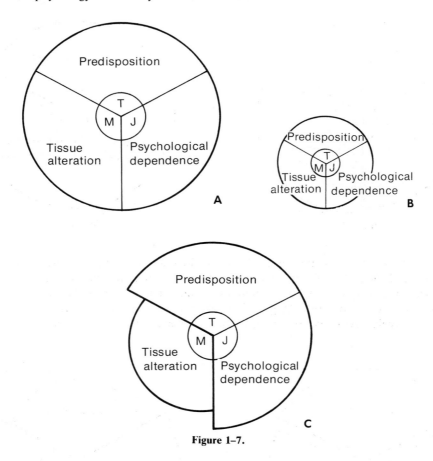

Figure 1–7.

between individuals and, in fact, can vary in the same individual on a temporal basis.

In summary, the existence of the three members composing the TMJ triad is necessary to precipitate TMJ dysfunction. The variables in this principle arise from the degree or contribution of each necessary to complete the triad for a particular individual. This variability in degree accounts for the difference between individuals as well as in the same individual at various times.

If the etiology of TMJ dysfunction is accepted to be the existence of a TMJ triad, then treatment should be directed toward removing one of its components or at least reducing its severity so that the triad is not complete. For example, drug therapy, i.e., tranquilizers, may be employed to reduce tension and stress (bruxism, clenching), thereby eliminating or reducing the psychological component (Fig. 1–6C). A mandibular orthopedic appliance may be utilized to reestablish the maxillo-mandibular relationship and reduce the destructive forces resulting from grinding or clenching of the teeth (Fig. 1–6D).

Thus we can understand how the TMJ triad explains much of the existing controversy over the various modalities of treating TMJ dysfunction that appear to have the same degree of effectiveness.

Let us now discuss each member of the triad relative to the physiological basis for the occurrence and treatment.

Figure 1-8.

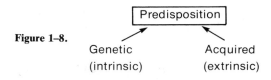

PREDISPOSITION

By definition[1] predisposition is "a condition of special susceptibility." When considering predisposition as a member of the TMJ triad we must further separate this component into two very distinct categories: genetic or intrinsic predisposition and acquired or extrinsic predisposition (Fig. 1–8).

GENETIC (INTRINSIC) PREDISPOSITION

Genetic (intrinsic) predisposition is considered to be a special susceptibility inherent in the individual through cellular specificity. Genetic predisposition would involve the muscles and their neuromuscular mechanisms, the ligaments and tendons, the skeletal structures, including the TM joints, and psychological factors. Familial consideration of symptoms related to TMJ dysfunction would aid in revealing genetic predisposition.

Muscular and Neuromuscular Predisposition

The muscles of the head and neck are either directly or indirectly involved with mandibular movement. The muscles of mastication—the masseter, temporalis, external (lateral) pterygoid, and the internal (medial) pterygoid—are primarily responsible for mandibular movement. The suprahyoid muscle group—the digastric, mylohyoid, geniohyoid, and stylohyoid muscles—are also involved in mandibular movements. The muscles of mastication are innervated by the mandibular division of the fifth (trigeminal) cranial nerve, which is also the sensory nerve for these muscles. Developmental deficiencies in any of these muscles would create conditions in which they are less able to cope with stressful situations foreign to their normal biochemical and physiological processes.

Congenital defects in skeletal muscles can range from general weakness to absence of the whole or part of muscles. It appears that any muscle can occasionally be absent, with absence of the sternocostal portions of the pectoral muscles being most common,[2] followed by slightness or absence of the trapezius.[3] Congenital absence of the pterygoids and masseter has also been reported.[4] Although these instances are relatively uncommon and usually discovered early in life, they exemplify conditions possibly existent in certain individuals.

The most common example of congenital weakness involves the levator palpebrae,[5] which clinically manifests as a slight narrowing of the palpebral slit to ptosis of the eyelid. These conditions may indicate liability to myotonic dystrophy and should be held suspect in clinical examinations. In some cases, movement of the jaw is accompanied by an elevation of the ptosed eyelid. This combined movement has been termed "jaw winking phenomenon" of

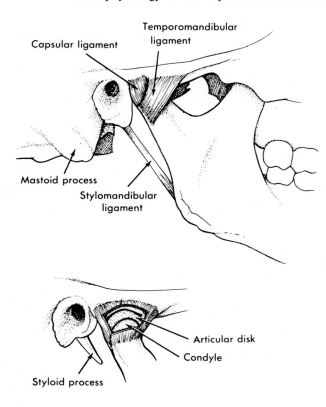

Figure 1–9. Ligaments and articular disk of the temporomandibular joints. (From Grieder, A., and Cinotti, W. R.: Periodontal Prosthesis. St. Louis, C. V. Mosby Co., 1968. Reprinted by permission.)

Marcus Gunn.[6] The eyelid is elevated when the jaw is opened strongly and descends when it is closed. Finally, facial diplegia can presumably result from a primary aplasia of jaw muscles or be secondary to a neural or spinal deficiency.[7]

LIGAMENTS

Ligaments determine the direction in which muscle action is transmitted to the moving surfaces of joints and maintain the integrity and stability of the joint. Increased vulnerability to joint dysfunction can result from a constitutional and/or congenital variation of ligaments. A generalized connective tissue weakness due to deficiencies in the collagenous proteins can result in joint weakness. Inadequate form and size of ligaments also predispose joints to dysfunction. Internal derangement of joints can arise from instability of the joint due to ligament damage or weakness.[8] Collectively, these situations contribute to premature degeneration of the joints.

JOINT DEVELOPMENT

Although condylar growth ceases by approximately the twenty-first year, remodeling of the articular surfaces continues throughout the lifetime in response to stresses placed on them.[9] Because of the bilateral nature of the TM joints, unilateral alteration in the growth patterns or remodeling can affect normal joint function. If the development of the joint is not coordinated with growth of the muscles and development and eruption of teeth, an inherent functional deficiency exists. The resulting altered relationship will affect the ability of the joint to function. This is especially critical during those periods when the joint is subjected to abnormal stressful situations.

CALCIFIED TISSUES

The integrity of the alveolar bone and the teeth within it are two significant principles in considering a patient's predisposition to TM joint dysfunction. Since bruxism is a major factor in TM joint dysfunction, the ability of the alveolar bone to endure traumatic and parafunctional forces may determine whether a patient will suffer from periodontal disease or TM joint dysfunction. If the alveolar bone is strong and resistant to resorption, the TM joints will absorb the brunt of the destructive forces of bruxism and clenching. Conversely, if the alveolar bone is more susceptible to resorption, periodontal disease will develop as the primary problem, not TM joint dysfunction.

The skeletal portions of the TM joints are governed by genetic controls similar to those governing the alveolar bone. The ability of the joint structures to withstand destructive forces initiating degenerative changes will depend on where it lies in the ladder of susceptibility. The destructive forces will seek the least resistant member of the TM joints and related structures.

PSYCHOLOGICAL STRESS

In susceptible individuals, psychological stress cannot be readily coped with, resulting in symptoms of anxiety neurosis and depression.[10] Personality traits resulting in intense personalities contribute to bruxism and clenching of the teeth, resulting in more severe stress placed on the TM joints and related tissues.

ACQUIRED (EXTRINSIC) PREDISPOSITION

Acquired or extrinsic predisposition can be defined as a special susceptibility brought about by traumatic injuries to the TM joints and related structures or by some pathological alteration of the systemic milieu vital to the normal functioning of the TM joints and related structures.

TRAUMATIC INJURIES

Trauma to the structures or growth centers of the TM joints can be as innocuous as a blow to the jaw causing a depressed growth rate of one condyle relative to the other, or as severe as fractures of the condyle. Trauma to the growth centers of the developing condyle can result in asymmetry of the two condylar heads. This would predispose the TM joints to dysfunction by initiating uncoordinated bilateral movements. Trauma can also result in monoarticular arthritis, usually called a sprain or a dislocation.[11]

A forward dislocation can actually tear the capsular ligaments as well as permanently detach the meniscus.

Condylar head fractures, although rare, can occur and may result in partial ankylosis of the condylar head and glenoid fossa.

These situations obviously change the relationship of the condyle and glenoid fossa, resulting in an altered maxillo-mandibular relationship.

Trauma to Ligaments

The capsular ligament (articular capsule)[10] and temporomandibular ligament surround the joint and determine the direction in which the joint can move. This fibrous capsule is composed mainly of collagen, which is relatively avascular. Although ligaments are designed to tolerate intermittent forces associated with joint motion, they can be stretched and permanently distorted as a result of a constant forceful load. In fact, exposure to abnormal nonphysiological pressures or tensions can actually damage or tear ligaments. Because of the limited blood supply, the repair of damaged ligaments is slow or nonexistent (see Fig. 1–9).[12]

Analogous to damage of the TM joint capsule are the problems associated with the ligaments of the knee joint. There seem to be structural variations which predispose knees of certain athletes to traumatic injury. Variations in form and size of the ligaments, as well as a generalized connective tissue weakness, have been reported.[13] Once ligaments are damaged, instability of the joint and internal derangement occur.

The range of external forces causing damage to ligaments can be as severe as whiplash-type damage caused by automobile accidents to more innocuous forces of parafunctional joint movements and even prolonged dental visits.

Trauma To Muscles

Acquired predisposition to TM joint dysfunction through traumatic injuries to those muscles associated with normal function would result in pathological alterations, causing aberrations in normal muscle function. Traumatic muscle disease at one extreme can result from an external force, such as a violent exertion causing a tear in muscle fibers or groups of fibers. The trapezius and sternomastoid are more susceptible to tearing or rupture than are other muscles of the head and neck.[14] However, myopathy can be a result of local trauma, such as vigorous massage, causing focal pathology within the muscle.[15] Needling muscles, that is the penetration of muscle fibers with hypodermic type needles, can produce focal inflammatory myopathic changes which could ultimately lead to ischemic necrosis of these areas.[16]

Factors determining the manner in which a muscle reacts to extrinsic force are as follows:[17]

MUSCLE GROUP. Generally, the muscles associated with gross movements are composed of larger muscle fibers and are less susceptible to external destructive forces. Conversely, muscles associated with fine, delicate movements are composed of small fibers of greater numbers and are more prone to degenerative changes.[17]

DEVELOPMENTAL MATURITY. The younger the groups of muscle fibers exposed to trauma, the less resistant they are to pathologic change.

Acute or chronic durations of forces to muscle will significantly alter the response these muscles exhibit to destruction.

REGENERATION OR DEGENERATION. Whether a muscle reacts to trauma by regeneration, i.e., replacing the damaged fibers, or by degeneration, in which the damaged fibers are replaced by some type of scar tissue, depends on the type of trauma and the nature of the muscle affected. Complete regeneration is obviously the more favorable repair process, since the normal architecture is unchanged, resulting in normal muscle contraction with no signs of limited function. Regeneration is usually limited to areas of minor damage which are discrete in size. Degenerative repair, on the other hand, may leave the damaged area replaced with scar tissue or even a calcified nodule. This will interfere with normal contraction and neuromuscular response of these tissues, thus altering their normal function.

The most common cause of muscle damage results from violent exertions in which opposing muscle groups are brought into action simultaneously. Prolonged exercise or exertion in the untrained muscle, such as repeated strong contractions, may cause local ischemic areas.

PATHOLOGICAL CHANGES

All pathological states attributable to nutritional, hormonal, or metabolic alterations of normal tissues can ultimately be traced to biochemical changes of the individual cell. In muscles, we are concerned with those changes related to the individual muscle fiber. In the TM joint, we are concerned with the ability of the bony structures to resist transient alterations in nutritional and hormonal requirements necessary for cellular balance.

Nutritional Requirements

When the term nutrition is used, one usually thinks of undernutrition. The dietary intake is important during development of tissues to insure proper growth and development of tissues, especially in the skeletal and neuromuscular systems.[18] Deficiencies during the developmental phase can severely affect bone and muscle growth, as seen in vitamin D and vitamin C deficiencies, respectively. Muscle tissue is uniquely susceptible to nutritional deficiencies, especially when we consider that half the total body weight is represented by muscle tissue. Few tissues are more complex with regard to metabolic interactions and structural organization for maintenance and functional activity.

The following are important nutritional factors that should be considered when diagnosing and treating TM joint dysfunction.

Protein

Proteins are required by the animal body mainly to replace tissue proteins broken down in normal metabolic processes as well as for building new tissues. The source of protein is important. Grade I proteins are animal proteins found in meat, fish, and eggs. They contain amino acids in approximately the proportions required for protein synthesis and muscle maintenance and development.[19] Although some plant proteins are Grade I, most are classified as Grade II. Grade II proteins have different proportions of amino acids, and some lack one or more of the essential amino acids. Protein needs can be met with a mixture of Grade II proteins, but the intake must be large since there is significant amino acid wastage.[20] It is essential to evaluate the patient's dietary intake to ensure that adequate levels of Grade I proteins are being consumed.

Vitamin C (Ascorbic Acid)

Scurvy is the disease most commonly associated with vitamin C deficiencies. Degeneration of skeletal muscle has been recognized as a feature of human scurvy and is considered secondary to intramuscular hemorrhage and trauma. Although scurvy is virtually nonexistent in our society, subclinical vitamin C deficiencies can alter normal muscular activity. The masseter muscle has a relatively high susceptibility to vitamin C deficiency.[21]

Vitamin D

Vitamin D is concerned primarily with the absorption of calcium (Ca) and phosphate (PO_4) from the intestinal tract as well as the formation and maintenance of the calcified tissues of the body. The main action of vitamin D is facilitation of intestinal absorption of calcium, although this vitamin has a direct effect on bone. Vitamin D deficiency causes the protein matrix (collagen) of new bone not to calcify. This is responsible for the most common disease of children with vitamin D deficiency, rickets.

A deficiency also affects the growth and development of jaws and joint structures. Muscles would be affected secondarily by vitamin D deficiency by causing a lowered serum Ca level. Lowered serum calcium affects the normal contractions of muscles, as explained below.

Vitamin E

In 1928 a paralysis in the offspring of rats with a vitamin E deficiency was reported.[22] These animals responded dramatically to vitamin E therapy, which returned the affected muscles to normal. Since that observation, vitamin E has established itself as a prominent factor in preserving the integrity of skeletal muscle fibers.

Calcium

Calcium, in conjunction with phosphorus, constitutes the inorganic solid phase of bones and teeth. A constant concentration of calcium ions in the extracellular fluids is essential for normal neuromuscular function, blood clotting, and a variety of enzymatic reactions.[23]

The mineral in bone is mainly in the crystalline phase of hydroxyapatite, although more immature bone contains considerable quantities of amorphous (noncrystalline) Ca and PO_4 mineral. Throughout life the mineral in the skeleton is being actively turned over by a constant resorption and remodeling of bone. The balance of formation and resorption is maintained by two hormones, parathyroid hormone and calcitonin. Skeletal growth dependence on normal serum calcium levels is emphasized if we consider growth of the condyle to be by endochondral ossification, similar to the epiphysis of large bones. Condylar growth continues until approximately the twenty-first year. However, the contours of the articulating surfaces of the condyle and the articular eminence are reshaped throughout life in response to stresses placed upon them. Interference of this process by limited calcium availability can result in aberrations in condylar formation with the possibility of altered joint functions. Calcium metabolism is critically important when discussing TMJ dysfunction because normal serum levels are essential for maintaining the proper functioning of the skeletal and neuromuscular systems. The free, ionized calcium in body fluids is necessary for normal skeletal muscle contraction and nerve function. A decrease in extracellular calcium at the myoneural junction inhibits transmission, but there is an additional effect of low Ca on nerve and muscle cells.[24] There is an excitatory effect called tetany, which in its early stages may manifest itself as a subtle eyelid twitch. The discharge of Ca in a muscle cell is believed to trigger the interaction of ATP with the thick and thin myofilaments (see section on Neuromuscular Changes), which is one of the primary steps for muscle contraction. Conversely, muscle relaxation is a result of the depletion of Ca by the mitochondria of the muscle cell.[25] It is therefore apparent that calcium plays an important role in TMJ dysfunction by its direct effect on the skeletal and neuromuscular systems.

Phosphate

This essential constituent of all living organisms is relatively abundant in most food products. As a result, phosphate deficiency in man is rare. Organic phosphorus is involved in a large number of metabolic processes concerned with the conservation and transfer of energy. Inorganic phosphate is necessary for normal skeletal and dental formation and maintenance. It should be noted that phytates, an organic form of phosphorus found in unprocessed wheat, has a great affinity for calcium.[26] This is potentially hazardous to normal calcium absorption in the intestine, especially if the individual's calcium intake is limited. Consuming large quantities of whole wheat products containing significant levels of phytates will bind calcium, reducing the amounts of calcium absorbed through the intestinal wall. This can result in diminished calcium levels in the serum, affecting normal skeletal and neuromuscular integrity.

Other Nutritional Factors

Vitamin B_6

Deficiency in vitamin B_6 will cause interference with phosphorylase activity in the muscle cell. Phosphorylase is an enzyme necessary in the reaction for energy production in muscle contraction.

Potassium

Low potassium levels are more specifically related to abnormal cardiac muscle activity, although skeletal muscles are dependent on adequate potassium for normal neuromuscular activity.

Magnesium

Magnesium is necessary as a catalyst in many metabolic reactions, especially those of energy production necessary for muscle cell contraction. Deficiencies in magnesium can cause hyaline necrosis of a muscle cell resulting from defects in enzyme reactions.[27]

ENDOCRINE SYSTEM

The endocrine system is composed of a group of glands which secrete specific chemical substances (hormones) into the circulation. Hormones stimulate the development and activity of specific tissues, contribute to maintenance and homeostasis, and exert regulatory effects on enzymatic reactions. Changes in levels of circulatory hormones can alter an individual's response to stress on the muscles of mastication and related TM joint structures. This is dramatically apparent with changes in female hormones during menstruation or menopause, especially if one considers that 80 per cent of reported TM joint cases occur in women over 40 years of age.[28] Changes in the normal hormone levels are related to derangements of enzyme systems within the muscle cell, although the hormones' action at the cellular level is not completely known. Chemically, effects of hormonal imbalances are manifested by muscle weakness and paralysis, or by the opposite, spasm of the whole muscle or isolated groups of fibers. Morphological changes are, however, minimal.

Estrogens

Feminization in the adolescent female is caused by increasing amounts of estrogen secretion. Deficiencies in estrogens are characterized by nervousness, increased muscle tension, flashes, muscle pain, and fatigue. In women, muscular strength decreases a few days before the menstrual cycle and continues through the end of the cycle.[29]

Androgens

This hormone exerts masculinizing effects and promotes protein anabolism and growth. Testosterone, the most active androgen, is secreted by the testes and adrenal gland. However, adrenal androgens are only one-fifth as active as testicular androgens.

Thyroid Hormones

The thyroid gland maintains the level of metabolism in tissues optimal for normal function. Muscles are affected when thyroxine secretion is either increased or decreased. In hyperthyroidism we see tremor, eye symptoms, nervousness, weight loss, and sweating. Severe cases may mimic poliomyelitis. General muscle effects are weakness and fatigability. Hypothyroidism is also characterized by muscular weakness but with additional symptoms of stiffness, aches, cramps, and spasms.[30] More frequently, we see the muscle mass increasing in size and becoming firmer than usual.

Calcitonin

Calcitonin is secreted from the parafollicular cells of the thyroid gland. Calcitonin lowers plasma calcium and phosphate, apparently by inhibiting the resorption of bone. Excesses and/or deficiencies of this hormone have not yet proven to be clinically significant.

Adrenal Gland

The adrenal gland is actually two glands in one, the adrenal cortex and adrenal medulla. The adrenal medulla secretes epinephrine and norepinephrine. Although these hormones are not essential for life, they do prepare the individual to deal with stressful emergency situations. Their relationship to TM joint dysfunction seems to be minimal.

The adrenal cortex secretes steroid hormones. There are three groups of steroid hormones, the glucocorticoids (affect metabolism of carbohydrates and proteins), mineralocorticoids (essential for sodium balance), and androgens and estrogens (minor effects on reproductive system). Of the glucocorticoids, cortisol and cortisone act predominantly on organic metabolism in a catabolic manner. Absence or low levels of cortisol, as in adrenal cortical insufficiency, cause muscle weakness and muscle cramps.[31] These symptoms are caused by decreased blood flow. Increased levels of glucocorticoids, as in Cushing's disease, also cause generalized muscular weakness. This weakness is a result of muscular atrophy of the muscles due to the catabolic (antianabolic) effect of cortisone.

Parathyroid Gland

There are usually four glands situated at the posterior surface of the thyroid gland. Parathyroid hormone regulates calcium metabolism and plasma calcium concentrations through a few mechanisms. One important mechanism is to promote bone resorption initiating the release of calcium and phosphate and to increase phosphate excretion by the kidney. The parathyroid glands maintain a stable calcium concentration despite wide variations in calcium balance and bone metabolism.

Hyperparathyroidism and hypercalcemia result in muscular weakness and fatigability,[32] due to disorders in calcium metabolism. Calcium is necessary for normal muscle contraction and relaxation. Changes in the levels of available calcium in the muscle cell will interfere with normal contraction and relaxation of the cell.

TISSUE ALTERATIONS

Of the three components that make up the TMJ triad, tissue alterations represent the variable most within the control of the practitioner. As previously stated, predisposition establishes the susceptibility of the patient acquiring TMJ dysfunction. The psychological component "primes" the patient to enable the tissue component to initiate the processes that start the TMJ dysfunction cycle. The pathological alterations in the skeletal, dental, and neuromuscular structures are the end result of the TMJ triad. We must again emphasize that the degree of change in these tissues necessary for the precipitation of TMJ dysfunction is a factor of the patient's tissue tolerance and adaptability. As a result, the interrelationships of the involved tissues, as well as the level of alteration, is an important factor in the evaluation of patients.

The basic assumption to follow is that TMJ dysfunction can only exist (providing predisposition and the psychological factors are present) if there is some degree of habitual bruxism or clenching of the teeth while there exists an altered maxillo-mandibular relationship. This produces one or a combination of the following situations: (1) wear of the teeth; (2) dissolution and resorption of alveolar bone; (3) pathologic alterations of the TM joints; and (4) muscular spasm and resultant pain.

The discussion will first review those anatomical, physiological, and biochemical principles which are necessary to the understanding of how these tissues react to continual stress. Those theories related to the cause of TM joint pain will also be discussed.

TEMPOROMANDIBULAR JOINT AND SKELETAL RELATIONSHIPS

Detailed morphological and anatomical descriptions of the temporo-mandibular joints and alveolar processes have been presented in detail elsewhere.[33] The mandible is suspended from the cranium within a muscle sling. These muscles, referred to collectively as the muscles of mastication, are responsible for the functional as well as the parafunctional movements of the mandible. The mandible articulates with the cranium through two freely movable joints, the temporomandibular joints. The right and left TM joints stabilize the skull upon the vertebral column. Each TM joint is actually two joints in one.[34] The upper joint is situated between the mandibular fossa of the temporal bone and the articular eminence and the articular disc. The upper joint is a gliding joint when translatory movements take place. The lower joint is located between the inferior surface of the articulator disc and the head of the condyle. This is a hinge joint, and it functions through rotation.

Although freely movable in all directions, the joint is stable when the teeth are in contact, during rest position, and momentarily during movements.[35] This stabilization is primarily important during function of the joint and is achieved through the muscles and their neuromuscular mechanisms and by virtue of the anatomical design of the joint itself. The border movements of this joint are determined not only by the skeletal structures but also by the capsule and muscular components. When the physiological limits of these tissues are reached, neuromechanisms are activated; information sent to the brain initiates protective mechanisms to prevent damage to these tissues.

Function of the joint within physiological limits will not cause pathological alterations in the TM joints. It is when these tissues are required to function beyond the capacity for which they were designed that pathological alterations occur. Bone, for example, is plastic in nature. Physiological stress placed on bone enhances its integrity and ability to function under demands for which it was designed. Parafunctional forces, however, will induce bone resorption and dissolution.

Stress placed on alveolar bone during bruxism or clenching may induce bone loss, clinically indicative of traumatic occlusion. Clenching and bruxism with no alveolar bone loss, but existent weakness of the muscles, joint capsule, and/or ligaments will usually precipitate the TMJ dysfunction syndrome, since the tissues are absorbing the destructive forces and not the alveolar bone.

Although the osseous structures of the TM joints are susceptible to the same systemic influences as is the alveolar bone, the design of the joint makes it more capable of absorbing parafunctional pressures. This is why we see many patients with alveolar bone resorption from bruxing and clenching but with no joint problems. Conversely, we see many patients who clench and brux suffering from TM joint dysfunction but with no signs of alveolar bone loss.

The connective tissue surrounding the TM joints is susceptible to change and, in fact, is responsible for more mobility and less stability of the TM joints with increased stress. Ligaments and tendons are composed of collagen, acellular in nature, with a minimal blood supply. Although these tissues are very strong, they can be damaged. Depending on the severity of the pathological changes, we can expect to see a very slow healing process or possibly irreparable damage.

ARTHRITIC CHANGES

Other changes seen in the TM joints affecting the joint proper can be related to arthritic type changes. Three forms of arthritis affect the TM joints—rheumatoid, pyogenic, and osteoarthritis.

Rheumatoid Arthritis

Arthritis deformans, commonly known as rheumatoid arthritis, involves the temporomandibular joint in approximately 17 per cent of those patients who have the disease in other joints of the body.[36] The incidence of the disease is greatest in females below 40 years of age. Men are affected one-third less than women and usually have a history of streptococcal infections at some other location. The inflammation can result in cartilage being replaced by bone, fibrous adhesions in the joint space, and subsequent ankylosis. The joints of the wrist, feet, fingers, and knees should be examined for pain, swelling, and tenderness. There are usually bilateral disturbances when symptoms occur.

Pyogenic Arthritis

This arthritis is a direct result of bacterial infection by such organisms as staphylococci, streptococci, or gonococci. The infection can result secondary to a systemic involvement or directly by injecting cortisone or a sclerosing solution into the joint with a contaminated needle. Another route can be via the middle ear, the mastoid air cells, or parotid gland as a result of infected teeth.[37] Destruction of the articular cartilage usually occurs within a few days, with damage of ankylosis through immobilization of the joint during healing.

STRESS × DURATION = DYSFUNCTION AND PAIN   **Figure 1–10.**

Osteoarthritis

The degenerative joint disease is the most common pathosis of the TMJ.[38] Although the exact etiology is unknown, it is associated with aging and joint trauma. In contrast to rheumatoid arthritis, the individuals are usually more than 40 years of age. Repetitive trauma due to excess stress or degenerative tissue changes as a result of aging can be responsible for osteoarthritis. The most common trauma results from an altered maxillo-mandibular relationship causing displacement of the condylar head. This altered relationship results when the teeth are in occlusion. As a result, bruxism or habitual clenching becomes a significant factor. With the teeth out of occlusion, the right combination of pressure and duration that would cause significant levels of stress on the joints and related tissues is not present. Osteoarthritis usually destroys the articular disc and the connective tissue of the articulating surfaces. The bony components of the joint are remolded so that the articular eminence and the head of the condyle are flattened. The symptoms, as one might expect, are pain in the region of the TM joints, which may or may not be accompanied by clicking and/or crepitus.

OCCLUSAL RELATIONSHIP

The relationship of the occlusal surfaces of the maxillary and mandibular teeth is a critical factor when discussing the pathophysiology of TM joint dysfunction and related pain. It is the occlusion of the teeth that determines the degree to which the maxillo-mandibular relationship is altered when the teeth are in contact. The dysfunction and pain are a product of the stress and duration of forces placed on the TM joints and relaed musculature (Fig. 1–10). The stress can be considered to be the degree to which the maxillo-mandibular relationship is altered and the degree of bruxism and clenching (Fig. 1–11).

Treatment should be directed toward removing or diminishing the stress duration. Medications such as tranquilizers would help to diminish the duration of stress or the degree of bruxism or clenching. Treatment with a maxillary or a mandibular orthopedic appliance is designed to return the altered maxillo-mandibular relationship to a more physiological state. In addition, since the acrylic is more resilient and therefore more easily worn than the enamel of the teeth, less force is distributed to the alveolar bone, TM joint, and related musculature. In essence, an attempt is being made to compensate for the occlusal derangements responsible for altering the maxillo-mandibular relationships. The amount of bruxism may not necessarily decrease, but with the muscles and condyles functioning within their physiologic limits, a greater degree of stress is necessary to precipitate

STRESS = ALTERED JAW RELATIONSHIP
        × BRUXISM and/or CLENCHING   **Figure 1–11.**

comparable levels of pain and dysfunction than when not wearing an orthopedic appliance. Changes in the occlusion pathologically altering the maxillo-mandibular relationship can be classified into the following three categories:

1. Congenital or developmental.
2. Loss of posterior occlusion.
3. Iatrogenic changes.

Congenital and Developmental

The growth and development of the mandible and maxilla have been discussed elsewhere in great detail.[39] Deviations from the normal development of the jaws and sequential eruption of the teeth can result in less than ideal occlusions and jaw relations. Although esthetically displeasing, the Class II or Class III occlusions usually do not present much of a functional problem. The altered occlusion does, however, present problems when the teeth are together for extended periods of time.

Some of the more destructive situations are the unilateral and bilateral crossbites and rotated or malposed teeth. These conditions alter the jaw relationship, thus causing a "locking" of the jaws when the teeth are in contact.

More subtle developmental conditions could be delayed eruption of certain teeth, especially the six year molar or one other molar. This would create a spatial alteration of one condyle to the other. There would be in effect two different vertical dimensions—a left and a right. The growth of the condyle and associated soft tissue structures would compensate for the occlusal disharmonies. Again, none is particularly critical unless the teeth are together for extended periods of time, as in bruxism and clenching.

Loss of Posterior Occlusion

The posterior teeth when in occlusion determine the position of the condyle in the glenoid fossae. Loss of first molars prior to eruption of the second molars can result in a collapse of the vertical dimension. This will permit the second molars to erupt in an anterior position, with an increased possibility of propagating an infraocclusion in which the vertical dimension necessary to maintain a proper condyle-fossa-musculature relationship is not achieved. Whether unilateral or bilateral, the condylar head will have a posterior-superior displacement. Again, it must be remembered that problems will not occur unless the teeth are together for extended periods. Therefore, what may appear to be a well-balanced occlusion may in fact be pathological in nature when considering the TM joints, capsule, and musculature. A careful examination of the occlusion, as well as radiographic analysis of the TM joints, is necessary.

Loss of posterior teeth via extractions can be equally troublesome if such a tooth was maintaining vertical dimension. Unilateral loss can establish a torquing or rocking about the last tooth in the arch on the side where the posterior step is now missing.

This collapse of vertical dimension can be further increased if the muscles are in spasm. If the patient clenches or bruxes, the muscles can be in spasm, further shortening the vertical dimension on the affected side.

This can present potential problems to the dentist replacing the missing teeth. If the spasmed muscles have not returned to a physiological length prior to bite registration, a maxillo-mandibular relationship reflecting the shortened muscle will be recorded. This will perpetuate the conditions established already by the missing teeth.

Iatrogenic Changes

The concept discussed previously carries through when discussing iatrogenic alteration of the occlusion. A filling with a premature contact in a first molar placed prior to second molar eruption can, through proprioceptive mechanisms, cause altered closing patterns to be established. This altered relationship will be perpetuated during eruption of the second molars. Thus a permanently altered jaw relationship can be established. Any combination of a number of procedures can, if not properly executed, produce a nonphysiological maxillo-mandibular relationship.

Perhaps one of the most common sequences of events resulting in acute TMJ pain can be attributed to sudden changes in occlusion. This can result from quadrant dentistry and from fixed and removable prostheses. The occlusion is changed in such a way as to create changes in proprioceptive mechanisms, resulting in tissues that are more susceptible to stress from bruxing or clenching. Consequently, the tissue factor has been introduced.

NEUROMUSCULAR CHANGES

When considering tissue changes in relation to TMJ dysfunction, the neuromuscular system is a complex and important component through which TM joint dysfunction and pain can manifest themselves.

Changes in the muscles of the head and neck precipitate many of the symptoms associated with TM joint dysfunction and related pain. Generally, the acute symptoms of TM joint dysfunction are muscular in nature, while the more chronic, long-standing symptoms can also include connective tissue components (tendons and ligaments) of the TM joint and related musculature. Of course, acute symptoms related to traumatic injury can include both musculature and connective tissue components. These changes may result in muscular spasms, which are responsible for the dysfunction and associated pain.

The seemingly unrelated symptoms of joint clicking, trismus, head and neck pain, vertigo, ear stuffiness, and so forth, are all related directly or indirectly to pathological muscle alteration.

The interrelationships between muscle spasm, dysfunction, and pain can be understood only if a working knowledge of muscle function is readily at hand. Skeletal muscle is composed of individual fibers (myofibrils), which are arranged in parallel between their tendinous ends (Fig. 1–12).

Each muscle fiber is a multinucleated single cell. Each muscle cell is composed of fibrils, which are further divisible into protein filaments. These filaments are composed of the contractile proteins myosin, actin, and tropomyosin B. The characteristic cross striations are identified by letters (Fig. 1–13). The sarcomere is the area between two Z lines. The sarcolemma is the plasma membrane of the muscle cell.

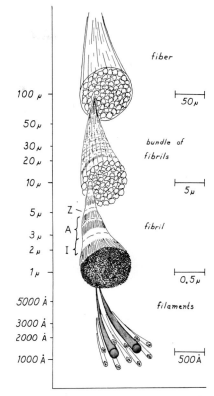

Figure 1–12. Histological picture of muscle fibers. (From Ruch, T. C., and Patton, H. D.: Physiology and Biophysics. Philadelphia, W. B. Saunders Co., 1965.)

The sarcotubular system is composed of the T-system and the sarco-plasmic reticulum. The T-system is involved in the transmission of action potentials (electrical discharge associated with contraction) to the fibrils of the muscle, which then initiates a contraction.[40] The sarcoplasmic reticulum is concerned with calcium movement and muscle cell metabolism. The

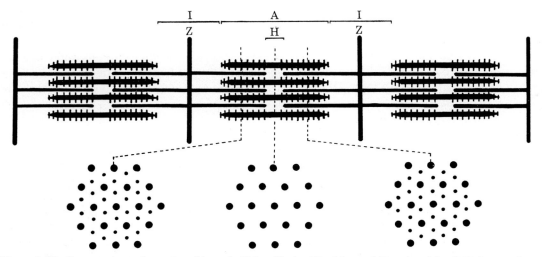

Figure 1–13. Cross-sections of muscles. (From de Vries, H. A.: Physiology of Exercise, 5th ed. Dubuque, Iowa, W. C. Brown, 1976. Reprinted by permission.)

resting cell membrane of a muscle fiber carries a positive external (extracellular) charge with a relative intracellular negative charge. Depolarization is characterized by Na^+ ions pouring into the cell as a result of increased cellular permeability. Repolarization is caused by K^+ efflux out of the cell.

Contraction is believed to result from a sliding of the myosin and actin filaments over each other. The mechanism for sliding seems to result from the breaking and reforming of cross-linkages between the actin and myosin filaments. Adenosine triphosphate (ATP) is the souce of energy for muscle contraction. Myosin is the catalyst for the hydrolysis of ATP to ADP (adenosine diphosphate). The action potential releases Ca from the sarcoplasmic reticulum. The Ca in turn activates adenosine triphosphate activity of myosin, which initiates the contraction.

Muscle contraction involves shortening of the contractile elements. It is, however, possible to have a contraction without appreciable decrease in muscle length. This is possible because the elastic elements are in series with the contractile elements. A contraction without decrease in muscle is referred to as an isometric contraction. Contraction with shortening is an isotonic contraction.

Tetany or tetanic contraction can occur with rapidly repeated stimulation. Activation of the contractile mechanism occurs repeatedly before relaxation has taken place, resulting in a fusing of the contractions into one continuous phase. This phenomenon is critical, especially during continual clenching or bruxing movements. The tension developed by these repeated contractions is considerably greater than during a single muscle contraction.

VASCULAR SUPPLY AND LYMPHATIC FLOW

The skeletal muscle system has a rich blood supply consisting of an intricate capillary network. Capillaries are arranged so that each muscle fiber is placed in relation to four or five capillary vessels (Fig. 1–14).

The muscle mass of adult males is estimated to have 62,000 miles of capillaries, with a total surface area of 6300 square miles.[41] Strong contractions can cause muscle fatigue by obstructing the capillary flow.[42]

During inactivity many of the muscle capillaries are closed. With increases in metabolic demands (activity) capillaries open and the blood flow is increased. Increased muscle size, as seen typically in the masseter muscle during TMJ dysfunction, can be caused by two factors. Initially, the increase in bulk of a highly trained muscle is due to increases in the number of open

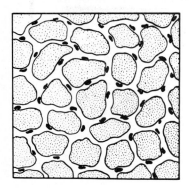

Figure 1–14. Capillary relation to muscle fibers. The black dots represent capillaries. (From Adams, R. D.: Disease of Muscle; A Study in Pathology, 3rd ed. New York, Harper and Row, 1975. Reprinted by permission.)

capillaries which, during a more inactive state, are closed. With increased activity of longer duration an increase in the size of individual fibers is noted and attributed to increase in sarcoplasm.[43] With prolonged heavy exercise the number of myofibrils also increases.

During the physiological exchange of fluids across capillary walls, the fluid leaving the capillary is usually greater than that volume entering the capillary. The excess fluid is taken up by the lymphatic network and eventually drains into the venous system. This process maintains a constant interstitial fluid pressure as well as a continuous turnover of tissue fluids.

An abundant supply of lymphatic vessels is found in the connective tissue sheaths and tendons of muscles but not within the body of the muscle. Their purpose is to collect and convey lymph from the muscles and return it back to the venous system. Lymphatic flow is increased during activity, but, as in capillary circulation, the flow can be impeded by excess pressure exerted by a constantly contracted muscle. Decreases in lymphatic drainage can contribute to muscular pain during long periods of activity by causing a buildup of interstitial fluids, increasing the hydrostatic pressures. In addition, there is an accumulation of waste products that would normally be drained by the lymphatic as well as the venous capillary system.

PROPRIOCEPTION

The central nervous system (CNS) coordinates information from receptors located in muscles, joints, and tendons. These sensory receptors are called proprioceptors. The proprioceptic mechanisms in the periodontal ligaments, muscles of mastication, and temporomandibular joints are well developed. These receptors feed back the results of movements as sensory information to the CNS.

Proprioceptors are responsible for the kinesthetic or muscle sense of an individual. This enables the individual to know where the mandible is and what it is doing at any given time without a visual experience. In addition, information about the tension and/or length of the muscle is quickly transmitted from muscle proprioceptors to the CNS. Two types of receptors serve the "muscle sense"—the muscle spindles and the Golgi tendon organ (Fig. 1–15). The muscle spindle reports changes in the length of the muscle. It consists of a connective tissue sheath that contains several intrafusal muscle fibers. The intrafusal bundle is located deep in the muscle mass and is formed by several thin striated fibers. The muscle spindle contains sensory and motor fibers.

Two types of sensory end organs are found in the muscle spindle, the annulospiral ending and the flower spray ending. Both are deformed by stretching the intrafusal muscle fiber. They lie parallel with the skeletal muscle fibers (extrafusal fibers). External stretch lengthens both intra- and extrafusal fibers. The annulospiral ending is deformed and sends a discharge over a fast-conducting nerve, while the flower spray sends discharges over a slower conducting nerve. The flower spray needs a much greater stretch to elicit a response. The efferent response is a motor response, causing a contraction of the skeletal muscle.

The Golgi tendon organ found in the musculotendinous junction is a simpler receptor than the muscle spindle. It discharges sensory impulses with

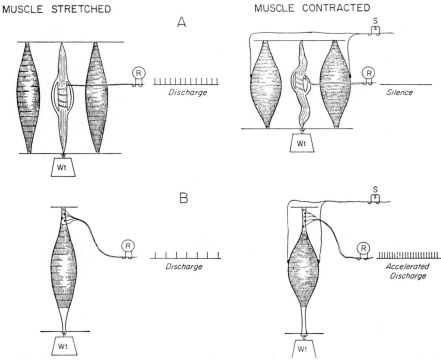

Figure 1–15. Relation of muscle spindles and tendon organs to muscle fibers. *A,* Spindle is arranged "in parallel" with muscle fibers so that muscle contraction slackens tension on spindle. *B,* Tendon organ is arranged "in series" with muscle fibers so that both passive and active contractions of muscle cause receptor to discharge. (From Ruch, T. C., and Patton, H. D.: Physiology and Biophysics. Philadelphia, W. B. Saunders Co., 1965.)

both stretch of a muscle and its contracture. It records the degree of stretch a tendon is experiencing. This receptor is in series with the muscle and tendon, not parallel as is the muscle spindle. Since deformation is caused by tension on the muscle, either on active contraction of the muscle or its stretching, it responds to both conditions similarly.

The muscle spindle facilitates or may cause contraction, whereas the tendon organ seems to be a protective mechanism inhibitory to the muscle of origin.

Stretching of a muscle receptor, either a tendon organ or a muscle spindle, sends an afferent impulse to the CNS. When a muscle contracts, the response of the two receptors is different. The tendon organ will be deformed, whereas the muscle spindle will shorten or relax.

STRETCH REFLEX

The stretch reflex, also called the myotatic reflex, employs a single sensory neuron. This reflex is initiated by stretch of the annulospiral receptor of muscle spindle and subsequently causes the stretched muscles to contract. The net effect of this reflex is to oppose any stretch of the muscle, thereby enabling the muscle to maintain a constant length.[44] Inhibitory impulses are transmitted to the motor neurons of the antagonist muscles, allowing the reflex to be more effective. It should be noted that the spindle can be stimulated many times as strongly by a *sudden* increase in the degree of stretch as by a continuous stretch.

In the mandible this phenomenon is referred to as the stretch, myotatic, or jaw jerk reflex.[45] When the jaw-closing muscles are stretched the muscle spindle mechanism sends information to the brain stem, causing a reflexively induced contraction of the jaw-closing muscles. With the teeth together the proprioceptive mechanisms of the periodontal membrane stimulate the jaw-opening muscles to prevent excessive contraction of the jaw-closing muscles.

The proprioceptors in the muscles and tendons of the mandible are highly developed, giving information concerning the movements and position of the mandible in space. Activation of the myotatic reflex also reciprocally inhibits the motor neurons of their antagonists while facilitating their synergists.[46] This type of reciprocal inhibition may also occur between different bellies of the same jaw muscles, as seen in the frontal and posterior bellies of the temporal muscle.

Additional sensory information is derived from the proprioceptive nerve endings found in the joints themselves. This information is related to the speed and direction in which the joint is moving.

During clenching or bruxing the muscles are contracted in a repetitive manner, sometimes for hours. This can in itself produce muscle soreness common to TMJ dysfunction (see further on). However, of even more impact is the continual contraction of the jaw muscle during bruxing and/or clenching when there is an altered maxillo-mandibular relationship (see above). For example, let us consider the individual with no posterior occlusion who, through various clinical and radiographic analyses, has been determined to have a posteriorly displaced condyle. This would cause the pterygoid muscles to be stretched when the teeth are in occlusion. With an absence of clenching or grinding of the teeth, the lack of posterior occlusion and collapsed bite would be of little consequence.

If, however, we have contact of the teeth for extended periods of time (clenching, bruxing), these muscles would attempt to shorten themselves through the stretch reflex mechanism. Since the muscle cannot shorten, the reflex would essentially perform repeated isometric contractions. Further stress would be placed on these muscles if there were a concomitant series of short jerky contractions, as seen during bruxism. This series of events can lead to muscle fatigue and subsequent muscle soreness.

A constant force on the joint and periodontal membrane proprioceptive mechanisms will cause the nerve endings to reversibly deteriorate to a level where they contribute minimally to the reflex control of the jaw muscles.

The pain and discomfort of the TMJ and related muscles experienced by individuals suffering with TMJ dysfunction can be considered to be related to muscular alterations.

TMJ PAIN

As explained previously, TMJ dysfunction results in pain of the joint and related musculature. The majority of pain is, however, muscular in origin, and its etiology is the overexertion of the muscles either by continual contractions in a normal physiological state or, if in a stretched pathological length, a combination of contractions and stretch reflex-relaxation reactions.

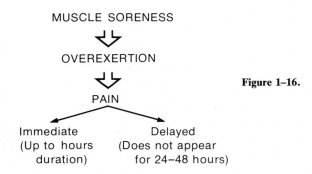

Figure 1–16.

Although the conditions necessary to initiate pain have been explained, the mechanism through which continual contraction actually produces pain must now be developed. Generally speaking, overexertion of muscles will produce pain. Postexertion muscular pain can be divided into the following two types: pain during and immediately after exercise, which can persist for hours (immediate pain), and a more localized soreness that does not appear for 24 to 48 hours (delayed pain) (Fig. 1–16). The delayed type of pain is usually referred to as myositis.[47]

The immediate pain experienced with muscular overexertion can be largely attributed to diffusible end-products of cellular metabolism acting upon pain receptors within the muscular tissues. The probable metabolites are potassium (K^+) ions and lactic acid (LA). K^+ are known to diffuse outward across the cell membrane into the tissue spaces during contraction. This ion stimulates the sensory nerve endings and is subsequently realized as pain by the brain.

Lactic acid is a direct product of muscular contraction when the energy requirements are greater than the oxygen available and the source of energy goes from an aerobic (with O_2) to an anaerobic (lack of O_2) reaction. Both potassium diffusion and lactic acid production are known to occur, but with exertion of shorter duration. The immediate pain can be relieved by total cessation of exercise or at least short periods of rest.

Of the two products, K^+ diffusion and lactic acid accumulation, lactic acid plays a dominant role in production of immediate muscle soreness. As stated above, lactic acid is produced because there is less oxygen available than needed to sustain aerobic energy production. The endurance of muscle tissue is directly related to the O_2 available to sustain aerobic energy production. Lack of oxygen results from a decrease in total circulation to the muscle. For example, an isometric contraction of only 60 per cent of maximal strength results in almost complete occlusion of the blood vessels that supply the muscle tissue.[47] This results when the pressure of the contracted muscle exceeds systolic arterial pressure. Decrease in blood flow not only diminishes the O_2 supply but also decreases removal of waste products such as lactic acid from the tissue. The accumulation of lactic acid is an irritant to nerve endings and lowers the pH of the muscle tissue as well. Both conditions result in a decreased contractibility of the muscle.

Further increases in tissue pressure result from increased osmotic pressure within the muscle. The accumulation of lactic acid, potassium, and other waste constituents increases the osmotic pressure. A retention of fluid follows with subsequent edema. Edema also excites sensory nerve endings, causing pain.

Fatigue can also be used to explain the phenomenon of immediate muscle pain and decreased contractility.[48] Fatigue can also be related to a depletion of energy stores or at least their diminished availability. Furthermore, the end-products of metabolism alter the physiochemical state causing a breakdown in tissue homeostasis.

The method in which the energy for contraction is produced is critical, since it will determine the character of the end-products accumulating in the muscle. The immediate source of energy in a contracting muscle is adenosine triphosphate (ATP) and, to a lesser extent, creatine phosphate (CP). Creatine phosphate functions as a phosphate donor to furnish ADP with a phosphate group producing ATP.* Figure 1–17 shows this to be a very inefficient source of energy.

When carbohydrates (CHO) such as glucose are used as the substrate, oxygen need or need not be present to produce energy in the form of ATP (see Neuromuscular Changes). CHO utilization in muscle cells takes place in the sarcosomes of the sarcoplasm.

In the presence of oxygen, the breakdown of CHO goes to completion, yielding 40 ATP for each 2 ATP expended (Fig. 1–17). The only byproducts, CO_2 and H_2O, are readily diffusible in the blood. This process is the aerobic form of energy production.[49]

When no O_2 is available, the anaerobic process takes over. This process is less efficient, producing only 4 ATP for each 2 ATP expended, and, because the reaction does not go to completion, intermediate metabolites of the reaction, lactic acid, are produced.

The theories of delayed or latent pain following muscle overexertion are indirectly related to the waste products or edema, as seen with the immediate pain reaction.[50]

A theory proposed as early as 1900[51] suggested that microscopic tears in the muscle and/or connective tissue are responsible for the latent pain experience. Although *violent* trauma or severe overexertion can result in rupture of muscle or tendon tissue, the majority of patients suffering with latent soreness and pain cannot attribute this to the torn tissue theory.

A more plausible and scientifically founded theory seems to be the spasm theory of delayed localized soreness (DLS).[52] Two explanations for the precipitation of muscular spasm and resultant soreness have been proposed. The first is related to the fatigue of muscle tissue. Muscle fatigue can result from repeated contractions with very short rest intervals (1 to 2 seconds). There is then seen a decrease in the amplitude of contraction of contractility of the muscle, accompanied by increased fatigue. This results in an inability to achieve complete relaxation of the muscle, which results in

---

*Also known as the alactacid oxygen debt.

$$Phosphocreatine^{(PC)} \longrightarrow Creatine^{(C)} + P$$

$$(Anaerobic)\, CHO + 2\ ATP \longrightarrow LACTIC\ ACID + 4\ ATP$$

Figure 1–17.

$$(Aerobic)\, CHO + 6\ O_2 + 2\ ATP \longrightarrow 6\ CO_2 + 6\ H_2O + 40\ ATP$$
$$\downarrow \qquad \downarrow$$

Readily Diffusible Products

contracture (spasm) of the muscle. The second explanation is related to soreness being produced by tonic, localized spasm of motor units.

The theoretical basis for the spasm theory is built upon the local changes in muscle tissue seen with excessive levels of muscle activity. Exercise above a minimal level, i.e., a level causing decreases in blood flow through the muscle tissue (see Vascular Supply and Lymphatic Flow), will cause local areas of ischemia due to oxygen debt in the active muscle.

Ischemia results in diffusion of potassium (K^+) ions into extracellular tissue. The increase in potassium raises the ionic concentration, which in turn elevates the osmotic pressure. The increase in osmotic pressure irritates free nerve endings, causing a pain sensation. The pain sensation initiates a reflex tonic muscle contraction, which prolongs the ischemia, completing the cycle (Fig. 1–18).

The increased motor activity observed can be recorded by electromyographic means. The rates are upwards to 300 per second, which spread through the muscle.[53] The spasms are relieved by stretching, possibly through activation of the Golgi tendon organs and the myotatic stretch reflex. Cessation of spasm reduces the degree and duration of pain. If tears in the muscle or tendon tissues were responsible for the latent pain response, the stretch-relaxation exercises would not reduce the muscle contracture or pain.

Further support of the spasm theory for latent muscle pain is supported by the following findings:[54]

1. Static stretch relieves and prevents pain.
2. Latent muscle soreness shows significantly higher EMG electrical activity.
3. Stretching of the muscles causes a reduction in EMG activity with concomitant symptomatic relief.
4. Muscular soreness has been produced and relieved under experimental conditions.

By observing the muscle electromyographically the rise in activity was used to predict pain as the decline in activity was used to predict relief.[55]

If we now evaluate those activities most likely to cause muscle soreness we can correlate them to the resultant pain. It also becomes readily evident that these activities are very similar to activities of jaw muscles when contracting during bruxism or clenching, especially with an altered maxillomandibular relationship. These activities are as follows:

1. Vigorous contraction of a muscle in a shortened state.
2. Muscular contraction involving short jerky movements.

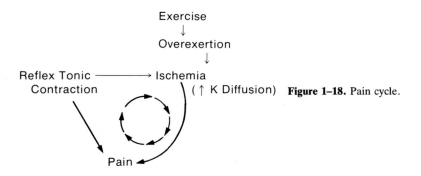

Figure 1–18. Pain cycle.

3. Muscle contraction involving repetitious movements over extended periods of time.

Furthermore, repetitious movements cause more soreness if a slight rest interval is allowed between these movements because a greater total workload can be demanded.

Awareness of the activities resulting in muscle soreness (TMJ pain) and an understanding of the events which take place within the muscle tissue altering the normal physiological processes enable the clinician to prevent and more effectively treat patients in acute or chronic TMJ pain. It should be noted that the sequence of events responsible for immediate muscle soreness are the same as those responsible for the latent pain response. The difference is that, during initial muscular activity, oxygen debt energy production and its accumulation of by-products proceed to a level which results in tissue changes initiating a degenerative cellular response. The ensuing cellular death and ischemic changes manifest themselves 24 to 48 hours later as a latent muscular soreness and dysfunction. The dysfunction is the spasm or "stiffness" the affected muscles experience due to tonic contracture related to the increased EMG activity.

Muscular dysfunction can then be attributed to two different situations. The first is the reflex action causing a self-perpetuating mechanism for increased tension, as seen in bruxism (see Proprioception) usually associated with trismus or degrees of joint stiffness with little or no specific pain. The second cause is the increased muscular tension or contracture seen secondary to ischemic changes, resulting in a delayed pain reaction. This type of dysfunction is associated with high levels of pain. Although the mechanism is similar with regard to the initiating events, the duration of activity will determine whether a latent pain response ensues.

PSYCHOLOGICAL COMPONENT

The third component of the TMJ triad, and probably the most difficult to understand, is the patient's psychological factors. The personalities of patients suffering with TM joint dysfunction fit a certain profile, suggested to be tense, depressed, resentful, obsessive, and perfectionistic.[56] An excellent discussion of the psychological aspects of TM joint dysfunction is given by Grieder and Cinotti.[57]

Aside from the genetic aspect of the intense perfectionist personality traits, there is a group of individuals who marginally fit the description of Moulton and others.[58] These marginal persons, however, can experience transitory periods of stress which can produce oral manifestations such as bruxism. There can then be varying degrees of this psychological component, degrees which are dynamic and depend on the adaptive capacity for a given individual, time, and circumstance. That is, patients not normally susceptible to bruxism of clenching can be subjected to transitory periods of stress which will induce them to respond by parafunctional oral habits (bruxism).

As stated above, although predisposition and tissue alterations in certain individuals may be prominent, absence of the psychological component resulting in the lack of muscle tension and bruxism will not precipitate as TM joint dysfunction. This is obvious in many individuals manifesting malocclusion and an altered maxillo-mandibular relationship with an absence

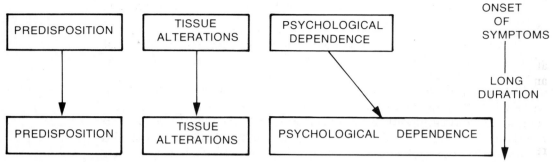

Figure 1–19. As duration increases, psychological dependence becomes proportionally more significant.

of symptoms indicative of TM joint dysfunction. However, these persons are uniquely susceptible to acquiring TM joint dysfunction symptoms. The onset of pain and dysfunction could be precipitated by such psychological events as marital or financial difficulties or the death of a loved one. Stress builds within the individual, and, since our society cannot condone outward expressions,[59] bruxism or clenching develops, which is an oral manifestation resulting from inhibition of open expression.

The person who presents the real difficulty when dealing with the treatment of TM joint dysfunction is not the one who experiences transitory periods of stress, or even the more genetically entrenched personality traits making a patient extremely susceptible to acquiring symptoms of TMJ dysfunction. Rather, the problem is with those who can be classified as long-term sufferers of TM joint dysfunction, that is, patients who have been incapacitated for long periods with pain and dysfunction. These patients usually have a long history of unsuccessful attempts at diagnosis by both medical and dental practitioners. These long-term sufferers of TM joint dysfunction usually develop anxiety neurosis and severe depression.[59]

These individuals are those with well-entrenched personality traits, not those within the marginal transitory zone. Those susceptible to the transitory stressful periods usually will have their symptoms resolved with treatment, but, if treatment is not begun, a cycling effect will develop and with time the psychological component can dominate.

When these patients present to your office for treatment it is difficult to determine which initially predominates, predisposition tissue alterations, or the psychological factors. Treatment to correct TMJ dysfunction, if initiated early, may have resolved all problems. However, when you examine these individuals, treatment may be futile without prior emotional rehabilitation by a psychologist or psychiatrist.

Early diagnosis is extremely important so that emotional degeneration can be prevented and treatment utilizing more conventional methods can be instituted.

References

1. Stedman's Medical Dictionary, 22nd ed. Baltimore, The Williams and Wilkins Co., 1981.
2. Adams, R. D.: Disease of Muscle; A Study in Pathology, 3rd ed. New York, Harper and Row, 1975.
3. Ibid.

4. Ford, F. R.: Disease of the Nervous System in Infancy, Childhood and Adolescence, 2nd ed. Springfield, Illinois, Charles C Thomas, 1944.

5. Adams, op. cit.

6. Gunn, R. M.: Congenital ptosis with peculiar associated movements of the affected lid. Tr. Ophthalmol. Soc. U.K., *3*:283, 1882–1883.

7. Henderson, J. L.: The congenital facial diplegia syndrome; clinical features, pathology and aetiology. Brain, *6Z*:381, 1939.

8. Ricklin, Peter, Ruttimann, A., and Del Buono, M. S.: Meniscus Lesions: Practical Problems of Clinical Diagnosis, Arthrography and Therapy. New York, Grune and Stratton, 1971.

9. Holmdahl, D. E., and Ingelmark, B. E.: The contact between the articular cartilage and the medullary cavities of the bone. Acta Orthop. Scandinav., *20*:156, 1950.

10. Cinotti, W. R., Grieder, A., and Springob, H. K.: Applied Psychology in Dentistry, 2nd ed. St. Louis, C. V. Mosby, 1972.

11. Schwartz, L., and Chayes, C.: Facial Pain and Mandibular Dysfunction. *In* Shira, R., and Alling, C. C. (eds.): Traumatic Injuries Involving the Temperomandibular Joint Articulation. Philadelphia, W. B. Saunders Co., 1968.

12. Ricklin et al., op. cit.

13. Ricklin et al., op. cit.

14. Mercer, W.: Orthopedic Surgery, 6th ed. New York, Arnold, 1964.

15. Hathaway, P. W., Dahl, D. S., and Engle, W. K.: Myopathic changes produced by local trauma. Arch. Neurol., *21*:355, 1969.

16. Ibid.

17. Mason, K.: Effects of Nutritional Deficiency on Muscle. *In* G. H. Bourne (ed.): The Structure and Function of Muscle, 2nd ed., Vol IV. New York, Academic Press, 1973.

18. Mason, op. cit.

19. Ganong, W. F.: Review of Medical Physiology, 11th ed. Los Altos, Calif., Lange Medical Publications, 1983.

20. Ibid.

21. Dalldorf, G.: The lesions in the skeletal muscles in experimental scorbutus. J. Exp. Med., *50*:293, 1929.

22. Evans, H. M., and Burr, G. O.: Development of paralysis in suckling young of mothers deprived of vitamin E. J. Biol. Chem., *76*:273, 1928.

23. Krane, S. M.: Calcium. Phosphate and Magnesium. *In* H. Rasmussen (ed.): International Encyclopedia of Pharmacology nad Therapeutics, Section 51, Pharmacology of the endocrine system and related drugs: Parathyroid hormone, thyrocalcitonin and related drugs. Pergamon Press, 1970.

24. Krane, op. cit.

25. Lehninger, A. L.: Biochemistry, 2nd ed. Worth Publications, 1975.

26. Hegsted, D. M.: Calcium, Phosphorus and Magnesium. *In* M. G. Whol and R. S. Goodhart (eds.): Modern Nutrition in Health and Disease, 4th ed. Philadelphia, Lea and Febiger, 1968.

27. Mason, op. cit.

28. Grieder, A., and Cinotti, W. R.: Periodontal Prosthesis, Chap. 9. St. Louis, C. V. Mosby, 1968.

29. Karpovich, P. V.: Physiology of Muscular Activity, 6th ed. Philadelphia, W. B. Saunders, 1965.

30. Adams, op. cit.

31. Adams, op. cit.

32. Vicale, C. T.: The diagnostic features of muscular syndrome resulting from hyperparathyroidism, osteomalacia owing to renal tubular acidosis and perhaps to related disorders of calcium metabolism. Trans. Am. Neural Ass., *74*:143, 1949.

33. Du Brul, E. L.: Sicher's Oral Anatomy, 7th ed. St. Louis, C. V. Mosby, 1980.

34. Grieder and Cinotti, op. cit.

35. Moss, M. L.: Functional Anatomy of the Temporomandibular Joint. *In* L. Schwartz (ed.): Disorders of the TMJ. Philadelphia, W. B. Saunders, 1960.

36. Grieder and Cinotti, op. cit.

37. Grieder and Cinotti, op. cit.

38. Grieder and Cinotti, op. cit.

39. Du Brul, op. cit.

40. Lehninger, op. cit.

41. Krogh, A.: The Anatomy & Physiology of Capillaries. New Haven, Yale University Press, 1922.

42. Merton, P. A.: Voluntary Strength and Fatigue. J. Physiol., *123*:553, 1964.

43. Adams, op. cit.

44. Ruch, T. C., and Patton, H. D. (eds.): Physiology and Biophysics, 20th ed. Vol. 4. Philadelphia, W. B. Saunders, 1982.

45. Kawamura, Y.: Mandibular Movement: Normal Anatomy and Physiology and Clinical Dysfunction. *In* L. Schwartz and C. M. Chayes (eds.): Facial Pain and Mandibular Dysfunction. Philadelphia, W. B. Saunders, 1968.

46. Kawamura, Y.: Neurophysiologic Background of Occlusion. J Am. Soc. Periodontol., 5:175, 1967.
47. de Vries, H. A.: Physiology of Exercise, 5th ed. Dubuque, Iowa, W. C. Brown, 1976.
48. Ibid.
49. Ibid.
50. Dorpot, T. L., and Holmes, T. H.: Mechanisms of skeletal muscle pain and fatigue. Arch. Neurol. Psychiatry, 74:628, 1955.
51. Hough, T.: Ergographic studies on muscular soreness. Am. J. Physiol., 7:78, 1902.
52. de Vries, op. cit., 47.
53. de Vries, op. cit., 47.
56. Moulton, R.: Psychiatric considerations in maxillofacial pain. JADA, 51:408, 1955.
57. Grieder, A., Cinotti, W. R., and Springob, H. K.: Psychological Aspects of Temporomandibular Joint Dysfunction and Neuromuscular Dysfunction in Applied Psychology in Dentistry. St. Louis, C. V. Mosby, 1972.
58. Lupton, D. E.: Psychological aspects of temporomandibular joint dysfunction. JADA, 79:131, 1969.
59. Grieder et al., op. cit.

Selected Readings

Basmajian, J. V.: Muscles Alive. Baltimore, Williams & Wilkins, 1982.
Blaschke, D. D., Solberg, W. K., and Saunders, B.: Arthrography of the temporomandibular joint: Review of current status. JADA, 100:388, 1980.
Beard, C. C., and Clayton, J. A.: The effects of occlusal splint therapy on TMJ dysfunction. J. Prosthet. Dent., 44:323, 1980.
Bell, W. E.: Orofacial Pains, Differential Diagnosis, 2nd ed. Chicago, Year Book Medical Publishers, 1979.
Cherrick, H. M.: Pathology. In Sarnat, B. G., and Laskin, D. M. (Eds.): The Temporomandibular Joint, 3rd ed. Springfield, Ill., Charles C Thomas, 1979, pp. 180–204.
Detsch, S. G.: Bruxism, Emotional or Occlusal Problem, U.S. Navy Medical 69:26, March 1978.
Du Brul, E. L.: Sicher's Oral Anatomy, 7th ed. St. Louis, C. V. Mosby Co., 1980.
Greene, C. S., Olson, R. E., and Laskin, D. M.: Psychological factors in the etiology, progression and treatment of MPD syndrome. JADA, 105:443, 1982.
Hansson, T.: Temporomandibular joint changes related to dental occlusion. In Solberg, W. K., and Clark, G. T. (Eds.): Temporomandibular Joint Problems. Chicago, Quintessence Publishing Co., 1980, pp. 129–143.
Hiatt, J., and Gartner, I.: Textbook of Head and Neck Anatomy. New York, Appleton-Century-Crofts, 1982.
Kraut, R. A.: Treatment of osteoarthritis of the temporomandibular joint. Oral Surg., 51:355–356, 1981.
Lederman, K. H., and Clayton, J. A.: A study of patients with restored occlusions. Part I. TMJ dysfunction determined by a pantographic reproducibility index. J. Prosthet. Dent., 47:198, 1982.
Lipke, D. P., Gay, T., Gross, B. D., et al.: An electromyographic study of the human lateral pterygoid muscle. J. Dent. Res., 56B:230, 1977.
Manhold, J. H.: Physiologic and psychologic aspects of orofacial pain: An overview. Clin. Prevent. Dent., 3:18, 1981.
Mikhail, M., and Rosen, H.: History and etiology of myofascial pain–dysfunction syndrome. J. Prosthet. Dent., 44:438, 1980.
McNeill, C., Danzig, W. M., Farrar, W. B., et al.: Craniomandibular (TMJ) disorders—the state of the art. J. Prosthet. Dent., 44:434, 1980.
Scott, D. S.: Treatment of the myofacial pain–dysfunction syndrome: Psychological aspects. JADA, 101:611, 1980.
Solberg, W., Woo, M., and Houston, J.: Prevalence of mandibular dysfunction in young adults. JADA, 98:25, 1979.
Stanfield, J. P.: The influence of malnutrition on development. Practitioner, 226:1373, 1982.
Weinberg, L., and Lager, L.: Clinical report on the etiology and diagnosis of TMJ dysfunction–pain syndrome. J. Prosthet. Dent., 44:642, 1980.
Weinberg, L. A.: The etiology, diagnosis and treatment of TMJ dysfunction–pain syndrome. J. Prosthet. Dent., 42:654, 1979.
Weinberg, L. A.: The role of stress, occlusion and condyle position in TMJ dysfunction–pain. J. Prosthet. Dent., 49:532, 1983.

2

Oral Orthopedics

MYRON M. LIEB, D.D.S., F.A.G.D.

As the dental profession moves into its second century, more and more advances are registered toward the achievement of its objectives. From an initial emergency and cosmetic service, the profession has developed into an important arm of the health services, accepting as its responsibility the comprehensive task of saving teeth, promoting oral health and safeguarding the total health of the individual.

For many years we have been aware of the ravages of the destructive processes of caries and periodontitis. Many techniques have been developed, and better understanding of the nature of these processes has helped us in attaining our goals. The use of the newer adjuncts to oral hygiene, the advances in the field of nutrition, and the chemical reinforcement of the calcifying as well as the erupted teeth, together with early and regular care, all give good promise of the early control of caries.

The periodontal destructive process has been a greater challenge. Here, too, improvement in surgical and other techniques, advances in nutritional guidance and home care, and a better understanding of the role of trauma from occlusion have helped us to treat this destructive process. Here, as in every area of clinical practice, our attention has been focused on the fundamental importance of occlusion. Yet, despite all these advances, patients still lose many teeth through periodontal destruction and are still faced with many unsolved problems. These problems continue to plague us, no matter the age of the patient, no matter whether he has all his teeth, some of his teeth, or none of his teeth: Costen's syndrome, myofascial syndrome (MFS), TMJ syndrome, clicking joints, difficulties in breathing, swallowing, chewing, and speaking, and pains and muscle spasms in the face, head, and neck, to name a few.[1]

As a matter of fact, many people suffer from all kinds of head and neck pains of varying degrees of intensity. Except for those commonly (and incorrectly) associated with the temporomandibular joints, dentistry has done little about them beyond the empirical approach. Sadly enough, medicine too, despite exhaustive investigation, has been unable to be of more than palliative help. Thus, these patients wander dolorously about in this medicodental no-man's-land, beset and bedeviled by pain. Not a few of them are consigned to the limbo of psychosomatics, with little relief.

The more these problems are investigated, the more our attention is focused on occlusion of the teeth. We are being forced to recognize more and more that occlusion of the teeth is not the be-all and end-all of our endeavors. As we find that many of these problems arise more from abnormal tonicity of the muscles involved, we are forced to think of occlusion as more than a teeth-to-teeth relationship. We see now that malrelationship of the jaws has a consequent effect upon the whole neuromuscular system involved in the various static and active functions of the structures in the head, neck, and shoulders of our patients. Occlusion now comes to mean the relationship of all the parts of the dental apparatus: the jaws, muscles, joints, and all the surrounding structures, not the teeth alone. We must consider the relationship of the dental apparatus to its surroundings and investigate further the functions of the various parts. The relationship of structure is, of course, a structural concept, and, since posture and balance are orthopedic in nature, the term "oral orthopedics" was selected as descriptive of the entire discipline.

Oral orthopedics is not a revolutionary concept divorced from the mainstream of dentistry. It is not governed by arbitrary rules and formulas into which, like the fabled bed of Procrustes, we forcibly fit our patients. Nor does it consist of a series of theories and procedures which suddenly appeared out of nowhere, with Victor Stoll[2] as its Moses, bringing the revelations out of his own head, or from heaven, down to us. Many years of pioneering research by Stoll showed that mastication was only one of the functions of the dental apparatus. Stoll had gone back to the anatomy of Gray and Cunningham and the basic work of Sherrington,[3] Fulton,[4] Adrian,[5] and others. He burrowed into the field of physical medicine and drew upon his prior training and experience as an engineer. He came to realize and he showed how, directly and indirectly, the dental apparatus is involved in such other functions as respiration, speech, balance, posture, and orientation. As the cinefluoroscopic films of Klatsky and Fowler[6] demonstrate, the muscles involved in chewing and swallowing are not limited to the "four muscles of mastication," nor are the temporomandibular joints the only joints involved in these activities. Once one sees in these films the head rocking on the atlas and the cervical and thoracic vertebrae as well as the shoulder girdle, the sternum and clavicle, all moving during swallowing and mastication, one cannot but understand and appreciate the many structures involved and the neuromuscular systems concerned. Thus there are many structures related to the dental apparatus, all of whose activities must be coordinated and synchronized with a correctly aligned and functioning masticatory organ, if all these body functions are to proceed smoothly and without stress or strain.

To say this is but to affirm that oral orthopedics is a logical and natural forward step of long-established ideas in physiology, physics and mechanics, no less than in traditional dentistry. As far back as 1915–1918, Martin Dewey[7] and G. H. Wilson[8] were writing and teaching what has become known as "Dewey's Law"–"the movements of the mandible are not influenced in any way by the shape of the condyle, but the condyle may assume a certain shape because the mandible has assumed certain movements." Wilson went on to say that the mandible was not a lever of the third class nor of any class whatever. Despite similar assertions by many investigators since then and down to our own day (Marsh Robinson[9]), the misconception that the condyle-fossa relationship is the arbiter of mandibular movement, and that the condyle acts as a lever, persists. Men like Leon Williams[10] and George Monson[11] in this country and George Villain[12] of France wrote about and taught the geometrical analysis of the dental apparatus in the early 1920s. The equilateral triangle of Bonwill and the curve of Von Spee attest to the long-established use of geometry in dentistry. Perhaps Costen's classic work in the thirties directed many in the profession into the field of the temporomandibular joint, exaggerating its importance and neglecting the work of the men mentioned above. Nevertheless, interest has persisted to this day both here and abroad, with Boyle[13] in England as an example. It can therefore be seen that oral orthopedics is the natural outgrowth of much that has gone before.

Oral orthopedics is thus an advanced development in dentistry based on appreciation of the fact that improper relationship of the mandible to the maxilla not only can occur but actually is present in a large number of cases. It has been found that when such a relationship exists it results in an unbalanced occlusion, with the unhappy sequelae of that condition and often with other difficulties not hitherto recognized as having an oral relationship.

Oral orthopedics, then, may be defined as the concept of dental science and art concerned with postural relationships of the jaws, both normal and abnormal; analysis of the harmful influence of improper relationship of the mandible to the maxilla on dental and other related structures; the diagnosis and correction (as far as possible) of such malrelationship; and the treatment or prevention of disturbances resulting therefrom.

If correct occlusion is the foundation of dental science and art, as has been asserted, oral orthopedics, by providing a method for obtaining optimal occlusal relationships, supplies the maximal refinement of oral biomechanics for the benefit of the patient. The usual concept of balanced occlusion is insufficient to encompass the range of oral orthopedics. It is not enough merely to secure the best attainable relations of the teeth themselves. Fundamental to that is the requirement of obtaining optimal postural relations of the mandible to the maxilla.

Oral orthopedics can now be seen as embracing every field of dental practice, unifying the different phases into one comprehensive and correlated whole. It touches upon all scientific and artistic knowledge leading to a desired result. It is a well-linked chain of many parts working together for the benefit of one objective, namely, the normal working of the dental apparatus in coordination with all the other parts and functions of the body. A moment's reflection on this definition discloses how far along the road dentistry has progressed and how close it has come to realizing our objectives of saving teeth, improving oral health and safeguarding the total health of the individual.

Studies in anatomy, physiology, body mechanics, kinesiology, and neuromuscular function all lead to the ready realization that the proper relationship of the head upon the spine is essential to proper total body posture and balance. In turn, these are basic requirements for optimal general health. The suspended, heavy, highly dynamic mandible plays a most important role in establishing the posture of the head upon the spine. We are primarily concerned with the proper alignment of the mandible to the maxilla, which we call jaw relationship. Improper jaw relationship must mean impaired posture and balance, which is a stress-producing beginning for any function. Where improper jaw relationships exist, many compensatory adjustments must be made by all the parts involved in the activity. Although the activity may appear to be smooth and efficient, we know now that the functions are being performed at the cost of considerable strain on the functioning parts.

To quote Mabel Todd:

"In holding up its own weights the body may exert muscular effort far beyond what is really called for; and it can continue to do this because of its reservoir of energy. But in so doing, if the parts are held out of alignment and away from the axis of gravity, peculiar strains are put upon the spinal structure, which may give way with results of a quite unforeseen and disastrous nature. Sometimes the end-results are remote from the site of strain; and, moreover, symptoms may be misleading because of the nature of referred and reflected pain."[14]

Whether these strains and stresses will produce intraoral breakdown, extraoral pain, or disturbed functions will depend in large measure upon the resistive, adaptive, and recuperative powers of the individual patient. Stoll was among the first to point out the relationship between Selye's[15] "general adaptive syndrome" (GAS) and the many pain syndromes, not only in the head and neck but frequently distributed elsewhere in the body, concomitant with these complaints and simultaneously relieved. The most important stress is produced by malalignment of the jaws. An overall emotional or psychic stress makes these syndromes all the more likely to occur. Thus noci-stimuli travel afferently and efferently up and down the neuro-muscular systems involved and frequently are the direct and indirect cause for the atypical, sometimes bizarre, neuralgias and other pain syndromes mentioned above.

To provide a rational procedure for analysis of the structural development, as well as for the relationship of the maxilla and mandible, the following method of analyzing these jaws is presented.

A GEOMETRIC ANALYSIS OF THE HUMAN MAXILLA AND MANDIBLE (THE DENTAL MASS), INDIVIDUALLY AND RELATED: PART ONE*

From the time of Edward H. Angle's[16] first presentation of a systematic classification of malocclusion in 1893, down to the present, there have been many and varied other classifications of occlusion. Angle related his classification fundamentally to the relationship of the mandible to the maxilla. He used the permanent first molar relationship as his criterion. His primary concern, jaw relationship, has largely been forgotten almost from the first. Indeed, this may be due in large part to his mistaken assumption that the upper first molar is the most stable of all the teeth and could be assumed to be in its "normal" correct position. We have known better for many years, but the classification is still almost automatically decided by how the lower first molar relates to the upper first molar. Of late, the relationship of the upper canine to the lower canine and first premolar has been added to the first molar criterion, but it is still largely automatic and the jaw relationship is assumed to be as the molars and canines disclose.

Simon[17] argued in 1923 that since growth of the face and jaws occurred

---

*This analysis was compiled and written by Myron M. Lieb, D.D.S., Arthur A. Friend, D.D.S., and William Kaplan, D.D.S.

in all three planes of space, abnormalities and irregularities in height, width and depth also may occur in any one or more of the three planes. He called these abnormalities Anteroposterior, Sagittal and Mediolateral. Simon based his classification on anthropometric and craniometric measurements. For his vertical analysis he chose the Frankfort Plane as the horizontal base. Perpendicular to it and dividing the face into two equal halves was his Sagittal Plane. And he chose as his criterion of anteroposterior relationships his Orbital Plane perpendicular to both. Unfortunately, the Frankfort Plane chosen by arbitration at an anthropological congress is rarely parallel to the ground in a correctly positioned head. The median raphe does not universally bisect the maxilla, and the upper canines in many normal occlusions are not bisected by the Orbital Planes. Nevertheless, Simon was the first to orient our thinking along the lines of using orientation planes for analysis of study casts. Although he made strong representations favoring functional analysis as well as structural analysis, his ideas were largely ignored for more than a quarter of a century. It is well to quote him:

"A wide experience has taught us that orthodontics does not occupy itself to any great extent with function but only with the form of dentures . . . the part which function plays is somewhat platonic. Function is always regarded as dependent on structure, and orthodontists generally consider it secondary. An orthodontist may urge his patients to use their dentures, especially after corrective treatment, but he does not subject them to a functional test. He never speaks of *articulation* but always of *occlusion,* his subject is a denture at rest not in action . . . The functional norm, as the physiologist would consider it, is empirically demonstrable; it approaches reality,"

and he added, in speaking of "ideal normal,"

"all we ever find are variations; an exact ideal normal does not exist, cannot exist. And this is our enigma; in theory we will never find the normal, in practice we forever feel its need and apply it constantly."

With time, a fuller realization of the importance of Simon's observations has redirected orthodontists' thinking and more importance is being placed on functional analysis.

In all systems of orthodontic classification the analysis of the study casts is a fundamental step in arriving at a diagnosis or more correctly an analysis of the occlusion. Nor has geometry been neglected. From the equilateral triangle of Bonwill to the curve of Spee and from Monson's sphere to Boyle's sphere both plane and solid geometry have been used to explain the structure of the two main elements of the masticatory apparatus—the teeth and jaws. In the following concept of the structural analysis of study casts several basic thoughts are fundamental, especially in relation to all of the foregoing:

1. Without structure there can be no function.
2. Without correct structure function cannot be correct.
3. Incorrect function may adversely affect not only correct structure, but also seriously affect developing structures.

These fundamental postulates must be kept in mind whenever we attempt to analyze any structure. To study the functions of that organ or organism, understanding its physical structure and the relationships of its component parts precedes the analysis of the functional activities involved. In the masticatory apparatus, it is incumbent upon us to *determine the relationship of the jaws to the cranium and to each other.*

In order to do that, it is necessary:

1. To establish whether the maxilla and mandible are in their correct relationship to the cranium.

2. To establish the relationship of the mandible to the maxilla in static occlusion (habitual intercuspation).

3. To establish whether the upper permanent first molars are in their correct position in the maxilla and whether their axial inclination is correct.

Analysis of study casts should reveal the answers to the above. After such analysis has been made structurally and statically, the clinician is prepared to undertake an analysis of the functional activity of the masticatory apparatus.

With all the above in mind the following is a detailed description of what has become known as the "Oral Orthopedic Analysis of Study Casts." We accept Simon's dictum as to the "enigma," but hope this presentation will give to all dentists, not only orthodontists, a definitive geometric analytical guide. Less reliance, therefore, will have to be placed upon subjective criteria, since geometry is quite objective. Lest any one cry "you cannot squeeze human beings into a mathematical formula!" we hasten to point out the following: far from being a Procrustean bed, the "system" outlined below provides a formula for analyzing each individual's study casts. Geometric analysis is not exclusively an engineering modality used for inanimate structures. The geometric analysis of the human body as a whole, and of the head in particular, is familiar to all art students. Geometry is really "Nature's language" enabling us to understand the structures of all things, from the merest hut to the World Trade Center, and from the single atom to the universe and its galaxies.

A number of people asked to draw a straight line on a blackboard would describe an acceptable "straight line." If the group were given a T-square, all the lines would be exactly straight. What we are trying to do is provide dentists with a T-square to draw out the details of the structures in the teeth and jaws. Used carefully, analysis by different dentists would all agree, with insignificant differences here and there. This schema, this T-square, uses three planes of orientation, the Horizontal, the Mid-Sagittal and the Transverse. Simon's Horizontal—the Frankfort Plane—could not be delineated on the study casts. Our Horizontal Plane is parallel to the Earth's surface and can be marked off on the models. It is predicated on the fact that a well-developed skull would sit on a table top resting on the upper alveolar ridge and the occiput (Fig. 2–1).

In the living human being with the head properly related to the rest of

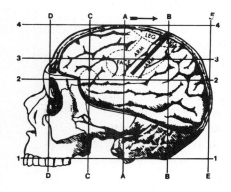

Figure 2–1.

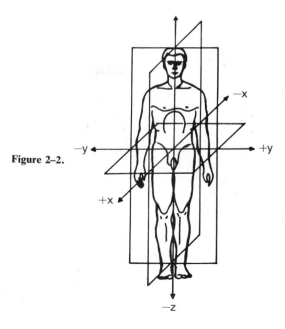

Figure 2–2.

the body in correct standing posture* (Figs. 2–2, 2–3) this plane can be visualized as passing through the anterior nasal spine and the lower border of the right and left tragi of the ears. It is parallel to the face of the Earth, and would be found to be parallel to the crest of the alveolar ridges (Figs. 2–1, 2–4).

---

*Correct standing posture can be defined as one in which the different segments of the body, head, neck, chest and abdomen are balanced vertically one upon the other so that the weight is borne mainly by the bony framework, with a minimum of effort and strain on muscles and ligaments; this is when the long axis of its segments, seen in profile, forms a vertical line instead of a zigzag. In addition the chest is held high, the scapulae in moderate eduction, the pelvis tilted forward normally and the lower limbs in full extension, with the weight poised over the arch of the foot.

Reference: Bowen and Stone, "Applied Anatomy and Kinesiology," Lea & Febiger, 1949, page 272.

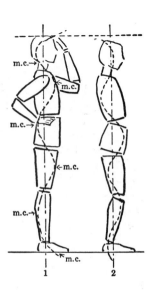

Figure 2–3. 1. Power balancing power through opposed muscle centers. Muscle centers coordinate cross line of gravity in movement when bones are balanced. 2. Bones opposing bones. When bones are unbalanced, weight opposes weight across line of gravity, thus throwing muscle centers under tension.

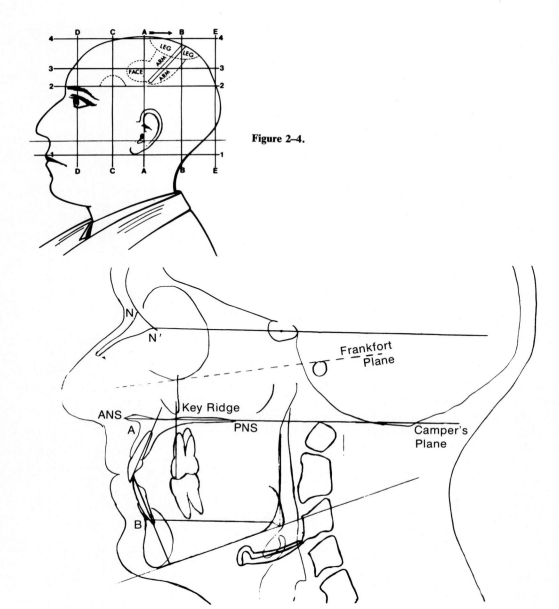

Figure 2–4.

Figure 2–5.

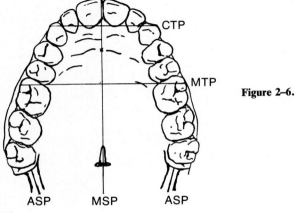

Figure 2–6.

38

I. PLANES OF ORIENTATION OF THE CORRECTLY DEVELOPED
MAXILLA WITH HEAD IN PROPER POSTURE:

A. The *Horizontal Plane,* parallel to the surface of the Earth, is parallel
to the Horizontal Plane of the skull which touches the alveolar ridges and
the occiput. The Horizontal Plane on the cephalograph is substantially
parallel (Fig. 2–5) to Camper's Plane (ANSPNS) and to a line drawn from
the lowest portion of the frontomaxillary nasal suture to the middle of the
sella turcica (WK).

B. *The Mid-Sagittal Plane* of the maxilla is perpendicular to the Horizontal plane and bisects the face and therefore the maxilla. In the upper jaw
it passes midway between the second palatal rugae and the fovea palatina.
It may or may not bisect the incisive papilla or coincide with the labial
frenum and median raphe (Fig. 2–6).

C. *The Maxillary Transverse Plane* is perpendicular to both the Horizontal and Mid-Sagittal Planes and in general bisects the left and right key
ridges at their lowest point (Fig. 2–5). The line formed by the intersection
of this Transverse Plane and the Mid-Sagittal Plane is called the Structural
Axis of the maxilla. On this axis, approximately four inches from the occlusal
plane, in the region of the glabella, is the Structural Center of the Dental
Mass (the upper and lower jaws and their contents). The inclination of the
upper teeth and the lower posterior teeth is such that their *central axes* all
converge toward this Structural Center. This Structural Center is also the
apex of a cone whose base is the occlusal plane; the lateral borders are
formed by the long axes of the molars and the anterior border is formed by
the axes of the upper anterior teeth. This cone is called the Dental Cone. It
is a section of a sphere whose center is the Structural Center and whose
radius is generally four inches (Figs. 2–7, 2–8).

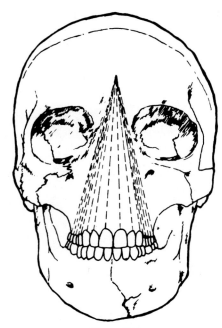

Figure 2–7.

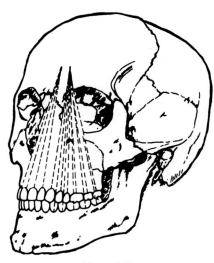

Figure 2–8.

D. *The Cuspid Transverse Plane* is also perpendicular to the Horizontal and Mid-Sagittal Planes, hence parallel to the Maxillary Transverse Plane. It is "x" millimeters (equal to the sum of ½ the mesiodistal diameter of the canine, the mesiodistal diameters of the first and second premolars and ½ the mesiodistal width of the mesiobuccal cusp of the upper first molar) anterior to the Maxillary Transverse Plane, usually bisecting the central lobe of the correctly positioned cuspid tooth. In an edentulous ridge this plane will lie in the region of the canine eminence (Fig. 2–6).

E. *Auxiliary Sagittal Planes* are parallel to the Mid-Sagittal Plane bilaterally and arise from the hamulus which is the most posterior and medial portion of the hamular notch (Fig. 2–6).

II. PLANES OF ORIENTATION OF THE CORRECTLY DEVELOPED BODY OF THE MANDIBLE WITH HEAD IN PROPER POSTURE:

A. *The Horizontal Plane* of the body of the mandible is parallel to the alveolar ridge. Cephalometrically, it can usually be described as parallel to a line drawn from Down's point "B" to the bisectant of the gonial angle. This plane is also parallel to the surface of the Earth (WK). This is so only when the mandible is correctly related to the maxilla (Fig. 2–5).

B. *The Mid-Sagittal Plane* is perpendicular to the Horizontal Plane and bisects the mandible. Its anterior edge will coincide with a line drawn between the genial tubercles and through the apex of the lingual spine. It may or may not coincide with the labial or lingual frena (Fig. 2–9).

C. *The Molar Transverse Plane* is perpendicular to the Horizontal and Mid-Sagittal Planes and will fall approximately midway anteroposteriorly between Down's Point "B" and the center of the retromolar fossa (Fig. 2–10).

D. *The Cuspid Transverse Plane* is parallel to the Molar Transverse Plane, hence perpendicular to the Horizontal and Mid-Sagittal Planes. As in the maxilla described above, it is situated the same "x" millimeters (in the mandible equal to the mesiodistal diameters of the first and second premolars and the width of the mesiobuccal cusp of the lower first molar) anterior to the Molar Transverse Plane (Fig. 2–10).

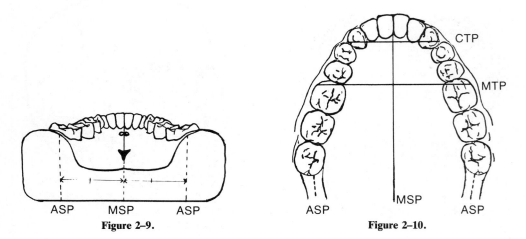

Figure 2–9.

Figure 2–10.

E. *Auxiliary Sagittal Planes* arise bilaterally as anteroposterior bisectants of the crest of the retromolar pads. These are projected parallel to the Mid-Sagittal Plane (Fig. 2–9).

The use of these orientation planes greatly facilitates the structural analysis of each jaw and the postural relationship of the lower jaw to the upper jaw in static occlusion (habitual maximal occlusal contact of the teeth or intercuspation). As will be shown below, these planes will also facilitate the positional analysis of each tooth in its respective jaw.

MODEL ANALYSIS

The following are the standards by which one can determine the structural correctness of a human maxilla and mandible using dental study casts.

I. Arch Form

A. The correct maxillary arch is developed sufficiently to accept all the teeth in their correct position, and is symmetrical, i.e., the right and left halves are substantially equal (Fig. 2–6).

B. The correct mandibular arch is developed sufficiently to accept all the teeth in their correct positions and is symmetrical, i.e., the right and left halves are substantially equal (Fig. 2–10).

C. The maxillary and mandibular dental arches will be harmonious with one another, i.e., they would have approximately the same general outline, with the maxillary arch approximately 10% larger than the mandibular arch anteroposteriorly.

II. Relationships of Teeth to Arches

A. Inclinations of teeth: Maxillary Dental Arch, Mandibular Dental Arch.

Maxillary Dental Arch

1. All anterior teeth have a slight labial inclination of the crowns (Figs. 2–7, 2–8, 2–11).

2. All posterior teeth have a slight buccal inclination of the crowns (Figs. 2–11, 2–12).

3. All the teeth anterior to the first molar have a slight mesial inclination (Fig. 2–11).

4. Beginning with the distal half of the first molar, all the posterior teeth have a slight distal inclination (Fig. 2–11).

5. The cusps of the posterior teeth and the incisal edges of the anterior teeth will be found mediolaterally and anteroposteriorly on a surface of a sphere with a radius of approximately 4 inches (with the central axes of all the teeth projecting toward the structural center of the dental cone, i.e., in the region of the glabella of the skull) (Figs. 2–11, 2–12).

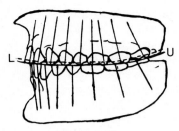

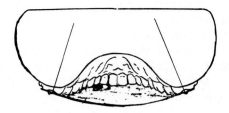

Figure 2–11.   Figure 2–12.

6. The lingual cusps of all upper posterior teeth are lower occlusally than the corresponding buccal cusps (Fig. 2–12).

Mandibular Dental Arch

1. All lower anterior teeth have a slight labial inclination, i.e., sufficient for the central axis of the lower central incisor to form a 90° ± 5° angle with the mandibular plane of the mandible and a 130° angle with the central axis of the correctly placed upper central incisor (evaluated on Cephalogram) (Figs. 2–5, 2–11).

2. All lower posterior teeth have a slight lingual inclination equivalent to the buccal inclination of the upper posterior teeth. The central axes of upper and lower posterior teeth are in the same plane (Fig. 2–13).

3. The bicuspids are positioned straight vertically (Fig. 2–11).

4. All molar teeth have a slight mesial inclination (Fig. 2–11).

5. The cusps of the posterior teeth and the incisal edges of the anterior teeth will be found mediolaterally and anteroposteriorly on a surface of a sphere with a radius of approximately 4 inches, with the central axes of the posterior teeth only projecting toward the Structural Center of the Dental Cone (Fig. 2–11).

6. The buccal cusps of all lower posterior teeth are higher occlusally than the corresponding lingual cusps (Fig. 2–14).

B. General Observations

1. Anteroposteriorly and mediolaterally the cusps of the lower posterior teeth (with the exception of the lingual cusp of the lower first bicuspid) and the incisal edges of the lower anterior teeth describe a curved plane which conforms to the base of the Dental Cone. This is the lower occlusal plane (Fig. 2–11).

2. The upper occlusal plane, also a curved plane, is concentric with (therefore parallel to) the curved plane of the lower occlusal plane but at a

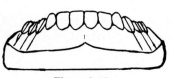

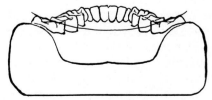

Figure 2–13.   Figure 2–14.

slightly lower level, i.e., equivalent to the depth of the cusps of the posterior teeth (Fig. 2–11).

3. In static occlusion all the upper teeth overlap the lower teeth labially and buccally, and the anterior overbite is equivalent to the depth of the posterior cusps. There is no anterior horizontal overjet.

4. All teeth in each arch are fully erupted and in correct mesiodistal and occlusal contact with their neighbors and opponents.

PROCEDURES FOR DEPICTING THE PLANES OF ORIENTATION ON STUDY CASTS

I. General Suggestions

A. All study casts should be accurate, not on art base forms, and include the following anatomic landmarks.
1. Maxilla:
   a. Buccal plate of bone up to the mucobuccal fold
   b. Both hamular notches
   c. Fovea palatina and rugae
2. Mandible
   a. Buccal plate of bone up to mucobuccal fold
   b. Genial tubercles
   c. Retromolar pads
   B. Accurate cephalometric x-ray which should include the key ridge.
   C. The locating and marking of the planes are done independently of the teeth since they relate solely to the structure of the individual jaw. (In a jaw wherein the teeth are correctly positioned these planes will always fall on the same areas of certain teeth. In malformed jaws and/or malpositioned teeth these planes will vary as to where they fall on certain teeth.)
   D. All markings of planes should be as accurate as possible; and measurements, using a pair of fine-pointed dividers, should be at approximately the alveolar ridge level of each jaw, at all times. This constant must be observed.
   E. All markings should be fine straight lines.

II. Procedural Steps

A. Maxilla—Adult:
1. Examine the arch form and note symmetry.
2. Examine the inclinations of the teeth and correlate with the cephalometric x-ray of anterior angular inclinations.
3. Locating and marking the Mid-Sagittal Plane (MSP).
   a. Mark the mid-point between the fovea palatina (Fig. 2–6).
   b. Mark the mid-point of the mesial aspect of the 2nd palatal rugae (Fig. 2–6).
   c. Join points 1 and 2 in a straight line and project anteriorly over the lingual surfaces and labial surfaces of the upper incisors to the

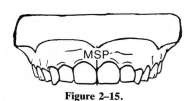

Figure 2–15.

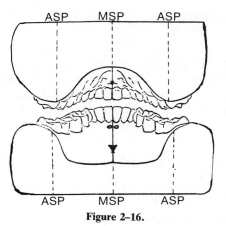

Figure 2–16.

mucobuccal fold. Project posteriorly over the posterior border of the model (Figs. 2–15, 2–16).

4. Locating and marking the Molar Transverse Plane (MTP).
   a. Locate, on the cephalometric x-ray, the key ridge and corresponding molar tooth (Fig. 2–5).
   b. Establish point at lowest portion of key ridge and draw perpendicular line to Camper's Plane (cranial horizontal plane) projecting it on above noted molar.
   c. Note position of this perpendicular on occlusal edge of molar on x-ray and mark this point on same molar on model.
   d. On model, project from this molar point a line perpendicular to the Mid-Sagittal Plane on to palate, projecting this line across palate, and on to both buccal plates to mucobuccal folds (Fig. 2–6).

5. Locating and marking the Cuspid Transverse Plane (CTP).
   a. The "x" millimeters which the Cuspid Transverse Plane is anterior and parallel to the Molar Transverse Plane is equal to the sum of ½ the mesiodistal width of the cuspid, the mesiodistal widths of the first and second bicuspids and ½ the mesiodistal width of the mesiobuccal cusp of the first molar (Fig. 2–17).
   b. After determining that exact distance, mark two points on the Molar Transverse Plane on the buccal alveolus. With the dividers set at the "x" millimeters distance, project a point anterior and at the same level for each of these points on the Molar Transverse Plane. Join these two new points in a straight line (which should be parallel to the

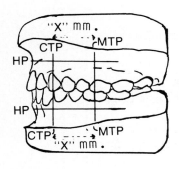

Figure 2–17.

Molar Transverse Plane), projecting from the occlusal plane to the mucobuccal fold.

  c. This is repeated on the opposite side of the model.

  d. These cuspid area lines can be projected across the palate forming a plane perpendicular to the Mid-Sagittal Plane and parallel to the Molar Transverse Plane (Fig. 2–6).

6. Locating and marking the Horizontal Plane (HP).

  a. Select a point on the Molar Transverse Plane on one side and project a perpendicular anteriorly to the Cuspid Transverse Plane on the same side, to the Mid-Sagittal Plane and finally to the Cuspid and Molar Transverse Planes on the opposite side. This plane should be at one level and perpendicular to all planes crossed (Fig. 2–17).

7. Locating and marking the Auxiliary Sagittal Planes (ASP) (Figs. 2–6, 2–16).

  a. Two additional heel markings are made by bisecting the hamular notch buccolingually (or marking the crest of the pterygomaxillary raphe anteroposteriorly) and projecting to the heel of the model where they are extended parallel to the projected Mid-Sagittal Plane. In a correctly developed maxilla these two sagittal planes will be equidistant from the Mid-Sagittal Plane.

  B. Mandible—Adult:

1. Examine the arch form and note symmetry.

2. Examine the inclinations of the teeth and correlate with the cephalometric x-ray of the anterior angular inclinations.

3. Locating and marking the Mid-Sagittal Plane (MSP).

  a. Bisect the lingual spine (from periapical film) (Fig. 2–9).

  b. Bisect the genial tubercles (from periapical film and/or study cast) (Fig. 2–9).

  c. Join points 1 and 2 in a straight line and project anteriorly over the lingual incisal and labial surfaces of the lower anterior teeth into the mucobuccal fold and posteriorly from point 2 to the lowest portion of the lingual alveolus (Figs. 2–9, 2–18).

4. Locating and marking the Molar Transverse Plane (MTP).

  a. With the dividers, measure the distance from the *upper* Mid-Sagittal Plane to the upper Molar Transverse Plane at the point of their intersection with the upper Horizontal Plane (Figs. 2–10, 2–17, 2–18).

  b. Take 90 per cent of this measurement and set your dividers for this computed distance.

  c. Select 2 points on the Lower Mid-Sagittal Plane on the labial alveolus in a relatively flat area of the alveolus, and mark off the computed distance, at relatively similar alveolar levels in the molar regions on both sides of the mandible.

  d. Connect the 2 points on each side in a straight line and project to the occlusal surface and mucobuccal fold. These two lines may be projected across the occlusal and lingual surfaces of the molar region onto the tongue area where they will join and establish the Molar Transverse Plane of the mandible which will be perpendicular to the mandibular Mid-Sagittal Plane were it to be projected to the heel of the study cast (Figs. 2–10, 2–17).

5. Locating and marking the Cuspid Transverse Plane (CTP).

  a. The "x" millimeters which the Cuspid Transverse Plane is anterior and parallel to the Molar Transverse Plane is equal to the sum of the

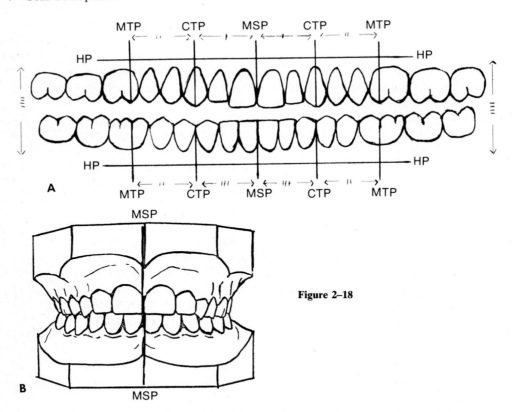

Figure 2–18

full mesiodistal widths of the first and second bicuspids and the mesiodistal width of the mesiobuccal cusp of the lower first molar. *It is equal to the "x" millimeters in the maxilla.*
   b. After determining that exact distance, follow the same procedure given for locating this plane in the maxilla (CTP).
6. Locating and marking the Horizontal Plane (HP).
   a. Follow the procedure outlined for establishing this in the maxilla (Figs. 2–10, 2–17, 2–18).
7. Locating and marking Additional Sagittal Planes.
   a. Two auxiliary heel markings are made by bisecting the retromolar pads buccolingually and projecting the lines anteroposteriorly over the heels of the lower study cast where they are extended parallel to the projected Mid-Sagittal Plane. In a correctly developed mandible these two Sagittal Planes will be equidistant from the Mid-Sagittal Plane (Figs. 2–9, 2–10).

PART TWO

In part one of this presentation we discussed the rationale and procedures used in analyzing each individual jaw's relationship to the cranium (Fig. 2–5) and the relationship of the two jaws to each other. In that presentation we described the use of the three orientation planes and their representation on each jaw, using study models of correctly formed jaws with the teeth in correct occlusion. In the following discussion we shall present the application of this geometrical analysis to the individual teeth in their respective arches and the relationship of both arches to each other when the teeth are in static occlusion (habitual maximal contact.)

I. ANALYSIS OF THE RELATIONSHIP OF THE MAXILLARY AND MANDIBLE TEETH TO THEIR RESPECTIVE ARCHES

A. If the lines denoting the specific vertical planes, in each jaw, coincide with the specific anatomic landmarks on the teeth previously described (Figs. 2–16, 2–17) the teeth are in their correct position in their individual arch anteroposteriorly.

B. *The Mid-Sagittal Plane* helps to establish whether homologous teeth are in their correct mediolateral position.

C. *The Horizontal Planes* help to determine whether the vertical position of each tooth is correct (whether they are in infra- or supraocclusion).

D. *The Cuspid* and *Molar Transverse Planes* determine the anteroposterior relationship of the teeth (Fig. 2–17).

E. For evaluation of axial inclination of the teeth the reader is referred to Part One, Roman Numeral II (see Figs. 2–11, 2–12, and 2–13).

F. Tooth arches should describe what is generally called a "Catenary Curve."

II. MAXILLOMANDIBULAR RELATIONSHIPS

A. *Correct Jaw Relationships*

1. When the upper and lower models (after accurate marking is performed) are articulated in static occlusion, the following conditions will be found to exist:

a. *The Mid-Sagittal Plane* (MSP) of the maxilla will be continuous and coincidental with the Mid-Sagittal Plane (MSP) of the mandible (Fig. 2–18).

b. *The Cuspid Transverse Plane* (CTP) of the maxilla will be continuous and coincidental with the Cuspid Transverse Plane (CTP) of the mandible (Fig. 2–17).

c. *The Molar Transverse Plane* (MTP) of the maxilla will be continuous and coincidental with the Molar Transverse Plane (MTP) of the mandible (Fig. 2–17).

d. The lines denoting the Horizontal Planes (HP) of the maxilla and the mandible respectively will be parallel to each other throughout their course anteroposteriorly and will be equidistant bilaterally (Fig. 2–17).

e. *The Auxiliary Sagittal Planes* (ASP) of the maxilla will be found contained within the Auxiliary Sagittal Planes (ASP) of the mandible, but on the horizontal aspect the right and left Auxiliary Sagittal Planes of the Maxilla will be found equidistant from the corresponding right and left Auxiliary Sagittal Planes of the mandible (Fig. 2–16).

2. All upper teeth will be in correct contact with the lower teeth and will also overlap the lower anteriorly and posteriorly equivalent to a distance equal to the depth of the cusps of the posterior teeth, thereby establishing the correct vertical dimension (Fig. 2–11) (see section on Model Analysis).

B. *Incorrect Jaw Relationships*

1. If the *Mid-Sagittal Plane* (MSP) of the mandible does not coincide with the Mid-Sagittal Plane (MSP) of the maxilla, but is found to the left of

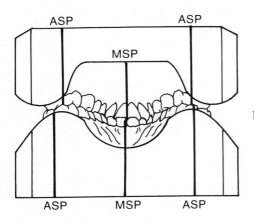

Figure 2–19.

the maxillary Mid-Sagittal Plane; and the CTP and MTP bilaterally remain coincidental, thereby showing no change anteroposteriorly of the mandible; and the Auxiliary Sagittal Planes (ASP) on the left side on heels of models are found further apart while those on the right side are found closer together, then there has been a bodily lateral shift of the mandible to the left (Fig. 2–19).

2. If the *Mid-Sagittal Plane* (MSP) of the mandible does not coincide with the Mid-Sagittal Plane (MSP) of the maxilla, but is found to the right of the maxillary Mid-Sagittal Plane; and the CTP and MTP bilaterally remain coincidental, thereby showing no change anteroposteriorly of the mandible; and the Auxiliary Sagittal Planes (ASP) on the right side are found further apart while those on the left side are found closer together, then there has been a bodily lateral shift of the mandible to the right (Fig. 2–20).

3. If the *Mid-Sagittal Plane* (MSP) of the mandible does not coincide with the Mid-Sagittal Plane (MSP) of the maxilla, but is found to the left of the maxillary Mid-Sagittal Plane; and the left CTP and MTP of the mandible are distal to the left CTP and MTP of the maxilla, while the right CTP and MTP of the mandible are mesial to the MTP and CTP of the maxilla or coincidental with them; and the left Auxiliary Sagittal Plane (ASP) of the mandible is closer to the left maxillary Auxiliary Sagittal Plane but the right

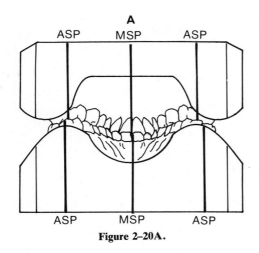

Figure 2–20A.

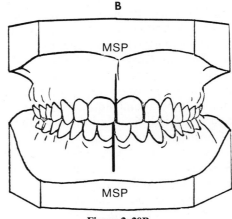

Figure 2–20B.

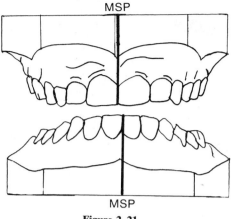

Figure 2–21.

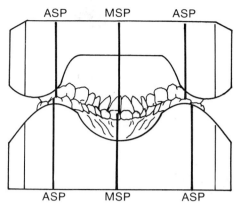

Figure 2–22.

Auxiliary Sagittal Planes are further apart, then there has been a bodily rotation of the mandible to the left (Figs. 2–21, 2–22, 2–23, 2–24). This is a horizontal rotation of the mandible around the vertical structural axis.

4. If the *Mid-Sagittal Plane* (MSP) of the mandible does not coincide with the Mid-Sagittal Plane (MSP) of the maxilla, but is found to the right of the maxillary Mid-Sagittal Plane; and the right CTP and MTP of the mandible are distal to the right CTP and MTP of the maxilla, while the left CTP and MTP of the mandible are either coincidental or anterior to the left CTP and MTP of the maxilla; and the right Auxiliary Sagittal Plane of the mandible is closer to the right Auxiliary Sagittal Plane (ASP) of the maxilla but the left Auxiliary Sagittal Planes are further apart, then there has been a bodily rotation of the mandible to the right (Figs. 2–25, 2–26, 2–27, 2–28).

5. If the *Mid-Sagittal Plane* (MSP) of the mandible coincides with the Mid-Sagittal Plane (MSP) of the maxilla, and the Auxiliary Sagittal Planes (ASP) of maxilla and mandible are equidistant on the horizontal but the Cuspid Transverse Plane (CTP) and Molar Transverse Plane (MTP) of the mandible *bilaterally* are distal to the CTP and MTP of the maxilla then the mandible is in a state of retrusion bodily (Fig. 2–29).

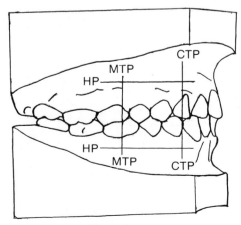

Figure 2–23.

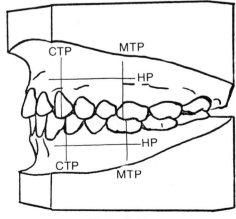

Figure 2–24.

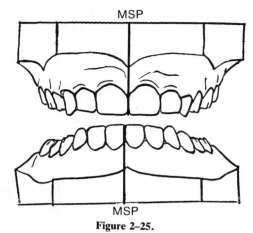

Figure 2–25.

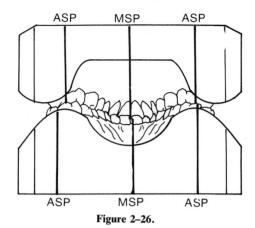

Figure 2–26.

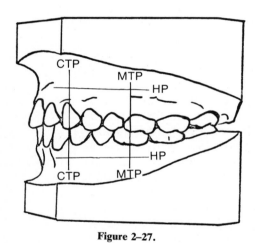

Figure 2–27.

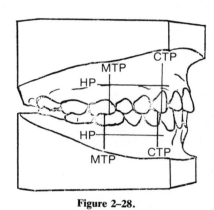

Figure 2–28.

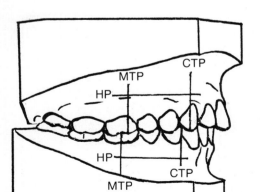

Figure 2–29.

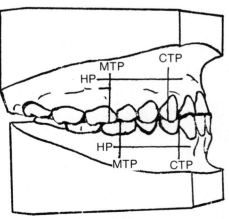

Figure 2–30.

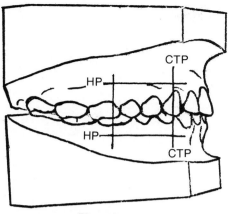

Figure 2–31.

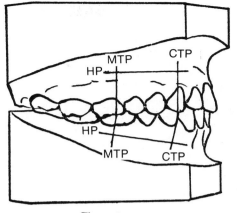

Figure 2–32.

6. If the *Mid-Sagittal Plane* (MSP) of the mandible coincides with the Mid-Sagittal Plane (MSP) of the maxilla, and the Auxiliary Sagittal Planes (ASP) of maxilla and mandible are equidistant on the horizontal, but the Cuspid Transverse Plane (CTP) and Molar Transverse Plane (MTP) of the mandible *bilaterally* are mesial to the CTP and MTP of the maxilla, then the mandible is in a state of protrusion bodily (Fig. 2–30).

7. If the *Mid-Sagittal Plane* (MSP) of the mandible coincides with the MSP of the maxilla, and the right and left Molar Transverse Planes (MTP) and Cuspid Transverse Planes (CTP) of the mandible coincide with the right and left MTP and CTP of the maxilla, and the maxillary and mandibular horizontal planes (HP) are parallel and bilaterally equidistant, and the ASP are equidistant on the horizontal, but the anterior overbite is greater than the depth of the cusps of the posterior teeth and the mandible and/or maxilla shows two planes of occlusion, then there has been a loss of vertical dimension, equally, anteriorly and posteriorly (Fig. 2–31).

8. If the maxillary and mandibular *Mid-Sagittal Planes* (MSP), Cuspid Transverse Planes (CTP), and Molar Transverse Planes (MTP) coincide and the Auxiliary Sagittal Planes are equidistant on the horizontal, with a correct anterior overbite relationship, but the Horizontal Planes (HP) of maxilla and mandible converge posteriorly, then the *mandible* has bodily tilted upward in the posterior region and the vertical dimension while remaining correct in the anterior region has been lost in the posterior region only, *unilaterally or bilaterally* (Fig. 2–32).

9. Varying combinations of the above stated possibilities may also occur and can be evaluated accordingly.

VARIATIONS

a. If the anterior overbite is greater than the depth of the cusps of the posterior teeth, with or without an anterior overjet and all the immediate conditions exist, then there has been an overall loss of vertical dimension, but it has been greater in the posterior region, *unilaterally or bilaterally,* than it has been in the anterior region (Fig. 2–33).

b. If the anterior bite is edge to edge or open, and all the immediate

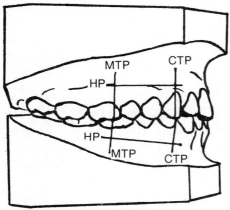

Figure 2–33.

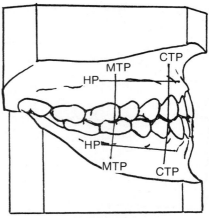

Figure 2–34.

conditions exist, then there has been a loss of posterior vertical dimension with an accompanying closure of the bite posteriorly and a corresponding opening of the bite anteriorly (Fig. 2–34).

This tilting of the mandible described above can be considered as a bodily vertical rotation of the mandible around a horizontal axis.

ANALYSIS OF PRIMARY AND MIXED DENTITION

This same method of analyzing the structure and the static relationship of the adult jaws can be successfully applied to the primary and mixed dentition. This is an accurate means of determining whether the developing occlusion and articulation are proceeding along correct lines. It may be useful, at this point, to review some pertinent stages of growth and development.

By the age of two and a half to three years, usually all the primary teeth have fully erupted. Normal or correct static occlusion requires that the mesial buccal cusp of the upper primary second molars occludes into the mesial buccal groove of the lower primary second molars and the upper primary canines fit between the distal inclines of the lower primary canines and the mesial inclines of the primary first molars.

If growth and development have been normal up to this point, we should find that the middle of the mesial buccal cusp of the upper primary second molar is directly below the lowest point of the Key Ridge in the cephalometric x-ray. As growth proceeds there occurs what Milo Hellman[18] called "mass mesial migration of all cellular elements." The teeth moreover move more rapidly than the maxillary bones; thus, at about age 10 or 11, the primary second molar is entirely mesial to the Key Ridge and the mesial buccal cusp of the permanent first molar occupies the position directly below the Key Ridge (Fig. 2–5). By about age 13 the transition from early primary to adult dentition is completed. Thus there is an interval of ten years on the average for this transition to be completed. If we measure, in the mixed dentition, the distance between the middle of the mesial buccal cusp of the primary second molar and the middle of the mesial buccal cusp of the permanent first molar we find the distance almost invariably to be ten millimeters. With a little arbitrary "judgment" we can say that the buccal segments of the maxillary arch move mesially approximately one millimeter per year. In the meantime the lower teeth migrate mesially slightly more rapidly, so that by 13 years of age the "leeway space" has been eliminated and the teeth are now positioned correctly. We now have both the teeth and jaws related correctly. The three orientation planes, as in the adult dentition described above, are thus used in the primary and mixed dentition.

Using the geometric analysis of the models of the primary or the mixed dentition we can now readily determine whether the teeth and the jaws are in correct relationship.

PRIMARY DENTITION: AGES 2½ TO 4 YEARS

The molar transverse plane is marked as a vertical line bisecting the mesial buccal cusp of the primary upper second molar and perpendicular to both the horizontal plane marked on the buccal alveolus and the midsagittal plane on the palate, precisely as described in the geometric analysis.

The cuspid transverse plane and the auxiliary sagittal planes are marked on the models as described in the "Analysis." Thus with the models held in static occlusion—if the upper and lower midsagittal planes and the molar and cuspid transverse planes are continuous and the horizontal planes are parallel to each other and the upper auxiliary sagittal planes are equidistant from the midsagittal plane and symmetrically medial to the lower auxiliary sagittal planes—we can safely assume the two jaws are in correct relationship. If the teeth in either jaw are not in the position described previously in relationship to the transverse and sagittal planes, then the teeth are in incorrect position. The midsagittal and auxiliary sagittal planes will reveal whether there is a lateral shift, or a rotation of the mandible, or both contributing to the incorrect position of any teeth.

ORAL ORTHOPEDIC CLASSIFICATION OF OCCLUSION

With the cast analysis in hand the clinician is now prepared to complete the examination of the masticatory apparatus. As the nature of the occlusion unfolds, the dentist checks all the structures and functions involved in the apparatus. The cephalometric x-ray is studied for the relationship of the palatal plane to the alveolar plane, both usually parallel to the horizontal plane and hence parallel to each other. The cervical spine should describe a graceful curvature, slightly convex anteriorly. The intervertebral spaces are substantially symmetrical. The hyoid bone generally is at the level of the fourth cervical vertebra. Deviations from these aspects in correct posture of the head upon the spine should be expected when analysis of the study casts discloses a malrelationship of the jaws.

Oral orthopedics sees the maxillary and mandibular bones as the major functioning units of the masticatory apparatus. Their proper development and correct relationship statically and functionally have a direct influence upon the proper physiologic functions of the whole apparatus. Correct jaw development and relationship is the fundamental requirement for normal muscle tone and the neural components involved in swallowing, breathing, chewing, speaking, and the posture of the head and neck. Disturbed or incorrect relationship of the jaws may lead to an imbalance of the neuromuscular systems involved in these varied functions.

To quote once more from Mabel Todd:

> In maintaining a balanced position amidst contending forces, stresses are set up within a structure, the degree of which varies with the position, the weight, and the resistant properties of the several parts. If strain occurs, its degree is proportional to, and varies with, the degree of the stress (Hooke's Law). To have a minimum of stress, and therefore of strain, within the body, not only must the structure as a whole be in balanced relation with the outside forces, but each part must be in balance with every other part within the system. This means that each part must be properly related to every other, remote as well as adjoining, if true mechanical balance is to obtain.[19]

The third, fourth, fifth, seventh, tenth, and twelfth cranial nerves are all closely related near their cortical nuclei as well as in some of the ganglia, where they are influenced and exert influences upon the autonomic (the sympathetic and parasympathetic) system. The deep spinal (sensory) root of the trigeminal descends at least to the level of the second or third cervical vertebra, where fibers emerge to merge with the cervical plexus. Only slightly further down, at level C3, C4, C5, the fibers of the brachial plexus arise. Noci-stimuli from any peripheral source can easily "jump" to the other parts of this neural system, giving us the wide variety of symptoms clinically observed.

Thus improper jaw relationships may not only produce mechanical trauma to the teeth and their supporting structures but also give rise to many of the symptoms affecting the structures innervated by the cranial nerves mentioned above. It is therefore essential for the clinician to be thoroughly familiar with the neural background involved in the various functions of the masticatory apparatus when assaying a diagnosis and formulating a treatment plan. Nor should the emotional and psychic state, including the life-style of the patient and its attendant stresses, be ignored. If dentists are to approach their patients with this holistic philosophy, they must be mindful of all these factors.

Throughout all his work Dr. Stoll stressed the importance of balance. "Balance," he wrote, "is one of the greatest principles of preservation in nature. Balanced occlusion is therefore a necessity for the health and efficiency of the dental apparatus. It may be defined as the coordination of all the structural elements of the dental apparatus properly aligned so that the normal physiological function can take place with equilibrium throughout all its parts, in harmony with all other parts of the body. Such balance minimizes shock to the nervous system and trauma and mechanical damage to the supporting tissues. It also minimizes lost motion and tends to stabilize the entire body mechanism."*

---

*The foregoing material was developed by the staff of the Institute for Graduate Dentists as part of the curriculum in the course in oral orthopedics. Particular acknowledgement is herewith extended to Doctors Arthur A. Friend, William Kaplan and Robert Ritt, co-members of the staff with the author. We were privileged to be taught and inspired by Dr. Victor Stoll, until his death in 1953. Institute for Graduate Dentists, 140 West 67th Street, New York, N.Y. 10023.

THE ORTHOPEDIC CLASSIFICATION OF MALOCCLUSIONS

Class A Correct occlusion
Class B Structural malocclusions

Class C Functional malocclusions
Class D Structuro-functional malocclusions

Class A

Correct occlusion may be said to obtain when the following elements are harmoniously developed and related for optimal functional efficiency:

1. Dental elements
   a) Structural components
      (1) Jaws
      (2) Teeth
      (3) Dento-facial relationship
      (4) Temporomandibular joint
   b) Functional components
      (1) Muscles of mastication
      (2) Tongue muscles
      (3) Lip muscles
      (4) Cheek muscles

2. Non-dental elements
   a) Posture
   b) The structures involved in
      (1) Respiration
      (2) Deglutition and ventilation
      (3) Speech
   c) Kinesiological tests give a positive response, indicating correct muscle tone

Malocclusion is said to exist when the structural components are incorrectly developed or related and the functions in which they participate are adversely affected or in turn may adversely affect the structures. Well-developed and harmoniously related structural components may also be adversely affected by aberrant function.

Class B

Structural malocclusions—the result of inharmonious development and relations of the jaws and incorrect relations of the teeth:

1. Incorrect development of the jaws as evidenced in static occlusion
   a) Correct maxillary development with mandibular underdevelopment
   b) Correct maxillary development with mandibular overdevelopment
   c) Correct mandibular development with maxillary underdevelopment
   d) Correct mandibular development with maxillary overdevelopment
   e) Bimaxillary underdevelopment
   f) Bimaxillary overdevelopment

2. Incorrect relations of teeth due to aberrations in
   a) Size
   b) Form
   c) Number
   d) Position

These may occur either in correctly developed and related basic structures or in any of the incorrectly developed or related basic structures in Class B1.

Class C

Functional malocclusions: incorrect relations of properly developed jaws caused or maintained by imbalance of muscle activity, with or without tooth malpositions:

1. Retrusions
2. Protrusions
3. Lateral displacements
4. Rotations
   (a) Vertically
   (b) Horizontally

5. Incorrect intermaxillary space
6. Combinations of any of the above
7. Kinesiological tests give negative reactions (weakened responses), indicating improper muscle tone.

Class D

Structuro-functional malocclusions: various combinations of Class B and Class C.

While in New York the Oral Orthopedic Group was pursuing further research and clinical application of their concepts and techniques, other dentists, in the Midwest, quite independently, were developing and practicing similar concepts. As has happened before, neither group was aware of the other's work. By fortuitous accident, we learned of the work of these dentists, members of the American Academy of Physiologic Dentistry and

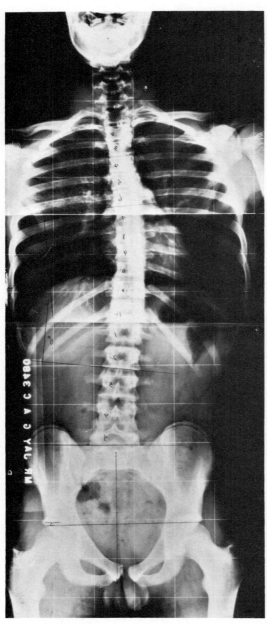

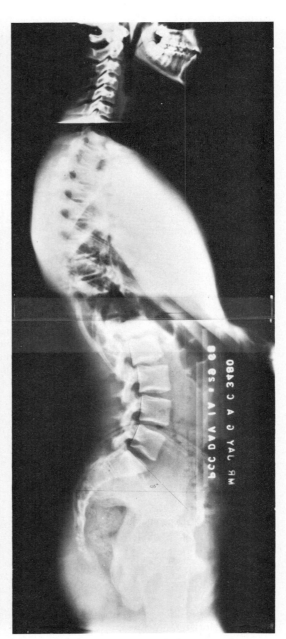

Figure 2–35. Anteroposterior view before treatment.

Figure 2–36. Lateral view before treatment.

the American Academy of Functional Prosthodontics. They organized their own research and dental laboratory facilities to help them carry out their concepts in their clinical practices. For 30 years they have been applying clinically their concepts, incorporating Selye's Stress Syndrome findings. They consider dental stress as a primary factor affecting near and remote structures. Not surprisingly, their experiences have paralleled those encountered in our practice of Oral Orthopedics.

With the kind permission of the Midwestern groups, and especially the Editor of their publication "Basal Facts," we present below synopses of several of their case histories and results.

Case 1

A 16-year-old boy with scoliosis and other defects of posture. His occlusion was diagnosed as being unphysiologic. His bite was corrected by the insertion of amalgam occlusal restorations in the mandibular second molars. This was to provide dominant molar support. It was with great difficulty that the patient was convinced to return for checkups. The results are pictured in Figures 2–35 to 2–38.

Case 2

A 21-year-old male with very bad posture.[20] He presented a deep overbite, primarily caused by all his lower posterior teeth being in linguoversion. In this case, upper and lower removable expansion appliances were used to upright all the posterior teeth. The improvement in posture is evidenced in Figures 2–39 to 2–42.

Case 3

This chronically ill and despondent housewife complained of severe headaches, backaches, and a host of other complaints. She could not lift her arms above her shoulders. She rejected medical suggestions that her problems were psychiatric in origin. Her occlusion had "collapsed" with several teeth missing. Temporary bridges, replacing the missing posterior teeth and giving her dominant molar support, were inserted. Considerable relief was experienced before she left the office. Although she had been advised to see her physician regularly, she had not done so in three years, because she felt so symptom-free. The only other treatment she has had were occasional chiropractic visits before each occlusal adjustment. She has not had all the spinal normalization looked for, because her visits to her dentist were sporadic. She now has a full-time job and "feels wonderfully alive again." Her case is pictured in Figures 2–43 to 2–47.

Our sincere thanks and appreciation to the Academy of Physiologic Dentistry, The American Academy for Functional Prosthodontics, and the Editor of "Basal Facts," Dr. A. C. Fonder, 303 West Second Street, Rock Falls, IL 61081.

Once again, we see demonstrated that the laws of mechanics and physiology are universal. They must be harmonized with everything clinical practice does if the patient is to derive the benefits of today's holistic treatment.

The following case studies, and their accompanying illustrations (photographs and radiographs) are examples of the effects of jaw malrelationships, and the Oral Orthopedic treatment.

Text continued on page 64

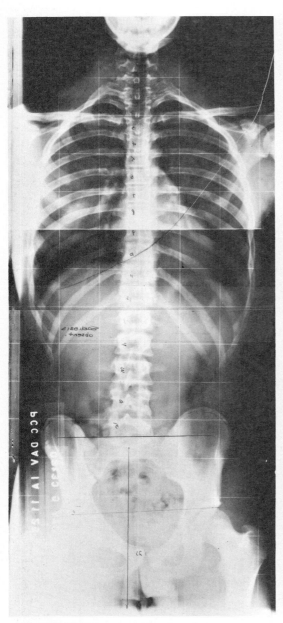

Figure 2–37. Anteroposterior view after treatment.

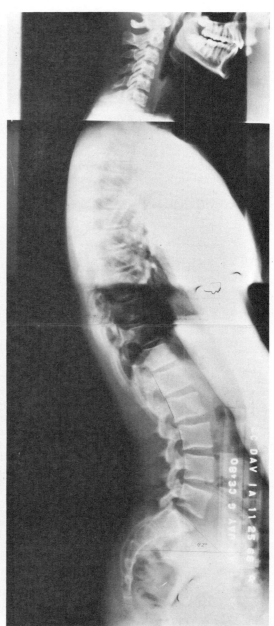

Figure 2–38. Lateral view after treatment.

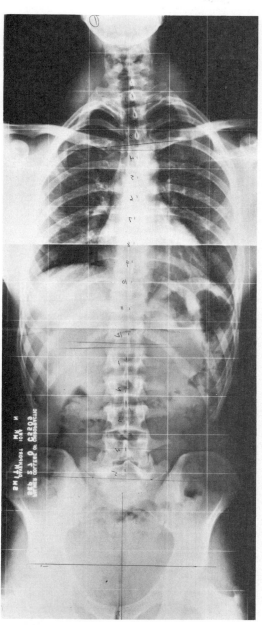

Figure 2–39. Anteroposterior view before treatment.

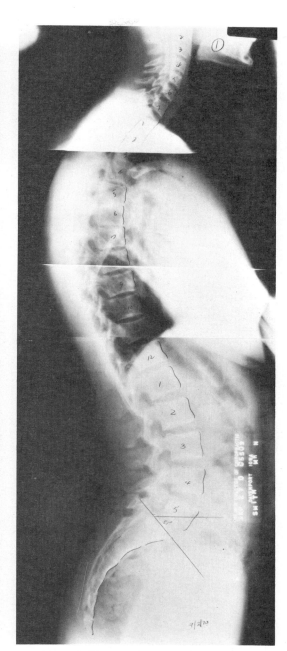

Figure 2–40. Lateral view before treatment.

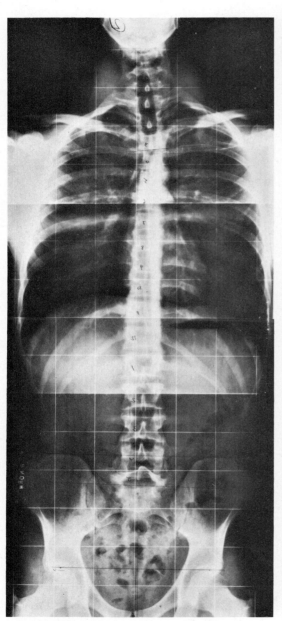

Figure 2–41. Anteroposterior view after treatment.

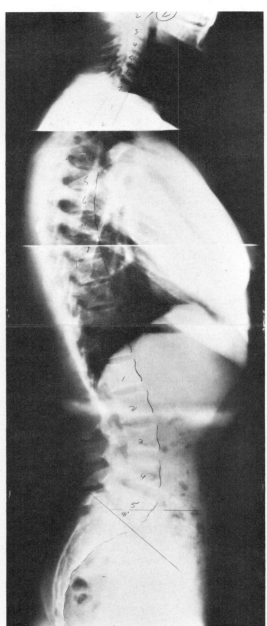

Figure 2–42. Lateral view after treatment.

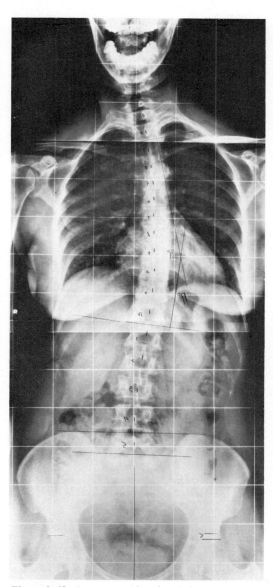

Figure 2–43. Anteroposterior view before treatment.

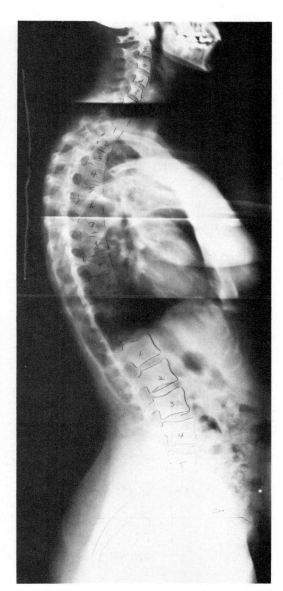

Figure 2–44. Lateral view before treatment.

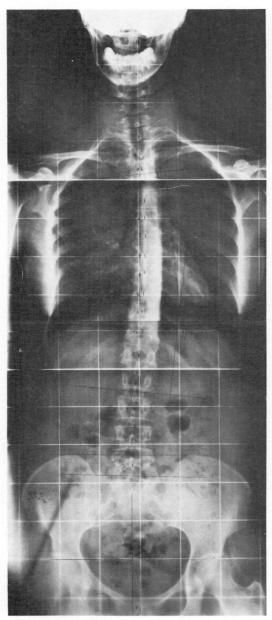

Figure 2–45. Anteroposterior view after treatment.

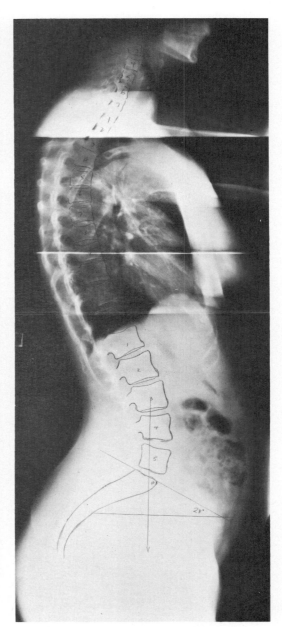

Figure 2–46. Lateral view after treatment.

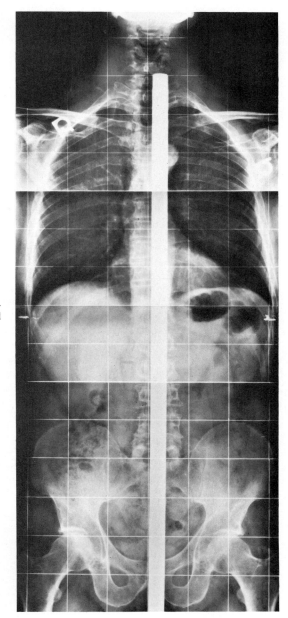

Figure 2–47. Anteroposterior radiograph showing minimal distortion, utilizing a greater energy source and target-film distance.

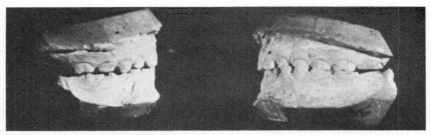

Figure 2–48. From Dental Concepts, *10*: Fall-Winter, 1966. Institute for Graduate Dentists, 140 West 67th Street, New York, NY 10023.

Case 4

A. W., age 5, female, presented with no significant medical history but with evidence of head pain of a generalized nature.[20] Her features never seemed to be at rest and were often contorted. She tended to shift her mandible from side to side. There was some difficulty in mastication and deglutition.

Dental examination showed a unilateral posterior cross bite. The patient could produce a normal posterior occlusion on either side at will. Figure 2–48 shows photographs of models indicating the cross bite on the left side. Treatment included orthodontic care together with repositioning of the mandible. The splint used for that purpose is shown on the model in Figure 2–49.

An interesting feature of this case is the effect of mandibular malposition on the balance of the skull on the spine and the lordosis of the cervical spine resulting apparently from muscle imbalance thus indicated (Fig. 2–50). The improvement in alignment of the cervical vertebrae which followed the orthodontic treatment with repositioning of the mandible is shown in Figure 2–51. The symptoms noted above were relieved.

Case 5

Mrs. L. L., age 40. Presented with complaint of pain in the temporomandibular joints and bleeding of gums, especially around the upper incisors.[20] There was clicking on opening and closing. There was a diastema, recently developed, between the upper right central and lateral incisors (Fig. 2–52).

There was no significant medical history, present health good. Dental examination revealed moderate periodontal disease, excessive anterior overbite, moderate posterior overclosure and retrusion of the mandible (Fig. 2–53).

A control prescription consisting of a removable lower lingual bar splint with acrylic cusps was constructed to restore correct vertical height, reduce the anterior overbite and permit mandibular repositioning (Fig. 2–54).

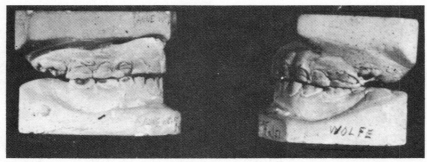

Figure 2–49. From Dental Concepts, *10*: Fall-Winter, 1966. Institute for Graduate Dentists, 140 West 67th Street, New York, NY 10023.

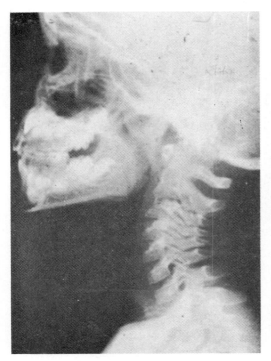

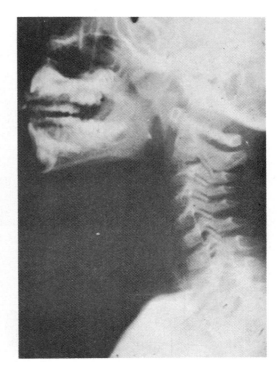

Figure 2–50   Figure 2–51

Figure 2–50. Lateral head and neck roentgenograms before treatment. Note marked lordosis of the cervical spine and compression of posterior intervertebral spaces. (From Dental Concepts, *10*: Fall-Winter, 1966. Institute for Graduate Dentists, 140 West 67th Street, New York, NY 10023.)

Figure 2–51. Lateral head and neck roentgenograms after treatment. Note marked improvement in alignment of cervical spine and increase in width of posterior intervertebral spaces. (From Dental Concepts, *10*: Fall-Winter, 1966. Institute for Graduate Dentists, 140 West 67th Street, New York, NY 10023.)

Four months later the upper incisors were firm, the diastema had closed and the gingivae were healthy. The pain in the temporomandibular joints was relieved and the clicking had subsided. (It was found later that the acrylic cusp coverage of the splint had worn somewhat, permitting partial overclosure and retrusion. Temporomandibular pain recurred but was relieved by re-establishment of the correct mandibular position.)

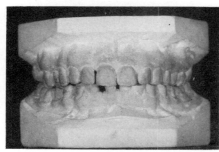
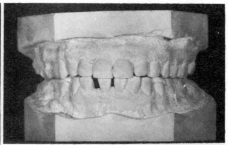

Figure 2–52.

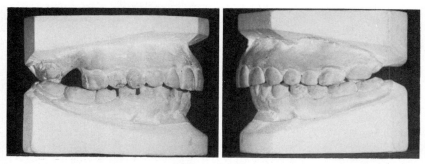

Figure 2–53.

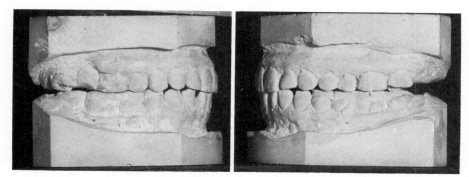

Figure 2–54.

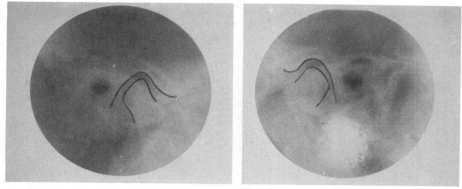

Figure 2–55.

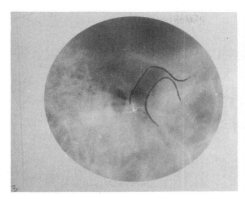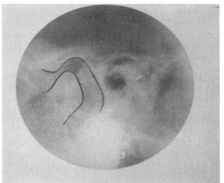

Figure 2–56.

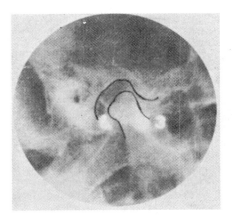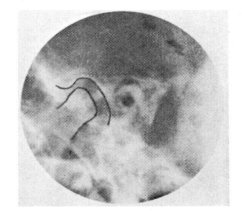

Figure 2–57.

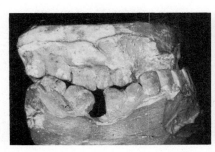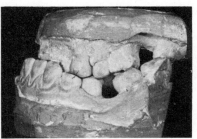

Figure 2–58.

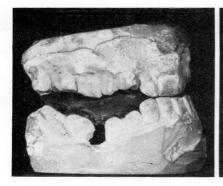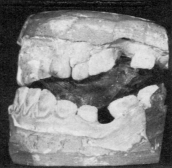

Figure 2–59.

Figure 2–55 shows temporomandibular roentgenograms taken at the time of the initial examination. Figure 2–56 shows the position of the condyles after repositioning of the mandible with teeth in static occlusion. Figure 2–57 shows the position of the condyles with the mandible in static occlusion, the roentgenograms being taken 18 months after those shown in Figure 2–56.

It should be noted that although the extent of malposition of the mandible was relatively slight the symptoms referable to it were quite severe and also that the slight change in mandibular position required for correction produced a marked alteration in the position of the condyles in the glenoid fossae.

Anatomical studies and clinical experience indicate that when jaw and tooth relationships are correct and the patient has developed a new pattern of jaw closure and function through muscle re-education, condyle-fossa relations as shown are entirely acceptable.

Case 6

J. S., age 63, male physician, general health good. Dental condition: several upper and lower posterior teeth missing, bite severely closed with development of functional Class III malocclusion. Moderate periodontal disease.[21]

With no warning in the way of previous discomfort the patient suddenly developed excruciating pain under the right eye, constant and so severe as to cause loss of sleep and inability to carry on daily routine. Consultation with several physicians was fruitless. The case was finally diagnosed as tic doulou-

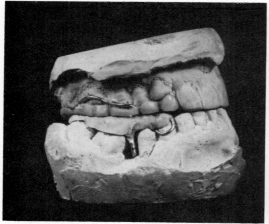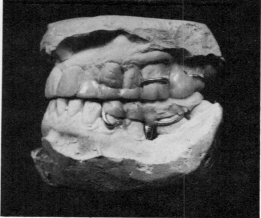

Figure 2–60.

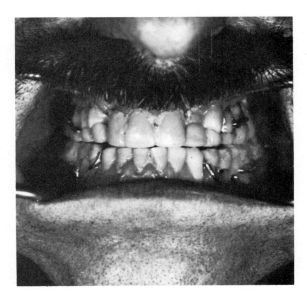

Figure 2–61.

reaux and the patient was advised to have an alcohol injection. He did not accept that diagnosis. Jaw realignment was then undertaken as a possible means of getting relief.

Casts reproducing the original mandibular malposture, shown in Fig. 2–58, were mounted on the Stoll analyzer and a correct relation set up (Fig. 2–59).

The wax bite was tried in the mouth. A temporary quick-curing acrylic splint was then processed, followed by removable splints in the form of partial dentures (Figs. 2–60, 2– 61). Within a few minutes after the insertion of the first splint the pain under the eye subsided. The patient had no pain from that time on and slept without opiate, and at once resumed his daily schedule. Leaving the splint out experimentally caused recurrence of pain.

(This case was discussed in Dental Concepts, 5:11, 1953.)

References

1. Costen, J. B.: Syndrome of ear and sinus symptoms depending upon disturbed function of the temporomandibular joint. Am. Otol., *43*:1, 1934.
2. Stoll, V.: Quoted in The Dentist and His Patient. New York, Revere Publishing Company, 1944, p. 176. See also Cervical Facial Orthopedia. Dental Concepts, 2:2, 1950.
3. Sherrington, C. S.: Integrative Action of the Nervous System. New Haven, Yale University Press, 1906.
4. Fulton, J. F.: Physiology of the Nervous System. New York, Oxford University Press.
5. Adrian, J. F.: Journal of Physiology, *61*:49, 1926.
6. Klatzky, M., and Fowler, E. P.: Cinefluoroscopic Films on Deglutition and Mastication, 1938.
7. Dewey, M.: JADA, 5:234, 1918.
8. Wilson, G. H.: Anatomy and physiology of the temporomandibular joint. NDA Journal, 7:414, 1920.
9. Robinson, M.: JADA, *33*:19, 1946.
10. Clapps, G. W.: Life of J. Leon Williams. New York, 1925.
11. Monson, G. S.: Occlusion and the teeth. JADA, 7, 1920.
12. Villain, G.: Trans. F.D.A.I., 1936.
13. Boyle, H. H.: Design of the Human Dentition. London, Staples Publishing Company, 1952.
14. Todd, M.: The Thinking Body. New York, Dance Horizons, 1968.
15. Selye, H.: The Physiology and Pathology of Exposure to Stress. Montreal, ACTA Inc., 1950.

16. Angle, E. H.: Treatment of Malocclusion of the Teeth, 7th ed. Philadelphia, S.S. White, 1907.
17. Simon, P. W.: Fundamental Principles of Systemic Diagnosis of Dental Anomalies. B. E. Lischer, trans. Boston, Stratford Press, 1926.
18. Hellman, M.: Factors Influencing Occlusion. Development of Occlusion. Philadelphia, University of Pennsylvania Press, 1941.
19. Todd, op. cit.
20. Dental Concepts, *10*:18, 1966.
21. Dental Concepts, *5*, 1953.

Additional References

Gelb, H., and Arnold, G.: The syndrome of the head and neck of dental origin. Arch. Otolaryngol., *70*:681, 1950.
Gelb, H.: A review of the medical-dental relationship in craniomandibular syndrome. N.Y.J. Dent., *41*:163, 1971.
Gelb, H., Calderone, J. P., Gross, S., and Kantor, M.: The role of the dentist and the otolaryngologist in evaluating TMJ syndrome. J. Pros. Dent., *18*:497, 1967.
Goodheart, G. J.: Kinesiology and Dentistry. J. Am. Soc. Prevent. Dent., *6*:76, 1976.
Eversaul, G. A.: Biofeedback and Kinesiology. Dental Applications. Las Vegas, Nevada, 1977 (privately published).
Dawson, P. E.: Evaluation, diagnosis, and treatment of occlusal problems. St. Louis, C. V. Mosby Co., 1978.
Clarke, N. G.: Occlusion and myofascial pain. Is there a relationship? JADA, *104*:443, 1982.
Funokoshi, M., Fujita, N., and Takehana, S.: Relations between occlusal interference and jaw muscle activities in response to changes in head position. J. Dent. Res., *55*:684, 1976.

3

Patient Evaluation

HAROLD GELB, D.M.D.

Although clinical research and observation have been conducted for many years by various investigators, there is currently disagreement about what symptoms and findings are characteristic of, and directly related to, the craniomandibular syndrome. If we are discussing symptoms of temporomandibular joint dysfunction, or the myofascial pain–dysfunction syndrome, then we allude primarily to pain and tenderness in joints and masticatory muscles, limited movement, clicking, and crepitation. However, if the scope is broadened to include the symptomatology of the head, neck, and jaws, we should then include the following wide variety of symptoms: subluxation, dislocation, conductive hearing loss, burning, pricking and tingling sensations, vertigo, clogged ears, tinnitus, radiographic changes, head, facial, neck, shoulder, and arm pain, and others.

Thus far the standard analysis of symptomatology has not provided a complete picture of the parameters or pathogenesis of the particular disorder we may be describing.

Suffice it to say that we should be in agreement when it comes to making a diagnosis, although our treatment of the patient may vary somewhat. Let us endeavor to escape a problem that has long ensnared the health professions, namely, *underdiagnosis coupled with overtreatment.*

In order to bring this point into sharp focus, it should be stated that head pain is civilized man's most common complaint. More than half the total visits to physicians' offices each year are for this problem. A recent research report involving a small dental population sampling of apparently "healthy" people revealed that 43 per cent had headaches, 17 per cent experienced neckaches, and 11 per cent suffered from both. Their frequency varied from monthly to daily occurrences.[1] As many more patients were examined, these percentages changed to 44.6 per cent and 21.9 per cent for the first two categories.[1a]

It is evident that a need exists to take a much closer look at the patients passing through our offices daily.

HISTORICAL PERSPECTIVE

As far back as 3000 B.C. "a dislocation of the mandible" was reported in Egypt.[2] Hippocrates described "a group of patients whose teeth are disposed irregularly, crowding one on the other and they are molested by headaches and otorrhea."[3] In 1771 Hunter recommended muscular exercise as an adjunct to the treatment of certain types of malocclusion.[4] A century later Sir Astley Cooper, a surgeon, described a subluxation of the temporomandibular joint as distinct from dislocation. He also observed that his cases were largely confined to females of lowered resistance with abnormal relaxation of joint ligaments.[5] Association between joint disturbances and faults in occlusion was observed over 50 years ago when Prentiss stated that the temporomandibular joint became pathological with the loss of teeth.[6] At about the same time, Wright[7] and Monson[8] related occlusal disharmonies to deafness. This gained further prominence when Goodfriend reported his results concerning deafness, tinnitus, vertigo, and neuralgia in 1933.[9]

In 1934 Costen[10] described a syndrome of ear and sinus symptoms predicated upon disturbed function of the temporomandibular joints observed primarily in patients with edentulous mouths and those with marked overclosure. Costen's theory remained unchallenged for approximately 15 years, at which time Sicher and Zimmerman[11] challenged his direct anatomical basis for relating the symptoms to pressure of the condyles on nerves or blood vessels behind the temporomandibular joint.

Cases of overclosure and posterior dislocation of the condyle were later reported to be caused by "lax" ligaments and also subluxation, and even the development of cases of complete luxation. These cases were treated by injection of sclerosing solutions into the joints. The theories stated above were mechanical in nature and concept. In recent years, however, theories have been proposed that take into consideration the neuromuscular mechanism and its capacity to be disturbed by morphofunctional imbalance.

Pain and dysfunction, evidenced by reduced mandibular movements, were the symptoms found most frequently in hundreds of cases treated by Schwartz,[12] but the symptom complex described by Costen was not found as such. These symptoms were precipitated by the sudden or continuous stretching of the masticatory musculature, yawning, excessive biting, prolonged dental treatment sessions, or proprioceptive changes caused by sudden or extensive alterations in the dental occlusion. Malocclusion was believed merely to be a contributing factor. Female patients were four times more numerous than males. Treatment was essentially spasmolytic, consisting of ethyl chloride spray and intramuscular infiltration with a local anesthetic of the affected masticatory muscles, followed by exercising of these muscles. Psychiatric evaluation and counseling were also included.

Campbell, another prominent investigator, conducted an 11-year study of 899 selected cases of temporomandibular arthroses with pain, and showed that 551 of these patients benefitted from dental care.[13] In this study, the ratio of females to males was 3.5 to 1, and a notable, though variable, pain pattern emerged. The pain was concentrated at the origins and insertions of the muscles, with the joint being the most common site.

Treatment was of a prosthetic nature, employing a temporary acrylic splint to discover the optimal jaw relations, followed by permanent occlusal reconstruction after close observation over a suitable period of time.

Both these studies revealed that the pain described by the patients was a constant, dull ache, in contrast to the sudden, sharp, intermittent pain of the neuralgias. Pains were also reported in areas remote from the temporomandibular joints themselves, namely, the jaws, neck, and shoulders. Collectively, the findings of hundreds of documented cases by several different investigators supported the theory that disturbances of occlusion, coupled with either extrinsic or intrinsic trauma, constituted the chief etiological factor in patients suffering from temporomandibular disorders. *Treatment by alteration of the occlusion and repositioning of the lower jaw was successful in over 75 per cent of all cases.*[14, 15, 16, 17, 18, 19]

It was Sicher[20] who originally concluded that the symptoms of local and radiating pain, clicking and crepitation of the joint, and restriction of joint movement were simply the symptoms of *arthritis.* He recommended that the term "Costen's syndrome," with its various implications, should be replaced by a diagnosis of temporomandibular deforming arthritis from mandibular overclosure or displacement. He also suggested that pain in the ear may arise from spasm of the masticatory muscles resulting from bruxism. Spasm may also occur as a result of painful stimuli from the joint. Sicher also stated[21] that localized pain in the joint may be caused by pressure of the condyle on the loose connective tissue behind it in the fossa, and that pain in the surrounding area is primarily muscle pain. The tenderness felt on palpation suggests that the painful stimuli may arise in the capsular ligament surrounding the joint. He found that pain in the temple area originated in the temporalis muscle, pain in the cheek and jaws originated in the masseter muscle, and pain in the throat derived from the pterygoid muscles. One other commonly seen symptom was earache. The work started by Schwartz was expanded by Laskin[22] at the University of Illinois. He propounded a psychophysiologic concept based on the theory that masticatory muscle spasm is the prime factor in the etiology of the signs and symptoms of this disorder. His investigations supported the role of muscle fatigue as the most frequently seen cause of these muscle spasms. This fatigue is believed to be related to psychologically motivated, persistent, tension-relieving oral habits. Since the role played by muscles is paramount, he suggested the term myofascialpain dysfunction syndrome (MPD) as a more accurate description.

Bell[23] said that temporomandibular joint disorders can be categorized into eight major groups (Table 3–1).

Most of these categories are easily differentiated and constitute a very small percentage of the total group. It remains only to differentiate between the pain-dysfunction syndrome, which is primarily a masticatory muscle problem, and temporomandibular arthritis, which is true arthropathy.

Temporomandibular joint arthritis, whether rheumatoid or degenerative, exhibits symptoms that are primarily of dysfunction. Only in the acute inflammatory stage is pain a symptom, indicating true arthralgia. Muscle involvement occurs as a secondary result of dysfunction or as a central excitatory effect of deep arthralgic pain.

Myogenic pain and muscle-induced masticatory dysfunction characterize the initial phase of the pain-dysfunction syndrome, but if the condition

TABLE 3–1. Categories of Temporomandibular Disorders*

---

1. Acute Masticatory Muscle Complaints
   a. Protective muscle splinting
   b. Masticatory muscle spasm (MPD syndrome)
      (1) Spasm of lateral pterygoid muscle
      (2) Spasm of elevator muscles
      (3) Spasm of lateral pterygoid and elevator muscles
   c. Masticatory muscle myositis
2. Complaints Involving Articular Disc Interference
   a. Class I Interference: Occurs at occluded position only
   b. Class II Interference: Occurs as translation begins and/or ends
   c. Class III Interference: Occurs during normal translation
   d. Class IV Interference: Occurs with overextended opening
   e. Spontaneous anterior dislocation
   f. Reciprocal click
   g. Closed lock (acute and chronic)
3. Complaints that Result from Extrinsic Trauma
   a. Noninflammatory traumatic conditions
   b. Inflamed retrodiscal pad ("retrodiscitis")
   c. Inflammatory traumatic conditions
      (1) Capsulitis
      (2) Traumatic arthritis
4. Degenerative Joint Disease
   a. Noninflammatory phase ("arthrosis")
   b. Inflammatory degenerative arthritis
5. Other Inflammatory Joint Disease
   a. Rheumatoid arthritis
   b. Infectious arthritis
   c. Metabolic arthritis
6. Chronic Mandible Hypomobilities
   a. Ankylosis
      (1) Fibrous
      (2) Osseous
   b. Contracture of articular capsule (capsular fibrosis)
   c. Contracture of elevator muscles
      (1) Myostatic contracture
      (2) Myofibrotic contracture
   d. Closed lock disc derangement
7. Complaints from Problems of Growth, Hyperplasia, Neoplasia
8. Postsurgical Complaints

---

*Reproduced with permission from Bell, W. E.: Clinical Management of Temporomandibular Disorders. © 1982 by Year Book Medical Publishers, Inc., Chicago. Additions made by author.

persists long enough or if it occurs in the presence of some preexisting arthropathy, the ultimate condition may be that of true acute inflammatory arthritis. Consequently, muscle therapy alone may produce no more than palliative results. It is very important, therefore, that a diagnostic distinction be drawn between an uncomplicated pain-dysfunction syndrome and acute inflammatory arthritis so that definitive treatment can be applied with reason and purpose (Fig. 3–1).[23]

It has been stated that all persons beyond the third or fourth decade of life develop changes in the joint characteristic of degenerative joint disease.[24] Osteoarthritis is easily the most common disease seen in the temporomandibular joint with increasing age.[25, 26] One clinical investigation of 1,350 healthy patients revealed evidence of degenerative changes of the temporomandibular joints in one third of the cases.[27]

On the other hand, Shore has stated that "temporomandibular joint arthrosis is a noninfectious, trophic, degenerative problem of the joint tissues initiated by intrinsic trauma and causing abnormal changes in the function of the joint."[28] It is not considered to be a disease of aging, since it

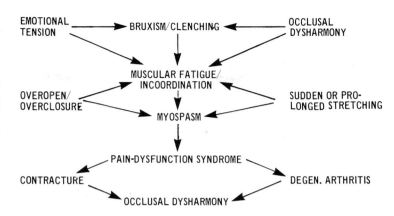

Figure 3–1. Etiology of the TMJ pain-dysfunction syndrome. (From McNeill, C.: Modern oral preventive techniques. J. Prosthet. Dent., *30*:572, 1973. Reprinted with permission.)

is most commonly seen in patients between the second and fourth decades of life. This disorder is caused by chronic intrinsic microtraumata within the joint structure itself. Arthrosis is a dysfunction, not a disease, and with proper care and treatment it can be reversed. It is important, therefore, to distinguish between myofascial pain–dysfunction, osteoarthritis, and arthrosis of the temporomandibular joints.

NEURAL PATHWAYS OF PAIN

Research by Wolff[29] and others many years ago established the concept of pain-sensitive structures both in and outside of the skull. These structures may be classified for discussion purposes as intracranial and extracranial, but they are closely integrated, and pain may be referred from one to the other in many instances. The extracranial structures include the superficial neck structures, the scalp, and the periosteum, while the intracranial group includes the meninges, nerves, and blood vessels within the skull, as well as the great venous sinuses and their tributaries, all in close proximity to the basal dura mater.

Pain impulses from the head and face area are carried by first order neurons of the trigeminal or fifth cranial nerve through the semilunar ganglion into the spinal tract nucleus of the fifth nerve, where the first synapse occurs. The pain fibers of the fifth nerve terminate in the nucleus caudalis. Pain fibers from the seventh, ninth, and tenth cranial nerves, as well as the upper three cervical spinal nerves, have their first synapse in the nucleus caudalis. The nucleus caudalis serves as the primary relay area for the pain impulses in man, which is most significant in understanding overlying symptoms. From this nucleus second order neurons carry impulses by three ascending systems to all levels of the spinal tract nucleus, the sensory nucleus of the fifth, the mid-brain, thalamus, and bilateral fibers associated with the lemniscal system. It is the medial part of the ventrobasal thalamus that is the target of the nerve impulses from the nucleus caudalis. From there third order neurons carry impulses to the somatosensory cortex.[30]

The peripheral branches of the trigeminal nerve, the ophthalmic, maxillary, and mandibular nerves, supply a fairly well-defined cutaneous area plus the deep structure underlying it. They also supply branches to the

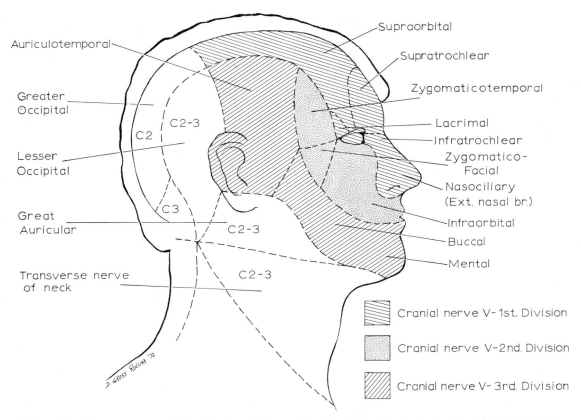

Figure 3–2. Cutaneous nerve supply of the face. (Adapted from Smith, B. H.: Anatomy of facial pain. Headache, 9:7, 1969.)

dura mater. There is not much overlap with the adjoining cutaneous fields of the cervical nerves (Fig. 3–2).

NEUROMUSCULAR CONSIDERATIONS

When dealing with the emotionally tinged problem of pain it is good to recall certain basic facts of neurophysiology. We first have to be sure of what we are talking about. Although all pain sensations are ultimately transmitted by nervous pathways, they may originate in various structures. Pain affecting the regions of head, neck, and jaws can be caused by pathologic processes involving the nerves, the muscles, or the connective tissues. Among these, muscle pain appears to be of special importance for our subject. Therefore we have to give some thought to the physiology of the masticatory musculature.

Generally speaking, the factors causing or predisposing to head pain are many. Nutritional or deficiency disease can impair the metabolism of the tissue cells, making them more susceptible to injury of a type that could give rise to pain. Other deficiencies, such as are seen with carbohydrates and oxygen, also predispose to metabolic disturbance. Once a focus of local pathology has become established, it usually irritates the surrounding nerves, causing pain.

Some of the common causes of nerve pain are as follows: (1) direct trauma; (2) indirect trauma on the perineural tissues causing pressure; (3) traction pressure on the vascular supply, leading to anoxia and ischemia; (4) extension of inflammation from neighboring tissues; and (5) invasion of a nerve by specific organisms or by a neoplasm.

When muscles are traumatized, compressed, overexercised, or in a state of sustained contraction or hypertonicity, they react with characteristic pain, which is often accompanied by spasm. Muscles may be subject to pain as a result of deficiencies, such as in carbohydrates, or from the accumulation of products of metabolism as a result of muscle function.

Connective tissues, such as deep fasciae, tendons, ligaments, and periosteum, may be the location of pain resulting from excessive traction or from injury from neighboring inflammatory processes. With regard to bone, the periosteum is very sensitive to traction tension. Cancellous bone is less sensitive to noxious stimuli, and compact bone hardly at all.

It is the task of careful examination to differentiate between these different types of pain. As a general rule, *neuralgic* pain is recognized by demonstrating tenderness at the points of exit of sensory nerves, such as at the trigeminal foramina. *Myalgic* pain is characterized by localized tenderness of the affected muscles and by their spastic contraction, such as in myalgia of the sternocleidomastoid, which hurts when it is pinched. Periosteal pain shows sensitive trigger areas, which may also appear thickened to the palpating finger.[31]

The body contains various types of muscle fibers. These fall into the following three distinct groups: skeletal, intestinal (smooth), and cardiac. The muscles associated with motor functions in the head and neck region are composed entirely of skeletal muscle fibers.

When dealing with muscle pathology, one must bear in mind certain physiologic characteristics of skeletal muscle, such as chemical action within the muscle fiber, its nutrition, and the phenomena of fatigue and tetanus. One of the most important facts is that skeletal muscle functions properly only when the normal distance is maintained between the origin and insertion of the fibers. Striated muscle loses tone and strength when the distance between these two points is shortened. On the other hand, muscle tone is increased beyond normal when the distance between origin and insertion is increased.[32]

Muscle has inherent properties, those residing in the muscle itself, and others controlled by impulses reaching it from the nervous system. Both play an important role in considering the resolution of the problems of dental pathology. Any given muscle may, on different occasions, act (1) as a prime mover, (2) as an antagonist aid in coordination, or (3) as an antagonist to neutralize an unwanted movement produced by another prime mover.

Muscles can contract either isotonically or isometrically. When they contract isotonically, they shorten but retain equal tension; if they contract isometrically, they increase tension but do not shorten, thereby retaining their strength. By contracting isotonically, muscles act as movers. By isometric contractions they act as holders, stabilizers, or positioners. In addition, muscles contract in preparing for their subsequent relaxation in order to brake or balance the moving contraction of their antagonists.[33]

Muscles are arranged in the body according to the best engineering principles, thus providing for conservation of energy. Furthermore, advantage is taken of effective leverage and assistance available from gravity. The following muscular functions influence the dental mechanism: posture maintenance, deglutition, mastication, and facial expression.

Regarding the problem of posture maintenance, we may consider the shoulder girdle, clavicula, sternum, and scapula as constituting the fixed base of operations. The head may be said virtually to teeter on the atlanto-occipital joint. Since the center of gravity of the head lies in front of the occipital condyles, it naturally follows that definite force must be applied to hold the head erect, a force which is provided by the large muscles of the back of the neck. Several groups of muscles are attached directly or indirectly to the anterior part of the head; their functions tend to add to the force of gravity and thus to the load on the posterior cervical muscles, thereby requiring greater bulk and strength on their part. The most important of these anterior cranial muscles are the masticatory and the supra- and infrahyoid groups. They constitute a sort of chain: with the mandible and hyoid bone, to which they are attached, they join the cranium to the shoulder girdle. It follows that within this chain the movements of the mandible and hyoid bone can occur independently of each other and of this functional chain itself (Fig. 3–3).[34]

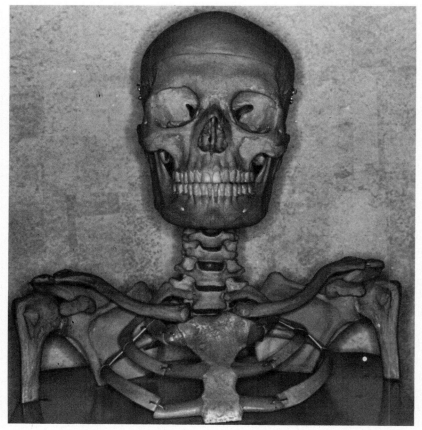

Figure 3–3. A muscular chain exists between the cranium and the shoulder girdle. The head virtually teeters on the atlanto-occipital joint, held erect by the large muscles of the back of the neck and the anterior cranial muscles (masticatory and supra- and infrahyoid muscle groups).

Campbell has stated his observations as follows:[35]

The temporomandibular meniscus must have something in common with the cartilage in the knee; at least both can be dislodged. If the muscles in the leg are subject to cramp, why not the masticating muscles, or even the muscles of facial expression? If the shoulders can ache with so-called fibrositis, then perhaps the tongue can ache likewise. The temporomandibular joint may have its own brand of tenosynovitis, which resembles that of the elbow. If intermittent claudication can cause pain in the lower leg, it is conceivable also in the face. If muscles can be torn elsewhere, why make an exception of the head and neck? Pain can be induced in muscles by vasoconstriction, by cold, anoxia, acidosis, or fatigue, all of which suggest that the blood supply cannot be ignored as a contributory factor. Sustained muscle tension without commensurate blood supply (incoming and outgoing) will starve the muscles of their metabolic requirements; nor will the muscle be flushed of the painful waste-products of metabolism.

If one group of muscles is in tension, then adjacent muscles are in tension: if one group relaxes, the adjoining muscles relax. Restoring muscles to their physiological resting length is a *three-dimensional concept;* it entails placing the origin and the insertion of the muscles in correct three-dimensional relationship.

Mandibular displacement is bound to upset the tonic harmony of the masticating muscles and maybe even of the muscles of expression. Indeed, the effect may spread to the shoulders and the chest. Surprising to relate, a few patients had intercostal pains which disappeared concurrently with the easing of the facial pain.[35]

Kraus has written as follows:

Muscle tension is probably the most frequent single or contributing cause of muscular derangement of the temporomandibular joint. This is equally true for a host of non-traumatic or post-traumatic orthopedic difficulties. Muscle tension is unfortunately built into our civilized and mechanized way of life. It does not necessarily have to be produced by emotional problems or even be associated with them. It is the result of a consistently repeated normal response to the unreleased fight and flight stimuli.

Among the endocrine and other organic reactions caused by emotional irritation, the tensing of skeletal muscles probably ranks first in frequency. It may be reinforced by endocrine imbalance produced by the same stresses, and by conditioned reflexes to which we are exposed when identical irritations occur with identical warning signals (such as the ringing of the telephone), and can be further aggravated by emotional difficulties, situational problems, and posture peculiarities.[36]

There are numerous similarities between facial pain of the type related to manibular movement and the pain associated with other muscle dysfunctions elsewhere in our bodies. The continuous or intermittent dull ache made more painful by movement, the limitation of joint movement, and the past history of other mild episodes of a similar nature can be found in many other conditions such as low back pain, frozen shoulder, fibrositis, and tennis elbow.[37]

MYOFASCIAL TRIGGER AREAS

Bonica[38] describes a group of disorders characterized by the presence of a hypersensitive area, called the trigger area, together with a specific pain syndrome, muscle spasm, tenderness, stiffness, limitation of motion, or weakness. This trigger area is generally located in one of the muscles or in the connective tissue. Occasionally autonomic dysfunction occurs in a so-called area of reference, also known as the target area, which is usually located at some distance from the trigger point. Various myofascial syndromes have been described by Bonica.[39] These syndromes are considered to be the most common musculoskeletal disabilities of the shoulder girdle, neck, and lower back.

Freese and Scheman have written as follows:

> Myofascial pain is the term applied to those pain syndromes originating in myofascial structures.
>
> A myofascial trigger area is a small, circumscribed, very hypersensitive area in myofascial tissues from which impulses arise to bombard the central nervous system and produce referred pain. It should be emphasized that it is a physical sign, not a symptom, and the patient is usually unaware of it.
>
> The zone of reference is the region in which pain, hyperalgesia, muscle spasm, and certain autonomic concomitants are produced by a myofascial trigger area. Patients can localize referred pain with surprising accuracy, distinguishing between reference zones even a half inch apart.[40]

These syndromes have been beautifully portrayed graphically (Figs. 3–4 to 3–11) by Travell and Rinzler.[41] Having charted the zones of reference for the commonly affected skeletal muscles throughout the body, they found the reference zones to be either "essential zones," those zones which were not found in all the subjects, or those reference zones of myofascial trigger areas in the head and neck, which are of extreme interest to the dentist treating these problems. Travell and Rinzler also described trigger areas in the masseter and temporal muscles that refer pain to other areas of the face and head. In the majority of cases the precipitating factor is thought to be motion that causes stretching of the muscle containing the abnormal focal area of pain, setting off a self-perpetuating pain–spasm–pain cycle, which frequently persists after removal of the precipitating cause.

Travell has classified the causes of the myofascial trigger mechanism as either precipitating or predisposing.[42] The factors that precipitate the condition are as follows:

(1) sudden trauma to musculoskeletal structures.
(2) unusual or excessive exercise.
(3) chilling of the body.
(4) immobilization.
(5) an acute myocardial infarction or appendicitis, with localized reflex spasm of extremities, as in popliteal thrombosis.
(6) rupture of an intervertebral disc with nerve root pressure.
(7) acute emotional distress.

The conditions that predispose to the myofascial trigger mechanisms are the following:

(1) chronic-muscular strain, produced by repetitive movement frequently performed over a long period of time.
(2) general fatigue.
(3) acute infectious illness, e.g., infectious mononucleosis, acute hepatitis, or an acute upper respiratory infection (postinfectious myalgias).
(4) a chronic focus of infection.
(5) nutritional deficiencies.
(6) a progressive lesion of the nervous system.
(7) nervous tension.

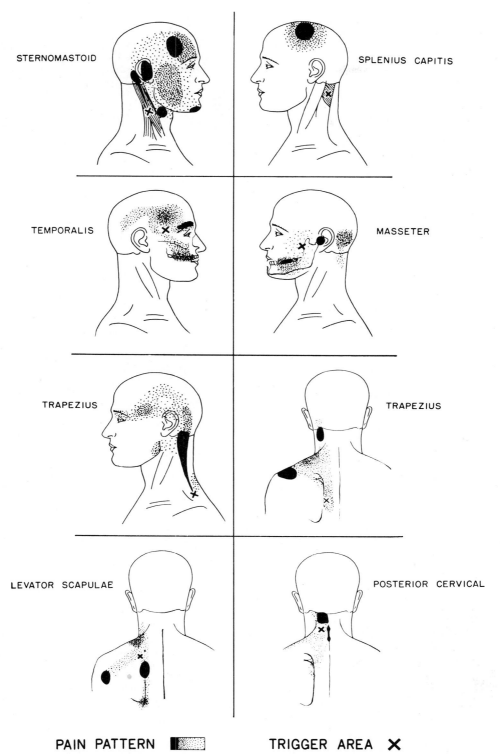

PAIN PATTERN ▮▨▒░   TRIGGER AREA ✕

Figure 3–4. Zones of reference in the head and neck. Solid black areas indicate so-called essential zones, while the stippled areas indicate spillover zones; the heavier the stippling, the more frequently this area is a zone of reference. (From Travell, J., and Rinzler, S. H.: Scientific exhibit: myofascial genesis of pain. Postgrad. Med., *11*:425–427, 1952. Used by permission of McGraw-Hill Book Company.)

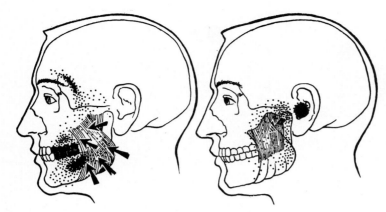

Figure 3–5. Pain reference patterns of the masseter muscle: Left, Superficial layer. Right, Deep layer. Trigger areas are indicated by arrows, and their pain reference zones by the stippled and black regions. (From Travell, J.: Temporomandibular joint pain referred from muscles of the head and neck. Prosth. Dent., *10*:745, 1960. Reprinted with permission.)

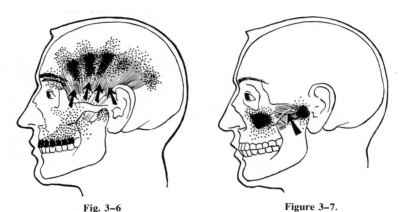

Fig. 3–6   Figure 3–7.

Figure 3–6. Composite pain reference pattern of the temporalis muscle. Trigger areas are indicated by arrows, and their reference zones by the stippled and black regions. (From Travell, J.: Temporomandibular joint pain referred from muscles of the head and neck. Prosthet. Dent., *10*:745, 1960. Reprinted with permission.)

Figure 3–7. Composite pain reference pattern of the external pteryoid muscle. (From Travell, J.: Temporomandibular joint pain referred from muscles of the head and neck. Prosth. Dent., *10*:745, 1960. Reprinted with permission.)

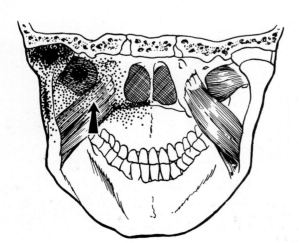

Figure 3–8. Composite pain reference pattern of the internal pterygoid muscle. A partial coronal section is shown with a view of the external and internal pterygoid muscles from the back of the mouth. Trigger areas at the arrow in the internal pterygoid muscle refer pain to the stippled regions. (Based on drawing by Netter, F.: Anatomy of the mouth. Clin. Symp. *10*:76, 1958.)

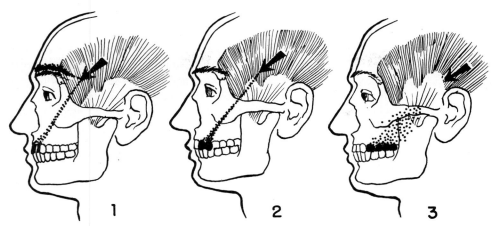

Figure 3–9. Specific trigger areas at three sites in the temporalis muscle, as observed in a case of facial neuralgia. Trigger areas were located at arrows, and pain was referred to the black and stippled zones. (From Travell, J.: Temporomandibular joint pain referred from muscles of the head and neck. Prosth. Dent., *10*:745, 1960. Reprinted with permission.)

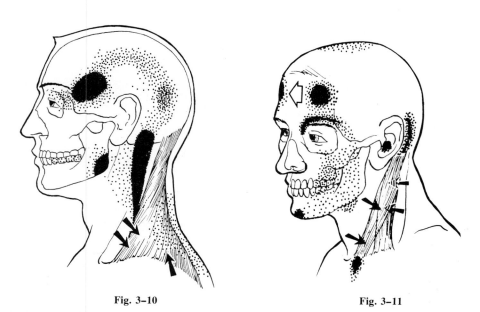

Fig. 3–10   Fig. 3–11

Figure 3–10. Composite pain reference pattern of the trapezius muscle, suprascapular region. Trigger areas are indicated by arrows, and pain reference zones by the stippled and black regions. (From Travell, J.: Temporomandibular joint pain referred from muscles of the head and neck. Prosthet. Dent., *10*:745, 1960. Reprinted with permission.)

Figure 3–11. Composite pain reference patterns of the clavicular and sternal divisions of the sternocleidomastoid. The sternal division refers pain mainly to the forehead bilaterally, to the posterior auricular region and deep in the ear, and infrequently to the teeth. Trigger areas are indicated by arrows, and pain reference zones by the stippled and black regions. (From Travell, J.: Temporomandibular joint pain referred from muscles of the head and neck. Prosth. Dent., *10*:745, 1960. Reprinted with permission.)

(8) syndromes of the menopause and male climacteric.

(9) hypometabolism with creatinuria.

"By its very nature, referred pain obscures the etiology of the disease process," Alling and Burton write. "Therefore, a thorough history and physical examination of the head and neck must be carried out, and the clinician must guard against an empirical approach to the wrong problem. A knowledge of the recognized patterns of referred pain as outlined below will be of diagnostic value."[30]

FROM	TO
upper incisors	supraorbital region
upper 2nd premolar	zygomaticofacial area
upper 1st or 2nd molar	infraorbital region
upper 2nd or 3rd molar	anterior to auricle
upper canine or 1st premolar	lateral and inferior to the ala of the nose
lower incisors, canine or premolar	lateral and inferior to the corner of the mouth
lower 2nd or 3rd molar	external auditory meatus and parotid region
lower 3rd molar	submandibular area

Other patterns of referred pain to the orofacial area are:

FROM	TO
Sternocleidomastoid	TMJ
	Preauricular area
	Postauricular area
	Tip of chin
Masseter muscle	Mandibular teeth
	Auricular area
Temporalis muscle	Maxillary posterior teeth
Medial pterygoid muscle	Retromandibular area
	Infra-auricular area
Lateral pterygoid muscle	TMJ
Occipital muscle	Temporal area
	Frontal area
Trapezius muscle	Temporal area
	Frontal area
Heart	Lower area
Sphenoid sinus	Nose
	Palate
	Canine teeth
Other paranasal sinuses	Multiple areas

Kraus and associates[43] have expressed the view that insufficient exercise may provide inadequate outlet for nervous tension and stress. This in turn produces increased muscular tension, often resulting in various types of disorders, which they have characterized as "hypokinetic disease." This concept may apply equally to jaw function. The histories of patients with temporomandibular joint pain and mandibular dysfunction indicate that they tend to use their jaws as a primary mode in tensional release to a greater degree than do other people. This is discussed in greater detail in Chapter 4.

CRANIAL CONSIDERATIONS

Osteopathic concepts in the cranial field should be of considerable interest to practicing dentists. They differ from the usually held concepts, which maintain that the cranium, with its associated dentofacial area, is a dry-bone, a static structure, when in reality it is a dynamic mobile complex. The temporomandibular fossae and the mandible, as well as both maxillae, are capable of a minimal but definite degree of normal movement. Correction of diagnosed malalignments can be of immeasurable help to those dentists interested in resolving the symptomatology of patients suffering from the craniomandibular syndrome.[44]

Sears[45] many years ago reported that "dentists are finding that delicate adjustment of the occlusion, plus osteopathic correction of temporal bone lesions, is much more satisfactory."

If only the dental and medical professions would grasp the significance of these few facts, that sutures in the human cranium never fuse unless there is bone disease, that the TMJ is particularly vulnerable to temporal malalignment, and that lesions of the cranial bones as to position or motion are quite universal in occurrence. They result from birth trauma, toddler's tumbles, adolescent roughhousing, school athletics, adult head bumps, whiplash injuries, and even rotation of the temporal bones internally by the V-shaped dental head rest.

Normal functional mobility of the component parts of the cranium occurs within limits determined mainly by the following three factors: (1) each cranial bone must have enough plastic resiliency in itself and enough pliability in its sutures to move normally without strain; (2) contiguous bones must be similarly free to accompany such excursions or to be able to compensate for it; and (3) the dural membranes must be unrestricted so as to permit such suppleness within normal limits.

A deeper insight into this problem is reported in Chapter 17.

DIFFERENTIAL DIAGNOSIS OF CRANIOFACIAL DISORDERS

Practicing physicians and dentists realize that symptoms in the head and neck areas may involve a multitude of etiologic factors. Surprisingly, symptoms experienced by the patients we see are not much different than those originally reported by Costen.[10] Costen described his symptom complex as occurring uniformly in disturbed temporomandibular joint function. The symptoms were described as follows: (1) ear symptoms, such as loss of hearing, stuffy sensation in the ears, tinnitus, earache, and dizziness without nystagmus; (2) pain in the form of headache about the vertex or occiput or behind the ears and a burning sensation in the throat, tongue, and side of the nose; (3) miscellaneous symptoms, such as dryness of the mouth and herpes of the external ear canal and buccal mucosa; and (4) trismus. The possible causes can be said to fall into the following three main groups:[46]

I. General systemic disease, such as cardiovascular, renal, or arthritic diseases.
II. Local pathology, such as in the ears, nose, sinuses, throat, or cervical spine.

III. Abnormalities of the craniomandibular system, the major topic of this chapter. (It is imperative that we first rule out by consultation with various medical specialists the following etiologic possibilities under Groups I and II before proceeding to Group III.)

  A. *Aural, nasal, and nasopharyngeal disease.* It is necessary to rule out the existence of probable nasopharyngeal conditions, such as lymphoid hypertrophy, cysts, or tumors. Audiometric tests should be taken to determine the precise type of hearing loss that may be present. The dentist must also be advised what portion of a detected perceptive hearing loss may be due to physiologic loss of hearing with age.

  B. *Adenopathy,* especially of the parotid gland, and infections from erupting and impacted third molars, as well as residual infections.

  C. *Disorders of neural origin,* such as isolated or associated paralyses of cranial nerves.

  D. *Collagenous disease,* such as rheumatoid arthritis or osteoarthritis, and scleroderma, which may affect the temporomandibular joint.

  E. *Bone dyscrasias,* including osteoporosis.

  F. *Traumatic disorders,*[47] no matter how long they have been present.

Burns[48] states that normal circulation to the brain is secured by means of (1) variations in the systemic blood pressure, (2) the nerves governing meningeal circulation, and (3) the vasomotor nerves to the blood vessels of the brain. When trauma occurs between the thoracic inlet and the cranial base it can disturb sympathetic nerves, cranial nerves, veins, arteries, and lymphatics. As a consequence, cerebral congestion, faulty cerebrospinal fluid metabolism, weakened tissues, deranged function, and the discomfort of headaches and neuralgia occur. Damage to vessels and nerves that pass through the foramina transversaria makes for a varied syndrome of neurologic and neurovascular trouble which would not show on the x-ray film. The patient may then be advised to consult a psychiatrist, even though the trouble is primarily structural.

This would tend to explain why whiplash victims are less active and alert, why mental activity becomes laborious, why there is insomnia and a reduction in customary skills, and why the patient is less stable in relation to environmental demands and manifests irritability, forgetfulness, fear, and inefficiency.

"Whiplash injury (of the neck)," Leopold and Dillon write, "is psychologically unique in that both its suddenness and its unconscious meaning (that the control—the head and neck, which have been injured—could be severed from the body) tend to mobilize greater anxiety in ordinarily stable and well-integrated individuals than do other disease processes and injuries to other parts of the body.... It is suggested that the emotional aspects are an integral part of the whiplash injury; that they are not dependent on the accompanying circumstances stressed in the literature; and that they are not significantly related to pre-existing psychologic disease."[49]

The previous evaluation is good in most respects except that it is built upon a false premise: that the injury is confined to the head and neck area. When the whole body sustains such a shock, it is no wonder that even "stable and well-integrated people" with no "pre-existing psychologic disease" are seriously disturbed. From this viewpoint, we would have to agree with Burns[48, 50] that such problems are primarily more physical than mental, considering the full significance of the greater lesion complex.

1. Acute trauma
   a. Sprains resulting from prolonged opening of the mouth
      (1) Long dental appointments
      (2) Extractions or tonsillectomies
      (3) Laughing, vocalizing, or yawning
   b. Sprains from mastication
      (1) Brittle, fibrous, or tough foods
      (2) Unilateral mastication
   c. Sleeping habits
2. Chronic trauma
   a. Prolonged acute conditions
   b. Malocclusions
      (1) Natural
      (2) Faulty restorative treatment
      (3) Orthodontic treatment
      (4) Missing teeth
3. Miscellaneous
   a. Osseous nodules
   b. Ankylosis
   c. Fractures
   d. Unknown

G. *Neoplasms* involving the temporomandibular joints:[51]
1. Benign
   a. Cyst
   b. Osteoma
   c. Chondroma
   d. Myxoma
   e. Benign giant cell tumor
   f. Fibrous
2. Malignant
   a. Fibrosarcoma
   b. Chondrosarcoma
   c. Metastatic carcinoma
   d. Metastatic myosarcoma
   e. Multiple myeloma
   f. Metastatic adenocarcinoma
   g. Transitional cell carcinoma

H. *Arthritides*
1. Rheumatoid
2. Osteoarthritis
3. Traumatic
4. Infectious

I. *Psychogenic factors*

In regard to psychogenic factors there is still a tendency to dismiss the symptoms of patients suffering from the temporomandibular dysfunction syndrome or of cervicofacial neuralgia as being of psychoneurotic origin.[52, 53] Hankey,[17] in a chance sampling of 100 patients, found only three who could definitely be diagnosed as psychoneurotic, and nine more who suffered from anxiety neurosis of mild degree. Although the pain threshold of many may have been low, their pain was very real. Of the 18 per cent of his patients who complained of pain only, without reference to the joint, none was psychopathic. "With the physical correction of the anatomic derangement, psychosomatic precipitation of painful episodes should become impossible," he wrote. The psychological state of the remainder of the 100 patients was average. This aspect is discussed in greater detail in Chaper 8.

Selye's[53] experimental work in physiology, pathology, and biochemistry led him to set forth stress as the common factor in the production of a great variety of apparently unrelated diseases involving the various organs and tissues in the body. These diseases are classified as diseases of the general adaptation syndrome (GAS), which is evidenced in three stages: the alarm reaction, the resistance reaction, and the exhaustion reaction. Each phase affects not only a local part, but also the body as a whole through its actions upon the nervous and endocrine systems. Not only are different organs and systems involved, but changes in the tissues occur as well, resulting in alterations in permeability of membranes, water balance, distribution of electrolytes, osmotic pressure, diffusion and internal environment of the cells, and the metabolic processes. Stress can be induced by such factors as trauma, heat, cold, loss of blood, emotional upsets, and so forth, which are examples of nonspecific agents.

Abnormalities of the craniomandibular system include the following:[54]

1. Local temporomandibular joint syndrome—pain on movement and limited motion of the temporomandibular joint, clicking on movement, crepitation, and hypermobility.

2. Peripheral symptoms—headache, vertigo, mild catarrhal deafness, tinnitus, stopping or stuffing sensation in the ears, pain in or about the ears, burning or pricking sensation of the tongue, throat, and nose, dryness of the mouth, tics of the face and neck, certain "neuralgias" of the neck and back, as well as pain over vertex, occiput, and postauricular areas.

3. Bruxism, including subjective symptoms—gnashing (wear facets) and clenching of the teeth with associated muscle fatigue, pain, and soreness of the temporomandibular joints and the periodontal membrane. This topic is covered most adequately in the textbooks on this subject, as well as in periodicals and in Chapter 14.

4. Tenderness on palpation—of the temporomandibular joints, the muscles of mastication, and the muscles of the neck and back.

Other factors to be considered in a differential diagnosis are:[40]
1. Facial neuralgias
   a. Trigeminal
   b. Glossopharyngeal
2. Vascular headaches (migraine)
3. Sinus disease
4. Temporal arteritis
5. Pulpally involved teeth
6. Coronary occlusion
7. Fracture of the styloid process
8. Elongation of the styloid process (Eagle's syndrome)
9. Ossification of the styloid ligament

10. Lesions of the tongue
11. Injury of the auriculotemporal nerve (Frey's syndrome)
12. Otitis externa
13. Carcinoma of the nasopharynx

Habits

Tension-related oral habits can be factors in causing dysfunction of the head, neck, and jaws. Consequently, a deeper look into their clinical manifestations is of utmost importance to the clinician attempting to treat this vexing problem.

Although gnashing and grinding of the teeth are not a necessary part of the mastication of food, they are prevalent at other times, when such activities are known as occlusal neurosis, bruxism, and, when habitual, as bruxomania. The phenomenon has been attributed to both psychosomatic and local factors (traumatic occlusion) or a combination of both. The frequent observation that, under emotional stress, the skeletal musculature exhibited general and sustained hyperfunction, emphasizes the susceptibility of this region to neurotic muscular contractions.

"Occlusion of the teeth," Jankelson writes, "a physiological act, occurs every 60 to 70 seconds, preliminary to deglutition. If the mandible cannot complete that act, because of the restraint of wedging tooth surfaces, struggling movements are initiated. These movements may take two observed forms—clamping, an attempt to force the mandible through to stable occlusion despite the restraint; or grinding, an attempt to make space by wearing away the restraining surfaces."[55]

Eisenman[56] states that whereas the normal palate is round it can be seen that habits such as thumbsucking and mouth breathing can move the palate into a distorted position during growth, producing more or less an apex, and in this developed abnormal position there is a collapse or narrowing of the maxillary arch, a probable factor in the production of septal deviation.

In cases of premature bite distortion or loss of teeth, palpation of the pterygoid process of the sphenoid bone, behind the upper third molars, may produce bilateral or unilateral tenderness. In normal breathing, the horizontal plate of the palatine bone has a floating or rocking action which can be palpated by the index finger.

When there is fixation of the pterygoid process and the horizontal plate of the palatine bone with resultant pain over the pteryoid processes, it is an indication that a shift has taken place producing fascial stress and strain which involves such important structures as the carotid sheath.

Other traumatic habits frequently cause joint disturbances and need attention. Included among these are lying in the sling position (lying prone on elbows with hands cupped under chin) while watching television, the barber "jaw set," the "sympathetic clipper movement," and similar habits. Also, joint strain may be related to accidents, sleeping position, jaw manipulation during general anesthesia (intubation), and prolonged dental procedures.[57]

Abnormal swallowing and tongue thrusting, of which there are various types, are aptly described by Garliner.[58] These are discussed in greater detail in Chapter 15.

A recent study of a largely "healthy" population revealed a high incidence of occlusal habits. The most prevalent habit was clenching, reported by a third of the patient sample. The second most frequently asserted symptom was morning awareness, followed by bruxism and a resultant sore mouth. Existing in much smaller percentage were anterior bracing and muscle hypertrophy.[1]

A more detailed list of noxious habits that contribute to periodontal disease as well as craniomandibular symptoms can be found in a chapter written by the author for Garliner's Myofunctional Therapy.[58]

Articular Remodeling

Moffett has demonstrated that although the form of a joint is established genetically in prenatal life, it is altered frequently by function during the postnatal period.[59] These alterations take place in the contour of the joints and in the architecture of the bone cartilage. The different types of remodeling have been identified in joints on the basis of the changes seen in articular contour. They are seen as progressive remodeling, which results in an advancement of the joint surface toward the articular cavity; regressive remodeling, which is a localized movement of the joint surface away from the articular cavity; and circumferential or peripheral remodeling, which results in an increased diameter of the articular surface and is commonly seen in patients with degenerative arthritis. Moffett views the temporomandibular joints as dynamic structures with a capacity and even a tendency for morphologic adaptation to changing functional stresses.

Blackwood[60] noted that joint remodeling is initiated by mechanical stimuli. Arthrotic lesions can develop from functional stimuli such as occlusal changes if the demand placed on remodeling activity in the temporomandibular joint tissues exceeds their capacity to respond. Despite many statements to the contrary, the occurrence of TMJ remodeling and arthrosis is probably higher in those individuals with depleted dentitions.[61]

Oral Orthopedics

The principles of oral orthopedics were explained in Chapter 2. Orthopedics is defined in Stedman's Medical Dictionary as the "correction or cure of deformities and diseases of the spine, bones, joints, muscles, or the parts of the skeletal system in children or in persons of any age."[62]

Posselt has defined orthopedics as the treatment of inherited or acquired deviations from normal form and position of some extremity or joint, e.g., the mandible, including its muscles. Treatment includes the use of biteplates and other appliances for treating muscles and temporomandibular joints until pain is eliminated, the logical first step before permanent treatment.[63] The orthopedic system of classification of malocclusion has been described in Chapter 2.

Anamnesis

It is a well-known scientific fact that the empathy and sympathy of the patient are established via a thorough anamnesis and clinical examination. The uniqueness of the communication with the temporomandibular joint patient demands at this time that in your history-taking and clinical examination you educate as well as perform. You perform by asking, "Have you ever had a headache?" You educate by explaining what headaches are. The chart for history-taking or the chart for performance and education during anamnesis is listed here.

COMPLETE PATIENT HISTORY

Name _____ No. _____   Patient's physician _____

Age _____ Sex _____ Date _____   Address _____

Occupation _____   Tel. _____

Address _____   Referred by _____

Tel. (home) _____   Address _____

(bus.) _____   _____

Tel. _____

HEAD PAIN AND TEMPOROMANDIBULAR JOINT EXAMINATION

CODE: ✔, Positive; X, Negative

MEDICAL HISTORY

A. Musculoskeletal Diseases
   1. External traumatic arthritis
   2. Infectious arthritis
   3. Osteoarthritis
   4. Rheumatoid arthritis
   5. Scleroderma
   6. Bone dyscrasias
B. ENT Symptoms
   1. Epidemic parotitis
   2. Middle ear infection
   3. Nasopharyngeal conditions
   4. Osteomyelitis
   5. Sinusitis
   6. Cysts
   7. Polyps
C. Vascular Diseases and Blood Dyscrasias
D. Traumatic Disorders and Blood Dyscrasias
   1. To TMJ—(R) (L)
   2. To other head areas
      (date) _____
E. Headaches and Head Pain (location, character, frequency, duration)
   1. Migraine (Physician)
   2. Neuralgias

F. Medication
   1. Type of Drug
   2. Allergy
G. Additional Medical Information — Past and Present
   1. Surgery — especially hysterectomies (full or partial)
   2. Psychic — past and present
   3. ENT — past and present
   4. Orthopedic — pay attention to fractures and sprains of extremities
   5. Endocrine — female patients with temporomandibular joint syndrome seem to be more disposed to hypothyroidism. In order to establish this deficiency, the patient is asked these questions:
      a. Do your nails break easily?
      b. Is your skin dry?
      c. Do you tire easily?
      d. Does the cold weather bother you?
      e. Do you have cold hands and cold feet?
      f. Do you have difficulty controlling your weight?

   6. Nutritional state

DENTAL HISTORY

A. Previous TMJ Treatment and Results
B. Family History of Similar Conditions
C. Pain Symptoms

   1. Date of onset (R) _____ (L) _____

   2. Area of onset _____

   3. Type — lancinating, paroxysmal, dull, superficial, deep

   4. Quality — burning, aching

   5. Frequency _____

   6. Duration — constant, intermittent

   7. Period of greatest intensity _____

   8. Status of pain — increased, decreased, unchanged

   9. Onset — abrupt, gradual
      a. tearing
      b. blurring
      c. vomiting
   10. Disappearance — abrupt, gradual

   11. Factors alleviating pain _____

   12. Longest pain-free period _____

   13. Triggering devices — eating, yawning, speaking, singing, shouting

   14. Pain in specific teeth _____ (Pulp test for vitality, percussion)

   15. Additional pain information _____

D. Oral Symptoms (other than pain)
  1. Jaws clenched upon awakening
  2. Clenching and grinding during sleep
  3. Clenching and grinding during waking hours
  4. Muscle fatigue _____
  5. Gingival bleeding and swelling
  6. Facial swelling _____

E. Vertigo, Syncope, Meniere's Disease (pseudo)
  1. When _____
  2. Frequency _____

F. Ear Symptoms
  1. Tinnitus (R), (L)
  2. Popping or whooshing noises on opening and closing (R), (L)
  3. Stuffiness of ear (R), (L)
  4. Changes in hearing ability (R), (L)
G. Additional Information (mandibular deformity)

H. Other Primary Complaints _____

CLINICAL EXAMINATION

A. Subjective Pain
  1. Vertex   (R)   (L)
  2. Occipital   (R)   (L)
  3. Preauricular   (R)   (L)
  4. Auricular   (R)   (L)
  5. Upper back   (R)   (L)
  6. Middle back   (R)   (L)
  7. Lower back   (R)   (L)
  8. Scapula area   (R)   (L)
  9. Supraorbital   (R)   (L)
  10. Cervical region (R)   (L)
  11. Shoulder   (R)   (L)
  12. Arm   (R)   (L)
  13. Fingers   (R)   (L)
  14. Chest   (R)   (L)
B. Muscle Examination (tenderness and pain on palpation)
  1. Temporal (Fig. 3–12):
    a. Anterior fibers (R), (L)
    b. Middle fibers (R), (L)
    c. Posterior fibers (R), (L)
  2. Masseter (Fig. 3–13):
    a. Zygoma (R), (L)
    b. Body (R), (L)
    c. Lateral surface of angle of mandible (R), (L)
  3. Internal pterygoid: insertion (R), (L) (Fig. 3–14)
  4. External pterygoid: insertion (R), (L) (Fig. 3–15)

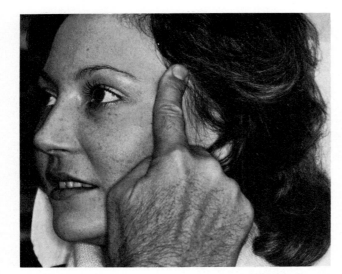

Figure 3–12. Palpation of middle fibers of the temporalis muscle.

Figure 3–13. Palpation of the body portion of the massseter muscle.

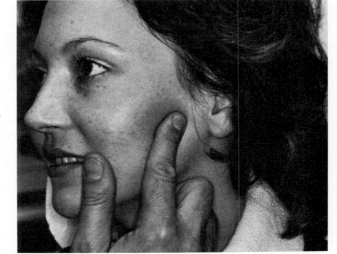

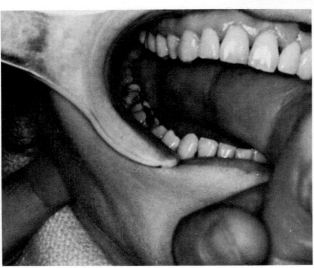

Figure 3–14. Palpation of the internal pterygoid muscle intra- and extraorally simultaneously.

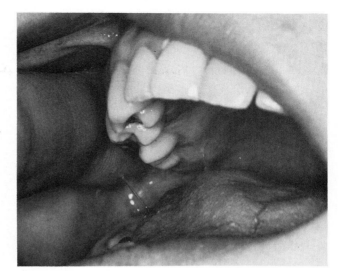

Figure 3–15. Palpation of the external pterygoid muscle (area of inferior head).

5. Sternocleidomastoid (Fig. 3–16):
   a. Origin (R), (L)
   b. Body (R), (L)
   c. Insertion (R), (L)
6. Trapezius (Fig. 3–17):
   a. Origin (R), (L)
   b. Body (R), (L)
   c. Insertion (R), (L)
7. Posterior cervicals (R), (L) (Fig. 3–18)
8. Mylohyoid (R), (L) (Fig. 3–19)
9. Coronoid process (R), (L) (Fig. 3–20)
10. TMJ (R), (L) (Fig. 3–21)
11. Intercostals (R), (L) (Fig. 3–22)
12. Sternum

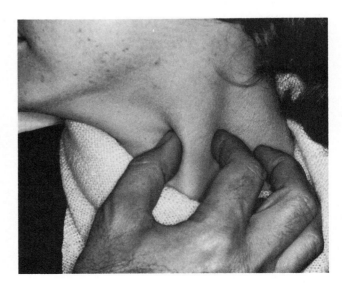

Figure 3–16. Palpation of body of the sternocleidomastoid muscle.

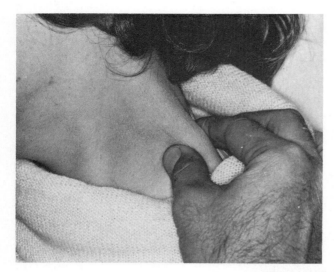

Figure 3–17. Palpation of the trapezius muscle.

Figure 3–18. Palpation of the posterior cervical muscle.

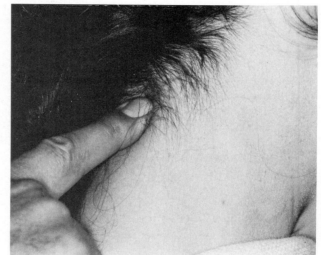

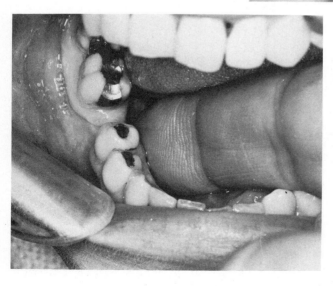

Figure 3–19. Palpation of the mylohyoid muscle.

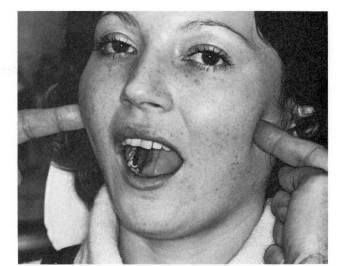

Figure 3–20. Palpation of the coronoid processes.

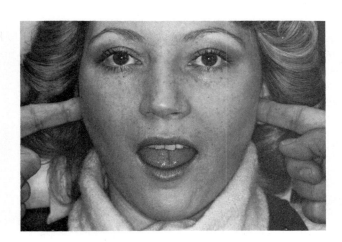

Figure 3–21. Palpation of right and left temporomandibular joints as patient opens and closes.

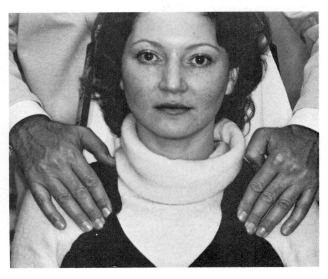

Figure 3–22. Palpation of the intercostal muscles.

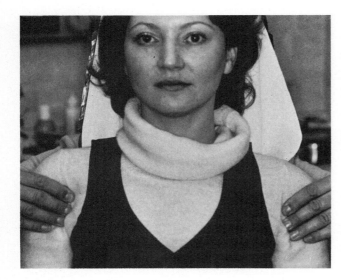

Figure 3–23. Palpation of the deltoid muscles.

13. Deltoid (R), (L) (Fig. 3–23)
14. Upper back muscles (Fig. 3–24)
15. Middle back
16. Lower back (Fig. 3–25)
17. Calves (Fig. 3–26)
18. Hypertrophy of any muscles

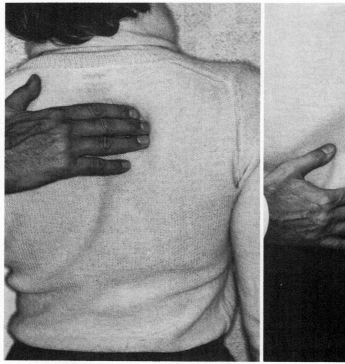

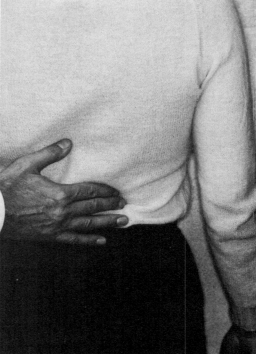

Figure 3–24. Palpation of upper back muscles.　　　Figure 3–25. Palpation of lower back muscles.

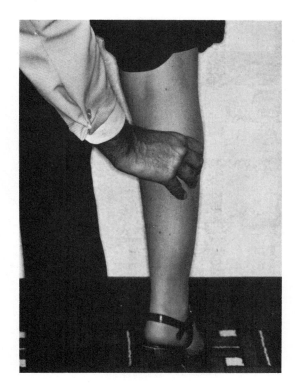

Figure 3–26. Palpation of calf for muscle tenderness.

C. Ear Examination
   1. Anterior wall tenderness (R), (L) (Fig. 3–27)
   2. Excessive wax (R), (L)
D. TMJ Symptoms Other Than Pain
   1. Noises (stethoscopic exam) (Fig. 3–28)
      a. Crepitation (R), (L)
      b. Rubbing (R), (L)

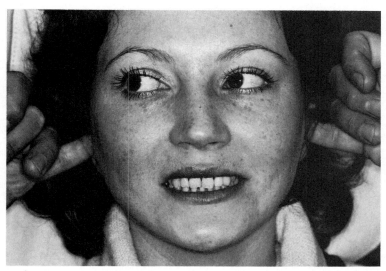

Figure 3–27. Palpation of condylar heads through external auditory meatuses using small fingers (nails face posteriorly).

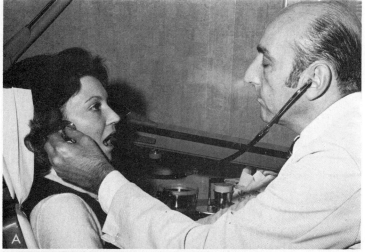

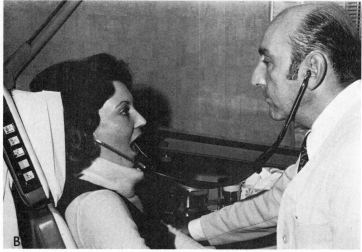

Figure 3–28. *A,* Listening to opening and closing clicks and crepitation with stethoscope (Ford or Bowles). *B,* Listening to opening and closing clicks and crepitation with double ear plug stethoscope. (Courtesy of Dr. Paul Scheman.) Distributed by Masel Orthodontics, Philadelphia, Pa.

      c. Sagittal opening click:
         immediate (R), (L)
         intermediate (R), (L)
         full opening (R), (L)
      d. Sagittal closing click:
         immediate (R), (L)
         intermediate (R), (L)
         terminal closure (R), (L)
    2. Audible click: (R), (L)
  E. Functional Analysis of Occlusion
    1. Centric occlusion
    2. Lateral excursions (Figs. 3–29*A, B*)
    3. Balancing interferences
    4. Protrusion (Fig. 3–29*C*)
    5. Centric relation prematurities
  F. Summary of Roentgenographic Findings: Diagnostic radiographs must be taken of all affected patients to exclude joint pathology and for medicolegal reasons.

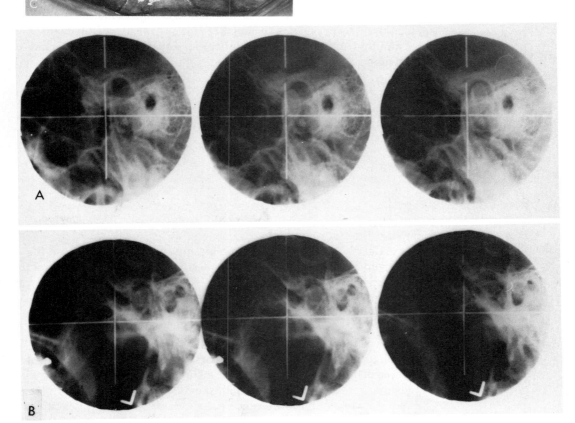

Figure 3–29. *A,* Patient moving jaw in right working bite excursion (lateral). *B,* Patient moving jaw in left working bite excursion (lateral). *C,* Patient moving jaw into protrusion. Notice excessive amount of interarch space posteriorly.

Figure 3–30. *A,* Right TMJ picture. *Wide Open*: condyle anterior to eminentia. *Rest Position*: condyle in 3–6 position. *Habitual Occlusion*: condyle in 1–2 position. *B,* Left TMJ picture *Habitual Occlusion*: condyle in 2–5 position. *Rest Position*: condyle in 5–8 position. *Wide Open*: condlye anterior to eminentia.

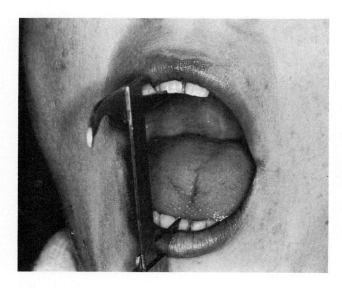

Figure 3–31. Using Boley gauge to measure widest interincisal opening in millimeters (Limited opening is said to exist if patient cannot open beyond 40 mm.)

    1. Intraoral (fourteen periapicals and four bitewings) or panoramic x-ray.

    2. Extra-oral cephalostatic temporomandibular joint pictures. No diagnosis can be made from these pictures alone. They are merely adjunctive aids. Six pictures are taken on each 8 × 10 or 5 × 7 plate. Both sides in occlusion, at rest and wide open (Fig. 3–30).

 G. Visualization: Discrepancies in facial symmetry, head posture, indications of mouth discomfort, speech difficulties and deviations of the midline on opening and closing (Fig. 3–31).

    1. Face

    2. Level of shoulders, hips, and breasts

    3. Sagittal pattern of mandibular movement

       a. Deviation from straight-vertical-opening-and-closing movements

Frontal View   Lateral View

       b. Widest interincisal opening _____ mm. (Fig. 3–31).

 H. Diagnostic Casts (See Chapter 2): The attempt is made to diagnose the patient's given relationship and any or all aberrations from the correct and most harmonious relationship, both structurally and functionally. These aberrations are corrected in realignment and retraining of the components mentioned above, based upon the findings of the following procedures:

    An incorporation of a three-dimensional approach to the overall diagnostic picture supersedes past endeavors, which focused their greatest attention on the variances in vertical dimension. By utilizing three planes of orientation, the horizontal, sagittal, and coronal (Fig. 3–32), it is possible to establish reference points for patients from which deviations from normal are more readily observed.[64, 65] By utilizing these three planes, we are able to analyze the dental mass within itself, as well as to determine its relationship to the head. This is described in

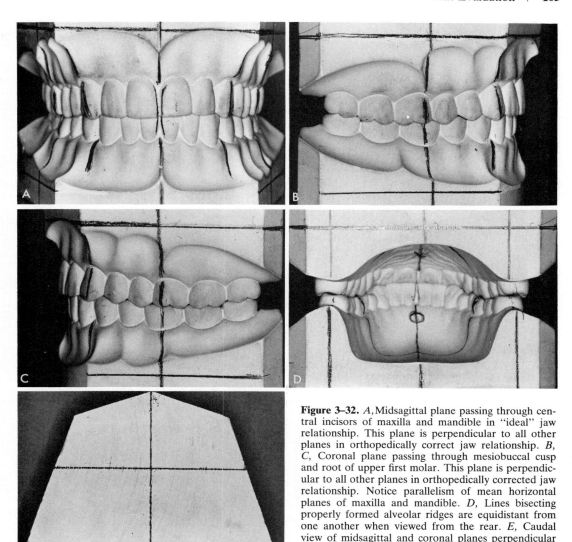

Figure 3–32. *A,* Midsagittal plane passing through central incisors of maxilla and mandible in "ideal" jaw relationship. This plane is perpendicular to all other planes in orthopedically correct jaw relationship. *B, C,* Coronal plane passing through mesiobuccal cusp and root of upper first molar. This plane is perpendicular to all other planes in orthopedically corrected jaw relationship. Notice parallelism of mean horizontal planes of maxilla and mandible. *D,* Lines bisecting properly formed alveolar ridges are equidistant from one another when viewed from the rear. *E,* Caudal view of midsagittal and coronal planes perpendicular to one another.

detail in Chapter 2. The landmarks on the upper cast are established first, according to these three planes, since it is fixed in the skull. The lower cast is mounted to it in the prevailing occlusion of the patient (Fig. 3–33). When the study casts are mounted on the Galletti articulator, the comparison of the line markings indicates the deviations from normal (Fig. 3–34). The deviations which are readily discernible from the casts are: (1) posterior collapse; (2) unilateral collapse; (3) anterior collapse; (4) loss of vertical dimension; (5) increased vertical dimension; (6) bodily shift of mandible; (7) rotation; and (8) prematurities. Study casts truly become an intrinsic part of patient education.

I. Abnormal Swallowing Habits[58]
  1. Incisal thrust
  2. Full fan thrust—molar to molar
  3. Bimaxillary protrusion thrust

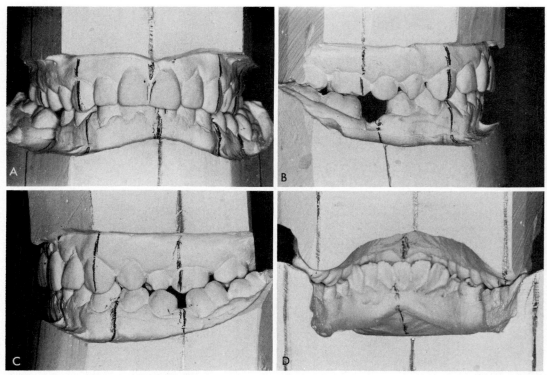

Figure 3–33. *A,* Frontal view of patient's study casts showing midline deviation to left; collapse of vertical dimension indicated by degree of anterior overbite. *B,* Right lateral view showing loss of vertical dimension due to missing lower first molar. *C,* Left lateral view showing loss of vertical dimension due to missing lower first molar. Note discrepancy of cuspid and molar coronal planes. *D,* Notice discrepancy between right and left ridge bisecting lines.

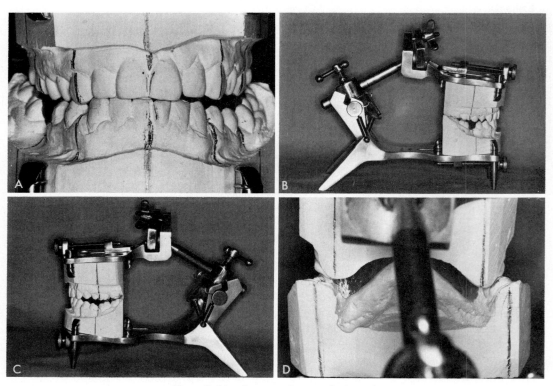

Figure 3–34. *See opposite page for legend.*

104

PHONATION: Sound made by laryngeal vibration.

SURD: Speech sound made without laryngeal vibration (phonation).

SONANT: Speech sound made with phonation.

SIBILANTS: High frequency sounds made by directing a stream of air through a minimal incisal separation or gap.
>   Surd forms of sibilants: "S," "SH," and "CH"
>   Sonant forms of sibilants: "Z," "ZH," and "J"
>   Incisal gap for sibilants: 1 to 1.5 millimeters.

NASAL SONANTS: Low frequency phonation with exit port through the nose because of oral closure. Examples: speech sounds "M" and "N."
>   Incisal gap for nasal sonants: 2 to 4 millimeters.

DIPHTHONGS: Rapid transition of one vowel sound to another vowel sound. Examples: "AE" and "IE" as in eight and nine, respectively.
>   Incisal gap: 5 to 10 millimeters.

ORAL FORMAT: The lip, incisal, and tongue arrangement necessary for the production of a given phonetic sound.

Figure 3–35.

---

   4. Class III thrust.
      a. Pseudo
      b. Skeletal
   5. Open-bite thrust
   6. Closed-bite thrust
   7. Posterior unilateral thrust
   8. Posterior bilateral thrust
   J. Phonetics (Fig. 3–35): Check closest speaking space (sibilants).
   K. Summary of General Examination
   L. Diagnosis
   M. Plan of Treatment
   N. Remarks: A tympanogram is taken on every patient suffering from the craniomandibular syndrome using a Grason-Stadler 1722 Middle-Ear Analyzer. This instrument was designed to provide a differential diagnosis of conductive deafness and to examine the reflex area of the middle ear muscles. Generally, a tympanogram impedance tracing provides a measure of (1) the volume of the ear canal (provided that ambient air pressure, humidity and temperature are known), and (2) the mobility of the middle ear system. The distance between the lowest points at the end of the susceptance curve and the zero horizontal axis of the tympanogram form is a function of the ear canal volume. The smaller the ear canal, the nearer to the zero axis will the curve be located. Tympanogram curves with high peaks are indicative of very mobile systems, curves with shallow peaks, of systems whose mobility is restricted. It was decided to use this instrument so that any changes in ear symptomatology could be recorded objectively, and not just subjectively. Chapter 7 will discuss this in greater detail.

Figure 3–34. *A,* Frontal view of patient's jaw relationship corrected. *B,* Right lateral view of patient's jaw relationship corrected. *C,* Left lateral view of patient's jaw relationship corrected. *D,* Posterior view of patient's jaw relationship corrected. Note confluence of right and left ridge bisecting lines.

PATIENT COMMUNICATION AND MOTIVATION[66]

The patient suffering from temporomandibular joint dysfunction generally has been referred to several different medical specialists, and even to some dentists, before the patient is properly diagnosed.

There are two possibilities regarding a patient presenting with a dysfunctional disorder of the jaws:

1. Patient professionally referred to a specialist.
    a. Reinforcement of the need has usually been made easier for you by the referring physician or dentist.
    b. Time for treatment is now; the patient has been suffering for weeks, months, and years.
    c. Source of treatment has been previously established by the referring practitioner.
    d. The fee is fair. It can be hindered by the referring practitioner and should be carefully noted.
    e. The place — the aura of the office and personnel as well as your own self-assurance — will come into play.
2. Patient presently within your own practice.
    a. The need is more difficult to establish because he has been seeking advice elsewhere and usually finds it difficult to comprehend that a dentist can help him. This presents a unique communication problem in dentistry. Another problem is that this patient has been in the practice for a length of time, and the practitioner's lack of diagnostic scope in this direction has not permitted earlier recognition.
    b. Time for treatment is difficult to establish because of the problems mentioned above. You must therefore reinforce the need. These are usually periodontally healthy patients.
    c. Source is right, needs meticulous documentation.
    d. The fee is fair and is usually easy to establish, since you are aware of their socioeconomic level.
    e. The place has already been established.

Most patients who have suffered for prolonged periods of time believe they have a brain tumor or cancer but that no one is willing to tell them. Many patients have been referred to psychiatrists because the other specialists to whom they were referred for treatment neglected to make the correct diagnosis. This generally occurs despite the taking of a brain scan, EEG, blood chemistry, and extensive roentgenograms.

Contact is made with the patient's problem *first* by telephone. At this time we get the patient's name, home address, business address, telephone number, name of referring doctor, and the nature of the complaint. If the symptoms are severe we schedule an appointment for the patient immediately. The receptionist also notes the attitude of the person making the call.

At the *first visit,* a complete medical and temporomandibular joint history is taken—diagnostic casts, lateral TMJ radiographs, and a clinical examination. We also hand out literature that explains the patient's problem in lay terms.

By the *second visit* we have assembled all of our diagnostic data and we communicate our findings to the patient. At this time, we establish the rela-

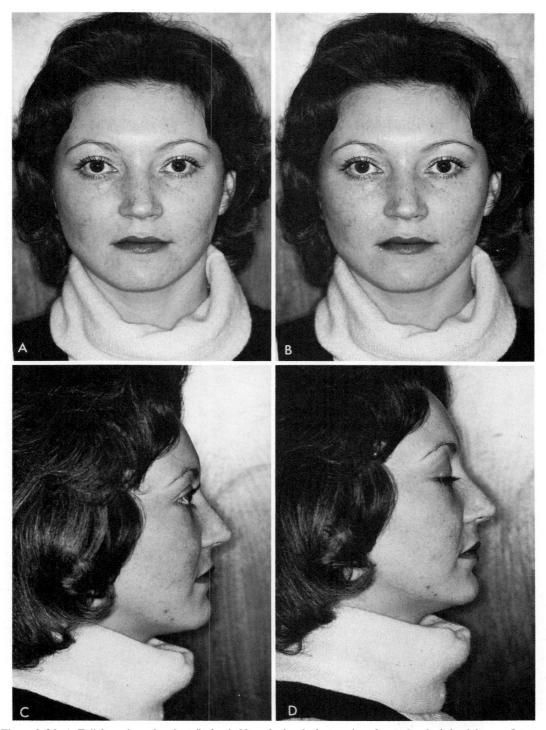

Figure 3–36. *A,* Full face view of patient (before). Note the level of eyes; size of eyes; level of cheek bones; flatness of cheek on left side; level of the lobes of the ears; and the angle of the lips, *B,* Full face view of patient (after, with wax bite in place). Note difference in level of eyes (also size and opening), cheek bones, ear lobes, angle of lips and change in overall facial contour. *C,* Profile facial view (before). *D,* Profile facial view (after, with wax bite in place).

tionship between facial and body asymmetry, the three-dimensional correlation between a Class I type of occlusion and what the patient presented with, the roentgenographic findings, the results of palpation, and the use of phonetics. This enables us to determine the criteria for starting treatment.

Criteria for Starting a Case

I. Visualization
    a. Face—eyebrows, eyes, cheekbones, lips (Fig. 3–36)
    b. Midline deviation of the teeth (Fig. 3–31)
        1. Closed
        2. Open
    c. Level of shoulders and hips (Fig. 3–37)

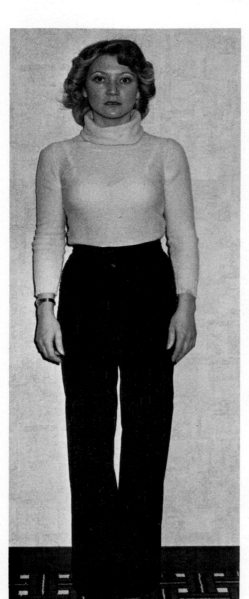

Figure 3–37. Notice that the right eye is higher and larger, while the right shoulder and hip are lower.

II. Palpation (Figs. 3–12, 3–26)
    a. Muscles of:
        1. Mastication
        2. Neck
        3. Back
        4. Legs (calves)
    b. Condyles through external auditory meatuses (Fig. 3–27)
III. Temporomandibular joint x-rays
    a. Cephalostatic lateral TMJ roentgenograms (Figs. 3–30, 3–38)
    b. Laminograms
IV. Diagnostic casts (jaw and tooth relationship)
    a. Three-dimensional analysis—mid-sagittal, coronal, and horizontal (Fig. 3–34)
    b. Wax bite of corrected jaw relationship
V. Phonetics—closest speaking space—surd and sonant forms of the sibilants. Words containing "s," "sh," "ch," "z," "zh," and "j."
VI. Applied kinesiology testing procedures (See Chapter 16)

If we look at the patient's face we find one eyebrow higher than the other, one eye higher and larger, the lips turned up to one side, one ear higher, and the midline generally off to the same side. This high side generally has the greatest loss of vertical dimension in the jaw. This is further corroborated by placing the small fingers in the external auditory meatus and feeling the backward thrust of the condyle greater on that particular side. The TMJ x-rays also verify this finding. Phonetics will indicate a greater free-way space on the collapsed side also. The diagnostic casts with a wax bite taken from the mounting on the Galetti articulator will also confirm the previous findings.

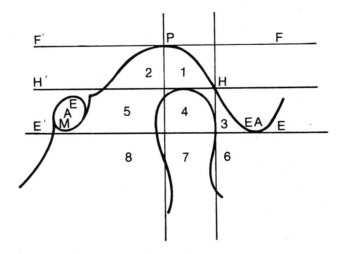

C = *lateral view of lateral pole of condyle.*
EA = *eminentia articularis.*

Figure 3–38. Structural relationship when taking cephalostatic lateral TMJ roentgenograms.

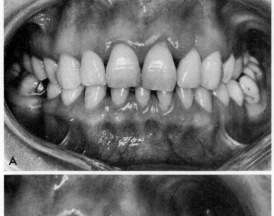
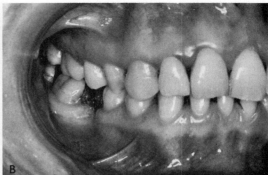
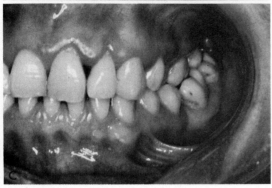

Figure 3–39. *A,* Frontal view of patient's habitual occlusion. Note midline shift to left, although right eye was higher. *B,* Right lateral view; habitual occlusion. *C,* Left lateral view; habitual occlusion.

Generally speaking, the shoulder is lower on that side, as well as the level of the breasts and the hips. It will usually be found that the leg is shorter on that side also. The exception to this rule occurs when the original loss of vertical dimension takes place on the right side (higher eye) (Fig. 3–36), but with time, owing to premature loss of teeth, dental procedures, and other complications, the loss of vertical height becomes greater on the left side (Fig. 3–39). The midline almost always shifts into the quadrant with the greatest loss of vertical dimension (Fig. 3–31). The condyle, now more pronounced, can be felt through the external auditory meatus on the left side, and it may even exhibit a *click* on closing. It is verified by x-ray, study casts, and phonetics.

We can now explain and show this to our patients. It is most important, therefore, to keep a hand mirror and pencil in every operatory. The three-dimensional correction of the patient's jaw relationship is shown, and the wax bite of the correction is tried in his or her mouth (Fig. 3–40). Immediately, any pain that the patient had on palpation through the external auditory meatus is gone, as well as a closing click, if it were present. In addition, many of the back muscles (upper, middle, and lower), which have been found to be the most frequently involved muscle group in patients with craniomandibular disorders, will no longer be tender to palpation.[67] This may also hold true for the masticatory and neck muscles, as well as the iliac crest.

If we find that some of the back muscles are still tender, we can try placing a ¼ inch heel lift into the shoe of the shorter leg to see if greater relief can be obtained (Fig. 3–41). Generally speaking, these lifts are used to ascertain their effect on symptoms and postural asymmetry.[67]

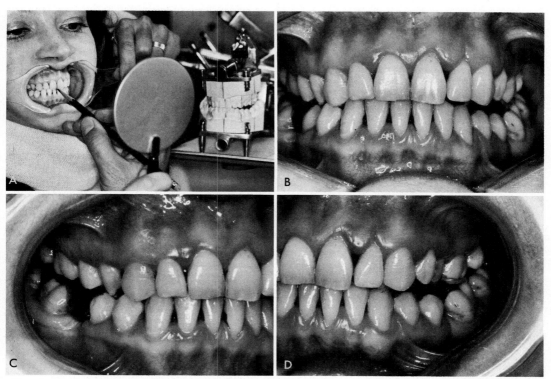

Figure 3–40. *A*, Hand mirrow and pencil in each operatory to guide patient gently into corrected orthopedic mandibular position using newly made wax bite. *B*, Frontal view of wax bite of corrected orthopedic mandibular position tried in patient's mouth. *C*, Right lateral view: orthopedically corrected jaw relationship with wax bite in place. *D*, Left lateral view: orthopedically corrected jaw relationship with wax bite in place.

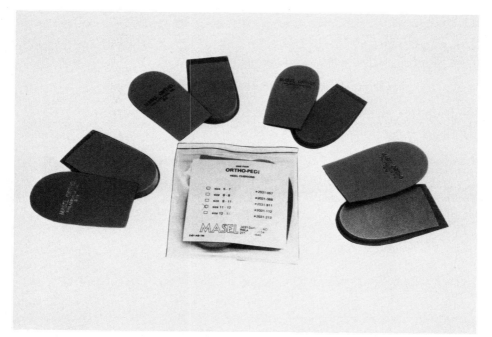

Figure 3–41. Ortho-Pedi Heel Cushions are used at the time of consultation visit to see if postural correction will reduce tenderness in various muscle groups. (Courtesy of Masel Orthodontics.)

This imbalance can be made more apparent to the patient by limping purposely on one foot, and relating this to the side on which he has the greatest loss of vertical dimension. Ask the patient, "You wouldn't expect me to shorten the good leg, would you? I am going to have to add to the sole and heel of the short leg." Patient understanding and acceptance of the problem is unbelievably high.

It is at this time that we present our consultation résumé, which explains what we are going to do, approximately how long it will take, and what the fee will be (Fig. 3–42). We sign this form and the patient countersigns it.

We are now ready to proceed to actual treatment on the *third* visit. Generally, the patient feels 30 to 40 per cent better between the first two visits just knowing that someone has recognized the cause of the problem.

What this means for us as dentists is that, for the first time, we have

---

TEMPOROMANDIBULAR JOINT PATIENTS

The treatment you are to receive is mainly orthopedic in nature and will correct your jaw relationship. This, in turn, will allow muscles which are in spasm to relax and will reduce pain.

The use of an orthopedic appliance helps to establish a correct jaw-to-jaw relationship. This, of course, affects the relationship of lower to upper teeth. After temporomandibular joint therapy is completed, dental treatment is usually required to permanently establish the corrected jaw relationship. The type and amount of dental care required varies with each individual and is not included in your temporomandibular joint therapy.

Your temporomandibular joint therapy includes the following: an orthopedic realignment of the jaw relationship, muscle treatments which may involve exercise, injection and/or electrogalvanic stimulation and techniques helpful in the control of stress and tension.

The fee for temporomandibular joint treatment is $_____.

This fee includes all necessary care for a period of up to six months. Treatment for temporomandibular joint dysfunction beyond the six months will be $_____ per visit.

I have been fully informed of the diagnosis and proposed temporomandibular joint treatment for _____ and hereby grant permission to Dr. _____ and his staff to render the proposed treatment. I have also been informed of the Federal Truth in Lending Statement and agree to abide by the financial arrangements of this office.

_____
Patient's signature

_____
Parent's signature

_____
Date

Figure 3–42.

clinical criteria to know where we are going at all times. If properly diagnosed, the proper jaw relationship must be *produced* and not just *obtained.*

It becomes apparent that the procedures utilized in the past, namely transferring cases from the mouth to the articulator and back again, were finishing techniques in the main. It is my belief, and that of many of my colleagues treating dysfunctional TMJ problems, that many of these cases that are being restored today are clinically symptomatic but are just being overlooked.

References

1. Rieder, C. E.: The incidence of some occlusal habits and headaches/neckaches in an initial survey population. J. Prosthet. Dent., *35*:445, 1976.
1a. Rieder, C. E.: Personal communication (1983).
2. Ruffer, M. A.: Studies in the Palaeopathology of Egypt. Chicago, University of Chicago Press, 1921.
3. Weinberger, B. W.: Introduction to the History of Dentistry. Volume I. St. Louis, C.V. Mosby, 1948, p. 390.
4. Hunter, J.: The Natural History of the Human Teeth. London, J. Johnson, 1771.
5. Cooper, A.: Treatise on Dislocations. London, Churchill, 1842, p. 393.
6. Prentiss, H. J.: Preliminary report upon temporomandibular articulation in human type. Dent. Cosmos, *60*:505, 1918.
7. Wright, W. H.: Deafness as influenced by malposition of the jaws. JADA, 7:979, 1920.
8. Monson, G. S.: Occlusion as applied to crown and bridgework. JADA. 7:399. 1920.
9. Goodfriend, D. J.: Symptomatology and treatment of abnormalities of the mandibular articulation. Dent. Cosmos, *75*:844, 1933.
10. Costen, J. B.: Syndrome of ear and sinus symptoms dependent upon disturbed function of the temporomandibular joint. Ann. Otol. Rhinol. Laryngol., *43*:1, 1934.
11. Zimmerman, A. A.: An evaluation of Costen's syndrome from an anatomic point of view. In Sarnat, B. G., The Temporomandibular Joint. Springfield, Charles C Thomas, 1951.
12. Schwartz, L. L.: A temporomandibular joint pain—dysfunction syndrome. J. Chron. Dis., *3*:284, 1956.
13. Campbell, J.: Distribution and treatment of pain in temporomandibular arthroses. Br. Dent. J., *105*:393, 1958.
14. Staz, J.: The treatment of disturbances of the temporomandibular articulation. Off. J. Dent. Assoc. S. Africa, 6:314, 1951.
15. Walsh, J. P.: Temporomandibular arthritis, mandibular displacement and facial pain. Off. J. Dent. Assoc. S. Africa, 5:430, 1950.
16. Lindblom, G.: Disorders of the temporomandibular joint. Acta Odont. Scand., *11*:61, 1953.
17. Hankey, G. T.: Discussion: affections of the temporomandibular joint. Proc. Roy. Soc. Med., *49*:983, 1956.
18. Posselt, U.: Physiology of Occlusion and Rehabilitation. Philadelphia, F. A. Davis Co., 1962, p. 88.
19. Soderberg, F.: Malocclusion—arthrosis—otalgia. Acta Otolaryngol. (supplement), *95*:85, 1950.
20. Sicher, H.: Temporomandibular articulation in mandibular overclosure. JADA, *36*:131, 1948.
21. Sicher, H.: Structural and functional basis for disorders of the temporomandibular articulation. J. Oral Surg., *13*:275, 1955.
22. Laskin, D. M.: Etiology of the pain-dysfunction syndrome, JADA, 79:147–153, 1969.
23. Bell, W. E.: Clinical Management of Temporomandibular Disorders. Chicago, Year Book Medical Publishers, 1982.
24. Bennett, G. A.: Joints. *In* Anderson, W. A. D. (ed.): Pathology, 6th ed. St. Louis, The C. V. Mosby Company, 1971, pp. 1766–1770.
25. Blackwood, H. J. J.: The Development, Growth, and Pathology of the Mandibular Condyle. Unpublished M.D. Thesis, Queens University of Belfast, 1959.
26. Schwartz, L. L., and Marbach, J. L.: Changes in the temporomandibular joint with age. J. Am. Soc. Periodontics, *3*:184, 1965.
27. Boman, K.: Temporomandibular joint arthrosis and its treatment by extirpation of the disk: a clinical study. Acta Chir. Scand., *95*:1, 1947.
28. Shore, N. A.: Temporomandibular Joint Dysfunction and Occlusal Equilibration, 2nd ed. Philadelphia, J.B. Lippincott Company, 1976, p. 166.
29. Wolff, H. G.: Headache and Other Head Pain, 2nd ed. New York, Oxford University Press, 1948.

30. Alling, C. C., and Burton, H. N.: Diagnosis of chronic maxillofacial pain. J. Ala. Med. Sci., *10*:73, 1973.
31. Gelb, H., and Arnold, G. E.: Syndromes of the Head and Neck of Dental Origin. Arch. Otolaryngol., *70*:681, 1959.
32. Harris, H. L.: Effects of loss of vertical dimension on anatomic structure of the head and neck. JADA, *25*:175, 1938.
33. Sicher, H.: Positions and movements of the mandible. JADA, *48*:620, 1954.
34. Brodie, A. G.: Anatomy and physiology of head and neck musculature. Am. J. Orthodont., *11*:831, 1950.
35. Campbell, J. Distribution and treatment of pain in temporomandibular arthroses. Br. Dent. J., *105*:393, 1958.
36. Kraus, H.: Muscle function and the temporomandibular joint. J. Prosthet. Dent., *13*:5, 1963.
37. Berry, D. C.: Facial pain related to muscle dysfunction. Br. J. Oral Surg., *4*:222, 1967.
38. Bonica, J. J.: Management of myofascial pain syndromes in general practice. JAMA, *164*:732, 1957.
39. Bonica, J. J.: The Management of Pain with Special Emphasis on the Use of Analgesic Block in Diagnosis and Therapy. Philadelphia, Lea & Febiger, 1959.
40. Freese, A. S., and Scheman, P.: Management of Temporomandibular Joint Problems. St. Louis, C. V. Mosby Co., 1962.
41. Travell, J., and Rinzler, S. H.: Scientific exhibit: myofascial genesis of pain. Postgrad. Med., *11*:425, 1952.
42. Travell, J.: Referred pain from skeletal muscle, the pectoralis major syndrome of breast pain and soreness and the sternomastoid syndrome of headaches and dizziness. N.Y. J. Med., *55*:331, 1955.
43. Kraus, H., Prudden, B., and Hirschorn, K.: Role of inactivity in production of disease. J. Am. Geriatr. Soc., *4*:463, 1956.
44. Magoun, H. I.: Osteopathic approach to dental enigmas. J. Am. Osteopathic Assoc., *62*:110, 1962.
45. Sears, V. H.: Lecture to the Sutherland Cranial Teaching Foundation, Kirksville, Mo., 1959.
46. Gelb, H.: A review correlating the medical-dental relationship in the craniomandibular syndrome. N.Y. J. Dent., *41*:163, 1971.
47. Hughes, G. A.: Clinical diagnosis and treatment of common temporomandibular disturbances. Meeting IADR, Rochester, N.Y., June, 1948.
48. Burns, L.: Effect of bony lesions on behavior. J. Am. Osteop. A., *24*:582, 1925.
49. Leopold, R. L., and Dillon, H.: Psychiatric considerations in whiplash injuries of neck. Pa. Med., *63*:385, 1960.
50. Burns, L.: Effect of bony lesions on behavior. J. Am. Osteop. A., *24*:499, 1925.
51. Moulton, R. E.: Psychiatric considerations in maxillo-facial pain. JADA, *51*:408, 1955.
52. Lupton, D. E.: Psychological aspects of temporomandibular joint dysfunction. JADA, *79*:131, 1969.
53. Selye, H.: The physiology and pathology of exposure to stress. Montreal, ACTA, Inc., 1950.
54. Posselt, U.: The temporomandibular joint syndrome and occlusion. Comp. Am. Equil. Soc., 1964, p. 51.
55. Jankelson, B.: Physiology of human dental occlusion. JADA, *50*:664, 1955.
56. Eisenman, M.: Occlusal dysharmonies as related to cranial nerve syndromes. Presented at the Annual Convention of the Eastern Osteopathic Association, New York, March 27, 28, 1954.
57. Waite, D. E.: Disorders of the temporomandibular joint. Plast. Reconstr. Surg., *34*:162, 1964.
58. Garliner, D.: Myofunctional Therapy. Philadelphia, W. B. Saunders Co., 1976.
59. Moffett, B.: The morphogenesis of the temporomandibular joint. Am. J. Orthod., *52*:401, 1966.
60. Blackwood, H. J.: Cellular remodelling in articular tissue. J. Dent. Res., *45*:480, 1960.
61. Oberg, T., Carlsson, G. E. and Fajers, C. M.: The temporomandibular joint. A morphologic study on human autopsy material. Acta Odont. Scand., *29*:349, 1971.
62. Stedman, T. L.: Stedman's Medical Dictionary, 18th ed. Baltimore, Williams & Wilkins Co., 1953.
63. Posselt, U.: Physiology of Occlusion and Rehabilitation. Philadelphia, F. A. Davis Co., 1962, p. 186.
64. Course in clinical oral orthopedics. New York, Institute for Graduate Dentists, 1953.
65. Haupl, K., Grossman, W., et al.: Textbook of Functional Jaw Orthopedics. St. Louis, The C. V. Mosby Co., 1952, pp. 231–238.
66. Gelb, H.: The temporomandibular joint syndrome: patient communication and motivation. Dent. Clin. North Am., *14*:288, 1970.
67. Travell, J. G., Simons, D. G.: Myofascial Pain and Dysfunction. The Trigger Point Manual, Baltimore, Williams & Wilkins Co., 1983, p. 651.

4

Muscular Aspects of Oral Dysfunction

HANS KRAUS, M.D.

Millions of years ago human beings made the mistake of climbing down from the trees and assuming an upright stance, and this has been blamed as the main cause for most back and neck pain. However, less than a hundred years ago, much more dramatic changes occurred in the environment and life of the human race than the transition from a quadrupedal to a bipedal stance. From the quiet of the countryside, where our existence was dependent on heavy physical labor and where stressful stimuli were rare, we have come to live in highly populated areas and overpopulated cities, where physical work is not only unnecessary most of the time, but where it is hard to get enough physical activity even if desired. At the same time, there is a tremendous amount of nervous irritation inherent in overpopulation; noise, traffic, telephones, deadlines, and business and family pressures add to the tensions of our lives. This radical change in our ecology has seriously disturbed the balance between physical action and response to stimuli (Fig. 4–1). This imbalance, underexercise on one hand and overstimulation on the other, contributes a host of chronic degenerative diseases which we have characterized as hypokinetic disease.[5, 13]

ACTION OF THE MUSCLES

Inactivity of muscles produces weakness and stiffness, leading directly to muscular problems. Over-irritation will lead to emotional imbalance. If both underexercise and over-irritation coincide, and if the physical response to stimuli is inhibited or prevented, the chronic, repeated inhibitions of the fight-or-flight response contribute to disease. The normal response of animals and humans to stimuli results in a number of reactions which prepare for physical action. These reactions include an outpouring of epinephrine, an increased heart beat, an increase in blood pressure, shifting of blood from stomach and intestines to the peripheral muscles, an increase in respiration,

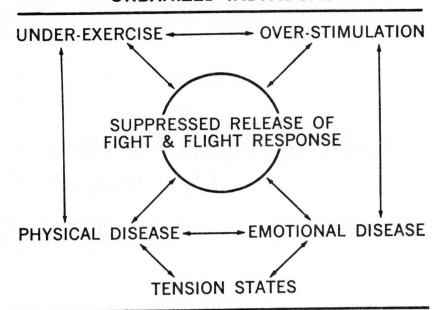

Figure 4–1. (From Kraus, H., and Raab, W.: Hypokinetic Disease: Diseases Produced by Lack of Exercise. Springfield, Ill., Charles C Thomas, 1961.)

and tension of muscles. All of this is useful in primitive life as a preparation to attack or to flee.[5, 13]

If this reponse is inhibited, all these reactions, among them the tensing of muscles, accumulate and, after weeks, months, and years, enhance hypokinetic disease.[5, 13]

Continued disuse of muscles will result in weakness and disuse atrophy. Accumulated tension will, in time, produce tension syndromes.[13] It is this aspect of unhealthful living conditions, of a noxious ecology, that applies not only to the muscles of the back, neck, and extremities but also to the masticatory muscles.[7, 9, 19, 20] The basic qualities of muscle function[6] include the ability of the muscle to contract and to produce power, to overcome resistance and gravity, to lift weights, to produce locomotion, to clench teeth, and to bite (Fig. 4–2). Equally important is the ability of the muscle to give up this contraction—to relax—and then to yield to passive stretch. Relaxation and ability to yield to stretch together form total elasticity. The ability to give up tension and to relax is called physiological elasticity, and the ability to yield to passive stretch after giving up contraction is called physical elasticity. Both physiological elasticity and strength in proper relation, in proper interplay, and under sensory regulation produce coordination.

The fact that muscles contract and produce strength is generally understood, and exercises to strengthen them are commonly used. These exercises require a certain amount of exertion, either lifting weights, or overcoming resistance.

It is different with total elasticity. Since the physiological elasticity of our muscles is constantly reduced to the tension of everyday life, most exercise progams require relaxation. This part of exercise is commonly

PHYSIOLOGY	DYSFUNCTION	THERAPY
I. Strength	Weakness	Strengthening exercises
II. Total elasticity Physiological elasticity	Spasticity	Relaxing exercises
	Spasm	Local relaxing exercises and relief of pain
	Tension	General relaxing exercises and relief of sources of tension
Physical elasticity	Contracture	Stretching exercises
III. Coordination	Incoordination	Exercises I and II and coordination training

Figure 4–2. Basic qualities of muscle function. (From Kraus, H.: Therapeutic Exercise. 2nd ed. Springfield, Ill., Charles C Thomas, 1963).

forgotten or neglected. If muscles do not completely relax—they rarely do in our overtense life—they remain in a constant state of residual tension.[17] Episodes of aggravation or stress can increase the tension to the point where it becomes painful muscle spasm. In this state, the contracted muscle causes pain which, in turn, causes further contraction; thus a vicious circle results whereby any motion becomes more painful and every pain and motion produces more muscle contraction and increases the problem (Fig. 4–3).

When the muscle remains in spasm for a period of time, or if it remains tense for a period of time, it loses part of its elastic property and contracture occurs; that is, it loses part of its physical elasticity. It will then not yield or

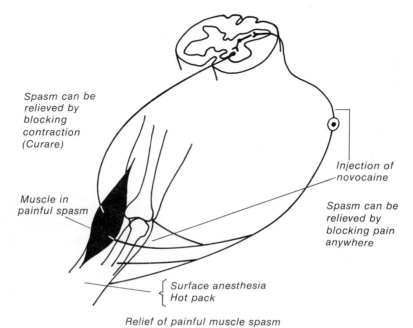

Relief of painful muscle spasm
Figure 4–3. Effects of stress on the muscles.

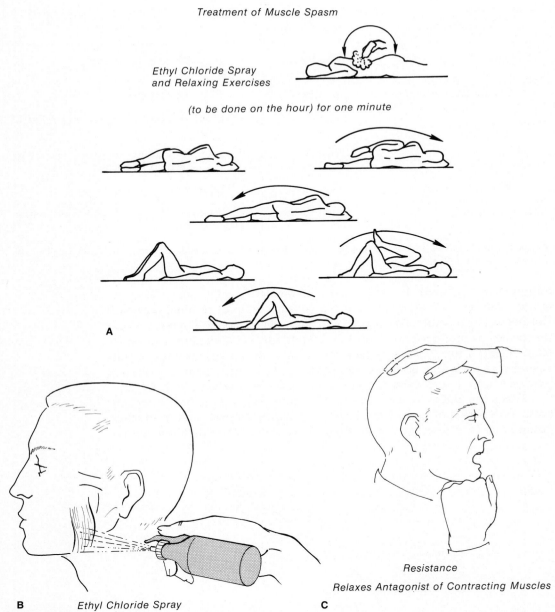

Treatment of Muscle Spasm

*Ethyl Chloride Spray
and Relaxing Exercises*

(to be done on the hour) for one minute

A

B   *Ethyl Chloride Spray*   C

Resistance
Relaxes Antagonist of Contracting Muscles

Figure 4–4. *A, B, C,* Treatment of muscle spasm. (From Kraus, H.: Therapeutic Exercise. 2nd ed. Springfield, Ill., Charles C Thomas, 1963).

will yield only incompletely to stretch. Treatment of muscle spasm consists basically of relieving pain. This is most effective if performed locally. We prefer the application of ethyl chloride spray to the painful muscle area, combined with gentle guarded limbering exercises.[6, 7, 10, 11, 12] Ethyl chloride spray applied to the skin will temporarily relieve pain and permit gentle motion (Fig. 4–4). As motion increases and the pain shifts, future spraying will be needed, and the procedure should be continued until maximum relief and range have been attained. Preceding this procedure by the use of tetanizing current for ten minutes and then sinusoidal current for ten minutes helps to limber up the muscle and greatly enhances the treatment. Tetanizing current is applied to the area in the muscle spasm, fatiguing the muscle, and sinusoidal current then gets it back to gradual rhythmic movements that cannot be duplicated as regularly and as well as by active motion. Ethyl chloride and gentle active motion follow. This procedure frequently relieves the spasm.[13] Several sessions on successive days are necessary, and in the interval the patient has to avoid whatever originally caused the attack or may contribute to it. In neck and back pain this may include prolonged sitting or standing, focusing, reading in bed, straining, and nervous tension. Tranquilizers are indicated whenever the source of tension cannot be eliminated. While they do not relieve the pain, tranquilizers help shield the patient from the source of the pain—tension. In cases of anxiety and in cases of emotional problems, psychiatric help may be needed.

The same principles apply to the treatment of facial and oral muscle spasm.[17, 18, 19, 20, 21]

TRIGGER POINTS

The frequent result of chronic muscle tension and especially of muscle spasm is trigger points, little nodules of degenerated muscle tissue.[4] They were first described at length by Max Lange in 1920.[13] Even before this, however, trigger points had been described by a number of people as far back as 1880. In the 1950s trigger points were biopsied (Fig. 4–5).

Trigger points occur on various parts of the body (Fig. 4–6).[1, 2, 3, 15, 19, 20, 21, 23] They can occur in the posterior neck muscles, in the suboccipital muscles, in the masseter, in the temporal muscles, in the shoulder girdle muscles, in low back muscles, and in hip muscles. Besides triggering pain, they may produce peripheral nerve entrapment. Trigger points in the scalenus muscles can produce scalenus spasm and scalenus syndrome; trigger points in the piriformis muscles produce nerve compression of the sciatic nerve. Once one muscle has been affected by trigger points, the whole system of synergists and antagonists is affected, and muscle dysfunction then leads to more episodes of spasm, tension, and more trigger points. Thus trigger points produced by muscular dysfunction cause pain in the neck and shoulder girdle muscles, with radiation to the extremities.

TREATMENT

Pain and Muscular Dysfunction

The local treatment of muscle spasm has been described before. Tetanizing, sinusoidal current is followed by ethyl chloride spray and gentle limbering motions. In cases of oral dysfunction, gently opening and closing the mouth, opening against gentle resistance, will often result in relief. Oral and facial pain will spread to occipital, cervical, and shoulder girdle muscles, causing trigger points, muscle spasm, and sometimes scalenus syndrome. Scalenus syndrome includes peripheral nerve entrapment at the brachial plexus, often leading to misdiagnosis of cervical disc disease. Trigger points

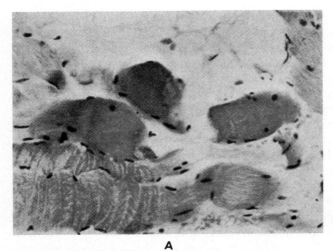

A

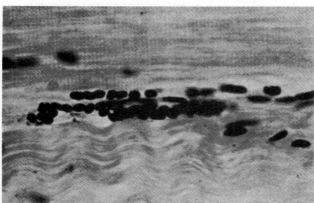

B

Figure 4–5. *A, B,* Biopsy specimens of trigger points. *A,* From Glogowski G., and Wallraff, J.: Ein Beitrag zur Klinik und Histologie der Muskelharten (Myogelosen). Z. Orthop. Grenzgreb., *80*:238, 1951. Reprinted by permission.)

in the sternocleidomastoid muscle may cause vertigo, leading to an impression of Meniere's disease.

Trigger Points[13, 15, 18–23]

Trigger points are best treated by injection of lidocaine or, if the patient is allergic to lidocaine, by injection of saline into the tender areas. The trigger point must be identified by palpation. Injection into the facial muscles with a 25 gauge needle should be made under sterile conditions after the spot of the trigger point has been marked with a little scratch on the surface of the skin. Fanning out in a complete circle to make sure that all areas of the trigger point have been touched is necessary. Following injection, three or four days of treatment with sinusoidal current for 15 minutes, combined with ethyl chloride spray and very gentle exercises, are important to produce optimum results.

Local treatment is only the beginning. Bite correction, when necessary, is essential, as is investigation and treatment of other sources of trigger points.[19, 20, 21] Relief of tension by teaching relaxation, the use of hypnosis,

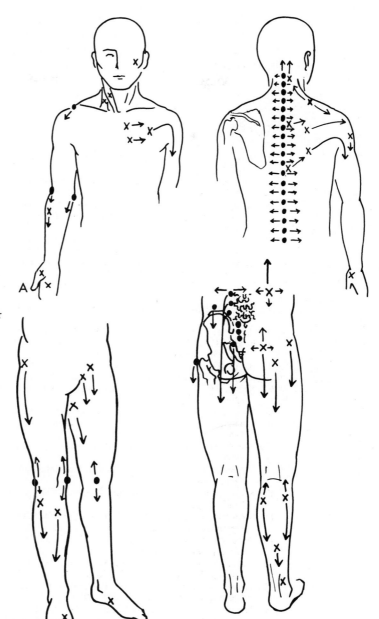

Figure 4–6. *A, B,* Location of trigger points on various parts of the body.

hypnotherapy, a change of working and living habits, where necessary, temporary use of tranquilizers, and psychiatric care may be indicated.

A factor frequently producing trigger points is endocrine imbalance.[16, 18] Even borderline hypothyroidism or borderline estrogen deficiency can be powerful contributing factors, and whenever the question of endocrine imbalance arises, endocrine evaluation and medication is essential. Equally important is the correction of bad working habits, such as straining when using the typewriter or squeezing the telephone between the ear and shoulder. Such problems as reading or watching television in bed may contribute to muscle tension, muscle pain, and trigger points. Only if all these factors are considered and properly managed can permanent results be obtained.

References

1. Bonica, J. J.: Management of myofascial pain syndromes in general practice. JAMA, *164*:732, 1957.
2. Bonica, J. J.: Clinical Applications of Diagnostic and Therapeutic Nerve Blocks. Springfield, Ill., Charles C Thomas, Publisher, 1959.
3. Brugger, A., and Gross, D.: Uber vertebrale, radiculare und pseudoradiculare Syndrome, Teil 11. Documenta Geigy. Acta Rheumatologica, no. 19, pp. 9–11, J. R. Geigy S. A., Basel, Switzerland, 1962.
4. Glogowski, G., and Wallraff, J.: Ein Beitrag zur Klinik und Histologie der Muskelharten (Myogelosen). Z. Orthop. Grenzgeb., *80*:238, 1971.
5. Kraus, H.: Principles and Practice of Therapeutic Exercise. Springfield, Ill., Charles C Thomas, Publisher, 1949.
6. Kraus, H.: Therapeutic Exercise. 2nd ed. Springfield, Ill., Charles C Thomas, Publisher, 1963.
7. Kraus, H.: Muscle function and the temporomandibular joint. J. Prosthet. Dent., *13*:950, 1963.
8. Kraus, H.: Pseudo-disc. South. Med. J., *60*:416, 1967.
9. Kraus, H.: Muscle function of the temporomandibular joint. Dent. Clin. North Am., 533–538, November, 1966.
10. Kraus, H.: New treatment for injured joints (abstract). JAMA, *104*:1261, 1935.
11. Kraus, H.: Neue distorsions behandlung. Wie. Klin. Wschr., *48*:1014, 1935.
12. Kraus, H.: The use of surface anesthesia in the treatment of painful motion. JAMA, *116*:2582, 1941.
13. Lange, M.: Die Muskelharten (Myogelosen). Munchen, J. F. Lehman, Verlag, 1931.
14. Michele, A. A., and Eisenberg, J.: Scapulocostal syndrome. Arch. Phys. Med., *49*:7, 383, 1968.
15. Norris, H. F., Jr., and Benh, J.: Panner: hypothyroid myopathy. Arch. Neurol., *14*:574, 1966.
16. Palchick, Y. S.: Tension headaches. Reprinted from the Summit County Medical Bulletin, May, 1961.
17. Schwarz, G. A., and Rose, E.: Neuromyopathies and thyroid dysfunction. Arch. Intern. Med., *112*:555, 1963.
18. Schwartz, L. L., and Chayes, C. M.: Physical Methods. *In* Facial Pain and Mandibular Dysfunction. Philadelphia, W. B. Saunders Co., 1968, p. 281.
19. Schwartz, L., and Chayes, C.: Facial Pain and Mandibular Dysfunction. Philadelphia, W. B. Saunders Co., 1968.
20. Shore, N. A.: Occlusal Equilibration and Temporomandibular Joint Dysfunction, 2nd ed. Springfield, Ill., Charles C Thomas, Publisher, 1963, pp. 165–168.
21. Travell, J., and Weers, V. D.: Postural vertigo due to trigger areas in the sternocleidomastoid muscle. J. Pediat., *47*:315, 1955.
22. Travell, J.: Basis for multiple uses of local block of somatic trigger areas (procaine infiltration and ethyl chloride spray). Miss. Valley Med. J., *71*:13, 1949.

5

Pain in the Head: A Neurological Appraisal

SIMON E. MARKOVICH, M.D.

Pain is the symptom most commonly described by our patients.

We all, at one time or another, have had our own personal encounter with suffering. The personal definition of pain ranges from superlative words of agony to the deep-suffering tone of the stoic. Pain is nearly always accompanied by a change in affect and/or a disturbance in general performance. Without a clear definition of the problem, all patients approach their physician as "the healer of pain." The patient does not ask "What do I have?" He demands to have his pain eliminated.

The most common complaint is described in the head, and it is called "headache" unless it is confined to specific anatomical areas (the mouth) or to another well-defined structure of the face (sinus, etc.). When not well circumscribed, head pain is a very difficult symptom to describe, particularly when the apparent immediate cause is not clear or visible.

CLASSIFICATION OF HEADACHES

Since the Ad Hoc Committee on Classification of Headaches of the National Institute of Neurological Diseases and Blindness made its report,[1] many articles have been published emphasizing results based upon some form of therapy. Different forms of headaches were reported, without much clarification as to the pathophysiology of these varying conditions.

Most of this knowledge is condensed into the classic book *Headache and Other Head Pains*, by H. G. Wolff.[2]

More recently, others have reclassified headaches,[3, 4] giving an account of their frequency of appearance. Interestingly enough, the so-called "vascular" and "traction-inflammatory" groups constitute about 10 per cent, while "muscle-contraction" headache occurs in about 90 per cent of the patient population (Table 5–1).

In spite of the overwhelming preponderance of nonvascular, the mi-

TABLE 5–1. Classification of Headaches

TYPE	INCIDENCE	CAUSE-CHARACTERISTICS
Traction-inflammatory	2%	Diseases of eye-nose Throat-teeth Mass lesions Cranial neuralgias Arteritis Temporomandibular joint dysfunctions Infections Allergy Cervical osteoarthritis Chronic myositis
Vascular	8%	Migraine Cluster Ophthalmoplegic Hemiplegic Associated facial Toxic Hypertensive
Muscle contraction type	90%	Anxiety Depressive Cervico-occipital

graine headaches, or "sick headaches," are the most actively investigated, nationally and internationally.

The effort in elucidating the neurohumoral, pathophysiological, and pharmacological events of migraine attacks and their treatment and prevention is worthwhile, since these "vascular conditions" have devastating effects when left untreated.

Less interest has been shown in the "garden variety" of headache to which most practitioners often attach an "affective" label of "anxiety and depression."[5, 6]

It is also common experience that those enthusiastic dilettantes who treat all headaches as migraine find themselves in the awkward position of hearing their patients complain that the "treatment is worse than the condition," since their headaches increase with ergotamines and similar type drugs. Often they recur owing to unnecessarily strong medication, usually narcotics, with the unfortunate conversion of the disease into a complicated addiction-dependency situation that few patients can successfully cope with.

This manuscript is intended to deal with what I consider to be pathophysiological considerations in the management of the most common pains in the head.

It is not the sophisticated super-specialist, but rather the well-trained general practitioner, who sees the majority of these cases, and he or she is the one most qualified to make the appropriate diagnosis, and to use the most effective management to effect rapid relief and success in the treatment of these unfortunate patients.

In my experience,[7, 8] the most common headache is the type caused by the "neuromuscular skeletal imbalance." The head in the human species has changed its position from the quadruped to the erect, thereby changing the basic relationship between the cervical spine and the head, with its important functional structures, and the rest of the body.

Although these concepts are elaborated upon in Chapter 4 and in an excellent monograph by the same author of that chapter,[9] it is, in my opinion, not redundant to call attention again to the very delicate interaction and extremely sensitive "biofeedback or servo-mechanisms" that are constantly adjusting the functions of body balance, hearing, vision, and the like with the posture of the head and neck.

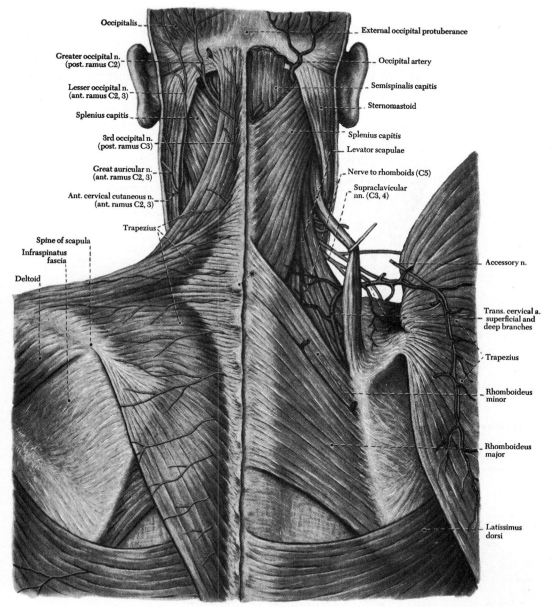

Figure 5–1. Muscles, nerves, and vessels of the back (1st and 2nd layers). On the left, the skin and cervical fascia have been removed to expose the first layer of back muscles. Piercing the trapezius close to the midline are the medial branches of the posterior primary rami of the cervical and thoracic spinal nerves. On the right, the trapezius has been cut and reflected from its vertebral and nuchal attachments. Part of the levator scapulae is retracted laterally, to show the second layer of back muscles and their blood and nerve supply. (From Detailed Atlas of the Head and Neck. R. C. Truex and C. E. Kellner. Oxford, Oxford University Press, 1948.)

These regulatory, homeostatic mechanisms can be disturbed by a variety of conditions originating at any level, including the inflammation and/or irritation of the cephalic projection of the upper cervical nerves (cervico-occipital neuralgias). The many manifestations of these syndromes can at times be treated successfully at one single point, resulting in the disappearance of the entire symptomatology, much to the surprise of the physician and the delight of the patient.

CAUSES OF HEADACHE

It has been my experience that the most common cause of headaches originates in the "vicious circle" generated by the abnormal and painful

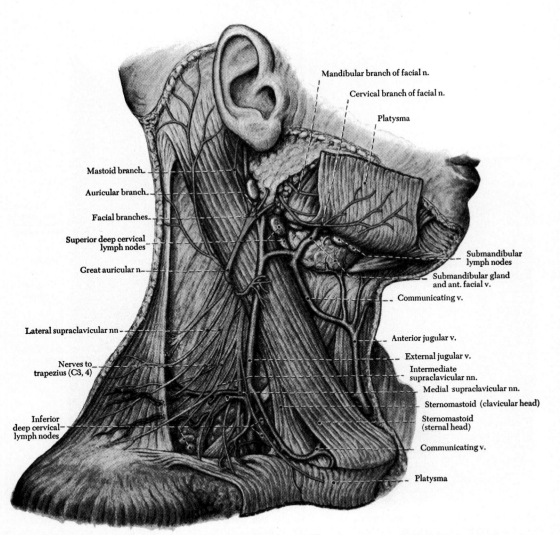

Figure 5–2. Superficial vessels and nerves of the neck (2nd layer). The platysma muscle is divided and reflected to expose the tributaries of the external jugular vein. The sternomastoid muscle is shown separating the anterior from the posterior triangle. (From Detailed Atlas of the Head and Neck. R. C. Truex and C. E. Kellner. Oxford, Oxford University Press, 1948.)

contraction of the cervical-nuchal muscles, mainly the trapezius muscle. These contractions generate a type of "ischemic irritation"[10, 11] that includes the entrapment of the second cervical nerves (greater occipital and lesser occipital) as they travel through the bulk of the muscle, ascending into the back of the head to innervate the posterior scalp region, the temporal areas, and the lobes of the ears, sending terminal branches into the angle of the jaw, the back of the eye and the vertex of the head (Figs. 5–1, 5–2, 5–3).

This creates a distinct clinical syndrome (Table 5–2), which is easily confused with atypical "vascular migraine" because of the unilaterality of the symptoms and frequent complaints of pain in the back of the eye with or without visual disturbance (Table 5–3).

A second common entity is the temporomandibular joint pain–dysfunction syndrome, first described by Costen in 1934.[12] This condition has been proved to be more common than expected, with many protean manifestations, and it has become known as the "Great Imposter" (Table 5–4).[13]

The two syndromes mentioned above have many symptoms that may reflect the same imbalance of neuromuscular skeletal functions that we have

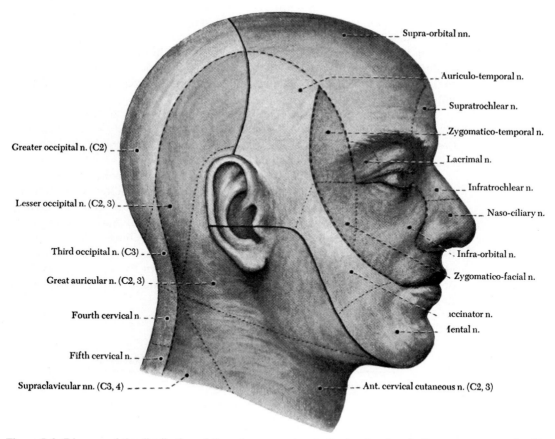

Figure 5–3. Diagram of the distribution of the cutaneous nerves to the head and neck. Sensory nerves to the skin overlying the shaded area are cutaneous branches of the medial divisions of the posterior primary rami of the upper cervical spinal nerves. The skin area supplied by the cutaneous branches of the anterior primary rami of the cervical spinal nerves is shown. The remainder of the face area receives sensory fibers from branches of the ophthalmic, maxillary, and mandibular divisions of the trigeminal nerve. (From Detailed Atlas of the Head and Neck. R. C. Truex and C. E. Kellner. Oxford, Oxford University Press, 1948.)

TABLE 5–2.   Cervico-occipital Neuralgia*

Dull chronic pain
Muscle spasms

Radiation { Eye
Ear
Neck

Paresthesia: Scalp
Tinnitus
Nausea

*From Markovich.[7, 8]

TABLE 5–3. Migraine Headaches*

Unilateral
Prodromatas
Sequential profile
Brief attacks

Associated symptoms { Nausea
Visual
Scotomas
Vomiting

Photophobia irritability
Neurological symptoms
Familial history

*From Markovich.[7, 8]

already commented upon. The fact that a cervical nerve irritation can create a painful condition in the angle of the jaw or in the temple explains the possible common "irritative" source of both syndromes.

If the practitioner takes a careful history, searching for the sequence of events, the location of symptoms, the frequency, duration, and characteristics of the pain, and the precipitating factors, it is possible, with a careful examination of the patient, to arrive at the correct diagnosis without the abuse of costly and specialized consultations and work-ups.

In making the differential diagnosis, one should be very careful in evaluating the primary areas of painful dysfunction and the secondary or radiating pain that, at times, appears in a nonanatomical distribution in or outside the head.

For mechanisms as cause of headaches from the cervical spine, I refer the reader to the excellent articles by Blumenthal.[14, 15] The author not only brought his ideas up-to-date, but he related in detail the technique and locations of blocking "trigger points" (Figs. 5–4, 5–5).

He also mentions the classic post-traumatic headache syndrome of Barre-Lieou.[16] This is a constellation of symptoms associated with blurring of vision, mydriasis, blepharospasms, dizziness, salivation and other vasomotor symptoms, pain and dysfunction of the neck, head, face, and muscles, nervousness, vomiting, memory impairment, and swelling and stiffness of the hand and fingers on the ipsilateral side, all encompassed within one alleged syndrome. The majority of symptoms known to appear in any kind of headache point to the confusing interaction of many systems involved in the appearance of such protean manifestations.

TABLE 5–4. Temporomandibular Joint Dysfunction*

Unilateral dull aching
Gradual onset
Aggravated by chewing
Click—crepitation in joint
Tenderness—muscle spasm
Bruxism
Deviation of jaw
Pain, opening, closing
Women 4:1

*From Markovich.[7, 8]

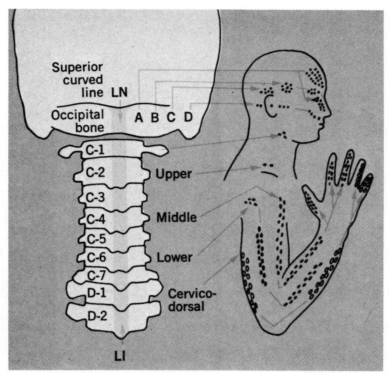

Figure 5–4. Headache and pain in the head and face originate in weak fibro-osseous attachments of tendons to the occipital bone (A, B, C, D) as weak fibers relax under normal tension and allow tension-overstimulation of sensory nerves of the cervical spine. Such pain is almost always referable to a specific location, a valuable aid in diagnosis. LI, interspinous ligament; LN, nuchal ligament. (Adapted from Kayfetz, D. O., et al.: Whiplash injury and other ligamentous headache—its management with prolotherapy. Headache, *3*:21, 1963.)

This is, in my opinion, the reason why so many practitioners, after the recitation of these complaints by the patient followed by a cursory examination, decide to dump these cases into the "anxiety-depression bag" and prescribe addictive-narcotic or strong tranquilizer therapy, thereby worsening the original condition and causing it to become chronic.

MANAGEMENT

The basic premise for successful management of a headache patient is to make an accurate diagnosis and then to treat the patient accordingly. The physician should be aware of his limitations and should first be able to relieve the patient of his pain (Table 5–5).

The different techniques may range from nerve blocks and injection of triggerpoints to the restoration of the neuromuscular skeletal balance, using physical therapy or biofeedback techniques, carefully combined medications, and/or transcutaneous electrical nerve stimulation (TENS).

The physician should also provide for the restoration of the physical and emotional balance by psychotherapy, with the aim of returning the patient to his regular and familiar social and working environments.

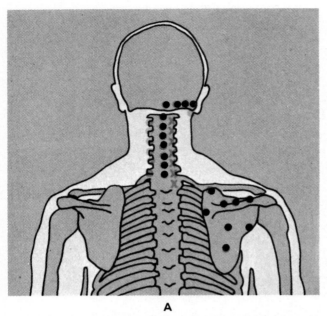

A

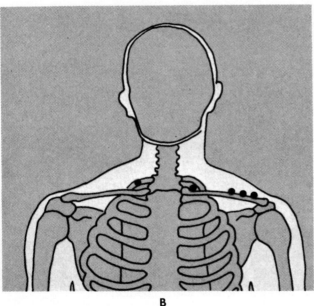

B

Figure 5–5. Trigger points (●) that often elicit muscle spasm and pain in patients with headache. *A,* Prone patient. Laminar and articular points. *B,* Supine patient. Points at scalenus, sternomastoid, and trapezius insertions. (Adapted from Kayfetz, D. O., et al.: Whiplash injury and other ligamentous headache—its management with prolotherapy. Headache *3*:21, 1963.)

TECHNIQUES TO REDUCE PAIN

In reviewing the literature, some techniques such as acupuncture, transcendental meditation, conditioning exercises, and the like seem to enjoy more popular appeal because they are considered to be less invasive or traumatic. None has been proven to be specific for any form or type of painful syndromes.

TABLE 5–5. Headaches—Differential Diagnosis*

	VASCULAR MIGRAINE	TRACTION TMJD	NEURALGIA CERV.-OCCIP.	TRIGEMINAL NEURALGIA
Pain	Severe paroxysmal	Severe dull	Throbbing paroxysmal	Excruciating paroxysmal
Quality	Throbbing	Dull ache	Muscle spasms	Stabbing
Location	Unilateral	Facial	Occipital	Facial
Aura	Visual	None	None	None
Duration	Few hours	Permanent	Days	Brief
Associated symptoms	Vomiting	Bruxism	Ear pain	Trigger zones
	Neurologic	Malocclusion	Eye pain	
	Irritability	Ear pain	Paresthesias	
	Protophob	Clicks	Anxiety	

*From Markovich.[7, 8]

ELECTRICAL STIMULATION

I have been particularly interested in the use of electrical stimulation as a technique to reduce pain, decrease the muscle spasms, and restore the neuromuscular system to its normal balance.

My results with the treatment of cervico-occipital neuralgias and the TMJ pain syndromes have been very promising, in spite of the reluctance of many patients to allow electrical currents to be applied to their heads.[7, 8]

We use a mild electrical current and/or fluori-methane spray to stimulate the cervical nerves or the muscles. Both have the advantage of easy control over the duration of the discomfort, and they may be repeated without any damage to the tissues.

In this way, we are able to differentiate among the atypical facial pains and the TMJ pain and to evaluate the associated muscle spasms.

Application of Electrical Stimulation

The modalities of management used vary according to the condition of the patient.

If the patient complains of severe pain, I attempt to reduce or block the pain with lidocaine (Xylocaine) 1 per cent, injected into the trigger zones. Often, more than one area is found. The block should be as circumscribed as possible in order to recognize its effects. Massive injections into the muscles are avoided (Fig. 5–6).

The association of steroids (dexamethasone) is advisable, and I consistently use a small amount (4 to 8 mg. of Decadron—1–2 ml.) to reduce the inflammatory reactions, with excellent results.

When using an electrical current, the electrode remains over the area for a few minutes (3 to 15 min.), resulting in considerable relief of pain and reduction of muscle spasm.

New approaches to the management of pain have resulted from the understanding of basic mechanisms of pain production and from the discovery that the brain synthesizes its own opiate-like substances.[17, 18] To reinforce the effects of transcutaneous electrical neural stimulation (TENS), the patient is given medication, usually consisting of a combination of analgesic, muscle relaxant, and tranquilizer drugs.

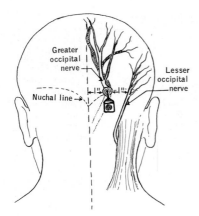

Figure 5–6. Technique of occipital nerve block. The greater occipital nerve is injected just above the superior nuchal line one inch from the midline. The nerve is just medial to the occipital artery, which can be palpated as it crosses the superior nuchal line. The lesser occipital nerve is blocked one inch lateral to the greater occipital nerve. (From Finneson, B. E.: Diagnosis and Management of Pain Syndromes. 2nd ed. Philadelphia, W. B. Saunders Co., 1969.)

Since the analgesic effects of psychotropic drugs of the tricyclic group has been confirmed[19, 20] I have been using amitriptyline in small doses (10 to 25 mg.) two or three times a day. This medication has been shown also to be effective in the prevention of migraine.[20, 21] Propranolol is also recommended in the prophylaxis of vascular headaches.[19, 20] The value of TENS in the relief of a variety of painful syndromes has been reviewed and confirmed in the literature.[20, 21, 22]

The patient is re-examined within the following 24 to 48 hours and, if the good results continue, no additional nerve blocks or electrical stimulation are repeated. The patient is told to continue with the medication regularly every six or eight hours (three times per day) to prevent the recurrence of pain, and the patient is re-examined in one week.

Most of my patients have had excellent responses, up to 80 per cent relief of pain. Twenty per cent of the patients are given two or more treatments. Rarely have I had patients who required more than three blocks or consecutive electrical treatments.

A few patients return in about three to four weeks complaining of pain in a slightly different distribution. In the majority of cases, an injection of the "secondary trigger point" and/or repeat electrical stimulation of the area is enough to improve the condition.

Many of these patients remain on the "preventive medication" for one to three months, regularly. After three months I begin to reduce the dosage in an effort to discontinue the drugs in the months to follow, with the advice to report any recurrence of the headache.

During this period, attention is given to the restoration of physical and emotional balance, and the patient is encouraged to visit a psychiatrist if the anxiety-depressive syndrome remains despite the disappearance of the headaches.

My results with the use of high-voltage galvanic currents in reeducating the muscles and reducing their irritability and painful spasm seem to correlate with the results obtained by others.[17, 22]

The effect of electrical currents in the trophism of tissues has been reviewed extensively, and the present concepts are encouraging. These techniques have been used without deleterious effects or risks in any part of the body.[23]

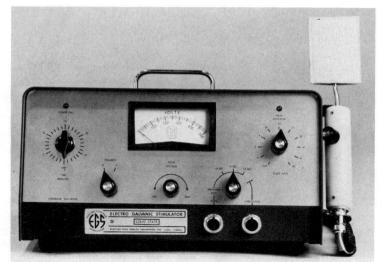

Figure 5–7.

High-Voltage Electrogalvanic Treatment

I have obtained the same excellent results with electrical stimulation using two different modalities.

One of these is a high-voltage electrogalvanic instrument that delivers twin short pulses in a unipolar fashion (Figs. 5–7, 5–8, 5–9). This instrument activates the muscle at frequencies that we can vary from low (4 per sec) to high tetanic (80 per sec.) After a minute or so, relaxation of the spastic

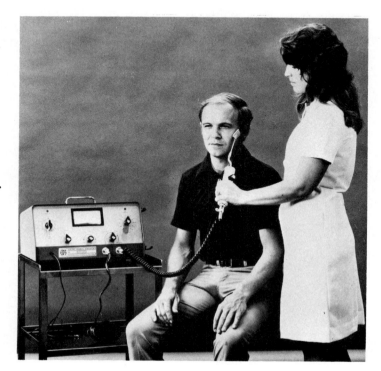

Figure 5–8.

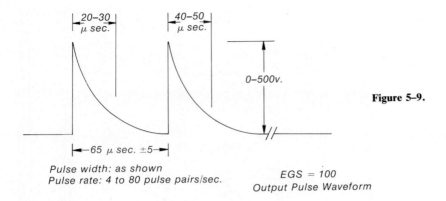

Figure 5–9.

Pulse width: as shown
Pulse rate: 4 to 80 pulse pairs/sec.

EGS = 100
Output Pulse Waveform

temporal or masseter muscle is obtained, with much relief of the pain. The electrode is applied over the skin but can also be used inside the mouth without any discomfort or damage to the oral tissues.

We usually give a 15-minute treatment over the selected area. At times, two electrodes are placed on the same side or opposite sides to alternate the treatment (every 10 sec.), or one large electrode with a continuous flow of current is used.

In most patients, the effect of the current is reinforced with the same type of medication as previously described given every six to eight hours to prevent the recurrence of the painful spasm of the muscles.

More recently, I have used a new modality of TENS instrument, a "pain suppressor" which interferes with the sensation of pain in the brain without the active response of the muscles (Figs. 5–10, 5–11, 5–12). The results obtained are quite encouraging. This new modality apparently acts as a central inhibitor of pain, restoring the balance of the neuromuscular system. All these patients are referred to dentists in the community for restoration of the malocclusion and/or adjustments in the position of the jaw

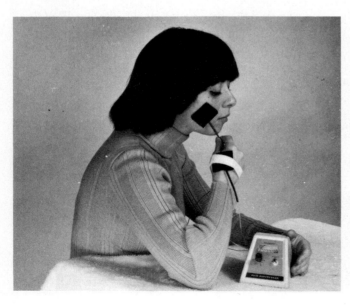

Figure 5–10.

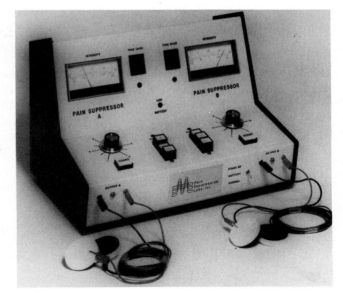

Figure 5–11.

by bite plates or splints. This, I believe, is absolutely necessary to avoid recurrence.

The duration of the condition, the lack of results and treatment, and the occasional mismanagement and poor interest of the previous treating physician create a feeling of mixed insecurity in the patients.

If the use of amitriptylines and the disappearance of the symptoms are not enough to restore the patient's confidence and motivation to return to his or her usual activities, I invariably make a referral for psychodynamic evaluation and supportive therapy.

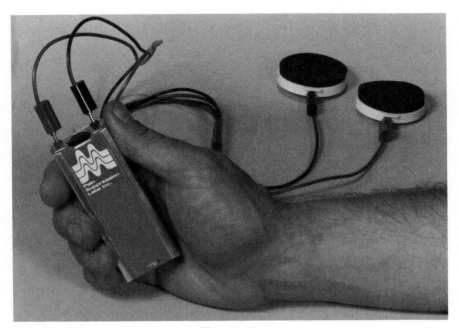

Figure 5–12.

I agree that the basis for good results in medicine is the rapport, empathy, and a trusting relationship between the patient and the treating physician. However, in my opinion, it is as dangerous to become an "amateur psychiatrist" as it is to use psychopharmacological manipulation without a real grasp of the potential dangers of such techniques.

I believe that, as we refine our diagnostic techniques and the armamentarium of drugs and therapeutic modalities, and most particularly, when we learn how to use them accurately and scientifically, we may be close to success in the erasure of this elusive, immeasurable sensation of human suffering that we call *pain*.

References

1. Classification of headaches. JAMA, *173*:717, 1962.
2. Wolff, H. G.: Headaches and Other Pains, 2nd ed. New York, Oxford University Press, 1962.
3. Diamond, S., and Baltes, B.: The diagnosis and treatment of headaches. Chicago Med. Sch. Q., *32*:41, 1973.
4. Diamond, S., and Baltes, B.: Clinical clues to different types of headaches. Postgrad. Med., *56*:69, 1974.
5. Dalessio, D. J.: Mechanisms and biochemistry of headaches. Postgrad. Med., *56*:56, 1974.
6. Basbaum, A. I., and Fields, H. L.: Endogenous pain control mechanisms. Review and hypothesis. Ann. Neurol., *4*:451, 1978.
7. Markovich, S. E.: Head Pain. Greater New York Dental Association Annual Meeting, 1975 (unpublished data).
8. Markovich, S. E.: Painful Neuromuscular Dysfunction Syndromes in the Head. A Neurologist's View. American Academy of Craniomandibular Disorders, Annual Meeting, 1976 (unpublished data).
9. Kraus, H.: Treatment of Back and Nerve Pain. New York, McGraw-Hill Book Company, 1970.
10. Sicuteri, F.: Vasoneuroactive substances in migraine. Headache, *6*:109, 1966.
11. Sicuteri, F., Franchi, G., and Michelacci, S.: Biochemical mechanisms of ischemic pain. Adv. Neurol. Symp. Pain, *4*:39, 1974.
12. Costen, J. B.: Syndromes of ear and sinus symptoms depending upon disturbed function of the temporomandibular joint. Ann. Otol., *43*:1, 1934.
13. Morton, H. D.: The great impostor (editorial). JAMA, *23*:2395, 1976.
14. Blumenthal, L. S.: Injury to the cervical spine as a cause of headache. Postgrad. Med., *56*:147, 1974.
15. Blumenthal, L. S.: Tension headaches, in Vinken, P. J., and Bruyn, G. W. (eds.): Handbook of Clinical Neurology, vol. 5. Amsterdam, North Holland Publishing Company, 1968.
16. Gavral, L., and Neuwirth, E.: Posterior Cervical Sympathetic Syndrome of Barre-Lieou. N.Y. State J. Med., *54*:1920, 1954.
17. Diamond, S., and Baltes, B. J.: Chronic tension headaches treated with amitryptiline. A double blind study. Headache, *11*:110, 1971.
18. Snyder, S. H., and Childers, S. R.: Opiate receptors and opioid peptides. Ann. Rev. Neurosci., *2*:35, 1979.
19. Gomersall, J. D., and Stuart, A.: Amitriptyline in migraine prophylaxis. J. Neurol. Neurosurg. Psychiatry, *36*:684, 1973.
20. Fields, H. L.: Pain II: New approaches to management. Ann. Neurol., *9*:101, 1981.
21. Raskin, N. H., and Appenzeller, O.: Headache. Philadelphia, W. B. Saunders Company, 1980.
22. Chapman, C. R., and Benedetti, C.: Analgesia following transcutaneous electrical stimulation. Life Sci., *21*:1645, 1977.
23. Liboff, A. R., and Rinaldi, R. A. (eds.): Electrically mediated growth mechanism in living systems. Ann. N.Y. Acad. Sci., *238*:1, 1973.

6

Endocrine Disorders and Muscle Dysfunction

LAWRENCE S. SONKIN, M.D., Ph.D.

Endocrine disorders have been mentioned as possible causal factors in temporomandibular joint (TMJ) pain and spasm by a number of European authors.[1-5] A statement by Laszlo Schwartz and his co-workers in 1959,[6] "Pain involving the temporomandibular articulation arises most often in its musculature," provides the key to understanding the possible connection of endocrinopathies with TMJ symptoms, since virtually all endocrine disorders may cause skeletal muscle dysfunction.

The menopause has been discussed as a possible cause of TMJ symptoms by Schlegel,[1] Hary and Matekovits,[2] and Ganshorn.[4] These authors noted between 78 and 80 per cent of cases occurring in women, and that the age of onset seemed to peak at puberty and again in the menopausal period.

The study by Hary and Matekovits[2] demonstrated a correlation between estrogenic deficiency and the appearance of temporomandibular joint disorders in 43 women with a previous history of normal menstrual cycles, who had been castrated for cancer of the cervix or for breast cancer. The age group of the patients was between 18 and 50. The following temporomandibular joint symptoms were observed: 39 per cent had pain, 11 in the joint and 6 in the periarticular region; 12 others noted noise on joint movement; abnormalities in opening the mouth occurred in 28 cases, and restriction of the opening occurred in 1; excessive mobility of the temporomandibular articulation was noted in 18 patients, and indentations at the joint in 4; 5 patients had diviation of the jaw from the midline on opening. The majority of temporomandibular problems arose in 21 patients during the first 2 years following castration, whereas only 2 cases appeared after the fourth year subsequent to treatment. None of these patients had received an adequate maintenance program of hormone therapy. Only 3 of the 29 patients with TMJ symptoms could recall any difficulties in the joint prior to castration. The authors concluded that of 43 patients with therapeutic castration, 29 (67 per cent) showed subjective or objective TMJ disturbances. They felt that there was a correlation between hormonal disturbances caused by castration and the TMJ symptoms. The age of the patients did not seem to be a factor.

Loewit and colleagues[3] measured gonadotrophin levels, estrogens, 17-hydroxycorticosteroids, and 17-ketosteroids in 23 women between the ages of 17 and 34 who had presented with TMJ symptoms. The authors noted a high incidence of abnormal gonadotrophin and estrogen levels in these patients. However, the results are open to question, since no clinical abnormalities were described among these patients other than TMJ symptoms and no normal controls were presented.

Ganshorn[4] recommended a therapeutic trial with estrogens for TMJ disorders in menopausal women.

A study of 43 patients with TMJ syndrome and suspected endocrine disorders was presented in the first edition of this book. Ten cases of metabolic dysfunction, including hypothyroidism, hyperthyroidism, estrogen deficiency, premenstrual tension, hyperparathyroidism, and symptomatic low metabolism responsive to thyroid hormone therapy, were described.

The following discussion will review the relationship between endocrine disorders and muscle dysfunction, as well as the structural, physiological, and biochemical abnormalities that have been reported.

THE PHYSIOLOGY AND BIOCHEMISTRY OF MUSCLE CONTRACTION

Familiarity with biochemistry and physiology of muscle contraction is essential to the understanding of some of the effects of hormones on muscle function.

Price and Van de Velde[7] and Gergely[8] have provided material for a simplified schematic diagram (Fig. 6–1). This diagram includes the phosphorylcreatine shuttle recently postulated by Bessman and Geiger[9] to explain insulin-independent energy transport in contracting striated muscle.

The signal for voluntary muscle contraction is conducted from the motor cortex of the brain by spinal tracts and motor nerve to the myoneural junction at the muscle cell surface, resulting in release of acetylcholine, and depolarization of the membrane with respect to inner potassium ion and outer sodium ion charges on the cell membrane (not shown in sketch). An impulse for contraction then travels by way of a tubular system to the subcellular myofibril (1), where the tubule encircles a saccular mesh, the sacrolemmal reticulum, with which it forms a unit called the triad (2). The stimulus causes rapid migration of calcium ions (Ca^{++}) by an undetermined mechanism from the sarcolemmal reticulum into the myofibril (3). Here the Ca^{++} passes between parallel filaments of actin, which form a hexagonal grid around myosin filaments. Ca^{++} action is blocked by Mg^{++} (4). Ca^{++} activates ATPase in the myosin heads, or meromyosin (5). These heads are also thought by Bessman and Geiger to contain the M band creatine phosphokinase (CPK) of muscle (7). The activated ATPase splits ATP and initiates a series of reactions resulting in muscle contraction (6). Bessman and Geiger have postulated, "When muscle contracts the interdigitation of actin and myosin brings the (myosin) heads into the region of free phosphorylcreatine around the I band (1), thereby providing substrate for the transfer of phosphate to bound ADP on the heads and permitting relaxation to occur." M band CPK provides phosphate, split from phosphorylcreatine,

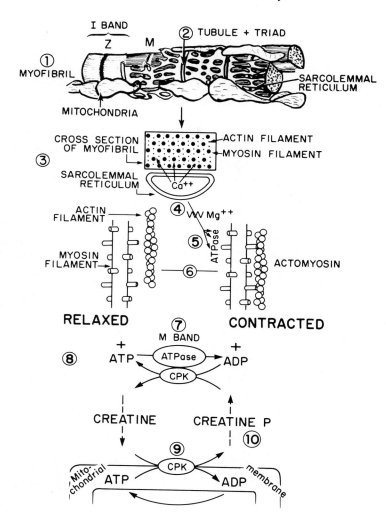

Figure 6–1. Physiology and biochemistry of muscle contraction. See text for explanation. Upper diagram (1 to 6) from Gergely, J.: Biochemical aspects of muscle structure and function. *In* Walton, J. N. [ed.]: Disorders of Voluntary Muscle. 2nd ed. London, Churchill Livingstone, 1981. Lower diagram (7 to 10), from Bessman, S. P., and Geiger, P. J.: Transport of energy in muscle: the phosphorylcreatine shuttle. Science, *211*:448, 1981. Reprinted with permission.)

to re-form ATP from ADP (*8*). A separate enzyme system in the mitochondrial membrane restores the phosphorylcreatine (*9*), which is then available on demand by contracting muscle (*10*).

MUSCLE ABNORMALITIES IN INDIVIDUAL ENDOCRINE DISORDERS

THYROID DISORDERS[10]

Hyperthyroidism

Hyperthyroidism (hyperactivity of the thyroid gland) causes an increased blood concentration of thyroid hormones, either L-thyroxine (T4) and triiodothyronine (T3), or T3 alone (T3 thyrotoxicosis). The overproduction may result from diffuse hyperplasia of the gland, *Graves' disease.* A few of its manifestations include weight loss, increased appetite, rapid pulse, cardiac arrhythmias, palpitations, nervousness, sweating, intolerance to heat, protrusion of the eyeballs, and weakness of ocular movements with lid lag, known as exophthalmic ophthalmoplegia.

Weakness and muscular atrophy were first described by Bathurst in 1895.[11] Askanazy[12] and Hed and colleagues[13] described degenerative histological changes, including fatty infiltration, increased interstitial connective tissue, hyaline degeneration, loss of striation, round cell infiltration, fragmentation and atrophy of muscle fibers, and increase in sarcolemmal nuclei, resembling changes seen in muscular dystrophy. Indeed, latent muscular dystrophy, myasthenia gravis, and periodic paralysis may be precipitated or aggravated by the thyrotoxic state.[14]

Electromyographic studies have shown evidence of myopathy and occasional neurogenic disease.[15, 16]

The first evidence of a chemical basis for myopathy in thyrotoxicosis came from the laboratory of Richardson and Shorr,[17] who described an increased creatine excretion in the urine of patients with thyrotoxicosis and reduced retention of ingested creatine. This substance is an essential component of muscle energy metabolism, since it is combined with phosphate by creatine phosphokinase (CPK) to form creatine phosphate, which, along with adenosine triphosphate (ATP), is an essential fuel in muscle contraction (Fig. 6–1). These workers demonstrated that therapy of hyperthyroidism with propylthiouracil or iodine rapidly abolishes the leak of creatine and ultimately corrects the muscle dysfunction. The studies were confirmed shortly thereafter by Thorn and Eder.[18, 19]

More recent studies have revealed that serum CPK level is normal or low in patients with thyrotoxicosis and elevated in hypothyroid patients.[20] Direct studies of muscle content in thyrotoxicosis have revealed reduction in creatine, creatine phosphokinase, and ATP, as well as water and potassium, with an increase in muscle sodium content.[21, 22] These losses may be caused by increases in membrane permeability which occur under the influence of high thyroxine concentration.[23]

Studies on mitochondria have been carried out by Peter,[24] who demonstrated an increased number of normally functioning mitochondria in the muscles of severely thyrotoxic patients. This, he felt, could account for the increased metabolism of such patients.

Studies by Karlberg and co-workers[25] have revealed a role of the beta sympathetic and adenyl cyclase systems in thyrotoxic myopathy. They demonstrated elevated levels of muscle fat and plasma cAMP in hyperthyroid patients and reduced levels in hypothyroid patients. Propranolol infusion, which blocks the activity of the beta sympathetic system, rapidly reduced cAMP levels and was effective in preventing periodic paralysis in hyperthyroid patients.

Temporomandibular joint symptoms might be anticipated as a manifestation of the myopathy and tension that accompany the thyrotoxic state. Two such patients are described below.

Thyrotoxicosis

Case 1: Single white female age 32, fashion designer.

1. 12–18–62: Chief complaint—"hyperactive thyroid."
2. Past history revealed chronic recurrent stiffness and inability to open jaw periodically for the past 5 years.

In September, 1962 the patient put 20 drops of an iodine preparation by mistake into each nostril. Immediately thereafter, she began to feel weak, overstimulated, developed palpitations, began to eat a "lot of liver" and lost 2 lb.

    3. 12–17–62: Radioactive iodine uptake at another hospital was reported to reveal toxic levels. Three hour postprandial blood sugar 138 mg./dl., protein-bound iodine, (PBI) 5.8, 5.9, 6.4 μg./dl. (normal, 3.5 to 8 μg./dl.)

    4. Physical examination: Pulse 104, weight 109.5 lb., blood pressure 110/70. Eyes appeared normal, patient hyperactive (somewhat fluttery), thyroid gland of normal size. Blood cholesterol 200 mg./dl., PBI 6.1 μg./dl.; BMR declined by patient and her physician. Impression: thyrotoxicosis with normal PBI, possibly due to low thyroid-binding globulin, or high T3.

    5. Patient returned to care of private physician who started methimazole therapy on the following day. Therapy stopped after 5½ weeks because the patient had heavy vaginal bleeding.

    6. 2–9–63: Consulted TMJ specialist because of recurrence of jaw pain.

    7. 2–15–63: Eyes more proptotic—2 mm; BMR −1, cholesterol 228 mg./dl., radioactive iodine (RAI) uptake 67 per cent, conversion ratio (CR) 77 per cent (high).

    8. 2–21–63: RAI therapy 3.54 mCi.

    9. 4–19–63: Complaint: muscle spasms and tension. Pulse 128. Clinically appears thyrotoxic. Prescription: methimazole, 10 mg. every 8 hr.

    10. June 1963: RAI uptake 30 per cent. CR 74 per cent. T4 4.0 μg./dl.; pulse 120. TMJ pain persists. Proptosis slightly increased 1 to 1.5 mm.

    11. 8–5–63: Upset because dentist is impatient with her. Told her she was acting out hostility. Patient shaky and sweaty.

    12. 10–2–63: RAI uptake 47 per cent, conversion ratio 73 per cent, PBI 4.2, 5.5 μg./dl.

    13. 1–9–64: Bite feels fine, still cracks and grates. No palpitations. Weight 107.5 lb. Pulse 96. Impression: Euthyroid ?

    4–9–65: Neurological consultation: "Back pain of emotional cause."

    4–22–65: Under care at headache clinic, improving; pain not constant. Pulse 96, weight 108 lb. PBI 3.5 μg./dl., T3 uptake normal. Impression: Euthyroid.

    5–12–65: Physiotherapy.

    14. 12–23–65: Back and jaw improved, pulse 108, patient hyperkinetic and voluble. RAI 36 per cent, CR 33 per cent.

    15. 7–25–67: "Sluggish," weight 123 lb., pulse 88.

    16. 11–13–67: Pulse 60, weight 129 lb. T4 by column 4.4 μg./dl., normal 2.9 to 6.9 μg./dl. Free T4 1.1 mμg./dl. (normal, 1–2.1 mμg./dl.). Thyroid binding globulin 12 μg./dl., (normal 10–26 μg./dl.) BMR −11, cholesterol 259 mg./dl.

    17. 1–21–73: T3 by radioimmunoassay 260 μg./dl., normal 150 to 250 μg./dl. Impression: Chronic T3 thyrotoxicosis, probable jodbasedow with slow remission following radioactive iodine therapy, secondary myalgia, temporomandibular joint syndrome, anxiety and depression remitting with remission of chronic T3 thyrotoxicosis.

    18. 5–8–81: Patient remains well.

Comment: This case is a fairly clear-cut example of T3 thyrotoxicosis, the diagnosis of which has been provable only since the late 1960s. The test for plasma T3 was done only as a research laboratory procedure until the early 1970s, at which time the diagnosis could be confirmed. The correlation between the patient's onset of acute TMJ symptoms, generalized muscle pain and spasm and active thyrotoxicosis seems to be well documented and confirmed by a clinical course which I have been privileged to observe over a period of the past 21 years. In retrospect, it seems apparent that the patient was thyrotoxic through December 1965, at which point she still had a mild tachycardia, and her weight was still down to about 103.5 lbs.; however, the one test then available, which had always previously indicated the patient to be thyrotoxic (namely, the radioactive iodine conversion ratio), had returned to normal range, indicating that the patient was on her way into a remission, which has persisted ever since her visit in December 1965. The improvement in her back and temporomandibular joint symptoms at that time were clear-cut and she has never had a recurrence of either of these complaints.

Case 2: A 32-year-old, single black, female accountant.
1. Referred for diagnosis and treatment of thyrotoxicosis.
2. Chief complaint and present illness: Pain in neck, jaws hurt with chewing, on first opening the mouth in the morning, weakness in knees.
One year: menses every two weeks, dizzy on arising, headaches.
Six months: all muscles sore, notes beating of heart.
Weak on walking, sweats excessively, nervous, cries easily.
One month: lost 15 lb., short of breath, ankles swell.
Two weeks: skin itches all over at night.
Depressed, neck swelling, can't sleep.
3. Physical findings: pulse 112 (on propranolol, 10 mg. t.i.d.), skin warm and moist, excoriation marks present on both thighs, all muscles diffusely tender to pressure, tenderness along mandible and on finger pressure in external auditory canals, thyroid diffusely enlarged to about 50 g., faint systolic murmur over left lobe of thyroid. Moderate systolic murmur over heart.
4. Positive laboratory findings: RAI uptake 85 per cent, CR 89 per cent, T4 RIA 15.2 μg./dl. (normal, 4.5–12.5 μg./dl.), T3 uptake 65.4 per cent, (normal, 35–45 per cent), cholesterol 95 mg./dl. (normal, 125–300 mg./dl.), ECG: sinus tachycardia.
5. 11–10–76: Rx: RAI 5.63 mCi., continue propranolol, 10 mg. q.i.d.
6. 12–9–76: Heart pounding, weak. Start methimazole, 10 mg. q.i.d.
7. 12–16–76: Fever, earache, coughing blood. Legs stronger, no more muscle pain. Physical examination: badly infected tonsils, temperature 101°F, pulse 140, right tonsillar lymph node large and tender. Lab: WBC 11,700; differential, 66 polymorphonuclear leukocytes, 22 bands, 12 lymphocytes. Throat culture: Hemolytic *Staphylococcus aureus*. Impression: Staphylococcal tonsillitis, not related to thyroid therapy. Rx: continue thyroid therapy plus potassium, penicillin V, aspirin, and gargles.
8. 12–24–76: Itching rash for 24 hours. Throat better. Penicillin discontinued. Rash clear the following day.
9. January 6, 1977: Feels like a different person, not depressed, "more relaxed to think," has gained 9 lb., all itching is gone, no palpitations, all muscle and jaw pain has cleared.
Physical exam: Pulse 80, weight 145 lb., muscles and TMJ are no longer tender. Patient is able to keep her mouth wide open without discomfort.

Comment: Although this patient had no enzyme changes and had normal CPK, aldolase, and LDH levels, her symptoms clearly suggested myopathic Graves' disease. The symptoms of temporomandibular joint involvement were unequivocal, as was the remission of this syndrome with the treatment of her Graves' disease.

Hypothyroidism

This disease results from a reduced secretion of thyroxine and triiodothyronine by the thyroid gland. Serum hormone levels are usually low. Primary failure of the thyroid gland is associated with a compensatory elevation of the pituitary thyroid stimulating hormone, and patients have been recognized in whom the elevation of the serum thyroid stimulating hormone (TSH) level may be the only direct laboratory measurement that suggests hypothyroidism. When thyroid failure is secondary to inadequacy of pituitary function the TSH concentration will be in a low or normal range.

The disorder may be manifested clinically by moderate weight gain, dryness of the skin, hair, and fingernails, intolerance to cold, fluid retention, puffiness and non-pitting edema of the face, eyelids, extremities and tongue, hoarseness, constipation, menstrual disorders, depression, fatigue, and need for an excessive amount of sleep. The extreme form of this condition is called myxedema because of the mucinous edema which accumulates in body tissues. Its congenital form may be associated with mental retardation. Patients may develop psychosis, called myxedema madness, and coma. Pain, stiffness, and tenderness of muscles in hypothyroidism were recognized by Ord as early as 1884.[26]

Gross abnormality in muscle appearance and structure has been described in the *Kocher-Debré-Semelaigne syndrome,*[27] which is characterized by a diffuse muscular hypertrophy, causing an athletic appearance in hypothyroid children. The muscles are stiff, weak, and slow, resulting in impaired motor activity. Najjar studied muscle biopsy specimens from these patients and could detect only quantitative increase in muscle fibers rather than qualitative changes.[28]* The muscle disorder is reversible by thyroid therapy. The syndrome is a rarity and its manifestations differ from those seen in hypothyroid myopathy.

Myopathy is probably experienced by all hypothyroid patients to some degree. It is manifested by weakness, cramps, and aching and tender muscles. Hypothyroidism is frequently overlooked in the diagnosis of patients presenting with generalized muscle symptoms. It is important to evaluate all such patients for hypothyroidism, which may be mild and occasionally difficult to diagnose. Nocturnal calf pain may be a symptom. Golding has described aggravation of pain by phenylbutazone, which he attributes to its antithyroid effect and peripheral antagonism of thyroxine.[31]

Myotonia, manifested by slow contraction and relaxation of muscles, is a sign that had been found to be diagnostically useful as early as 1924.[32] The response has been recorded by a galvanometric technique in a test called the *fotomotogram.* Although it provides a basis for understanding muscle pain and spasm, which may occur in hypothyroid patients, it is an unreliable test for hypothyroidism.[33]

Histological examinations of muscles in hypothyroid myopathy do not yield consistent results. Needle biopsies by McKeran and co-workers revealed only atrophy and loss of Type II muscle fibers.[34] Ahuja described eventual replacement of muscle cells by fat cells with restoration of normal structure as triiodothyronine was administered.[35] Astrom and co-workers have described a variation of fiber size, loss of striation, amorphous sarcolemmal material, hyalinization, vacuolar degeneration, round cell infiltration, and foamy PAS-staining material.[36] Increase of hyaluronic acid in muscle and collagen structures has been attributed to decreased degradation and excessive fibroblastic synthesis due to increased thyroid stimulating hormone.[37] Glycogen accumulation and mitochondrial deformation occur.[38]

---

*Ingwall and co-workers[29] demonstrated that creatine increases myosin heavy chain synthesis in muscle cultures, presumably due to its action as a genetic inducer of DNA activity. The increased creatine content in myxedematous muscle demonstrated by Shorr and associates[30] would fit with the above observation as a possible explanation for muscle hypertrophy in this disorder.

Chemical abnormality in hypothyroid myopathy was first described by Shorr and his group, who in 1935 reported the appearance of large amounts of creatine in the urine of hypothyroid patients treated with thyroid hormone.[30] They also demonstrated a spontaneous creatinuria in hypothyroid patients with muscular pain indicative of a more severe form of hypothyroid myopathy. This same effect was confirmed by Ahuja in his report of patients with fatty infiltration of muscle cells in hypothyroidism.[35]

Muscle 1–4 glucosidase, the acid maltase found to be deficient in glycogen storage disease type II (Pompe's disease),[39] is also low in hypothyroid myopathy[40] and increases within six months of thyroxine treatment.

Electromyography showed abnormalities in hypothyroid musculature in studies by Salick and co-workers.[41] They mentioned a proximal type of limb muscle weakness that responded satisfactorily to thyroid medication in hypothyroidism.

Neurological abnormalities may occur and include the carpal tunnel syndrome,[42] which probably results from myxedematous accumulation in the confined canal through which the median nerve passes to the hand. This is manifested by palmar numbness, weakness in the hand, and a positive *Tinel sign,* a shocklike sensation in the palm when the median nerve is percussed with a hammer in the region of the carpal tunnel. Nerve conduction times are slowed, especially those involving motor conduction.

Arthritic complaints in hypothyroidism have been described by several authors.[43, 44] Detailed clinical and pathological study of 12 patients by Dorwart and Schumacher[45] revealed synovial effusion in eight patients. Seven of these effusions were extremely viscous, and six contained calcium pyrophosphate crystals. Flexor tendon sheath thickening, joint laxity, and popliteal cysts were noted, but only two of the patients had proximal myopathy. X-ray study revealed chondrocalcinosis in seven of the patients, and needle biopsy showed a thickened synovium with mild inflammation. Loose bodies and narrowed joint spaces were observed in several of the patients. The joint effusions were absorbed with thyroid hormone therapy.

Newcombe and co-workers[37] demonstrated a direct effect of the pituitary thyroid-stimulating hormone (TSH) on synovial membrane adenyl cyclase. Recognizing that TSH is characteristically elevated in primary hypothyroidism, Dorwart and Schumacher suggested a direct role of TSH in the production of synovial effusion in hypothyroidism.

It seems clear that a careful evaluation for hypothyroidism should be undertaken in patients presenting with otherwise unexplained joint abnormality involving any articulation, including the temporomandibular joint. The following case reports are the first to illustrate this relationship.

Cretinism

Case 3: A 42-year-old, single, white male, New York Hospital clinic patient.

1. Hypothyroid at birth.
2. Parents refused to administer desiccated thyroid extract since he was better behaved when thyroid was not administered.
3. Physical findings best presented by Figure 6–2.
4. Patient's speech garbled, in part because of mental retardation, in part because of tightness of the muscles around the jaws. Despite this patient's excellent muscular development his movements were slow, uncoordinated, and weak.

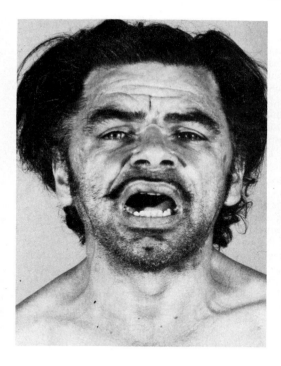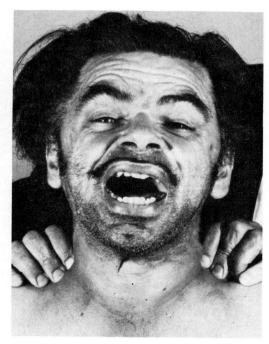

Figures 6–2 and 6–3. Spasm around TMJ in untreated patient with cretinism partially relieved by massage of trapezius muscle.

5. The restricted mouth opening could be improved by massage of the trapezius muscles (Figs. 6–2, 6–3).

Comment: This unfortunate young man's mental retardation may or may not have been benefited by early and steady use of thyroid replacement. He is presented as an example of the effects of muscular hypertrophy in hypothyroidism on movement of the temporomandibular joint. Figure 6–3 reveals that proper massage of the muscles of the neck can relax these muscles in part. He certainly is no candidate for temporomandibular therapy now.

Hypothyroidism of Acute Onset Following RAI Therapy for Thyrotoxicosis

Case 4: 60-year-old married, white female commercial artist.*
1. Two years: mild diabetes.
2. One month: enlargement of thyroid, 4 lb. weight loss, mild heat intolerance. Referring physician noted increased thyroxine by radioimmunoassay 18.8 μg./dl., T3 uptake 42.3 per cent (normal range, 25–33 per cent). RAI uptake, elevated to 52.6 per cent. Cholesterol, 186 mg./dl.
3. In July, 1976, patient was first seen by Dr. Park, who noted a weight of 101 lb., height 62 inches, blood pressure 150/80, pulse 80, thyroid was about two times enlarged. The speech was rapid at that time. Dr. Park felt that the patient showed evidence of thyrotoxicosis.

*This case is from the records of Dr. Benjamin Park, who kindly has permitted its publication in this series.

4. Confirmed by studies at the New York Hospital, which revealed a radioactive iodine uptake of 82 per cent, CR 67 per cent, T4 by radioimmunoassay was 22.8 µg./dl., T3 by radioimmunoassay 450 ng./ml. (upper limits of normal 170 ng./dl.), resin was 58 per cent.

5. On August 18, 1976, the patient was given a therapeutic dose of 3.32 mCi of radioactive iodine which was calculated to give a dose of 7000 rad to an estimated 35 g. thyroid gland.

6. October, 1976. The patient reported that she was feeling well. Weight 103 lb. Gland was smaller. Pulse 84. T4 by radioimmunoassay is still elevated 15.2 µg./dl. However, the T3 uptake was now in normal range, 39 per cent.

7. November 24, 1976: The paient's T4 was 3.9 µg./dl., which was borderline low for the New York Hospital laboratory. The TSH was greater than 100. T3 by radioimmunoassay was low, 45 ng./ml. RAI uptake was 1 per cent.

8. On December 3, 1976: Weight was increased slightly to 104.5, pulse 70, the thyroid was small, and it was Dr. Park's impression that the patient was showing early manifestations of hypothyroidism.

9. On January 13, 1977, the patient reported that she was tired, lacked energy and interest, was cold; she complained of dry skin, constipation, loss of appetite, and could not open her mouth well. Attempts to do so produced pain in the jaws. Physical examination revealed a weight of 112 lb., pulse 64, eyes were puffy, voice was low, she had tenderness on compression and palpation of the muscles around the temporomandibular joint as well as in the neck muscles. Neurological examination revealed delayed relaxation of the deep tendon reflexes. Impression: severe hypothyroidism.

10. The patient was begun at that time on sodium levothyroxine, 0.05 mg. daily for one week, increasing to 0.1 mg. thereafter.

11. On January 27, 1977, the patient stated that she was feeling considerably improved. Dr. Park described her state as revealing a world of difference. She was not as tired, had more pep, was thinking more clearly, not as cold, eyes were less puffy, she showed more interest. Her voice had returned to normal. There was still some stiffness about the neck and temporomandibular joint but this was strikingly diminished. Physical examination reveleaed the weight to be 112 lb., pulse 70, puffiness of the eyes and dryness of the skin was partly improved. At this time the patient was advised to increase the dose of sodium levothyroxine to 0.15 mg. daily for a week and then go to a maintenance dose of 0.2 mg. daily.

12. August 31, 1982. Patient reported to be in complete remission of hyperthryoidism and TMJ syndrome.

Comment: This beautifully documented case of Dr. Park clearly demonstrates the acute onset of temporomandibular joint syndrome in association with severe hypothyroidism after induction by RAI therapy. The rapid remission of the temporomandibular joint symptoms with treatment probably reflects the fact that the condition was treated after a relatively short duration of hypothyroidism. Chronically hypothyroid patients may not experience muscular and temporomandibular joint improvement for months after initiation of therapy. Indeed, some patients actually show a temporary exacerbation of pain, as chronically established hypothyroidism is corrected with thyroid replacement. I have observed four patients in my own practice who experienced increased myalgia on initiation of therapy. Two of these patients ultimately got over the muscle pain and their hypothyroidism could be completely corrected with an adequate replacement dose of thyroid. Unfortunately, two patients refused to go on with therapy and would not return for follow-up.

MENSTRUAL DISORDERS

Menopause

Upon entering the menopause many women experience pain and stiffness of joints and muscles with other manifestations of estrogenic deficiency, including hot flashes, sweats, tingling, headaches, vertigo, depression, inability to cope with responsibilities, loss of libido, vaginitis, cystitis, and dyspareunia. Osteoporosis is a common cause of back and neck pain during and after the onset of the female climacteric.[46, 47]

Studies by European workers have been discussed in the introductory paragraphs to this chapter.

Primary Amenorrhea

A physiological state of estrogenic deficiency exists in girls prior to the normal onset of puberty, which occurs approximately between the ages of 9 and 16. Lack of onset of menses following the sixteenth birthday warrants a diagnosis of primary amenorrhea and may be associated with high, normal, or low estrogenic levels, or with abnormally high androgen levels.

Primary and secondary estrogenic deficiency may produce, in the young adult, myofascial pain similar to that observed in the menopause.

Secondary Amenorrhea

Secondary amenorrhea is the arrest of menstruation following onset of function. The most common causes of secondary amenorrhea are pregnancy and menopause. It may be classified, like primary amenorrhea, according to high, normal, or low estrogenic function or elevated androgenic levels.

Secondary amenorrhea with decreased estrogenic function may occur in a premature menopause, surgical or radiological castration, ovarian tumors such as luteomas, abnormalities of the hypothalamic-pituitary system such as pituitary tumors, psychogenic trauma, malnutrition, anorexia nervosa, chronic debilitating disease, after prolonged use of birth control pills, with certain tranquilizers, or with elevated prolactin levels.

Malfunction of other endocrine glands, including adrenal hyperfunction, hypo- and hyperthyroidism, and pituitary malfunctions, may produce ovarian insufficiency.

As in primary amenorrheas, the classification of high, normal, and low estrogen causes of amenorrhea is especially pertinent to the discussion of muscle syndromes. The estrogen deficiency states are associated with muscle and joint dysfunction.

Shorr's Classification of Menstrual Disorders

A simple diagnostic technique for the detection of estrogenic deficiency states is the examination of stained vaginal smears devised by Shorr and his co-workers.[48, 49] They described four categories based on ovarian function as measured by sequential vaginal smears. These included atrophic smears with total absence of estrogenic function, hypofunctional anovulatory smears indicating low ovarian follicular function without ovulation, normal estrus type smears, and finally hyperfunctional ovarian bleeding manifested by high estrogen levels in the smears obtained sequentially throughout the month. This classification based on estrogen levels as determined in the vaginal smears is especially pertinent to a discussion of motor dysfunction which predominates in the atrophic and hypofunctional categories.

Atrophic smears are universally associated with amenorrhea. The *hypofunctional patient* may present with any menstrual pattern, including amenorrhea, infrequent menstrual periods, frequent but irregular menstrual periods, or heavy and frequent bleeding. These women with low estrogen function, however, may be subject to muscle syndromes regardless of their menstrual pattern.

Premenstrual Tension

Many women experiences at various stages of the menstrual cycle a variety of symptoms including tension, nervousness, depression, fluid retention, increased bruising, headaches, and muscle spasm. Depending on when these symptoms occur in the cycle, the endocrinologist may take various therapeutic measures to prevent them. When they occur just before, during, or after menstruation, it is reasonable to infer that they are associated with a physiological drop in estrogen levels. Relief may be obtained by administering estrogens for 21 days monthly, along with a progestin for seven to ten days at the end of the cycle. Withdrawal two days before the anticipated menstrual period usually results in vaginal bleeding at the correct time of the month. Other women experience symptoms from the mid-cycle immediately after ovulation until the onset of menstruation. These patients may be intolerant to progesterone produced by the corpus luteum after ovulation. An effort to prevent ovulation in such patients with higher doses of estrogen, from the fifth to the twenty-sixth days of the cycle and a progestin in the last seven to ten days of estrogen, may produce relief from the symptoms occurring in the last half of the cycle. One such TMJ patient who had a striking response to such a regimen is reported below.

Estrogen Therapy in a Female With Premenstrual Temporomandibular Joint Pain

Case 5: A 31-year-old single, white female, schoolteacher.

1. Chief complaint: Pain in the right side of the face premenstrually, 19 years.

2. Pain is relieved by TMJ therapy for two weeks, recurring prior to menstruation. Simultaneous pains in back. Menses normal every four weeks.

3. Neurological and ENT work-up at Montefiore Hospital Headache clinic revealed no abnormalities.

4. Physical examination: Build: asthenic. Weight 85 lb. Height: 65 inches. Blood pressure: 100/70. All other physical findings unremarkable.

5. Laboratory findings: All normal.

6. Therapy: Conjugated estrogens, 2.5 mg. daily for 21 days starting on the 5th day of menstrual cycle, norethindrone acetate with last five days of estrogens.

7. Pain cleared with first monthly cycle on estrogen. However it recurred when she started the five day course of the progestin.

8. Progestin changed to dydrogesterone, 10 mg. daily with last 5 days of estrogen. This resulted in remission of pain during the progestin course. Patient complains of discomfort only during the period when she is off all hormonal therapy.

9. Impression: Temporomandibular joint syndrome associated with muscle spasm, secondary to premenstrual tension associated with monthly drop in estrogen levels.

10. At 14th month of therapy patient states: "TMJ result sort of a miracle." Dr. Gelb states: "This was a basket case prior to her starting cyclical hormonal therapy."

11. 26 months post-initiation of therapy: Dismissed from dental care, bite plates removed, occasional charleyhorses, "too busy to notice anything."

Comment: This was a dramatic response to estrogen therapy. As noted in the foregoing section on hormonal mechanisms in producing and relieving muscle pain, we have no idea what the mechanism of pain and spasm is in estrogen deficiency states.

TESTOSTERONE DEFICIENCY

Papanicolaou and Falk[50] described general muscle hypertrophy induced by androgenic hormones almost 45 years ago. The reader may be intrigued by the fact that the effect was first noted in the temporal muscle of the male guinea pig. Pellegrino[51] has demonstrated that testosterone administered to rats causes, within hours, an increased penetration of glucose into muscle, hexose phosphorylation, and glycogen formation in the levator ani muscles. Carter, Cohen, and Shorr[52, 53] have demonstrated testosterone preparations to be a useful adjunct to estrogen hormone therapy of menopausal women. Testosterone can block the protein catabolic effects of thyrotoxicosis[54] and hyperadrenalcorticism[55] but requires insulin to stimulate muscle growth.[56] It is a potent stimulator of protein synthesis.[57] It is clear from clinical observations that testosterone may have a profound effect on muscle development. Hypogonadal males, cryptorchid males, and eunuchs characteristically experience reduced muscle strength and mass, which is reversible by testosterone treatment. Children of both sexes with hyperandrogenic syndromes are strong and muscular. Balance studies in hypogonadal patients have revealed a marked increase in nitrogen balance under the influence of testosterone therapy. Anabolic agents, developed to enhance nitrogen balance, increase muscle mass and weight loss in debilitated patients, and are derivatives of testosterone which retain its anabolic properties while eliminating most of its secondary sex stimulating effects.[58]

Aging men frequently experience a gradual drop in testosterone levels, which, however, usually remain within normal male range. Testosterone can be clinically useful in treating aging males who experience muscle weakness, pain, and spasm, especially if these are associated with evidence of marked fall in plasma total or free testosterone levels.

The infrequency with which temporomandibular joint symptoms occur in males raises the question whether testosterone plays some protective role in this disorder.

ADRENAL DISORDERS

Adrenal Insufficiency

The adrenal glands may fail as a result of inadequate pituitary ACTH stimulation or from primary damage (Addison's disease).

ADDISON'S DISEASE. The untreated state is manifested by weakness, hyperpigmentation of the skin and mucous membranes, weight loss, dehydration, low blood pressure, especially in the upright position, fall in blood sugar, occasionally resulting in coma, fall in serum sodium levels, frequently associated with salt craving, elevation of serum potassium levels associated with muscle weakness and spasm, depression, and mood changes that include apathy, negativism, and psychosis. Laboratory confirmation of the diagnosis is obtained by the demonstration of low plasma cortisol and aldosterone levels and low urinary 17-hydroxysteroid levels which cannot be stimulated by ACTH administration. Affected patients are remarkably intolerant to stress from various sources, including acute infections, salt deprivation, heavy sweating, blood loss, and acute pain. Simple procedures such as the withdrawal of 100 ml. of blood for diagnostic purposes, administration of a foreign polypeptide such as ACTH (which cannot produce an elevation of plasma cortisol from a nonexistent adrenal gland), or the administration of a cathartic for routine radiographic preparation may throw the patient into acute crisis, resulting in shock and death if mineralocorticoids and/or glucocorticoids are not administered promptly along with salt and intravenous fluids. During the acute crisis, these patients often develop severe muscular cramps and spasm, probably related to water and electrolyte disturbances.

Prior to the advent of cortisol therapy, several workers observed chronic contractures in the legs of chronically ill addisonian patients. Adams[14] mentions patients of his own and descriptions by Thorn.[59] In autopsied cases the muscle fibers seemed normal, and Thorn postulated an abnormality of sodium in the tendons as a cause of the contractures.

Cushing's Syndrome and Steroid Myopathy

Cushing mentioned muscular weakness and wasting in his earliest descriptions of the disease which bears his name.[60] The disease results from an ACTH-secreting tumor in the pituitary which stimulates the adrenals to produce excessive amounts of cortisol, usually in association with diffuse or adenomatous hyperplasia. An identical clinical picture may result from one or more autonomous nodules in the adrenal cortex which secrete excessive cortisol independent of hypothalamic-pituitary control. Patients characteristically gain weight owing to increased centripetal body fat, but they lose muscle mass. The extremities become thin, the skin may become stretched, and purplish striae may appear on the trunk and extremities. The face becomes rounded, pimply, and hairy. Hair on the head thins, and the extremities become thin and tapering. Patients often develop hypertension, diabetes, and bony demineralization which may lead to back pain and ultimately spinal fracture and hemiplegia. Hypokalemia, polycythemia and mood and mental changes are common. The patients usually complain of muscle weakness. Elevations of plasma cortisol with loss of the normal rhythmic daily 8:00 A.M. peak and 4:00 P.M. drop are diagnostic. Conventional histological muscle biopsies in these patients do not reveal characteristic abnormalities. However, electron microscopic studies have revealed striking changes in the mitochondria, which are haphazardly scattered, large, convoluted, and bizarre in appearance. Abnormalities have been noted in sarcolemma, nuclei, capillary basement membranes, and sarcoplasm. Glycogen deposition has been noted in the muscle cells.[61, 62] Lysosomal-like bodies have been reported in the sarcoplasm.

Nelson's Syndrome

Following bilateral adrenalectomy for Cushing's disease, occasional patients develop hyperpigmentation of the skin, increased ACTH production, and pituitary enlargement. Myopathy has been described in this syndrome by Prineas and co-workers.[63] It is characterized by proximal limb weakness and lipid droplets in Type I muscle fibers beneath the sarcolemma and in association with the mitochondria. The cause of this myopathy is not clear. It might be due to increased levels of β-lipotropin, a polypeptide formed in the pituitary that appears to be a precursor of ACTH and beta melanophore stimulating hormone. All of these substances are elevated in the blood of patients with Nelson's syndrome.

Primary Hyperaldosteronism

This syndrome occurs in patients with adrenal adenomas or hyperplasia. It is manifested by periodic paralysis and muscle spasm, hypertension, paresthesias, tetany, excessive thirst, and polyuria.[64] Loss of body potassium is associated with a marked increase of muscle sodium and urinary aldosterone during acute attacks. Attacks of weakness can be produced by glucose and insulin administration, a standard method of lowering potassium by sequestration into muscle and liver glycogen. Balance studies during this maneuver have revealed that the potassium loss and weakness were preceded by sodium retention and increased aldosterone production. Muscle function returned during sodium diuresis while potassium levels were still low. Paralysis could not be induced during low sodium intake.[65] When unprovoked hypokalemia is observed in hypertensive patients, primary hyperaldosteronism should be sought and can be demonstrated under standard conditions by low plasma renin levels and high aldosterone production and excretion. Hypokalemia alone is a common cause of muscle weakness and spasm.

17 α-Hydroxylase Defect

This congenital defect in adrenal hormone synthesis results in male pseudohermaphroditism, sexual infantilism, hypertension, and hypokalemic alkalosis. A case with hypokalemic myopathy has been reported.[66]

PRIMARY PITUITARY AND HYPOTHALAMIC DISORDERS

The pituitary gland, a small, rounded structure measuring about 10 mm. in diameter, lies in a bony fossa at the base of the mid-brain in the center of the sphenoid bone. The gland is made up of two separate glandular structures.

The neurohypophysis, or *posterior pituitary,* is a projection from the brain which secretes two hormones: *vasopressin,* an antidiuretic that causes reabsorption of water by the kidney, and *oxytocin,* which initiates uterine contractions in labor, stimulates milk flow, and is weakly antidiuretic. Inadequate secretion of vasopressin results in diabetes insipidus characterized by the secretion of large volumes of dilute urine and excessive thirst. Occasionally, excessive antidiuretic hormone secretion gives rise to increased water retention and hyponatremia with clinical water intoxication. The conditions are of interest in a discussion of muscle disturbance, since muscle weakness, cramps, and spasm can be associated with changes in tissue osmolarity.

The *anterior pituitary* secretes a number of stimulating hormones including follicle-stimulating hormone (FSH), which is responsible for ovarian follicle development in the female and spermatogenesis in the male. Luteinizing hormone (LH), otherwise known as interstitial cell-stimulating hormone, stimulates the development of the corpus luteum following ovulation in the female and the androgenic-producing Leydig cells in the testis. Prolactin is a stimulator of the breast and milk production and inhibitor of ovulation. Thyroid-stimulating hormone (TSH) and adrenocorticotrophic hormone (ACTH) are also produced. The anterior pituitary secretes at least two additional hormones, somatotrophin (GH), or growth hormone, and melanophore-stimulating hormone (MSH).

The adenohypophysis is under control of the *hypothalamus* at the base of the brain, which secretes a number of simple polypeptide releasing and inhibiting factors, including agents that cause release of corticotrophin, growth hormone, thyrotropin, prolactin, FSH, LH, and MSH. Three inhibiting factors have been recognized, including somatostatin, or growth hormone-inhibiting factor, prolactin-inhibiting factor, and melanocyte-stimulating hormone release inhibiting factor.

Acromegaly is a disease resulting from a pituitary tumor, often an eosinophilic adenoma, which secretes excessive prolactin and/or growth hormone. Patients affected by this condition are easily recognized in most cases because of striking physical changes. If the tumor appears prior to cessation of growth, the patient becomes a giant. After cessation of growth, a number of physical changes occur, including prognathism and enlargement of soft tissues and cartilaginous structures, resulting in a large nose and broad features. The skin often becomes thickened, and the facial creases increase in depth. The sinuses become enlarged with a resulting protruding brow. The patient may develop osteoporosis and rounding of the back. X-ray films of bones of the hands may reveal increased growth of the tufts of the tips of the fingers and an increase in the size of the sesamoid bones. The hands and feet gradually increase in size, resulting in an increasing glove and shoe size. Patients frequently develop visceromegaly, including enlargement of the heart and thyroid gland. About 35 per cent of patients become diabetic. Early in the course of the disease the muscles may become hypertrophied and muscular strength is often increased.[67] In the later stage of the disease the muscles become weak. Diagnosis of the condition can be confirmed by the demonstration of an enlarged sella turcica in about 80 per cent of patients. The ultimate diagnosis depends on the demonstration of increased growth hormone levels in the blood, either in spontaneous fasting samples or after a variety of provocative and suppressive tests.

Mastaglia and co-workers[68] demonstrated a patchy myopathy in the proximal muscles of acromegalic patients. This was confirmed by Picket and his co-workers.[69] Many patients had elevated CPK values and EMG changes. Similar studies by Lundberg and Osterman[70] failed to show these changes.

Ultramicroscopic studies have been inconsistent. Stern and co-workers[71] found little abnormality, whereas Cheah and associates[72] described mitochondrial abnormalities and demonstrated diminished muscle mass, which was related to a diminished DNA replication reversible by growth hormone administration.[73]

Of considerable interest to the dental surgeon is a report by Sudaka and Lespine[5] on patients with pituitary abnormalities and enlarged sella turcica who showed abnormalities of the temporomandibular joint attributed to both mechanical and secretory effects. It is surprising that the bite abnormalities resulting from the skeletal distortion of the jaw of acromegalic subjects does not cause TMJ complaints more frequently.

Pituitary insufficiency may produce any of the muscle problems previously mentioned by virtue of failure of the target organs, including gonads, thyroid, and adrenal glands. Failure of growth hormone may have direct effects on muscles, as mentioned previously. Flexor muscle spasm has been described in hypopituitarism with "little" evidence of hypothyroidism.[74] In our own experience muscle spasm can occur with minimal hypothyroidism, which does not seem to be ruled out in the above patients. The condition was associated with low blood sugar and sodium in one patient and was relieved by cortisone therapy, suggesting that the problem was caused by secondary adrenal insufficiency, another potential cause of muscle pain and spasm.

Muscle creatine was shown to be affected by pituitary dysfunction.[75] This may be secondary to hypothyroidism.

PARATHYROID DYSFUNCTION AND OSTEOMALACIA

Hyperparathyroidism Versus Osteomalacia

The disordered calcium metabolism of hyperparathyroidism may cause weakness of muscles, atrophy, fatigability, pain, and tenderness in muscle and bone[76, 77] In the first reported case of hyperfunction of the parathyroid bodies, Dubois, Shorr, and co-workers[78] described motor symptoms which could have been related to the osteitis fibrosa cystica present in the patient. Subsequently, workers described the presence of bone tenderness.[79] Vicale[80] described the muscle syndrome in a case of renal tubular acidosis, osteomalacia, and hyperparathyroidism. It is not clear from the early reports whether the muscle problems were related to abnormalities of calcium, phosphorus, or bone. Prineas and co-workers[81] described proximal muscle weakness in one patient with osteomalacia secondary to malabsorption, steatorrhea, and secondary hyperparathyroidism, with a low serum phosphorus, normal serum calcium, and elevated ionized calcium, and in another patient with primary hyperparathyroidism and osteomalacia. They likened the muscle syndrome to that seen in vitamin D–resistant rickets and renal osteodystrophy. They felt that the syndrome was not related to blood calcium elevation, a view shared by Smith and Stern,[82] who noted myopathy in only six of their 91 patients with primary hyperparathyroidism, but in 20 of 45 patients with osteomalacia who had no elevation of the serum calcium.

Landau and Kappas described muscle and bone wasting in a patient with parathyroid carcinoma.[83] They attributed the myopathy, which could be reversed by anabolic therapy with estrogens and testosterone, to a catabolic effect of parathormone on muscle similar to its effect on bone. This theory has never been developed further or confirmed. Richardson and co-workers described necrotizing lesions of skin and muscle in a hyperparathyroid patient with uremia. The lesions were attributed to ischemia resulting from calcification of blood vessels.[84]

Frame and associates[76] described several cases of myopathy in a series of patients with primary hyperparathyroidism, and attributed the malfunction to hypercalcemia. This idea received strong confirmation from Lemann and Donatelli,[85] who demonstrated severe weakness in patients with acute hypercalcemic parathyroid crisis. Henson[86] recorded muscle weakness as a presenting symptom in five and as a secondary symptom in six of 34 patients with primary hyperparathyroidism. Cure of the myopathy has been reported following surgical removal of an abnormal parathyroid tumor.[87]

Henson[88] has proposed the obvious explanation that a similar muscle syndrome results from different biochemical abnormalities in osteomalacia and hypercalcemia. He feels that the myopathy in osteomalacia may be a result of defective vitamin D metabolism and that severe hypercalcemia from a variety of causes, including severe hyperparathyroidism, may be an occasional but less frequent cause of a similar type of myopathy. Rasmussen[89] has suggested that the hypophosphatemia of osteomalacia is a most likely cause of weakness in this condition. The importance of high-energy phosphate as a fuel for muscle contraction has been recognized for many years. Rall and coworkers have demonstrated that all the energy required for muscle contraction can be accounted for by the breakdown of ATP and creatine phosphate.[90]

Osteomalacia may cause muscle cramps and rapid tendon reflexes. When the condition is suspected, the patient should have blood examinations of serum calcium, phosphorus, proteins, alkaline phosphatase, and bone x-rays to determine radiographic signs of osteomalacia. Occasionally bone biopsy is necessary to detect the widened osteoid seams of osteomalacia. Renal tubular acidosis should be sought by determining the patient's ability to secrete an oral acid load.

Hyperparathyroidism can be diagnosed by obtaining, in addition to the above studies, a measurement of the parathyroid hormone level from a competent laboratory.

Hyperparathyroidism: Case Report

Case 6: A 64-year-old widowed, white female, unemployed.

1. October 9, 1973. Chief complaint: Pains all over the body, especially ribs, back, shoulders, and temporomandibular joint region. Has to hold rail while walking downstairs. Duration 1½ years.

2. First developed headaches four years previously after dental extraction.

3. Visits to 15 different physicians recorded in patient's medical history. Patient is extremely critical of the care she received from most of the previous physicians. Forty years previously had thyroidectomy for hyperthyroidism with relapse. Had to receive X-irradiation to the neck to produce remission.

4. Received therapy with thyroid replacement until one year prior to this visit.

5. Past history: Rib fractures, 5–19–70 and 8–26–71.

6. Physical examination: X-ray dermatitis of neck. Thyroidectomy scar. Small thyroid nodule on right side of trachea. Laboratory values: SMA-12 revealed serum calcium level, 13.4 mg./d. (normal range, 8.5 to 10.5 mg./dl.); serum phosphorus, 2.7 mg./dl. (normal range, 2.5 to 4.5 mg./dl.); alkaline

phosphatase, 95 microunits/ml. (normal range, 25 to 85 microunits/ml). Repeat determinations of serum calcium: 11.4 and 12.2 mg./dl. Repeat serum phosphorus determinations, 2.2 mg./dl. Thyroxine level was normal, 5.5 μg./dl. Blood specimens examined at Mayo Clinic revealed serum calcium concentration to be 12 mg.dl.; phosphorus, 2.0 mg./dl.; magnesium, 2.3 mg./dl.; parathormone, 78 mg./dl., indicating an elevated parathormone level diagnostic of hyperparathyroidism.

7. Patient did not return. Sought the opinion of another endocrinologist. No further follow-up.

Comment: The clinical history of generalized bone pain, rib fractures, and associated temporomandibular joint symptoms occurring within the period that other body pains appeared could be explained by the laboratory findings of hyperparathyroidism with bone disease, manifested by consistently high serum calcium, low serum phosphorus, and elevated alkaline phosphatase and serum parathormone levels. This patient's highly suspicious and negativistic behavior was consistent with the mental disturbance that occasionally occurs with hyperparathyroidism. Unfortunately we have not had an opportunity to determine whether or not treatment would affect her bone and temporomandibular joint symptoms.

Hypoparathyroidism

Hypoparathyroidism is characterized by low levels of serum and urinary calcium and elevated serum and urinary phosphorus levels, which occur in the absence of renal disease, and is correctible by the administration of parathyroid hormone or vitamin D. Blood parathyroid hormone levels determined by radioimmunoassay are low. Most cases follow surgical removal of the parathyroid gland during thyroidectomy. Rarely, the disease is familial or of undetermined cause. Clinically, about 70 per cent of patients experience tetany, which may appear as facial muscle spasm, carpopedal spasm, numbness, and tingling, all of which may be aggravated by tissue akalosis, which reduced ionized calcium even further. *Trousseau's sign* is the appearance of rigid contracture of the fingers into the obstetrical position when the arterial blood supply is cut off for up to three minutes by an inflated pressure cuff on the arm. Increased neuromuscular irritability may be demonstrated by twitching of the face, eyelids, and mouth when the various branches of the facial nerve are tapped with a neurological hammer at their point of emergence from the facial area just anterior to the temporomandibular joint, *(Chvostek's sign)*. Patients may display varying degrees and forms of emotional disturbance and dementia. Muscle weakness, fatigue, palpitations, dysesthesias, as well as neural and psychiatric disorders may occur even years before the diagnosis is made. Laboratory examination may reveal calcifications of basal ganglia of the brain or in the cerebellum. The dental roots in the juvenile form of the disease are commonly hypoplastic. Coarse, scaling skin, monilial infections, pigmentation, thinning of the hair of the head and genital organs, and fingernail abnormalities and cataracts may occur.

Myopathy in this condition was described by Gomez and co-workers.[91] Other organs, including the brain, retina, and peripheral nerve, were involved. The mechanism for tissue involvement has not been explained. One other case of hypoparathyroid myopathy with elevated serum levels of CPK corrected by elevation of the serum calcium level with vitamin D therapy has been reported.[92] Wolf and co-workers have reported hypocalcemic myopathy.[95]

Pseudohypoparathyroidism

This rare and X-linked dominant hereditary disorder is characterized by clinical and chemical abnormalities resembling those of hypoparathyroidism but is not correctible by parathyroid hormone administration, since it appears to be caused by a renal tubular receptor defect to parathyroid hormone, and the blood parathyroid hormone level is commonly high. Patients characteristically show a short stature, round facies, strabismus, short digits, metacarpals, and metatarsals, and, frequently, mental retardation.

Subcutaneous calcifications are common in this disorder, and a single case of temporomandibular joint ankylosis has been described.[94]

MYOPATHY IN DISORDERS OF CARBOHYDRATE METABOLISM

Diabetes Mellitus

Diabetic amyotrophy, myopathy due to diabetes mellitus, was first mentioned in 1955 by Garland, who described patients with proximal muscle pain and weakness, fiber atrophy, and proliferation of sarcolemmal nuclei. Gregerson[96] suggested that the disease was, in fact, a manifestation of diabetic neuropathy, since most of his patients had sensory symptoms and did not show the purely motor syndrome described by Garland. Schwartz,[97] in his editorial comments in the 1970 Yearbook of Endocrinology, pointed out that Gregerson's inability to find cases with this pure syndrome did not negate Garland's observations.

Further support for the existence of myopathy is found in studies by Locke and others, who described bilateral symmetrical proximal weakness of the lower extremities associated with anterior thigh pain, muscle wasting, fasciculations, weight loss, and occasional involvement of the right upper extremities, which was self-limiting and frequently followed by improvement or recovery over a period of months to years.[98] Muscle biopsies showed atrophy of scattered muscle fibers, rounded and hyperchromatic nuclei which often clustered, and arteriolar sclerosis in about one fourth of the patients. Changes were unlike those seen in nerve fiber or anterior horn disease. Similar observations are reported by Gårde and Kugelberg[99] and by Bischoff and Esslen.[77] Bloodworth and Epstein[100] performed electron microscopic studies on a series of patients and described thickening of the capillary basement membranes, which was, however, not confined to myopathic areas and therefore was not felt to be causally related.

An association between glucose intolerance and TMJ syndrome has been reported.[101]

Insulin-Induced Hypoglycemia

High plasma insulin levels are produced by benign and malignant islet cell adenomas, rarely by islet cell hyperplasia of the pancreas. In 1939

Tannenberg[102] described pathological changes in the heart and skeletal muscles of rabbits caused by shock doses of insulin. The muscle cells were necrotic, contained infiltrations of polymorphs, lymphocytes, and macrophages, and showed evidence of regeneration of sarcolemmal nuclei.

Subsequently, Ziegler[103] demonstrated evidence of weakness in the hands of two of 22 patients treated with insulin shock therapy. These changes were probably of neurological origin, since 13 of his patients also had paresthesias. A later report by Mulder and co-workers[104] described studies of 20 patients with functioning insulinomas who developed paresthesias, muscle atrophy, slapping gait, twitching, and EMG evidence of reduced motor units. Biopsy in one of these patients showed relatively normal muscles in the gastrocnemius. Levratte and Brette,[105] on the other hand, reported in a single patient with islet cell carcinoma, weakness, muscle pain and muscle fibrosis.

The small number of patients involved and the short time of observation raises considerable doubt about the validity of this study and the general applicability of the author's conclusion that the responses were due to underlying psychological disorders.

OTHER MUSCLE SYNDROMES OF ENDOCRINE INTEREST

Myotonic Dystrophy

This congenital disorder is characterized by a variety of findings including myotonia and muscular dystrophy, cataracts, frontal baldness, and testicular tubular fibrosis in about 50 per cent of affected males. Affected females may have menstrual irregularities and early menopause.[106–111] Glucose intolerance and high plasma insulin levels may be present, but the characteristic microangiopathy of diabetes is relatively infrequent.[112] These patients often have low basal metabolic rates, but tests of thyroid function are otherwise normal. The hypometabolism is thought to be caused by reduced oxygen consumption by the affected musculature, although some cases of hypothyroidism have been reported in association with this condition.[108]

Symptomatic Low Metabolism Responsive to Thyroid Treatment

Patients are frequently encountered with a variety of symptoms suggesting hypothyroidism who in fact appear to be euthyroid when subjected to a battery of laboratory studies, including radioactive iodine uptake, blood thyroxin level, T3 binding tests, and, more recently, pituitary thyroid-stimulating hormone (TSH) measurements.

This condition is of great interest to the practitioner dealing with muscle problems since it may be a major cause of myofascial pain encountered in practice; it is illustrated by the two following case reports.

Symptomatic Low Metabolism of Uncertain Etiology
Responsive to Thyroid Administration

Case 7: Married white female, age 30.
1. Five years' back spasm, nails breaking, falling hair, TMJ pain.

2. Physical examination unremarkable.

3. Laboratory examination—all tests within normal limits. BMR −11, in lower normal range. Cholesterol, 242 mg./dl., in upper normal range. T4 by Murphy Pattee 5.8 μg./dl., TSH test not yet available as a routine laboratory test at the time this patient was seen.

4. Therapeutic trial undertaken with T4 in doses increasing to 0.2 mg. daily and T3 in doses increasing to 50 μg. daily, resulted after a period of 10 weeks in a rise in BMR from −11 to +3 and a fall in cholesterol from 242 to 190 mg./dl. The patient initially experienced insomnia on starting thyroid, which ultimately cleared. She lost two pounds of body weight without attempting to do so. Her back pain cleared in a period of a week after starting thyroid and her facial pain was gone in a period of three months. It has not recurred. Follow-up of serum cholesterol 5½ months after the initiation of therapy revealed a further drop to 162 mg./dl.

Comment: A positive diagnosis of hypothyroidism cannot be made for this patient in view of the fact that no TSH test was available, and T4 was normal. As mentioned in previous pages the normal T4 does not necessarily rule out mild hypothyroidism. Her response to the therapeutic trial seemed prompt, the maintenance of her state of improvement over a six month period speaks against a placebo reaction, and the improvements in the BMR and cholesterol provide objective evidence that the administration of thyroid hormones did produce a metabolic response in this patient, which confirmed her subjective improvement.

Case 8: An 18-year-old, single, white female student. This patient began to experience pain in the neck, shoulders and temporomandibular joint one year prior to her examination by me following a whiplash injury while seated in a car which was struck from behind. Her menstrual function was normal and physical examination was normal.

Laboratory examination revealed the BMR to be −27; cholesterol 205 mg./dl., and the thyroxine by radioimmunoassay, 11.2 μg./dl. TSH tests were not available at the time. The patient was offered a therapeutic trial of sodium levothyroxine (Synthroid) 0.2 mg. daily in gradually increasing doses. Two months after she had been on a complete replacement dose she was feeling considerably improved. Her basal metabolism rate was −6 and the cholesterol was 175 mg./dl. She was advised to remain on thyroid for the immediate future and possibly for life.

Comment: This is a fairly clear-cut metabolic response to thyroid in a patient who could not be chemically proved to be hypothyroid but was clearly hypometabolic as manifested by a BMR of −27. It is of interest that the cholesterol level did not appear to be exceptionally high at 205 mg./dl. which is within the normal range quoted for this age (150 to 275 mg./dl.). However, on treatment with thyroid she did have a moderate drop of 30 points, which along with her clinical response, indicated that she was responsive to thyroid; despite the normal level of T4, her bar rose 211 units.

Williams, in a discussion of this condition in 1962 prior to the development of many newer tests, mentioned symptoms including sensitivity to cold, brittleness of hair, constipation, and obesity associated with a low BMR.[113] He also listed other conditions in which thyroid treatment seems advantageous, including growth in children with retarded bone age but no demonstrable evidence of glandular disease, menstrual disorders, sterility, habitual abortion, and a few instances of hypogonadism. The two preceding case reports suggest that the list should include muscular symptoms of weakness, pain, and spasm, including the TMJ syndrome.

Williams described a sustained therapeutic effect in members of this group of patients from a therapeutic trial with two to three grains of thyroid daily. Some patients whom he examined required increasing doses of thyroid because of what appeared to be a placebo response and finally had to be withdrawn after a large dose proved to be of no avail. Other patients had no response to the trial whatsoever. He felt it was important, because of the subjective nature of many of the complaints, to evaluate the response by a double-blind study.

Keating[114] made a similar proposal following the identification by Kurland and co-workers[115] of four patients with this problem who responded well only to treatment with triiodothyronine, a condition which they called *hypometabolism.*

Ultimately, two double-blind studies were done by different investigators. In one, 18 patients were divided into groups of six subjects and given courses of either T3, T4, or lactose placebo for two weeks after two weeks of gradual buildup of dose.[116]

The other double-blind study also suffers from poor design.[117] It was conducted on one male and 19 female college students who complained of fatigue and were found to have moderately low BMR at a student health service. Ten students were improved when treated with T3 but did not respond to placebo. Nine students responded to placebo but not to T3. One student responded to both. BMR seemed higher in patients on T3 but the changes were interpreted as not being significant. Statistical analysis was not done. The author's conclusion that there was a failure to demonstrate a metabolic insufficiency syndrome does not seem justified, since a true placebo reactor should have shown similar responses to placebo and T3; however, only one patient showed responses to both treatments. Furthermore, the same paper describes a study of 12 subjects with low BMR and normal serum PBI levels whose symptoms suggested a thyroid deficiency state. These people were not treated by a double-blind technique. All of them responded well to desiccated thyroid therapy. The author stated that "Failure to respond to desiccated thyroid is not an invariable result when the serum PBI level is normal." The statement, without the triple negative, is that a response to desiccated thyroid may occur when the serum PBI level is normal. This is a contradiction by the author of her final conclusion.

Analysis of these two double-blind studies reveals a paucity of data and weakness in experimental design, which makes it doubtful that any conclusion can be drawn from them.

The performance of a double-blind study in hypothyroid treatment is a virtual impossibility in private medical practice. Most hospital clinics are not organized to conduct such trials. Furthermore, the character of response of hypothyroidism to treatment does not lend itself to double-blind study, because of the following reasons:

1. Thyroid-deficient patients may require treatment for months before the response is clear-cut. Acid maltase deficiency in hypothyroid muscle may require six months for correction.

2. Personal, mental or emotional problems and varying life situations may obscure the subjective responses to thyroid therapy for long periods of

time. A depression may persist, and its symptoms may blanket clinical manifestations of an improved metabolic state.

3. Many patients are chronically uncomfortable and require a relationship with a physician who knows what therapy is being prescribed.

4. A switch from thyroid to placebo occasionally results in a period of hypothyroidism which may last for 11 weeks in patients who do not require thyroid in the first place.[118] This problem can be minimized by gradually replacing thyroid with the placebo or by giving every patient a period of three months off all therapy between preparations. Such a protocol would greatly prolong the trial, increase its cost, and provoke even more dropouts than that experienced in Levin's study.[116]

5. The ethics of subjecting normal controls to thyroid withdrawal symptoms is open to question.

6. Identification of normal controls poses a problem, since a substantial number of patients receiving thyroid are unaware of symptoms until they have appreciated retrospectively the benefits of thyroid administration. There may be unsuspected responders in the control population.

7. The sizable number of normal controls required for a suitable study would greatly increase the cost of the study.

8. A cycle of muscle pain, trigger points, and spasm occurring in hypothyroidism often requires rehabilitation therapy in conjunction with hormone replacement, introducing another variable into an already complicated experiment.

Controlled therapeutic trials with thyroid hormones, at one time a standard diagnostic procedure, currently provide the only available means for measuring the *peripheral response* to thyroid hormones. Following the introduction of precise radioimmunoassay techniques for measuring thyroid hormone *production,* and following the publication of the above two defective double-blind studies, which challenged the concept of hypometabolism responsive to thyroid hormone supplementation, these trials have fallen into disuse.

In recent years there has been increasing awareness of discordant abnormalities of thyroid hormones in the blood.[119] Ambiguous values in measurements of pituitary-thyroid axis function occur in conditions such as the low T3 syndrome,[120, 121] peripheral resistance to thyroid hormone,[122, 123] inappropriate TSH secretion,[124] premyxedema,[125, 126] and decreased thyroidal reserve.[127] *Symptomatic low metabolism* responsive to thyroid therapy may be added to this list. Measurements of serum TSH and thyroid hormone levels in these conditions are unreliable indicators of peripheral metabolic function.

Evaluation of peripheral resistance to thyroid hormones must include measurements of the basal metabolic rate,[122, 123] but in the literature on other syndromes of ambiguous hormone secretion, metabolic state is usually evaluated by uncontrolled clinical impression. Most authors state that their patients are clinically euthyroid. Hesch, on the other hand, has observed that the biological effects of the low T3 syndrome are uncertain.[121]

It appears that clinical trials controlled by measurements of peripheral metabolic response, the BMR,[128, 129] and serum cholesterol levels should be revived when tests of thyroid hormone production are ambiguous or do not fit the clinical picture. The following section updates my experience with the application of such trials.

THE CONTROLLED THERAPEUTIC TRIAL WITH THYROID

Method

After a complete history, physical examination, and laboratory evaluation, patients suspected of suffering from symptoms of thyroid deficiency, despite normal blood measurements of thyroid function, are sent to the laboratories of the New York Hospital for determination of a basal metabolic rate. They are then placed on thyroid medication. The current regimen is usually sodium L-thyroxine in a dose of 0.15 or 0.2 mg daily. None of these patients is given a thyroid hormone dosage that produces any manifestation of hyperthyroidism.

For serial BMR the patients are requested to prepare themselves in exactly the same way and to avoid major changes of diet or lifestyle during the period of repeated observations. They are especially cautioned against changing cholesterol modifying diets or attempting weight reducing diets. Thus, *each patient serves as his own control.*

The second set of observations of BMR, cholesterol, and clinical response is made after the patient has been on a full replacement dose for a period of approximately two months. Additional BMR and cholesterol determinations are made if further confirmation is sought.

The relevant values in the trial are not the individual BMR and cholesterol values, but rather their change (ΔBMR, Δ cholesterol). These changes are then correlated with the clinical impression of whether or not the patient has responded to therapy and are plotted in Figure 6–4.

Observations

Figure 6–4 is a plot of the author's observations of 172 therapeutic trials including 11 therapeutic withdrawals performed on patients who had normal PBI or T4. Fifty-five of these patients had normal TSH. On the horizontal axis is plotted ΔBMR obtained from the difference in measurement before starting and while receiving thyroid. On the vertical axis is plotted Δ cholesterol calculated from two values obtained at the same time as the BMR. Clinical evaluation of response is plotted as a black circle if a clinical improvement occurred and as an open circle if there was no clear-cut clinical response.

Interpretation of the graph depends upon recognition that negative metabolic responses scatter randomly about the zero point, whereas positive metabolic responses distribute in the upper right hand quadrant, reflecting a rise in BMR and a fall in cholesterol level. The metabolic responses of patients with negative symptomatic response (open circles) scatter almost evenly around zero, whereas positive responses (black circles) are confirmed by highly significant metabolic responses.

A normal TSH was not useful in differentiating patients who would be responsive to thyroid hormone medication.

Discussion of Therapeutic Trials

The explanation for responsiveness of patients to thyroid hormone therapy despite normal measurements of thyroid hormone and TSH in the

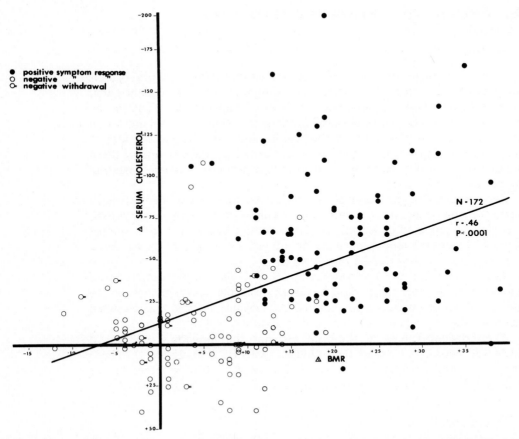

Figure 6–4. Results of therapeutic trials and withdrawals with varying combinations of T3 and T4 in 172 patients with symptoms suggesting possible thyroid hormone deficiency states. All of these patients had normal PBIs or more recently normal TSHs and/or T4 measurements. In none of these patients were symptoms of hyperthyroidism produced by therapy. The graph shows a distinct response in BMR and cholesterol in many of these patients. Furthermore, patients showing the most clear-cut responses in these two measurements showed positive clinical responses (black circles), whereas patients with no significant metabolic response in BMR and cholesterol showed no clinical response (open circles). This graph appears to support the validity of using the change in BMR and cholesterol in response to thyroid hormone medication for confirmation of a positive or negative clinical response to treatment in patients who cannot be proved to be thyroid deficient by any other technique.

blood is not entirely clear. Some patients with normal T4 levels may have mild compensated hypothyroidism or diminished thyroidal reserve responsive to thyroid hormones. However, in such a case an elevation of TSH would be expected.

Patients mentioned by Thompson and Thompson[130] experienced low metabolism as a result of chronic debilitation, muscular atrophy, depression, muscular dystrophy (see previous section on myotonic dystrophy), hypopituitarism, anorexia nervosa, and Addison's disease.

Abnormality in responsiveness or concentration of end organ receptors, antibodies against receptors, or abnormalities of intracellular carriers of thyroid hormones is an intriguing possibility.

Another possible explanation is that the population that showed responses to medication actually became mildly thyrotoxic. This raises the interesting question of whether patients can be chemically thyrotoxic without being clinically thyrotoxic. Many of these patients on doses of 0.2 mg. of T4 with or without supplemental doses of T3 had high serum T4 and T3 levels, as has been demonstrated by Braverman and co-workers.[131] It is difficult to accept the concept that such patients have thyrotoxicosis in the total absence of clinical manifestations of this disorder. However, whether or not one chooses the semantics of labeling such a disparity thyrotoxicosis, the patients with measurable metabolic improvement are frequently relieved of their complaints without sustaining undesirable thyrotoxic side effects, a reasonable criterion for successful therapy.

Data presented in Figure 6–4 update clinical observations extending over 20 years. Additional therapeutic trials are being completed. Undoubtedly, new insights will emerge as these data develop and as new tests of thyroid function become available for clinical use.

It appears that the use of serial BMR and cholesterol determinations in evaluating response to thyroid therapy is a more practical solution to the detection and treatment of symptomatic low metabolism than the double-blind type of protocol. Unfortunately, BMR and cholesterol determinations for the evaluation of thyroid problems have been falling into unwarranted disuse. There is a general trend in the medical community to consider the BMR an obsolete test. The data reported here provide evidence that the test is still useful when properly applied to the appropriate clinical problem.

A COMMON PROBLEM RESPONDING TO MULTIPLE ENDOCRINE THERAPY

Menopausal or amenorrheic women occasionally present with complaints of chronic muscle stiffness, pain, spasm, and trigger points in various muscles of the body. They often give a history of previous diagnoses of disc disease and sciatica, and some have had orthopedic surgery, spinal fusion, laminectomy, or surgery for bursitis. They often present symptoms suggestive of hypothyroidism. Complete clinical evaluation generally reveals few striking abnormalities. The T4 and TSH levels are usually normal, but the BMR may be low to borderline, and the cholesterol level slightly elevated to borderline. Occasionally, these parameters may appear to be within normal range. In younger patients vaginal smears by Shorr stain reveal estrogenic insufficiency, the usual finding, of course, with menopausal women. Treatment of the estrogenic deficiency with estrogens alone may not afford complete relief of all symptoms. The administration of a therapeutic trial of thyroid hormone in conjunction with estrogens may produce a striking symptomatic response confirmed by a significant elevation of the BMR and fall in the cholesterol.

The addition of methyltestosterone is sometimes helpful.

Cases 9 and 10 show the results of such trials on patients who were classified as "basket" temporomandibular joint cases by Dr. Gelb until their estrogen therapy was supplemented by thyroid replacement.

Responses to Mixed Hormonal Therapy

Case 9: 52-year-old married, white female, piano teacher.

1. First seen on 6–1–73 with a chief complaint of muscle spasm in jaws radiating to the temple and back of eyes. Back pain after half hour at the piano.

2. Past history of "never being well." Respiratory problems, asthma, and allergy since childhood.

1963—total hysterectomy for rectocystocele.

Treated at Montefiore Headache Clinic and referred for opening ethmoid and sphenoid sinuses which had no effect on headache.

1971—low estrogen count. Placed on estrogen therapy.

Prednisone, 20 mg. daily, begun at Montefiore Hospital Headache Clinic 5½ weeks with complete cessation of headaches, which returned when the patient was on 10 mg. daily.

Rejected for physical medicine and rehabilitation therapy because she was considered not to be treatable.

Felt better when local physician put her on ¼ gr. thyroid.

3. Review of system—cold intolerance, dry skin, overweight, constipated.

4. Physical examination: dry skin and hair, nose congested, markedly delayed relaxation of ankle jerk.

5. Laboratory: Estrogen smear showed low level. BMR −20, cholesterol 258 mg./dl. T4 not done since patient was receiving estrogens. TSH test not available at that time.

6. Diagnosis: hypothyroid, menopausal syndrome following hysterectomy with high-dosage estrogen requirement, TMJ, and generalized myalgia secondary to combined estrogen and thyroid deficiency.

7. Rx: Increase estrogen to 2.5 mg. daily for 49 days, rest 7 days.

6–6–73. Start and increase T3 to 25 μg. daily and T4 to 0.1 mg. daily.

8. Course: 6–22–73. Patient feeling better. Jaws ache but no bad spasm. Requires fewer TMJ injections, experiences less fatigue. Pulse 76, ankle jerk relaxation still delayed.

Increase T4 to 0.2 mg., T3 to 50 μg. daily.

8–8–73: The jaw feels better. Visits to dentist greatly decreased. Ankle jerk brisk! Pulse 80. Migraine and spasms controlled. Energy improved.

Laboratory tests: BMR increased from −20 to +7, cholesterol dropped from 258 to 150 μg./dl.

10–18–73. Aches, headaches have increased, complains of loss of libido causing domestic problems. Start methyltestosterone 10 mg. three times weekly, increasing as necessary to 10 mg. daily in addition to other hormonal therapy.

12–19–73. More energy, mouth opens widely, increase T4 to 0.3 mg., T3 50 μg., methyltestosterone 10 mg. three times weekly. Estrogen reduced to 1.25 mg. daily for 21 days each month.

August 1, 1974: Patient feels well for weeks at a time.

11–13–74: Patient is able to tolerate dentistry without TMJ spasm. Better coordinated, able to teach. "No more numbness in hands" revealed a carpal tunnel syndrome that she apparently never mentioned before. Voltages on the EKG appeared slightly higher than those at the time of her initial visit.

June 14, 1975: Feels "really good" since receiving new dental appliance.

Attack of allergy in nose and eyes started headaches and exacerbated jaw spasm.

9–12–75: Increased estrogen; headache and TMJ cleared. On seven-day withdrawal they reappeared and did not respond to resumption of oral therapy. Nose congested; Teldrin not helpful. Vaginal smear showed very low estrogen effect, despite 1.25 mg. conjugated estrogens daily. Rx: Estradiol valerate, 10 mg. IM. Symptoms improved.

May 1982: Patient continues thyroid, oral conjugated estrogens, and testosterone, plus IM estrogen weekly. She remains professionally active, and experiences occasional headaches. TMJ asymptomatic.

Comment: This case reveals the many subtle decisions which the clinical endocrinologist must make in dealing with symptomatic patients who have multiple endocrine deficiencies, especially when objective parameters are incomplete because of unavailability of diagnostic procedures or interference by concomitant medication. Despite these limitations it was possible to obtain objective support for the many decisions that had to be made. Among the useful parameters were, first of all, the very clear-cut physical finding of a delayed ankle reflex, which did not require any specialized equipment other than a neurological hammer for its demonstration. The use of the BMR and cholesterol was indispensible in confirming the fact that the patient did indeed have a metabolic response to therapy. Another important principle which this case demonstrates is the necessity for the endocrinologist to be willing to vary both dosages and preparation of estrogen hormones. A fascinating aspect of her clinical course was the fact that her entire syndrome went into relapse when she had a bad allergic episode in the late summer of 1975. An increase in estrogen was apparently effective in arresting the relapse.

Case 10: A 54-year-old housewife.
    1. 10–25–73: Chief complaint: Migraine headache of 20 years' duration.
    2. Five years Rx with Cafergot at Montefiore Headache Clinic.
    Cafergot in larger doses causes pain in the left side of the chest, shortness of breath, and pain in joints.
    Has used "every drug imaginable." Has seen "50 to 60 doctors."
    Nine months: partially relieved by TMJ therapy.
    Headaches have recently increased to daily.
    3. Past history: Hysterectomy 20 years ago followed by hot flashes.
    Relief of flashes by conjugated estrogens, 1.25 mg. for 21 days, monthly.
    Skin dry. Loses hair. Nails in bad condition. Terribly constipated. Infrequent muscle cramps.
    4. Physical examination: Skin sallow and dry.
    5. Laboratory: Cholesterol, 348 mg./dl.; T4 on estrogens, 7.2 μg./dl. as thyroxine, BMR − 17.
    10–29–73: Started therapeutic trial with sodium L-thyroxine, increasing to 0.2 mg. daily and triiodothyronine increasing to 50 μg. daily.
    12–12–73: Moving bowels normally for the first time in many years. Headaches increased in frequency. Cholesterol fell to 230 mg./dl.
    March 25, 1974: BMR has increased to − 2. Cholesterol remains lower at 260 mg./dl. Continues to have headaches.
    October 11, 1974: Feels fantastic. Has been able to remove bite plate. Headaches occur about every 2–3 weeks. Has been able to play 18 holes of golf for the first time in years.
    February 26, 1975: Headaches got worse when she ran out of T4.

Comment: This appears to be another good example of a patient with a long history of virtual invalidism produced by migraine headaches and temporomandibular joint pain. She received partial relief from estrogen therapy following surgical menopause but did not achieve complete remission of her symptoms and rehabilitation until she had been on adequate replacement doses of thyroid for a period of about one year. This case points out that improved muscular function may not occur for many months after the metabolic level has been raised.

SUMMARY AND CONCLUSIONS

Endocrine gland dysfunction may cause muscle pain and spasm. These symptoms can affect the temporomandibular joint. Ten examples of this relationship are detailed in this chapter and are summarized in Table 6–1. Palliation of symptoms resulted from treatment of two hyperthyroid and one hypothyroid patient. Two subjects with symptomatic low metabolism who could not be proved to be hypothyroid responded well to controlled therapeutic trials with synthetic thyroid hormone. One young woman with

TABLE 6–1. Patients with Endocrine Related TMJ Syndrome

Case	Sex	Age	Diagnosis	Treatment	Results
1. R.A.	F	32	T3 Thyrotoxicosis	^{131}I	Cured
2. F.W.	F	32	Thyrotoxicosis	^{131}I	Cured
3. S.C.	M	42	Cretinism	None	—
4. B.P.	F	60	Hypothyroid after ^{131}I	T4	Corrected
5. C.R.	F	30	Symptomatic Low Metabolism	T4 and T3	Improved
6. L.N.	F	18	Symptomatic Low Metabolism	T4	Improved
7. R.Z.	F	31	Premenstrual Spasm	Estrogens	Improved
8. A.K.	F	52	Combined Deficiency	Estrogens, T4, T3	Improved
9. C.S.	F	54	Combined Deficiency	Estrogens, T4, T3	Improved
10. R.S.	F	64	Hyperparathyroid	None	—

premenstrual TMJ pain responded dramatically to estrogen therapy. Two patients required mixed thyroid and estrogen therapy for relief. A patient with cretinism and TMJ spasm is described. One patient with hyperparathyroidism declined therapy, and a causal relationship could not be proved. The TMJ is yet another syndrome which can be added to the list of motor disorders associated with metabolic diseases.

References

1. Schlegel, D.: Endokrine Faktoren Bei Kiefergezenkbeschwerden. Dtsch. Zahnaertzl. Z., *17*:247, 1962.
2. Hary, M., and Matekovits, G.: Correlations between certain hormonal disorders and chronic temporomandibular joint diseases. SSO Schweiz. Monatsschr. Zahnheilkd., *80*:243, 1970.
3. Loewit, K., et al.: Hormonal disorders and arthropathies of the temporomandibular joints. Osterr. Z. Stomatol., *70*:122, 1973.
4. Ganshorn, M. L.: Studies on possible correlations between diseases of the temporomandibular joint and female sex hormones. Z. W. R., *84*:726, 1975.
5. Sudaka, R., and Lespine, J.: Quelque aspects pathologique de la selle turcique. Ses incidence sur l'articulation temporomandibulaire. Rev. Odont. Par., *75*:120, 1953.
6. Schwartz, L., Moulton, R., and Goldensohn, E.: Pain involving the temporomandibular articulation. Dent. Clin. North Am., 515, 1959.
7. Price, H. M., and Van de Velde: Ultrastructure of skeletal muscle fiber. In Walton, J. N. (ed.): Disorders of Voluntary Muscle, 2nd ed. London, Churchill Livingstone, 1981.
8. Gergely, J.: Biochemical aspects of muscle structure and function. In Walton, J. N. (ed.): Disorders of Voluntary Muscle, 2nd ed. London, Churchill Livingstone, 1981.
9. Bessman, S. P., and Geiger, P. J.: Transport of energy in muscle: the phosphorylcreatine shuttle. Science, *211*:448, 1981.
10. Ramsey, I.: Thyroid Disease and Muscle Dysfunction. Chicago, Year Book Medical Publishers, 1974.
11. Bathurst, L. W.: A case of Graves' disease associated with idiopathic muscular atrophy. Lancet 2:529, 1895.
12. Askanazy, M.: Pathelogisch-anatomische Beitrage zur Kentniss des Morbus Basedowii, inbesondere uber die dabei auftretende Muskelerkrankung. Dtsch. Arch. Klin. Med., *61*:118, 1898.
13. Hed, R., Kirstin, L., et al.: Thyrotoxic myopathy. J. Neurol. Neurosurg. Psychiatry, *21*:270, 1958.
14. Adams, R. D.: In Diseases of Muscle. New York, Harper and Row, 1975.
15. Havard, C. W. H., Campbell, E. D. R., Ross, H. B., and Spence, A. W.: Electromyographic and histologic findings in muscles of patients with thyrotoxicosis. Q. J. Med., *32*:145, 1963.
16. Peterson, I., Tengroth, B., et al.: Electromyographic study of the eye muscle in endocrine exophthalmos. Acta Ophthalmol. (Kbh), *39*:171, 1961.
17. Richardson, H. B., and Shorr, E.: Creatin metabolism in atypical Graves' disease. Trans. Assoc. Am. Physicians, *50*:156, 1935.
18. Thorn, G. W.: Creatine studies in thyroid disorders. Endocrinology, *20*:628, 1936.

19. Thorn, G. W., and Eder, H. A.: Studies on chronic thyrotoxic myopathy. Am. J. Med., *1*:538, 1946.
20. Craig, F. A., and Crispin Smith, J.: Serum creatine phosphokinase activity in altered thyroid states. J. Clin. Endocrinol., *25*:723, 1965.
21. Satoyoshi, E., and Kinoshita, M.: Some aspects of thyrotoxic and steroid myopathy. In Walton, J., et al. (eds.): Muscle Disease. (Excerpta Med. Int. Congr. Ser. No. 199.) Amsterdam, Excerpta Medica Foundation, 1970, p. 455.
22. Satoyoshi, E., Murakama, K. et al.: Myopathy and thyrotoxicosis, with special emphasis on an effect of potassium ingestion on serum and urinary creatine. Neurology, *13*:645, 1963.
23. Green, K., and Matty, A. J.: The effect of thyroid hormones on water permeability of the isolated bladder of the toad Bufo bufo. J. Endocrinol., *28*:205, 1964.
24. Peter, J. B.: Hyperthyroidism. Ann. Intern. Med., *69*:1016, 1968.
25. Karlberg, B. E., Henrikson, K. G., and Andersson, R. G.: Cyclical adenosine 3'5' monophosphate concentration in normal subjects and in patients with hyper- and hypothyroidism. J. Clin. Endocrinol. Metab., *39*:96, 1974.
26. Ord, W. M., Address in medicine on some disorders of the nutrition related with affection of the nervous system. Br. Med. J., *2*:205, 1884.
27. Debré, R., and Semelaigne, G.: Syndrome of diffuse muscular hypertrophy in infants causing athletic appearance and its connection with congenital myxedema. Am. J. Dis. Child., *50*:1351, 1935.
28. Najjar, S. S.: Muscular hypertrophy in hypothyroid children: Kocher Debré Semelaigne syndrome: review of 23 cases. J. Pediatr., *85*:236, 1974.
29. Ingwall, J. S., Morales, M. F., and Stockdale, F. E.: Creatine and the control of myosin synthesis in differentiating skeletal muscle. Proc. Natl. Acad. Sci. USA, *69*:2250, 1972.
30. Shorr, E., Richardson, H. B., and Mansfield, J. S.: Influence of thyroid administration on creatine metabolism in myxedema of adults. Proc. Soc. Exp. Biol. Med., *32*:1340, 1935.
31. Golding, D. N.: Hypothyroidism presenting with musculoskeletal symptoms. Ann. Rheumat. Dis., *29*:10, 1970.
32. Chaney, W. C.: Tendon reflexes in myxedema. A valuable aide in diagnosis. JAMA, *82*:2013, 1924.
33. Rives, K. L., Furth, E. D., and Becker, D. V.: Limitations of the ankle jerk test. Ann. Intern. Med., *62*:1139, 1965.
34. McKeran, R. O., Slavin, G., Andrews, T. M., Ward, P., and Mair, W. G. P.: Muscle fiber type changes in hypothyroid myopathy. J. Clin. Pathol., *28*:659, 1975.
35. Ahuja, M. M. S.: Myxedema myopathy: Report of cases with response to therapy. Indian J. Med. Sci., *20*:537, 1966.
36. Astrom, K. E., Kugelberg, E., and Muller, R.: Hypothyroid myopathy. Arch. Intern. Med., *5*:472, 1961.
37. Newcombe, D. S., Ortel, R. W., and Levey, G. S.: Activation of human synovial adenylate cyclase by thyroid stimulating hormone. Biochem. Biophys. Res. Commun., *48*:201, 1972.
38. Norris, F. H., and Panner, B. J.: Hypothyroid myopathy: Clinical electromyographical and ultrastructural observations. Arch. Neurol., *14*:574, 1966.
39. McArdle, B.: Metabolic and endocrine myopathies. In Walton, J. N. (ed.): Disorders of Voluntary Muscle. Edinburgh, Churchill Livingstone, 1974, p. 735.
40. Hurwitz, L. V., McCormick, D., and Allen, I. V.: Reduced muscle alpha glucosidase, acid maltase activity in hypothyroid myopathy. Lancet, *1*:67, 1970.
41. Salick, A. E., and Colachis, C. S., et al.: Myxedema myopathy: clinical electrodiagnostic and pathological findings in an advanced case. Arch. Phys. Med. Rehab., *49*:230, 1968.
42. Frymoyer, J. W., and Bland, J. H.: Carpal tunnel syndrome in patients with myxedematous arthropathy. J. Bone Joint Surg., *55A*:78, 1973.
43. Pearson, C. M.: Muscle and Hormones. In Williams, R. H. (ed.): Textbook of Endocrinology, 5th ed. Philadelphia, W. B. Saunders Co., 1974, pp. 994–1003.
44. Golding, D. N.: The musculoskeletal features of hypothyroidism. Postgrad. Med. J., *47*:611, 1971.
45. Dorwart, B. B., and Schumacher, H. R.: Joint effusions, chondrocalcinosis and other rheumatic manifestations in hypothyroidism. Am. J. Med., *59*:78, 1975.
46. Sonkin, L. S., and Cohen, E. J.: Treatment of the menopause. Mod. Treat., *5*:545, 1968.
47. Saville, P. D.: Treatment of postmenopausal osteoporosis. Mod. Treat., *5*:571, 1968.
48. Shorr, E.: An evaluation of the clinical applications of the vaginal smear method. J. Mt. Sinai Hosp., *12*:667, 1945.
49. deAllende, K. C., Shorr, E., and Hartman, C. G.: Contributions to Embryology. No. 198. A comparative study of the vaginal smear cycle of the rhesus monkey and the human. Carnegie Institute of Washington Publication 557. Contributions to Embryology, *318*, 1943.

50. Papanicolaou, G. N., and Falk, E. R.: General muscular hypertrophy induced by androgenic hormone. Science, *87*:238, 1938.
51. Pellegrino, C.: The effects of testosterone on the ultrastructure and glycogen synthesis in the levator ani muscle of the rat. In Walton, J. N., and Canal N. et al. (eds.): Muscle Disease. Exerpta Medica Int. Congr. Ser. No. 199. Amsterdam, Exerpta Medical Foundation, 1970, p. 704.
52. Carter, A. C., Cohen, E. J., and Shorr, E.: The use of androgens in women. In Harris, R., and Thimunn, K. (eds.): Vitamins and Hormones. Vol. 5. New York, Academic Press, 1947.
53. Shorr, E.: Treatment of some chronic muscular diseases. Conference on Therapy, Cornell University Medical College. Am. J. Med., *2*:630, 1947.
54. Kochakian, C. D.: Protein anabolic action of testosterone propionate in hyperthyroid castrated rats. Endocrinology, *66*:286, 1960.
55. Albright, F.: Cushing's Syndrome. Harvey Lect., *33*:123, 1942–1943.
56. Kochakian, C. D., and Costa, G.: The effect of testosterone propionate on the protein and carbohydrate metabolism in the depancreatectomized—castrated dog. Endocrinology, *653*:298, 1959.
57. Bartlett, P. D.: Rates of protein synthesis, amino acid catabolism, and size of nitrogen pool during nitrogen storage induced with testosterone propionate and testosterone propionate combined with growth hormone. Endocrinology, *52*:272, 1953.
58. Kochakian, C. D.: Anabolic and Androgenic Steroids. New York, Springer-Verlag, 1975.
59. Thorn, G. W.: The Diagnosis and Treatment of Adrenal Insufficiency. Springfield, Ill., Charles C Thomas, 1949, pp. 144–145.
60. Cushing, H.: The basophile adenomas of the pituitary body and their clinical manifestations. Bull. Johns Hopkins Hosp., *50*:137, 1932.
61. Afifi, A. K., Bergman, R. A., and Harvey, J. C.: Steroid myopathy: Clinical, histologic and cytologic observations. Johns Hopkins Med. J., *123*:158, 1968.
62. Pearce, G. W.: Electron microscopy in the study of muscle disease. Ann. N.Y. Acad. Sci., *138*:138, 1966.
63. Prineas, J., Hall, R., Barwick, D. D., and Watson, A. J.: Myopathy associated with pigmentation following adrenalectomy for Cushing's syndrome. Q. J. Med., *37*:63, 1968.
64. Conn, J. W.: Primary aldosteronism: A new clinical syndrome. J. Lab. Clin. Med., *45*:661, 1955.
65. Conn, J. W., Louis, L. H., Fajans, S. S., et al.: Intermittent aldosteronism in periodic paralysis: Dependence of attacks on retention of sodium, and failure to induce attacks by restrictions of dietary sodium. Lancet, *1*:802, 1957.
66. Yazaki, K. et al.: Hypokalemic myopathy associated with 17-alpha-hydroxylase deficiency: A case report. Neurology, *32*:94, 1982.
67. Maranon, G.: Les syndromes neuromusculaires. Bull. Acad. Med., *118*:293, 1937.
68. Mastaglia, F. L., Barwick, D. D., and Hall, R.: Myopathy in acromegaly. Lancet, *2*:907, 1970.
69. Picket, J. B. E., Layzer, R. B., Levin, S. R., Schneider, V., Campbell, M., and Sumner, A. J.: Neuromuscular complications of acromegaly. Neurology, *25*:638, 1975.
70. Lundberg, P. O., and Osterman, P. O.: Neuromuscular signs and symptoms in acromegaly. In Walton, J. N., Canal, N., et al. (eds.) Muscle Diseases. Exerpta Medica Int. Cong. Ser. No. 199. Amsterdam, Exerpta Medica Foundations, 531, 1970.
71. Stern, L. Z., Payne, C. M., and Hannapel, L. K.: Acromegaly: Histochemical and electron microscopic changes in deltoid and intercostal muscle. Neurology, *24*:589, 1974.
72. Cheah, J. S., Chua, S. P., and Ho, C. L.: Ultrastructure of the muscles in acromegaly before hypophysectomy. Am. J. Med. Sci., *269*:183, 1975.
73. Cheah, D. B., Brasel, J. A., Elliot, D., and Scott, R.: Muscle cell size and number in normal children, and in dwarfs (pituitary, cretins and primordial) before and after treatment. Bull. Johns Hopkins Hosp., *119*:46, 1966.
74. Stewart, A. C., and Sprunt, J. G.: Hypopituitarism and flexor muscle spasm. Acta Endocrinol., *53*:489, 1966.
75. Shapiro, B. G., and Zwarenstein, H.: On the relation of the pituitary gland to muscle creatine. Proc. R. Soc. Endinburgh, *56*:164, 1936.
76. Frame, B., Heinze, E. G., Jr., Block, M. A., and Manson, G. A.: Myopathy in primary hyperparathyroidism. Ann. Intern. Med., *66*:1022, 1968.
77. Bischoff, A., and Esslen, E.: Myopathy with primary hyperparathyroidism. Neurology, *15*:64, 1965.
78. Hannon, R. R., Shorr, E., McClellan, W. S., and DuBois, E. F.: A case of osteitis fibrosa cystica (osteomalacia?) with evidence of hyperactivity of the parathyroid bodies. Metabolic Study I. J. Clin. Invest., *8*:215, 1930.
79. Richet, C., Sourdel, M., et al.: Syndromes parathyroidomusculaires: Myopathies sclereuses liees à des troubles parathyroidiens. J. Med. Franc., *26*:377, 1937.
80. Vicale, C. T.: The diagnostic features of muscular syndrome resulting from hyperparathy-

roidism, osteomalacia owing to renal tubular acidosis, and perhaps to related disorders of calcium metabolism. Trans. Am. Neurol. Assoc., *74*:143, 1949.

81. Prineas, J. W., Stuart-Mason, A., and Henson, R. A.: Myopathy in metabolic bone disease. Br. Med. J., *1*:1034, 1965.

82. Smith, R., and Stern, G.: Myopathy, osteomalacia and hyperparathyroidism. Brain, *90*:593, 1967.

83. Landau, R. L., and Kappas, A.: Anabolic hormones in hyperparathyroidism: With observations on general catabolic influence of parathyroid hormone in man. Ann. Intern. Med., *62*:1223, 1965.

84. Richardson, J. A., Herron, G., Reitz, R., and Layzer, R.: Ischemic ulcerations of skin and necrosis of muscle in azotemic hyperparathyroidism. Ann. Intern. Med., *71*:129, 1969.

85. Lemann, J., Jr., and Donatelli, A. A.: Muscle weakness in parathyroid crisis. Ann. Intern. Med., *60*:477, 1964.

86. Henson, R. A.: The neurological aspects of hypercalcemia: with special reference to primary hyperparathyroidism. J. R. Coll. Physicians Lond., *1*:41, 1966.

87. Cholod, E. J., Haust, M. D., Hudson, A. J., and Lewis, F. N.: Myopathy in primary familial hyperparathyroidism: Clinical and morphological studies. Am. J. Med., *48*:700, 1970.

88. Henson, R. A.: Clinical aspects of some disease of muscle. In Bourne, G. H. (ed.): The Structure and Function of Muscle. IV. Pharmacology and Disease. New York, Academic Press, 1973, p. 456.

89. Rasmussen, H.: Parathyroid Hormone, Calcitonin, and the Calciferols. In Williams, R. H. (ed.): Textbook of Endocrinology. Philadelphia, W. B. Saunders Co., 1974, p. 755.

90. Rall, J., Homsher, E., and Mommaerts, W. F. M. H.: Heat production and phosphocreatine hydrolysis with unloaded shortening in Rana pipiens semitendinosus muscles. Fed. Proc., *32*:730, 1973.

91. Gomez, M. R., Engel, A. G., and Dyck, P. J.: Progressive ataxia, retinal degeneration, neuromyopathy, and mental subnormality in a patient with true hypoparathyroidism, dwarfism, malabsorption and cholelithiasis. Neurology, *22*:849, 1972.

92. Hower, J., Struck, H., et al.: Myopathy and elevated serum enzymes in a case of hypoparathyroidism. Z. Kinderheilkd., *116*:193, 1974.

93. Wolf, S. M., Lusk, W., and Weisberg, L.: Hypocalcemic myopathy. Bull. Los Angeles Neurol. Soc., *37*:166, 1972.

94. Goldberg, M. H., Slaughtern, T. W., and Harrigan, W. F.: Pseudohyperparathyroidism with temporomandibular ankylosis: report of case. J. Oral Surg., *25*:175, 1967.

95. Garland, A.: Diabetic amyotrophy. Br. Med. J., *2*:1287, 1955.

96. Gregersen, G.: Diabetic amyotrophy—a well-defined syndrome? Acta Med. Scand., *185*:303, 1969.

97. Schwartz, T. B.: Editorial comment. Yearbook of Endocrinology, 1970, p. 213.

98. Locke, S., Lawrence, D. G., and Legg, M. A.: Diabetic amyotrophy. Am. J. Med., *34*:775, 1963.

99. Gårde, A., and Kugelberg, E.: Myopatier vid diabetes (Abstr.). Nord. Med., *70*:1252, 1963.

100. Bloodworth, J. M. B., Jr., Epstein, M.: Diabetic amyotrophy: Light and electron microscopic investigation. Diabetes, *16*:181, 1967.

101. Oles, R. D.: Glucose intolerance associated with temporomandibular joint pain–dysfunction syndrome. Oral Surg., *43*:546, 1977.

102. Tannenberg, J.: Pathological changes in heart, skeletal musculature and liver in rabbits treated with insulin in shock dosage. Am. J. Pathol., *15*:25, 1939.

103. Ziegler, D. K.: Minor neurological signs and symptoms following insulin coma therapy. J. Nerv. Ment. Dis., *120*:75, 1954.

104. Mulder, D. W., Bastron, J. A., and Lambert, E. H.: Hyperinsulin neuronopathy. Neurology, *6*:627, 1956.

105. Levratte, M., and Brette, R.: Cancer langerhansien du pancreas avec hypoglycemie, doleur musculaires et myosite degenerative d'origine metabolique. Presse. Med., *56*:6340, 1957.

106. DeCourt, J. J., Lereboullet, R. H., and Tinel, G.: Testicular changes of myotonic myopathy (Steinert's disease). Ann. Endocrinol., *12*:1046, 1951.

107. Clarke, G. B., Shapiro, and Monroe, R. G.: Myotonia atrophica with testicular atrophy. J. Clin. Endocrinol., *16*:1235, 1956.

108. Caughey, E., and Myrianthopoulos, N. C.: Dystrophia myotonia and related disorders. Springfield, Ill., Charles C Thomas, 1963.

109. Drucker, W. D., and Blank, W. A.: The testes of myotonic muscular dystrophy. J. Clin. Endocrinol., *23*:59, 1963.

110. Huff, T. A., and Lebovitz, H. E.: Insulin dynamics in myotonic dystrophy. J. Clin. Endocrinol., *28*:992, 1968.

111. Renwick, J. H., Bundey, S. E., Fergusen-Smith, A., and Izatt, M. M.: Confirmation of linkage of the loci for myotonic dystrophy and ABH secretion. J. Med. Genet., *8*:407, 1971.
112. Danowski, T. S., Khurana, R. C., and Gonzales, A. R.: Capillary basement membrane thickness and the pseudodiabetes of myopathy. Am. J. Med., *51*:757, 1971.
113. Williams, R.: Hypometabolism ("Metabolic Insufficiency"). In Williams, R.: Textbook of Endocrinology, 3rd ed. Philadelphia, W. B. Saunders Co., 1962.
114. Keating, R.: Editorial: Metabolic insufficiency. J. Clin. Endocrinol. Metab., *18*, 531, 1958.
115. Kurland, G. S., Hamolsky, M. W., and Stone Freedberg, A.: Studies in non-myxedematous hypometabolism. J. Clin. Endocrinol. Metab., *17*:1365, 1957.
116. Levin, M. E.: "Metabolic Insufficiency," A double blind study using triiodothyronine, thyroxine, and a placebo. J. Clin. Endocrinol., *20*:106, 1960.
117. Sikkema, S. H.: Triiodothyronine in the diagnosis and treatment of hypothyroidism, failure to demonstrate the metabolic insufficiency syndrome (controlled study). J. Clin., Endocrinol., *20*:545, 1960.
118. Greer, M. A.: Effects on endogenous thyroid activity of feeding desiccated thyroid to normal human subjects. N. Engl. J. Med., *244*:385, 1951.
119. Ingbar, S., and Weber, K.: States associated with abnormal hormone concentrations in the blood. In Williams, R. (ed.): Textbook of Endocrinology, 6th ed. Philadelphia, W. B. Saunders Co., 1981, p. 154.
120. Carter, J. N., Eastman, C. F., et al.: Effect of severe chronic illness on thyroid function. Lancet 2:971, 1974.
121. Hesch, R. D. (ed.): The "Low T3 Syndrome." Proceedings of the Serono Symposia, Vol. 40. New York, Academic Press, 1981.
122. Refetoff, S., DeWind, L. T., and DeGroot, L. J.: Familial syndrome combining deaf mutism, strippled epiphyses, goitre, and abnormally high PBI: A possible target organ refractoriness to thyroid hormones. J. Clin. Endocrinol. Metab., *27*:279, 1967.
123. Kaplan, M. M., Swartz, S., and Larsen, R.: Partial peripheral resistance to thyroid hormone. Am. J. Med., *95*:352, 1981.
124. Weintraub, B. D., Gershenhorn, M. C., Kourides, I. A., and Fein, H.: Inappropriate secretion of thyroid stimulating hormone. Ann. Intern. Med., *95*:352, 1981.
125. Fowler, P. B. S., Swale, J., and Andrews, H.: Hypercholesterolemia in borderline hypothyroidism—stage of premyxoedema. Lancet, *2*:488, 1970.
126. Evered, D. C., Ormston, B. J., et al.: Grades of hypothyroidism. Br. Med. J., *1*:657, 1963.
127. Ingbar, S., and Woeber, K.: Mild hypothyroidism, metabolic insufficiency and decreased thyroidal reserve. In Williams, R. (ed.): Textbook of Endocrinology, 5th ed. Philadelphia, W. B. Saunders Co., 1974, p. 210.
128. Becker, D. V.: Tests of peripheral thyroid hormone action: Metabolic indices. In Werner, S. C., and Ingbar, S. H. (eds.): The Thyroid. Hagerstown, Md., Harper & Row, 1978.
129. DuBois, E. F.: Basal Metabolism in Health and Diseases. Philadelphia, Lea and Febiger, 1924.
130. Thompson, W. O., and Thompson, P. K.: Low basal metabolism following thyrotoxicosis. II. Permanent type without myxedema. J. Clin. Invest., *5*:471, 1928.
131. Braverman, L. E., Ingbar, S. H., and Sterling, K.: Conversion of thyroxine (T4) to triiodothyronine (T3) in athyreotic human subjects. J. Clin. Invest., *49*:855, 1970.

7

The Otomandibular Syndrome

HAROLD ARLEN, M.D., F.A.C.S.

In the "otomandibular syndrome" the patient complains of pain in and around the ear, fullness in the ear, hearing loss, tinnitus, and a loss of equilibrium. The patient may have one or more of the symptoms with no pathology in ENT examination and always has one or more of the muscles of mastication in a state of spasm. This chapter will describe this close relationship of disorder of mastication with disorders found in otolaryngology. The concept of an otomandibular syndrome will be described in terms of embryological development, symptomatology, and treatment.

EMBRYOLOGY AND ANATOMY

If we examine a cross-section of the head of an embryo of approximately 28 days, we find it composed of three parts—the pharyngeal or branchial arches, the pharyngeal pouches, and the branchial grooves or clefts. These parts of the human branchial system are best understood when considered from an evolutionary viewpoint. In fish and larvae amphibians, the branchial apparatus forms a system of gills for exchanging carbon dioxide and oxygen between the blood and water. The branchial arches form supports for the gills. The branchial apparatus develops in human embryos, but as no gills form, the branchial arches are the pharyngeal arches (Fig. 7–1). These are numbered in a craniocaudal manner, with the first one called the mandibular arch. The mandibular arch develops into two processes, the mandibular process and the maxillary process. The mandibular becomes the lower jaw and the maxillary becomes the upper jaw (Fig. 7–2).

From an evolutionary point of view, a double jaw was developed at the bony fish level, which developed into a structure called Meckel's cartilage. The dorsal end of Meckel's cartilage is closely related to the developing ear. It becomes ossified and forms the two middle ear bones, the malleus and the incus. The intermediate portion of Meckel's cartilage regresses and the

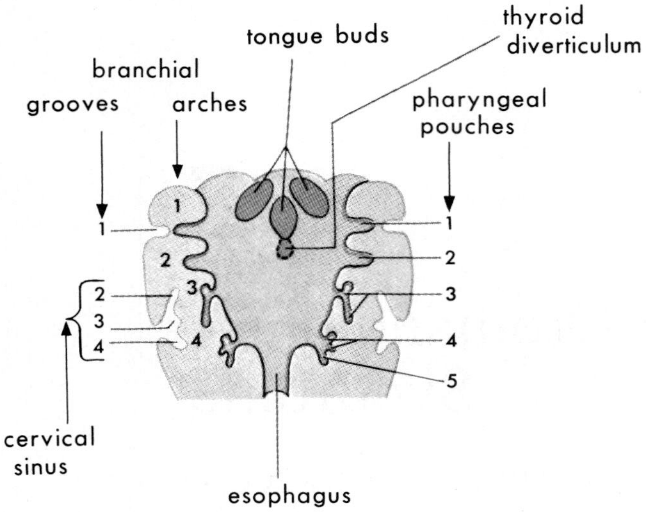

branchial
grooves   arches   tongue buds   thyroid
diverticulum   pharyngeal
pouches

cervical
sinus

esophagus

Figure 7–1. Adult derivatives of pharyngeal pouches. (From Moore, K.: The Developing Human. 2nd ed. Philadelphia, W. B. Saunders Co., 1977.)

perichondrium around it forms the anterior ligament of the malleus and the sphenomandibular ligament. The ventral portion of Meckel's cartilage disappears, and then by intramembranous ossification, a mandible develops.

The nerve of the mandibular arch is the trigeminal nerve. This nerve innervates the muscles of mastication, i.e., the temporalis, masseter, and both pterygoid muscles. It also innervates the mylohyoid and the anterior belly of the digastric. In addition to the muscles of mastication, the trigeminal nerve also innervates the tensor tympani and the tensor veli palatine muscles (Fig. 7–3).

The tensor tympani has its origin in the bony canal above the osseous portion of the auditory tube, adjoins the part of the greater wing of the sphenoid and the osseous canal in which it lies, and then, by a slender tendon which crosses the middle ear, distributes onto the neck of the malleus

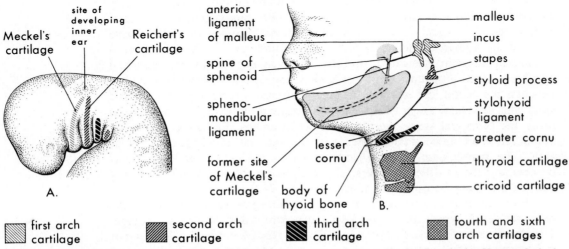

Figure 7–2. Head and neck region of a four-week-old embryo. (From Moore, K.: The Developing Human, 2nd ed. Philadelphia, W. B. Saunders Co., 1977.)

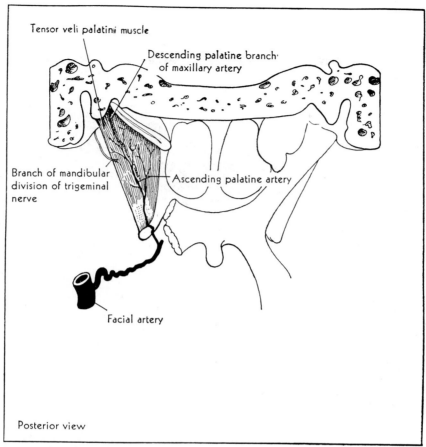

Tensor veli palatini muscle

Descending palatine branch of maxillary artery

Branch of mandibular division of trigeminal nerve

Ascending palatine artery

Facial artery

Posterior view

Figure 7–3. *Origin:* Scaphoid fossa and spine of sphenoid bone, lateral sides of membranous and cartilaginous portions of auditory tube. *Insertion:* Tendon winds around pterygoid hamulus and into aponeurosis of soft palate, posterior part of palatine bone. *Function:* Tenses soft palate, opens auditory tube during swallowing. *Nerve:* Small branch from mandibular division of trigeminal. (From Warfel, J.: The Head, Neck, and Trunk: Muscles and Motor Points, Philadelphia, Lea & Febiger, 1973).

(Fig. 7–4). The tympanic membrane is drawn medially upon contraction. The innervation of the tensor tympani is a branch of the nerve to the medial pterygoid muscle. In studying embryology, there are structures in the embryo called blastemas. The blastema gives off each structure in the human body. *The same blastema emerges as the tensor tympani muscle, as well as the medial pterygoid muscle.* This means that the same nerve that comes off the mandibular branch of the trigeminal innervates both muscles. The tensor tympani muscle is a remnant of that which moved the jaw at the reptilian stage, and it continues to maintain its identity with the fifth cranial nerve of the jaw apparatus. This suggests that early in embryologic development, neural patterns are established within the brain stem where the jaw bone and ear bone movements are integrated.

This is the key to the relationship between the jaw and ear dysfunction that is plaguing modern man, along with the deterioration of other parts of the jaw and dental apparatus. We really do not have to look for a mechanical impingement of the joint on a nerve. We simply look for a disturbance in neuromuscular function.

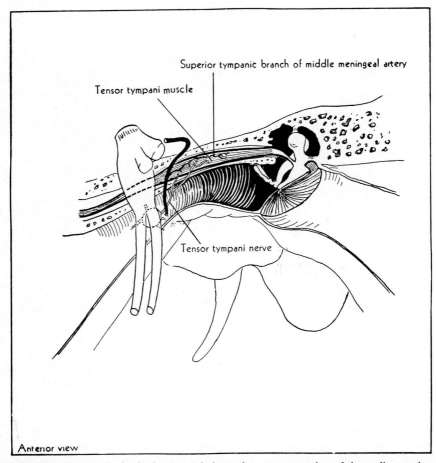

Figure 7–4. *Origin:* The muscle lies in the bony canal above the osseous portion of the auditory tube. Arises from cartilage of auditory tube, adjoining part of greater wing of sphenoid and osseus canal in which it lies. *Insertion:* By a slender tendon which crosses the tympanic cavity and inserts near the root of the handle of the malleus. *Function:* Tenses tympanic membrane by drawing it medially. *Nerve:* Branch of mandibular division of trigeminal through otic ganglion. (From Warfel, J.: The Head, Neck, and Trunk: Muscles and Motor Points. Philadelphia, Lea & Febiger, 1973).

The second muscle, the tensor veli palatini, is not related to mastication but is also innervated by the mandibular portion of the trigeminal. *This is the only muscle of the soft palate that is innervated by the trigeminal nerve, and it is also the only muscle which functions to open the eustachian tube.*

Excessive movement of the condyle can also be responsible for symptoms. Pinto[11] discovered a structure that resembles fibroelastic tissue with ligamentous qualities. It was found inserted into the neck of the malleus immediately above the anterior process and lying laterally to the chorda tympani nerve. This is not the tensor tympani muscle. The tiny ligament spreads from this point in a cone-shaped form forward, downward, and laterally, to insert into the medioposterior-superior part of the capsule and the meniscus of the temporomandibular joint. Therefore, movement of the capsule by grasping the exposed part of its posterior-superior border, or even movement of the meniscus of the temporomandibular joint, causes this tiny ligament, the ossicular chain, and the tympanic membrane to move.

SYMPTOMS

Patients with no demonstrable otolaryngological pathologic process and only a temporomandibular joint dysfunction generally have unilateral ear complaints. These complaints are pain, fullness, tinnitus, dizziness, and hearing loss. The patient generally points to an area just below the auricle and also says the pain seems to be radiating downward along the sternocleidomastoid muscle. Again, these symptoms are almost always *unilateral*. Patients have a difficult time actually locating the area of the pain. They explain that it is "deep" and may even·be found somewhere other than the ear, e.g., "in the neck." This is in sharp contrast to the ear symptoms that are found in most ear diseases, such as otitis externa or otitis media, in which the patient very carefully pinpoints the area of the pain. Pain due to mandibular movement is not a reliable sign for TMJ dysfunction, because it is also present in otitis externa and other definite ear diseases. As stated, pain in and around the ear is the most common symptom, but radiation to the temporal region, along with radiation along the ramus of the mandible, is also prevalent. Many patients complain of pain in the mastoid, in the posterior cervical region, and down to the shoulder. These are otlaryngological symptoms which motivate patients to come to the otolaryngologist rather than to the dentist. Fullness, blockage, or pressure sensations that are often felt cause these patients to say that they feel "something in the ear."

A high-frequency, hissing type of tinnitus is present in approximately one third of the patients.

Another symptom seen with great frequency is that of an abnormality of sound perception. This is described as a slight, episodic "waxing and waning" of sound.

Some patients have a subjective feeling of disequilibrium and nonspecific dizziness. Whe moving their head in different positions they feel off balance, but they do not show the typical vertigo associated with Meniere's disease or labyrinthitis.

EXAMINATION

Upon completion of the routine ENT examination, the otolaryngologist should then perform a TMJ examination. This consists of first examining the teeth to see if there is evidence of an obvious dental problem, such as missing teeth or loose dentures.

The first sign to be looked for is a deviation of the mandible upon opening and closing as follows:

1. Ask the patient to open his mouth. The patient with normal TMJ function opens and closes his mouth in straight up-and-down movement.
2. The jaw of the patient with TMJ dysfunction moves toward the affected side when the interincisal distance approaches 25 mm.

The area directly anterior to the tragus is then palpated bilaterally by the index finger, both in the closed and then the opened jaw position. A difference in sensation between one side and the other is a sign that there is a disease state either in the joint proper, such as arthritis, or in the function of the joint. Next, place the little finger in the external auditory canal with the fingernail facing posteriorly. Again, the patient is instructed to open and close the jaw. There are two signs to look for in this instance. One is pain or discomfort localized to one side. The other sign is an unequal abutment of the condyle against the finger. The side of greatest abutment is the side of the collapse.

During the jaw examination, abnormal sounds in the form of clicking or scraping should be listened for. If these sounds are not heard, then one should use a stethoscope directly over the joint. It is only with this examination that a joint could be considered noise-free and therefore more than likely without disease.

The most important aspect of the examination is palpation of the muscles of mastication. It is the spasm of one or more of these muscles that accounts for practically all the symptoms that these patients present to the otolaryngologist. (The examination for spasm of the medial pterygoid muscle is important because it indicates that the tensor tympani muscle is also in spasm. This helps account for the otological symptoms.)

The first intraoral muscle palpated is the medial pterygoid. It is palpated by pressing the finger laterally toward the medial surface of the mandibular ramus. The painful response of this muscle when in spasm is self-evident to both the patient and the examiner. Significant information is achieved by asking the patient to compare the two sides. In most cases, one side is much more painful than the other, thereby showing the side in spasm.

The same type of procedure is followed in the examination of the lateral pterygoid muscle. The index finger is placed in the upper buccogingival fold posteriorly to the maxillary tuberosity and then directed medially.

Two other muscles to examine are the temporalis and the sternoclei-domastoid. The whole temporal muscle is palpated carefully in the search for trigger points.

The sternocleidomastoid muscle, when palpated, generally has its tender point halfway between the sternum and the mastoid process.

There is no special order to be followed except that each clinician should develop a routine in order not to miss the palpation of an important muscle. The reader is referred to Chapters 3 and 11 for a complete discussion.

ETIOLOGY OF THE OTOMANDIBULAR SYNDROME

When dysfunction of the masticatory apparatus is present for any length of time, multiple muscles become spasmodic. Travell[4] has stated that this most common condition, which results in chronic muscular strain, predisposes the patient to muscle spasm. Another factor is a high-frequency barrage of noxious impulses, also resulting in chronic muscular strain. Therefore, it can be postulated that the tensor veli palatini is in spasm at the time that the muscles of mastication are in a chronic state of strain. Inasmuch as the tensor veli palatini is the only muscle that functions to open the eustachian tube, its dysfunction explains a large part of the otological symptomatology. This would include fullness in the ear, hearing loss, and disequilibrium.

In addition to dysfunction of the tensor veli palatini, spasm of the tensor tympani also contributes to the various otological symptoms already presented. Klockhoff and Westerberg[5] showed that impedance changes were caused by fluctuating tonic contractions of the tensor tympani muscle. This "tonic tensor tympani phenomenon" is associated with otalgia, a sense of fullness in the ear, tinnitus, hearing loss, disequilibrium, and a tension headache.

The otomandibular syndrome, with its above-mentioned symptoms, is present in the absence of the conventional clinical signs of middle ear pathology when spasm of one or more of the muscles of mastication manifests itself. It is generally the spasm of the medial pterygoid muscle that is responsible for the tonic tensor tympani syndrome inasmuch as they have exactly the same innervation.

DIFFERENTIAL DIAGNOSIS

At the beginning of this chapter it was stated that the problem of head and neck pain presented to the otolaryngologist was most difficult when the ENT examination was negative. However, another very difficult problem is the patient with definitive otolaryngologic disease combined with a disorder of the muscles of mastication. This results in a frustrating situation when the usual treatment does not reduce or eliminate the pain. At this point extensive tests are generally ordered because serious diseases are suspected. Therefore, it is essential that the already described examination be performed routinely on all otolaryngological patients either at the time of the original consultation or when the ENT pathology is resolved. If a patient is suffering from otitis externa, for example, it is impossible to perform an examination of the temporomandibular joint or the muscles of mastication.

OTOLOGICAL EXAMINATION

A review of the causes of pain in and around the ear will show the magnitude of diseases that are necessary to consider in a differential diagnosis. The external ear can show an external otitis, a foreign body in the ear canal, furunculosis, impacted cerumen, plus a host of other more remote diagnoses not to be considered within the scope of this volume. The middle ear or mastoid is painful in the presence of acute eustachian tube obstruction, acute otitis media, acute aero-otitis media, and acute mastoiditis. They can all result in complications which require the skills of an otolaryngologist for the diagnosis. One must also suspect a malignant or benign growth as well as the presence of a cholesteatoma. Diseases of the oral cavity, esophagus, and various other conditions, such as trigeminal neuralgia, sinusitis, and elongation of the styloid process can cause direct pain in the ear. One must also be aware of the referred causes of pain in the ear, such as from the larynx when cancer, ulceration, or arthritis of the cricoarytenoid joint is present. Another area could be from the pharynx, where there might be pharyngitis, tonsillitis, a peritonsillar abscess, or a retropharyngeal abscess.

The otolaryngologist, after physical examination of the ear combined with audiology, can generally diagnose the presence of cerumen, serous otitis media, otosclerosis, Meniere's disease, presbyacusia, noise-induced hearing damage, and the like in searching for the cause of a hearing loss.

If a patient complains of dizziness, it must be remembered that only a disturbance of the statokinetic system gives rise to true, whirling vertigo.

Dizziness can mean several things to the patient. A subjective sensation may be one of uncertainty, insecurity, giddiness, weakness, confusion, blankness, unsteadines, lightheadedness, or near syncope. If the statokinetic examination is within normal limits, such diseases as tabes dorsalis, pellagra, pernicious anemia, and cerebral anoxemia must be considered. Others might be hypoglycemia, petit mal, and a tumor of the cerebellopontine angle. The correct evaluation of a dizzy patient needs a broad approach, and the physician must be constantly aware of the possible influence of a systemic disease.

A feeling of fullness in the ear indicates an obstruction of the eustachian tube, which includes numerous possibilities. There would then be negative pressure in the middle ear cleft with or without effusion. These would include upper respiratory illnesses, sinusitis, and allergic rhinitis. In children, hyperplasia and chronic inflammation of the tonsils and adenoids or other lymphoid tissue in the nasopharynx, especially in Rosenmuller's fossa, can produce obstruction of the tube. However, the importance of spasm of the muscles of mastication in children in causing symptoms has not as yet been determined.

PSYCHOLOGICAL IMPRESSIONS

Patients with TMJ problems may have difficulty coping with other problems in their lives. Patients with TMJ dysfunction may be those who express their coping difficulties by tensing their muscles of mastication, e.g., by clenching and/or bruxing. It is also possible that they "tense" their tensor tympani muscles for significantly long periods of time when under stress. This could result in a complaint of an ear problem or a subjective experience of hearing loss in one ear. When stress is suspected as one of the factors resulting in a TMJ problem, the patient should be encouraged to obtain a psychological evaluation in order to determine the feasibility of relaxation training as an adjunct to dental and otological treatment nodes.

TREATMENT

The prime treatment factor is the release of any muscle spasm that might present. This can be done by dry needling, by the injection of saline, or by the injection of a local anesthetic into the trigger point of the muscles in question. The injection of a local anesthetic (always without epinephrine) appears to be the most effective. Generally 1 ml injected into a spasmodic intraoral muscle seems sufficient. The extraoral muscles, such as the temporal or sternocleidomastoid, for example, can be treated either by injection or by the use of galvinic stimulation. Any method that releases the muscle spasm is acceptable (Fig. 7–5).

The efficacy of the treatment is determined by the patient's subjective response. If pain is the presenting symptom, it is very often immediately relieved after the injection. The same can be true of other symptoms, such as hearing loss, disequilibrium, and the tinnitus. However, it must be made very clear to the patient that this relief is only temporary. If there is on one hand an occlusal problem, or, on the other hand, extreme emotional tension causing bruxism, for example, these factors have to be explained to the patient.

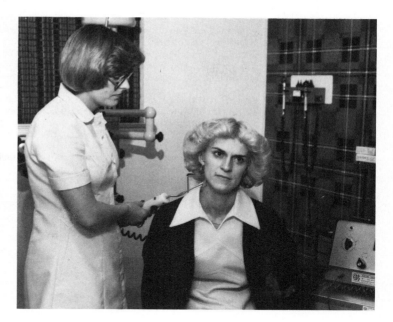

Figure 7–5. Releasing muscle spasm using electrogalvanic stimulation.

If the symptoms have been present for a great length of time with no previous relief, the gratitude of these patients is very satisfying to the clinician. The otolaryngologist, with the judicious use of proper consultation, should then determine whether dental and/or psychotherapeutic techniques are necessary for resolution of the problems.

CONCLUSION

A new otomandibular syndrome has been described in order to help explain otolaryngological symptoms in the absence of disease in the examination of the ears, nose, and throat. For both the dentist and the physician, the description of this syndrome can be extremely useful. It can guide the clinician toward a diagnosis that heretofore has been largely neglected. For the dentist, the aim is to broaden his thinking to include extraoral symptoms as being directly related to dental diseases. For the physician, the converse is true. Knowledge of this syndrome will orient the physician toward an expanded concept of etiology by including a possible dental explanation of the presenting symptoms.

Acknowledgment: Without the editorial assistance of Dr. Arthur L. Terr, this Chapter might not have conveyed all the aspects of the otomandibular syndrome.

References

1. Moore, K. L.: The Developing Human. Philadelphia, W. B. Saunders Co., 1973.
2. Paparella, M. M., and Shumrick, D. A.: Otolaryngology. Philadelphia, W. B. Saunders Company, 1973, vol. 2, p. 77.

3. Bernstein, J. M., Mohl, N. D., and Spiller, H.: Temporomandibular joint dysfunction masquerading as disease of the ear, nose and throat. Trans. Am. Acad. Ophthalmol. Otolaryngol., *73*:1208, 1969.
4. Travell, J.: Referred pain from skeletal muscle. N. Y. J. Med., *55*:331, 1955.
5. Klockhoff, I., and Westerberg, C. E.: The tensor tympani muscle and tension headache. Scandinavian Migraine Society. Proceedings. Annual Meeting. Uppsala, Oct., 1970. Sandoz, 1971.
6. Costen, J. B.: A syndrome of ear and sinus symptoms associated with disturbed function of the temporomandibular joint. Ann. Otol. Rhinol. Laryngol., *43*:1, 1934.
7. Sarnat, B. G.: The Temporomandibular Joint. Springfield, Ill., Charles C Thomas, 1951.
8. Gelb, H.: A review correlating the medical-dental relationship in the cranio-mandibular syndrome. N.Y. J. Dent., *41*:163, 1971.
9. Shore, N. A.: Occlusal Equilibration and Temporomandibular Joint Dysfunction. Philadelphia, J. B. Lippincott Co., 1959.
10. Schwartz, L.: Disorders of the Temporomandibular Joint. Philadelphia, W. B. Saunders Co., 1959.
11. Pinto, O. F.: A new structure related to the temporomandibular joint and middle ear. J. Prosth. Dent., *12*:95, 1962.

8

Does a "TMJ Personality" Exist?

HAROLD H. MOSAK, Ph.D.

INTRODUCTION

The temporomandibular joint syndrome has piqued the scientific curiosity of dental investigators for several decades, but only recently have psychologists devoted much attention to its understanding.

In part, this situation has existed because clinical psychologists until recently were trained in graduate programs in the diagnosis and treatment of psychopathology. The syndromes listed in the Diagnostic and Statistical Manual of the American Psychiatric Association held the attention of the clinical psychologist, while the study of "normal" people or even "normal" people with symptoms (e.g., the patient with TMJ dysfunction), was limited to psychologists whose atypical personal interests challenged them to wander into areas not treated in their curricula. A second reason for the relative lack of interest of the psychologist in the study of the TMJ syndrome was that one of the major theories of TMJ distress proposed that the source of the pain syndrome resided in some form of malocclusion. So explained, the problem was understood as being somatogenic and totally within the province of the dental, and sometimes medical, practitioner.

THEORIES OF TMJ SYNDROME

In surveying the literature it appears that there are three major families of theory that explain the syndrome and provide rationales for its treatment. The first family of theory, as already noted, describes the syndrome in purely physical terms. The root cause is usually understood to be an occlusive disorder with attendant muscular and facial-orthopedic components. Since treatment follows from theory, treatment has taken the form of grinding down teeth, splints, orthodontia, and equilibration. These interventions have been designed generally to eliminate the physical symptoms of the syndrome; it is anticipated that, with the elimination of these symptoms, the pain will subside or evaporate.

Psychological Status of the TMJ Patient

Yet anyone who has observed or treated the TMJ patient must be impressed with the patient's painful psychological situation. He is in chronic pain and often cannot eat or sleep. The ringing in his ears drives him to distraction. He has daily headaches, which render him nonfunctional. He is equally unable to work or to relax. He does not want to go anywhere or do anything and then feels guilty because he should want to. Depression has him in its grip; it clings to him like a wet shirt. In short order he becomes enveloped in his pain. It has achieved such a central position in his consciousness that he does not or cannot attend to life around him, and this failure or inability reinforces and exacerbates his guilt feelings and depression. In his self-absorption he alternates between the fear that he may be losing his mind and the unsettling half-certainty that he already has.

He becomes a cog in the health delivery system and is often passed from practitioner to practitioner, none of whom seems to help, at least on a permanent basis. He receives tranquilizers, which only dull the pain but give no permanent relief. He is treated physically but often to no avail.

His physicians give up, indicating that they have reached the boundaries of their, or perhaps anybody's, knowledge. The patient becomes confused, as one practitioner suggests that his teeth need building up with an appliance after another practitioner, at much expense to and discomfort for the patient, has just finished grinding them down. Thoughts of suicide are not uncommon as the patient wrestles with the unpleasant thought that only in killing himself will he find the solution for killing the pain. At some point, because of the intractability of the pain, he may be told, "It's all in your mind. It's nerves. Go see a psychiatrist or psychologist." Now the patient is caught in a dilemma. How can anything this painful be "all in my mind"? For some patients it merely confirms their worst fears about their mental health. Others reject the referral because they find a certain security in a physical diagnosis. For most patients there is something concrete about a physical condition, while the mind is a mystery. Moreover, psychotherapy is usually conceived (much of the time erroneously) by the lay public as a long-term procedure, and the TMJ patient wants immediate help. For this reason many patients are referred for hypnotic treatment in the hope that this will have more immediate results. For the patient who does seek psychotherapy the benefits are not only not immediately discernible, but he has now added an additional worry—how to pay for the treatment. His financial resources have become depleted as he has paid for dentists, physicians, medications, appliances, and even travel for medical purposes. In addition to the worry, he now must also incorporate the guilt for putting his family to so much expense when they could be using the money for their needs and pleasures.

The psychotherapist and the patient often work at cross-purposes. The patient wants to talk about his pain, while the therapist wants to discuss such topics as oedipal fixations, inferiority feelings, cognitive factors, and the patient's family and social life. Even when therapy proceeds smoothly, the psychotherapist, because of his training, very often has little understanding of pain and even less of the TMJ syndrome. He is ill-equipped to treat patients who cannot be described with such nomenclature as "obsessive-compulsive" or "schizophrenic."

In the light of all these experiences the patient feels anger toward the health delivery system, an anger he cannot easily afford to express directly because he is still dependent upon it. "With all the money I've spent, you'd think I'd have received some help by now. Am I being punished for something?" The litany is familiar to every practitioner.

Concurrent with his incorporation into and difficulties with the health care system, the patient both experiences and creates problems within the social sphere. As the psychiatrist Alfred Adler pointed out,[3] a person cannot be understood independently of his social context. Man operates not in a vacuum but in a social field. In this social field the patient becomes the center of attention of well-meaning friends, co-workers, and relatives, who initially provide sympathy, optimistic encouragement, and advice. "I have a friend who had the same thing you have, only worse." The patient, even if he devours the attention eagerly, is confused. He is pulled at from all sides. As he tries each suggestion in turn, his depression increases as in turn each fails to eliminate the pain.* Soon the world turns against the patient, and the patient turns against the world and himself. His friends tire of listening to him and his complaints. Not understanding the extent of his feelings of futility, they resent his not taking or acting upon their advice. They regard him as, and he indeed is, poor company. They shun him, and he feels like an outcast. His attempts not to complain leave him feeling miserable and still "out of it." He sits at home, an isolate in his own living room, unable to tell others about his feelings. "It won't help. They've heard it before a thousand times. I'm hopeless." There is no surcease. The patient sinks lower and lower into the mire of defeat.

If one were to discuss with patients their subjective feelings about the pain, one would find that the picture painted above is not overdrawn. A holistic approach requires that psychological factors be considered; the reductionistic theory based upon malocclusion fails to do justice to these psychological considerations. In this holistic view there is a suffering person who may or may not have an occlusive disorder. Adherents of the occlusive theory treat pain, while those advocating the following theories treat pain patients, a distinction made by Sternbach.[27]

This view has led to the development of two theories, both psychophysiological in nature. The first holds that there is a pre-existing TMJ personality, a personality which we might describe as pain-prone. Several investigators hold that psychological factors are more important than occlusal factors.[13, 16, 25] They consider the treatments of choice to be the prescription of muscle relaxants, psychotherapy, hypnosis, biofeedback, and behavior modification. Practitioners within this school of opinion rarely attempt treatment of the occlusive process itself. On the surface this position appears to be valid. We know, even in the absence of confirming research,

---

*I once had the opportunity to hear the story of a 21-year-old girl who had considered suicide because of her chronic excruciating pain. She had seen 200 physicians, dentists and psychiatrists (she offered to document this for me with their names) before obtaining relief from a holistic dentist.

that not all persons with malocclusions develop the TMJ dysfunction patient's symptoms. Observation tells us that people have varying pain thresholds as well as differing degrees of pain tolerance. At a deeper level within the context of this theory, it should be possible to distinguish one or more personality types or constellations whose experience of pain is greater than that of others. Mosak[21] has described a number of common life styles, among which "the controller" and "the victim" might a priori be considered especially vulnerable to pain and suffering. This classification of life styles will be used later in our study.

A second psychophysiological theory proposes that psychological factors do not *cause* the patient's responses to the TMJ condition but are instead the *consequences* of the syndrome. The proponents of this theory maintain that anyone who suffers from pain as intensely and constantly as the pain patient might be transformed psychologically into a pain patient by virtue of his subjective experiences. These two viewpoints constitute more than a "which came first, the chicken or the egg?" problem. The former point of view holds that a TMJ personality does indeed exist and, by implication, change in the personality configuration, perhaps through psychotherapy, must occur for the pain to be reduced. If one holds to the second theory, then, again by implication, alterations of the physical process should restore the patient to psychological stability. Following this point of view, treatment might consist of treating the occlusion by grinding the teeth, moving the teeth, equilibration and prostheses, treatment of various muscles or muscle groups,[12] or myofunctional therapy.[11] The correction of the existing physical factors, according to this view, would ameliorate or even eliminate the coexisting psychological symptomatology.

Which of these viewpoints is the more tenable is the question to which the present chapter addresses itself. Before proceeding, it is important to note that these viewpoints are not mutually exclusive. Some investigators believe that occlusal factors and personality factors join together in creating the condition,[14, 24] while others hold that the occlusal and personality factors combine and reinforce each other circularly so that a vicious circle is set up in which malocclusion (but not necessarily in terms of primacy) results in pain and stress, which results in greater tension and exacerbation of the malocclusion, which results in more distress and pain, and so on. Research becomes complicated.

METHODOLOGICAL CONSIDERATIONS

In mounting studies on these questions, several methodological considerations invite our attention. Previous studies fall into the following groups, according to the statistical treatment of the data:

1. Frequency studies. In this group of studies frequency of occurrence is the focus. We find statements such as, "In a sample of 75 subjects, 53 were found to . . ." and "78 per cent of the experimental group . . . while 22 per cent. . . ." Frequency count studies unfortunately tell us nothing about whether the results are statistically significant or could conversely have occurred through chance. If a large majority of the sample possesses some characteristic or trait, it is often assumed that the factor which has been isolated possesses an intimate or causal relationship to the variable under study. In a parody of such studies, Clifton illustrates the fallacy in attributing causality to such factors.[5] His paper, "The Dread Tomato Addiction," provides such astounding conclusions as 92.4 per cent of juvenile delinquents and 92.3 per cent of American Communists have eaten tomatoes. Furthermore, he states that:

... Those who object to singling out specific groups for statistical proof, require measurements within a total. Of those people before the year 1800, regardless of race, color, creed, or caste, and known to have eaten tomatoes, there has been 100% mortality.
... In spite of their dread addiction, a few tomato eaters born between 1800 and 1850 still manage to survive [in 1958], but the clinical picture is poor—their bones are brittle, their movements feeble, their skin seamed and wrinkled, their eyesight failing, hair falling, and frequently they have lost all their teeth.

2. *Measure of central tendency studies.* In nontechnical terms, the objective of these studies is to find an average of the variable(s) being studied. These measures do not lend themselves easily to the investigation of subjective variables (e.g., pain). We can measure optical deficiency or distortion and we can measure hearing loss, but the measures to elicit the intensity of pain still elude us. The use of mean scores presents further problems, since the mean may not resemble any datum within the group. Generations of students have joked about the average American family having 2.3 children. In a similar vein one psychology professor characterized the "average American" as "50% male, 9/10 white and only slightly pregnant." What is the "average TMJ patient" like?

3. *Test of significance studies.* Two groups, usually an experimental group and a control group, are compared in these studies. The usual methodology involves discovering variables on which one group scores higher than the other and then determining whether these differences are statistically significant or could have occurred in chance fashion. Many differences are found in comparing groups, and these differences are recorded in the literature as reaching high levels of significance. The nagging question which remains is whether the differences, though significant, are relevant. We might, for example, discover that TMJ patients have longer noses or smaller incomes than a control group might have, but what does this portend for the treatment of the patient? Should we shorten his nose or increase his income? Standen shows the absurdity of this type of argument.[26] "Executives," he writes, "have been found to have a large vocabulary; therefore, learn ten new words every day, and you will become an executive." Before the reader summarily dismisses the above as ludicrous, I should like to cite a study by Levitt and Lubin on the incidence of depression in a large population.[15] Among their conclusions is the following statement:

Investigations of depression are legion, but studies of its antithesis, happiness, are strikingly rare.... The happy person may be of either sex or any religion as long as he or she is well educated and well paid. Less satisfaction with one's life space is reported by those in lower socioeconomic strata.
In the ultimate analysis, a therapy for some forms of depression may be money.

Even when we discover that the difference between means approaches statistical significance, the results tells us nothing about the individual person. To know that the average income in the United States is greater than that in Italy does not permit us to make predictions about any single American or Italian.

4. Common factor studies. Overlapping with some of the categories above are the common factor studies. The thrust of these studies is to isolate a factor which the members of the investigated group share in common. If a group shares a germ in common or lacks an enzyme in common or shares an environment in common or exhibits commonality in some background factor, it is assumed that the commonly shared factor is a causative agent. The argument, Standen tells us, in principle, runs like this: a man gets drunk on Monday on whiskey and soda water; he gets drunk on Tuesday on brandy and soda water, and on Wednesday on gin and soda water. What caused his drunkenness? Obviously, the common factor, the soda water.[26]

5. Correlational studies. These studies measure the relationship between two variables. When two variables correlate, as one variable changes, the other changes in the same or the opposite direction, thus producing either a positive or a negative correlation. The most common error found in such studies is the one that students in introductory statistics classes make, i.e., to assume that correlation implies causation. Two variables may vary perfectly without a causal relationship existing between them. In studies where this error is committed and a causal relationship is imputed to be correlated variables, the author would still be confronted with the decision of whether variable A caused variable B or variable B caused variable A.

The above discussion is not intended to serve as a polemic against the use of statistics, nor is it a call to arms to dispense with them entirely. Only a note of caution is intended with respect to the understanding and use of statistics—that they be used responsibly and that the figures be treated not only as figures but as the products of underlying logical and mathematical rationales which can easily be abused. Bearing this in mind, the reader will observe that several of the above methods will be used in this study.

THE RATIONALE OF THE STUDY

Psychological tests very frequently are assumed to tap different levels of behavior, such as superficial, unconscious, or situational. The psychologist encounters the question of whether the test product elicited from the subject reflects the subject's enduring behavior, the core of his personality, or whether it reflects his behavior in "the here and now," behavior reactive to a current situation. For that matter, the test itself may be the immediate situation. More specifically, as it applies to the TMJ distress patient, is there a pre-existing personality disposition or is his distress reactive to the situation in which he finds himself? To explore this question we shall employ Alfred Adler's concept of the life style.[3, 4] Contrary to contemporary popular usage, which has diluted or distorted its meaning in such phrases as "the suburban life style" and "the hippie life style," Adler specifically limited his usage to the individual. Simply stated, the life style constituted the unique way in which every person perceives life and himself. Each life style contains the individual's convictions about his self and the environment *as he perceives them*. These convictions, all subjectively derived and therefore neither necessarily accurate nor in agreement with other people's perceptions, may be grouped in the following categories:

1. The self-concept. All convictions relating to the individual's self-perception and self-evaluation fall into this category.
2. The self-ideal. Convictions in this group take the format of "In order to have a place in life, I should (must). . . ."
3. The *Weltbild*. In this group we have convictions about life, the meaning of life, people, classes of people, and the physical environment.
4. The ethical convictions. These are the individual's conception of right and wrong and the consequences of doing right and wrong.

While people hold a large number of convictions, these tend to cluster around a central theme or themes.[20] Mosak[21] has described some of the more common life style central themes which will be used in the analysis of our data. Among these are the getter,[19] the controller,[17] the driver, the person who has to be right, the person who has to be superior, the person who has to be liked, the person who has to be good, the "aginner," the victim, the martyr, the baby, the inadequate person, the person who avoids feelings, the excitement seeker, and the social interest type.

One way in which the Adlerians determine the central themes in the life style is the interpretation of the person's early recollections.[2, 18] Adler,[3] in describing these as every person's "The Story of My Life," suggested that a process of selective retention in memory commits each of us to remember only those recollections from our childhoods which reflect our current postures toward ourselves and life. Thus, by examining a person's early recollections, we can determine the component convictions of the *enduring* personality. Since the life style crystallizes in the first six years of life and remains fairly constant after that, our analysis of early recollections provides a personality picture which is independent of current events. Some illustrations follow.

Getter. A friend gave me a doll. I was proud of it. It was a big doll I always wanted.

Controller. My brother took the emergency brake off my father's car. The car smashed into the garage.

Victim of others. My older brother crept into my crib and cut my hair off. When accosted by my mother, he said he was studying to be a barber.

Victim of self. I remember going to the beach and stepping on a jellyfish. I felt scared, petrified.

Baby. I was in a hallway in a crib, wet, cold, alone, and crying. It just seemed I was too old to be in a crib.

Right. The last day in the first grade all the parents came to see the children's achievements. I did something wrong and the teacher held me by the shoulders and shook me up. I was very upset.

To return to the present study, if TMJ distress were related to a pre-existing personality configuration, we should find that patients' early recollections distribute themselves within a single life style category or within a small number of such categories. If they do not distribute themselves in this manner, more likely inferences would be that (1) TMJ distress is independent of enduring or pre-existing personality variables, and (2) the distress which the TMJ personality experiences is the *result* of a physical process rather than the personality being distress-prone.

Forty-two subjects participated in this study, all of whom had been diagnosed as TMJ distress patients by dentists in a private practice.* As part of the initial diagnostic procedure, they were asked to relate their early recollections after being given the standard instructions.[18] While in clinical psychological assessment customary practice permits the patient to give as many recollections as he can, the patients in this study were limited to three recollections each. Table 8–1 gives the distribution of types for the recollections elicited.

While we might have expected 126 recollections to be given by 42 subjects, the total in Table 8–1 is at variance from the expected total because several subjects provided fewer than the three requested recollections, and several other subjects gave reports rather than recollections. The latter consists of a "One day I remember . . ." memory, while the former is of a more general nature, such as "I used to go to the movies every Saturday." While both provide useful data in psychodiagnosis, only the recollection may be used for determining personality type.[18]

Examination of Table 8–1 reveals that TMJ distress is not related to any single personality type. Seventeen different personality types are reflected in these recollections. Moreover, when we examine the 42 subjects rather than the 114 recollections, only eight subjects gave three recollections in the same category — two "pure" getters and one each of "pure" excitement seeker, center, special, need to be good, controller, and social interest types. We must conclude that TMJ distress patients do not cluster into any personality type categories in terms of psychogenesis. In spite of the group results, it is still possible, on the basis of these data, to entertain the hypothesis that, on an individual basis, a patient may unconsciously select the TMJ distress syndrome because it satisfies some element within his life style. Thus the victim may experience distress because he is, as a victim, distress-prone. The controller may suffer because the TMJ condition places life out of control, while the getter may use the syndrome in order to get attention, sympathy, special treatment or exemption from the tasks of life.[9, 10, 23]

*I am grateful to Dr. Harold Gelb and his staff for providing these patients for study.

TABLE 8–1.   Distribution of Early Recollections According to Personality Type

Controller	20
Getter	15
Need to be right	11
Center	9
Victim of others	9
Victim of self	7
Excitement-seeker	6
Observer	6
Social interest	6
Special	5
Baby	5
Need to be good	3
Inadequate	3
Confuser	3
Need to be superior	3
"Aginner"	2
Feeling avoider	1
Reports	17
No recollection	5
	136

TABLE 8–2.   Responses of 42 TMJ Patients to "The Question"

Somatic	19
Primarily somatic; partly psychological	4
Psychological	3
Primarily psychological; partly somatic	3
No answer	13
	42

Nevertheless, at this point in any analysis we have no conclusive information upon the question of somatogenesis or psychogenesis. A second study was conducted in an attempt to provide the answer to this question. In ordinary medical practice, differential diagnosis is generally performed through exclusion. If all the physical possibilities are ruled out, the patient may be informed that "It's all in your mind" or "It's your nerves." Diagnosis by exclusion is not conclusive, since the absence of physical findings merely tells us that no physical basis has been found, not that a physical cause may not exist. A substitute for this form of differential diagnosis consists of making a diagnosis upon the basis of purpose. The assumptions underlying such diagnosis are (1) that all behavior is purposive and that (2) somatogenic symptoms will have a somatic purpose, while psychogenic symptoms will have a psychological or social purpose. Derived from these assumptions, Adler formed "The Question,"[1, 6, 7, 8] which invites patients to respond to the question, "If I had a magic wand or magic pill which would eliminate your symptom(s) immediately and irrevocably, what would be different in your life?" If the patient answers, "I would go to school, travel, maybe become an LPN," the symptom would most likely be psychogenic. If the patient replies, "I wouldn't have to worry about chewing or eating" or "I wouldn't be dizzy with pain I couldn't tolerate," then the symptom is most likely somatogenic. The results are generally conclusive in distinguishing organic from psychological, with the exception of those symptoms which are somatogenic with a psychological overlay (e.g., cardiac neurotic symptoms) and psychological symptoms with organic sequelae (e.g., hysterical paralysis with subsequent atrophy).

When the 42 subjects of this study were asked "The Question," their responses could be categorized as in Table 8–2.

Of the 29 subjects who responded, 19 (66 per cent) replied in ways which indicated that their syndrome was somatogenic. If we add to this the number of those whose replies were primarily somatic, the percentage increases to 79.3 per cent. If we consider all situations in which a somatogenic component occurs, the percentage rises to 89.7 per cent. In only 10 per cent of the responses was the psychological component emphasized, although if we add mixed answers (primarily psychological, partly somatic), the percentage of all answers in which a psychological component occurs increases to 20.6 per cent.

DISCUSSION

The results of these two experiments would suggest that the TMJ distress syndrome is in most instances somatogenic. In 80 per cent of the subjects studied, the physical factor assumes predominance. Whether this physical factor is orthopedic, malocclusive, muscular, or caused by deviate swallow I leave to dental practitioners to determine. Cases for each have already been made in the literature. There is no evidence of a monolithic pre-existing TMJ personality, nor did we discover a small number of such vulnerable personalities.

Psychological symptoms associated with the TMJ syndrome appear to be the patient's response not only to the physical pain but also to his loss of the sense of mental well-being, to his deteriorating social situation, and to "the run-around I get from dentists and doctors." In this light the personality picture which the patient presents appears to be reactive to the condition rather than the cause of the condition. These reactions, however, may be selected unconsciously by the patient on the basis of his pre-existing life style as well as on a situational level. Thus, for example, the person with the life style of a victim may seize upon this syndrome to reinforce and reconfirm his conviction that life is out to victimize him. The controller may utilize his symptomatology to express how catastrophic it is when things are not in control.

On the surface it would seem that, granted these conclusions, the practitioner ought to direct his attention toward correcting the physical situation, intending that, as a consequence, the psychological symptoms would disappear. However, good practice transcends good theory. The patient is unconcerned with the issue of whether his symptoms are somatogenic or psychogenic. He knows he hurts; he feels that "the pain is killing me," and he would like to be free of his pain yesterday. For this reason the initial step of the practitioner should be directed toward alleviation of the pain. This can be accomplished through drugs, mechanical corrections, hypnosis, suggestion, and other methods. The preferences of the practitioner and the response of the patient will determine the method or combination of methods employed.

Since the psychological symptomatology is reactive in most cases, "here-and-now" therapy rather than major personality reconstruction might be a concurrent procedure for the holistic dentist. While the dentist or physician may not be a psychotherapist, he may still be able to provide psychotherapeutic assistance for his patient. There are three necessary (but not sufficient) conditions for any psychotherapy—faith, hope, and love or caring.[22] Even the practitioner untrained in psychotherapy can provide these ingredients. He can inspire faith, enhance hope, and show the patient that he cares. This posture, accompanied by whatever physical procedures the practitioner may deem most appropriate, may in many instances suffice. In refractory cases or cases requiring greater attention, or when the patient himself is moved to seek more "answers" about the self, referral for psychotherapy ought to be made. When the latter is done, both therapists should maintain close communication. Again, my preferences lie in the direction of avoiding long-term, intensive, insight psychotherapy for most patients in favor of therapy of brief duration aimed at changing the patient's reactions rather than the core of his personality. In auto mechanics' language, it may not be necessary to overhaul the engine; wiping the spark plugs or a good tune-up may be all that is required.

References

1. Adler, A.: Problems of Neurosis. New York, Harper Torchbooks, 1964.
2. Adler, A.: Significance of early recollections. International Journal of Individual Psychology, *3*:283, 1937.
3. Adler, A.: What Life Should Mean to You. New York: Capricorn Books, 1958.
4. Ansbacher, H. L.: Life style: a historical and systematic review. J. Individ. Psychol., *23*:191, 1967.
5. Clifton, M.: The dread tomato addiction. Astounding Science Fiction, *60*:97, 1958.
6. Dreikurs, R.: Can you be sure the disease is functional? Consultant (Smith, Kline & French), August, 1962.
7. Dreikurs, R.: Organic or functional disorders: a diagnostic aid. North Chicago, Ill., Abbott Laboratories, 1958, pp. 8, 9.
8. Dreikurs, R.: A reliable differential diagnosis of psychological or somatic disturbances. International Record of Medicine, *171*:238, 1958.
9. Dreikurs, R., and Mosak, H. H.: The tasks of life. I. Adler's three tasks. Individ. Psychologist, *4*:18, 1966.
10. Dreikurs, R., and Mosak, H. H.: The tasks of life. II. The fourth life task. Individ. Psychologist, *4*:51, 1967.
11. Garliner, D.: Myofunctional Therapy. Philadelphia, W. B. Saunders Co., 1976.
12. Gelb, H. et al.: The role of the dentist and the otolaryngologist in evaluating temporomandibular joint syndromes. J. Prosthet. Dent., *18*:497, 1967.
13. Laskin, D. M.: Etiology of the pain-dysfunction syndrome. JADA, *79*:147, 1969.
14. Lerman, M. D.: A unifying concept of the TMJ pain-dysfunction syndrome. JADA, *86*:833, 1973.
15. Levitt, E. E., and Lubin, B.: Depression: Concepts, Controversies, and Some New Facts. New York, Springer, 1975.
16. Lupton, D. E.: Psychological aspects of temporomandibular joint dysfunction. JADA, *79*:131, 1969.
17. Mosak, H. H.: The controller: a social interpretation of the anal character. In H. H. Mosak (ed.): Alfred Adler: His Influence On Psychology Today. Park Ridge, N. J., Noyes Press, 1973, pp. 43–52.
18. Mosak, H. H.: Early recollections as a projective technique. J. Projective Techniques, *22*:302, 1958.
19. Mosak, H. H.: The getting type: a parsimonious social interpretation of the oral character. J. Individ. Psychol., *15*:193, 1959.
20. Mosak, H. H.: The interrelatedness of the neuroses through central themes. J. Individ. Psychol., *24*:67, 1968.
21. Mosak, H. H.: Lifestyle. In A. G. Nikelly (ed.): Techniques For Behavior Change. Springfield, Ill., Charles C Thomas, 1971, pp. 43–52.
22. Mosak, H. H.: Adlerian psychotherapy. In R. J. Corsini (ed.): Current Psychotherapies. Itasca, Ill., F. E. Peacock, 1979, pp. 44–94.
23. Mosak, H. H., and Dreikurs, R.: The life tasks. III. The fifth life task. Individual Psychologist, *5*:16, 1967.
24. Ramsfjord, S. P., and Ash, M. M.: Occlusion, 2nd ed. Philadelphia, W. B. Saunders Co., 1971.
25. Schwartz, L. L.: Disorders of the Temporomandibular Joint. Philadelphia, W. B. Saunders Co., 1968.
26. Standen, A.: Science Is A Sacred Cow. New York, Dutton, 1950.
27. Sternbach, R. A.: Pain Patients: Traits and Treatment. New York, Academic Press, 1974.

9

Radiology and Radiography of the Temporomandibular Articulation

PART I: RADIOGRAPHY OF THE TEMPOROMANDIBULAR JOINT

Paul Scheman, D.D.S.

PROBLEMS AND SOLUTIONS IN VIEWING THE TMJ

Many authors and investigators have maintained that the articulation of the human temporomandibular joint constitutes the following two sets of surfaces: (1) the glenoid fossa and the capitulum (ginglymoid motion); and (2) the posterior-inferior surface of the tuberculum and the superior-anterior surface of the capitulum (arthrodial motion).[1-4] Many authors have maintained that the ginglymoid portion of the joint movement is in the glenoid fossa.[1-4] This is also considered the "centric" position of the capitulum.[5] The greater part of published radiographic interpretations of this joint accept this view as correct, and moreover measure and describe "condyle-fossa relationships" as a basis for arriving at a diagnosis and treatment plan for disease and dysfunctions of this joint.[6,7] On the other hand, there is the opinion that considers this to be a biconvex grinding joint with an interposed stabilizing biconcave disc.[8] Some writers have conceded that the glenoid fossa is not a functioning part of the articulation;[9,10] however, the concept of a "condyle-fossa relationship" persists. Even the bizarre opinion that the temporomandibular joint is the only one in the body that habitually "dislocates" has been expressed.[11,12] These views, if incorrect, are to the detriment of clinical practice and application.

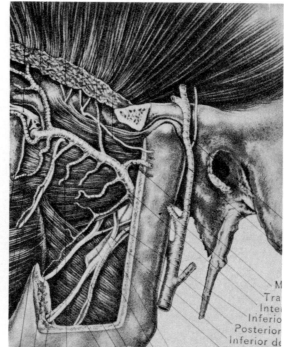

Figure 9–1. Dr. John B. Deaver, M.D., represented the disc (meniscus)* as concavo-convex, but that was in 1904. His view has the virtue of consistency. There are many more contemporary illustrations that represent the meniscus as biconcave but still insist that the capitulum articulates in the glenoid fossa. (From Deaver, J.: Surgical Anatomy. Philadelphia, P. Blakiston and Sons, 1904.)

---

*The word meniscus is the Greek diminutive for moon, "meniskos." This referred to a little or crescent moon which the disc would be if it were concavo-convex, as above.

Consider the following:

1. If the condyle articulates in the glenoid fossa, why is it that the interarticular disc is biconcave? For an articulation in which one element is concave (glenoid fossa) and the other convex (condyle, capitulum), the disc should be concavo-convex (Fig. 9–1).

2. Articulating surfaces should be covered with histologically appropriate fibrocartilage. This is absent in bone forming the glenoid fossa, but it is present in the articular eminence (tuberculum) and the condyle (capitulum) (Fig. 9–2).

3. Bones involved in articular movement should contain bony trabeculation capable of a directional response to the demands of functional stresses, i.e., specific directionality to reduce the impact sustained in function and dysfunction (a feedback mechanism) (Figs. 9–3, 9–4).

In the famous Chase photomicrograph of the TMJ these contradictions are apparent as long as the figure is viewed as it is usually printed (Fig. 9–5). If, however, the illustration is rotated as shown, all the contradictions disappear and we are presented with a biconvex joint (Fig. 9–6). The joint in this view consists of the condyle (capitulum) articulating with the articular eminence (tuberculum), and now the following characteristics are apparent:

1. The interarticular disc *is* a biconcave disc.

2. The articulating surfaces *are* covered with articular fibrocartilage, thicker over the surfaces most subject to functional pressure and thinning away over surfaces of lesser or no functional pressure.

3. The trabeculations of the tuberculum (articular eminence) and the capitulum (condyle) *are* as one would expect to find them in functioning forcebearing bones in an articulation.

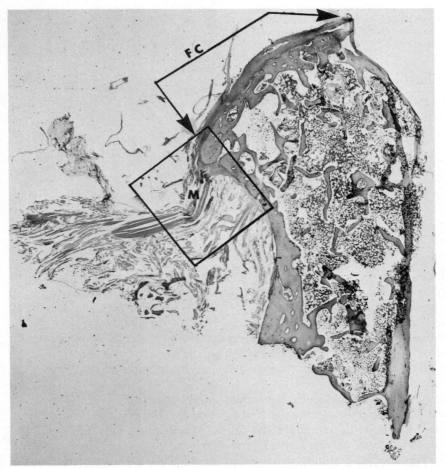

Figure 9–2. This section demonstrates the distribution of an articular type of fibrocartilage over the anterior face of the capitulum, FC. Note the integral insertion of the inferior belly of the external pterygoid muscle into the bone of the capitulum (M) (magnification × 5).

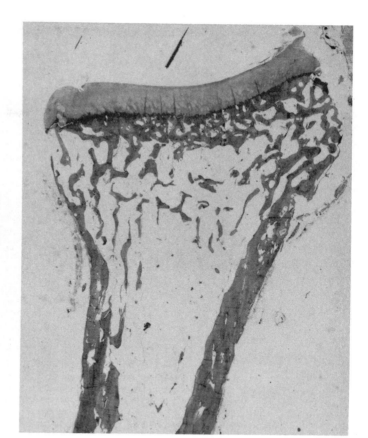

Figure 9–3. This section of a terminal phalanx of the hand illustrates the directionality of the bony trabeculae well. Note the alignment of the trabeculae to brace against the forces applied to the bone (magnification × 5).

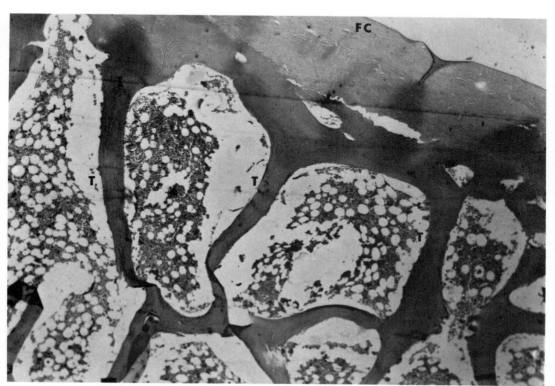

Figure 9–4. This part of a section of the capitulum of a TMJ illustrates the same principle as seen in Figure 9–3. The articular fibrocartilage (FC) is the reference plane, to which it may be noted the trabeculae (T) are perpendicular (magnified × 25).

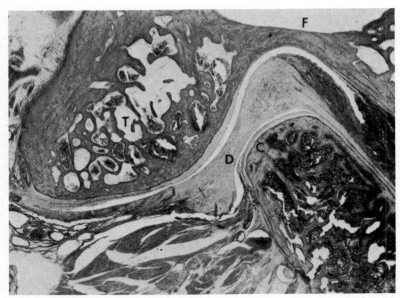

Figure 9–5. The famous photomicrograph by S. W. Chase, which gives the appearance of a "condyle-fossa relationship." However, note the contradictions: the tuberculum (T) and the capitulum (C) show functional trabeculations. The fossa (F) does not. The bone surfaces opposite the disc (meniscus) (D) are covered with fibrocartilage except in the area of the fossa (F), where there is a thin periosteum. These contradictions disappear if the photo is rotated as it is in Figure 9–6.

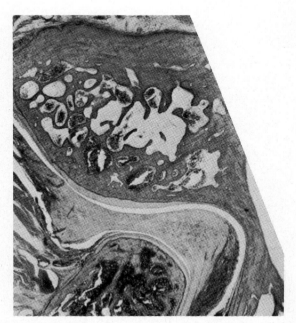

Figure 9–6. Viewed as a biconvex articulation with an interposed biconcave disc, all the contradictions as noted in Figure 9–5 disappear.

EXPERIMENTAL EVIDENCE THAT THE TMJ IS A BICONVEX JOINT WITH A BICONCAVE DISC

Investigations by the author are reviewed here to establish, on independent experimental grounds, that the TMJ is a biconvex joint.

CONGRUENCE OF ARTICULAR SURFACES

Not all joints necessarily have congruent (reciprocally matching) surfaces. In those that do, the congruency is the result of the functional relationship of the surfaces. In sections of dry specimens in which there is indisputable interdigitation of an intact dentition, it has been demonstrated that the surfaces of the capitulum and tuberculum are congruent but that the capitulum and fossa are not. Statistically, congruence of the capitulum and tuberculum is highly significant.

This study was done to determine objectively whether the articulating surfaces could be identified by means of congruence which is observed to exist between tuberculum and capitulum in PA radiographic views of the joint. Fossa-capitulum outlines in such views have not been visualized with equal precision. The hypothesis tested was that the joint surfaces which function together should have congruent curves along a frontal plane. Capitulum-tuberculum surfaces appear to be congruent; however, the capitulum and fossa likewise appear to be functionally related when the dry specimen is viewed from many angles. This study attempted to measure these contours by means of a contour gauge in order to test whether the contours derived from the capitulum are congruent with those derived from the fossa or those derived from the tuberculum.

Materials and Methods

Fifty human skulls (dry specimens) were examined, and of these, sixteen were selected for measurement. The criteria of selection were based upon whether the mandible belonged to the skull to be measured. This was determined by an examination of (1) the interdigitation of the teeth; (2) the matching of wear facets; and (3) the absence of any alternative intercuspation. These were accepted as evidence that the mandible and cranium were from the same person. Measurements on these selected specimens were made to determine separately the long axis of (1) the glenoid fossa, (2) the tuberculum, and (3) the capitulum. After the long axis had been determined and marked, a contour gauge was pressed into the surface along this axis and the curve so generated was traced on paper. Fossa curves were labeled F, tuberculum curves were labeled T, and capitulum curves were labeled C (Figs. 9–7 to 9–12).

A biometrician determined the congruence of these curves by two methods. The first method involved the superimposition of the original curves with photo-copies of the same curves when placed upon a transilluminator. The second method was accomplished by measurement and comparison of the radii of the curves. The biometrician was not aware of the origin of the curves nor of the purpose of the measurements.

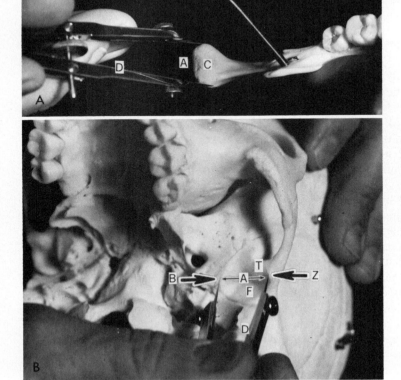

Figure 9–7. *A*, The dividers (D) measure the long axis (A) of the capitulum (C). *B*, The maximum distance from the lip of the articular facet on the zygoma (Z) to the lip of this facet on the temporal bone (B) measures the tuberculum (T). A similar measurement is made for the more posteriorly placed glenoid fossa (F).

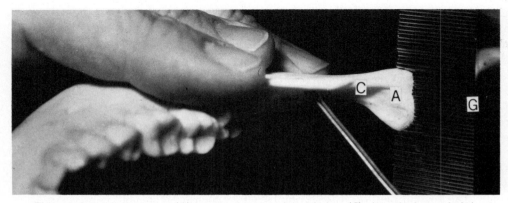

Figure 9–8. A contour gauge (G) is pressed against the capitulum (C) along the long axis (A).

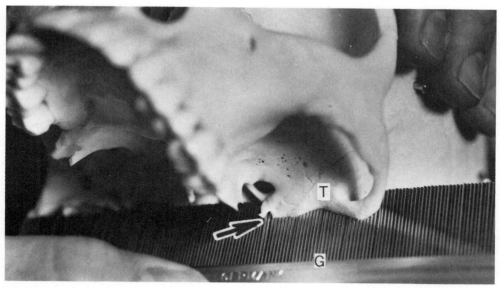

Figure 9–9. A contour gauge (G) records the curve of the tuberculum (T) along the longest axis. The same process is repeated for the glenoid fossa.

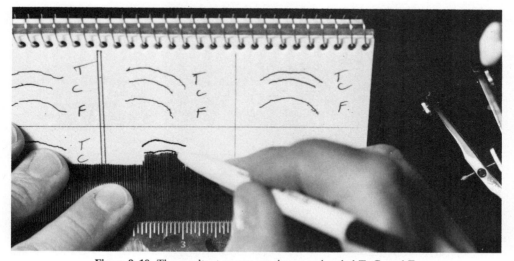

Figure 9–10. The resultant curves are drawn and coded T, C, and F.

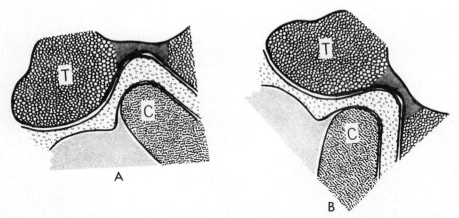

A

B

Figure 9–11. *A*, This tracing of an actual sagittal section of a human TMJ is shown in the conventional orientation. The capitulum (C) appears to articulate in the glenoid fossa. *B*, Rotation of the same tracing 30° as indicated gives the appearance of a capitulum-tuberculum (C-T) articulation with an interposed biconcave disc (see Fig. 9–6).

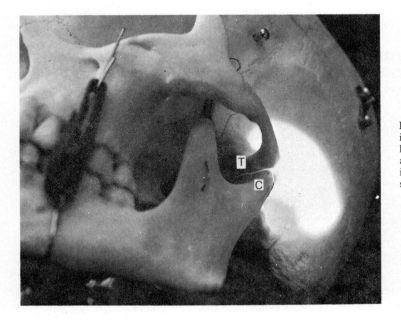

Figure 9–12. Note the specially illuminated view of the tuberculum (T)–capitulum (C) relation and the precision of the conformity of the interface of the joint surfaces.

TABLE 9–1. Data Derived from Comparison of Curves of Tuberculum, Capitulum, and Fossa by Means of Superimposition and by Measured Radii

Number of Measurements	SUPERIMPOSITION Congruence	% of Total	Number of Measurements	T = tuberculum F = fossa C = capitulum RADII Congruence	% of Total
60	T ~ C	57	54	T ~ C	57
16	T ~ F	15	15	T ~ F	16
29	F ~ C	28	26	F ~ C	27

Total: 105 measurements

P < .001   P < .001

Results

Using the above two methods, a congruence was shown to exist between the curves generated by the tuberculum and the capitulum. In all sets of measurements the data were significant. By the chi square test, P was less than 0.001. No such relationship could be shown to exist between the capitulum and the glenoid fossa (Table 9–1).

DIRECTIONALITY OF TRABECULATIONS IN THE JOINT SURFACES

As has been shown by Fukuda and Yasuda[21] and also by Frost,[22] directional alignment in the formation of bone trabeculae results in a structure which tends to reduce the effect of applied stress. This feedback mechanism gives strength to bones in the direction of stress, and thus reduces or resists applied forces. In this investigation, only the tuberculum and capitulum show this reactive phenomenon. The fossa is often a coalescence of tables of cortical bone from the middle cranial fossa and extracranial surface of the temporal bone (Fig. 9–5).

THE IDEAL TMJ RADIOGRAPH

The actual relationships in the TMJ are not easily demonstrated with present radiographic techniques. Since the capitulum and tuberculum have variable inclinations in three planes, one would have to know these in advance in order to correct the angulation of the incident ray to obtain a true cross-section of the structures.

Tomography may also permit us a more nearly correct representation of the structures of the joint. In tomographic methods, cycloidal tomographs have superior capabilities and need to be explored for use in dentistry. At the present time, PA projections and conventional tomography as well as lateral projections are useful to rule out intrinsic bone disease, but they are of little or no value in functional-dysfunctional studies. Thus, understanding the actual articulating surfaces of the TMJ is important to selecting the radiographic "window" that will produce a diagnostically productive radiograph.

Since the surfaces that are involved in continuous function, and therefore bear the stresses, are the antero-superior surface of the capitulum and the postero-inferior surface of the tuberculum, the most productive view would be taken through a port that is parallel and common to both. If the joint is viewed as two reciprocally rotating cylinders, as in an old-fashioned laundry wringer (which it is, on strong evidence), the ideal port would be parallel to the interface of the surfaces and along the long axis of the capitulum and tuberculum.

The problem that has faced TMJ radiographers, as has been stated, is the selection of a method of predetermining the inclination of the tuberculum and capitulum in three planes. It is well known that the wide variations in inclinations of these structures do not permit one to preselect "average" angles, if one has the objective of making a functional diagnosis, that is, the interpretation of mandibular or condylar position or malposition as recorded in a radiograph. If one is interested in intrinsic disease of the bony structures of the joint flat plates, however, even here there is extremely important information to be derived from a radiograph including tomography that is parallel to the functional surfaces. The yield of positive findings is greatly enhanced because the surfaces involved in functional stresses are brought into maximal view.

In actual practice an excellent compromise is to establish the angle of the capitulum (condyle) to the midsagittal by means of a vertex projection and of the frontal plane angulation by means of a PA projection. Lateral flat plate radiographs corrected for these angles will provide the needed "parallel window." Tomograms taken with these corrections will also show sections of the functional faces of the tuberculum and capitulum. Some investigators of radiographic techniques use only the vertex projection, which has the advantage of reducing the amount of x-ray exposure, and it is to be recommended for this reason. When this is done, a downward angle of 15° is used to avoid superimposition of the sphenoid bone and the petrous portion of the temporal bone.

THE MYTH OF JOINT SPACE MEASUREMENTS

In some published papers, the condyle-fossa relationship is seen as one involving the "joint space."[23] Measurements of the "anterior joint space" and "posterior joint space" determine whether the condyle is retruded, protruded, or otherwise displaced.[24, 25]

According to the method, the ideal to be achieved is a uniform joint space, and a dental treatment plan is designed to do this.

In fresh autopsy specimens the normal "joint" space as determined by measurements of discs is uneven. The joint space is a function of disc thickness, since the disc occupies the entire space. Hence, it is impossible for "uniform joint spaces" to be anything but an artefact (Fig. 9–13).

CONCLUSION

Since experimental evidence has been presented, some conclusions are in order.

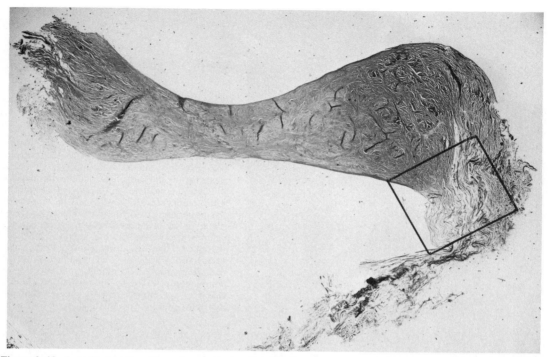

Figure 9–13. A sagittal section through an articular disc (meniscus). This section through the midplane indicates a marked variation in thickness in the anterior, left edge of the disc, the middle, and the posterior edge marked here with a square to indicate the bilaminar zone. It can be seen that the concept of an even anterior and posterior joint space is impossible when one considers that the joint space and the thickness of the meniscus are practically identical (magnification × 10).

The temporomandibular joint is a biconvex joint with a biconcave interarticular disc. This can be proven experimentally. Conventional TMJ radiographs are useful in ruling out intrinsic bone disease but are of little or no value in the determination of joint function or dysfunction. The concept of repositioning the condyle in its fossa so that even joint spaces are produced on an x-ray is faulty for two reasons. First, the condyle-fossa relationship does not exist as a functional entity. Second, the disc which occupies the entire joint space is uneven normally so that the joint space, assuming it can be correctly shown in radiograph, would be uneven (Figs. 9–14 to 9–24).

In this connection, the following is of interest. Chayes states: "The principal danger in interpretation of such films is the temptation to establish a geometric norm." "The presence of simple narrowing of a joint space without any other findings," Taueras maintains, "should be interpreted with caution. Such 'narrowing' may be nothing more than an artefact caused by the particular projection used . . . ." (Figs. 9–25 to 9–27).

By using different projections such as the Towne projection, it is possible to see the entire superior margin of both condyles and the margins of both glenoid fossa at the same time. In this way, the actual width of the joint space can be more definitely determined. It must be noted that even this fundamentally correct statement can relate only to the joint space in one plane (frontal).

Text continued on page 211

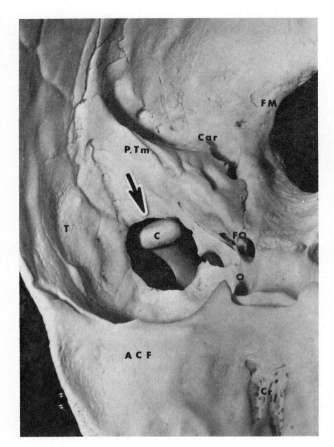

Figure 9–14. A view of the middle cranial fossa: (T) the temporal bone, (P.Tm) the petrous portion of the temporal bone, (FO) the foramen ovale for the passage of the mandibular division of the fifth cranial nerve, (O) the optic foramen. The anterior cranial fossa is at the bottom of the photograph (ACF). (Cr) is the cribriform plate. In the posterior cranial fossa the carotid canal (Car) and the foramen magnum (FM) are identified. Note the arrow pointing to the capitulum (C) which may be removed with the overlying structures containing the entire joint complex intact. This is done when the brain is taken in an autopsy and was the method by which the specimens in this study were obtained.

Figure 9–15. The block specimen taken through the middle cranial fossa is viewed from the inferior (caudal) side. The capitulum (C) with its attached superior belly of the external pterygoid muscle (Ps) has been turned out of the inferior surface of the meniscus or disc (D), with its attached inferior belly of the external pterygoid muscle (Pi). Note that this lettering (Pi) lies over a fascial separation between the two bellies and required little dissection to effect the separation. Note the cavity of the disc which is an accurate impression of the condyle and into which the condyle fits without intervening space. The middle third of the internal maxillary artery (A) is seen running in the fascial separation between the inferior and superior bellies of the external pterygoid muscle. This is further evidence that these bellies may have independent functional capabilities.

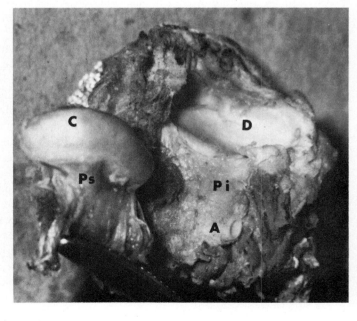

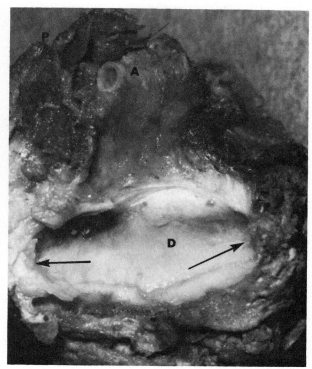

Figure 9–16. A close-up view of the under surface of the articular disc (D), showing the "condylar" shape of this structure. Note the internal maxillary artery (A) and the adjacent inferior belly of the external pterygoid muscle (P). Also, note on the right side that its attachment extends far to the medial of the articular disc. This arrangement gives this muscle enhanced effectiveness in lateral movements of the mandible. The arrow on the left points to the area of the lateral ligament, while the right arrow points to the medial insertion of the pterygoid muscle.

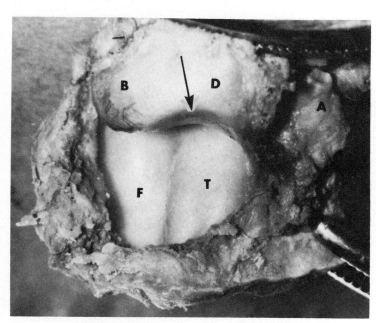

Figure 9–17. The articular disc has been peeled off and is held by a clamp (top). This is a view of the bony part of the TMJ. (T) is the tuberculum. Note the concave under portion of the articular disc (D) (arrow), which conforms to the tuberculum. Note the posterior edge of the disc proximal to the bilaminar zone (B) which completely fills the glenoid fossa; hence this space cannot be occupied by the capitulum. See Figure 9–18 for the location of the capitulum in this anatomical scheme.

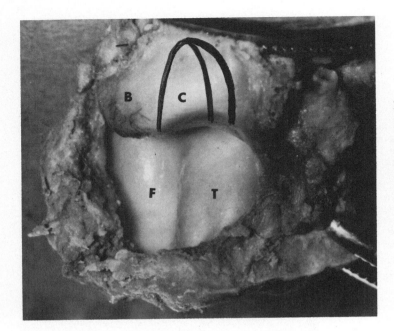

Figure 9–18. This is the same view as Figure 9–17, with a drawing of the relationship of the capitulum to the articular disc (C). Note that the bulbous bilaminar zone area (B) of the articular disc will fill the glenoid fossa (F) so that the capitulum lying in its closely fitting compartment in the underside of the articular disc will be in functional relation to the tuberculum (T) and not to the fossa (F).

Figure 9–19. The cranial portion of the temporomandibular articulation is seen here with the temporal portion of the zygoma (Z); the articular tubercle (A) is often a misnomer for the tuberculum (T). The fossa (F) is seen here to contain many foramina which coincide with the many blood vessels contained in the bilaminar zone, as can be seen in Figure 9–20. Note the tuberculum (T) is a cylindrical structure to match the cylindrical structure of the capitulum.

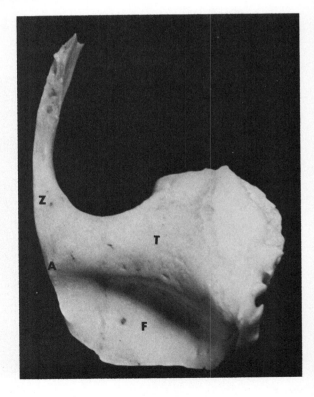

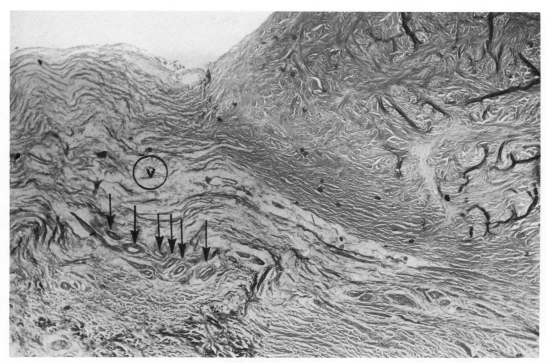

Figure 9–20. The posterior portion of the articular disc showing the numerous blood vessels (circled V and arrows) that are found in this region. There are also nerves in this region, not visible here but made apparent through the use of the specific stains. The articular disc itself, particularly in the stress-bearing areas related to the capitulum and tuberculum, are devoid of blood vessels and nerves. Compare with Figure 9–13.

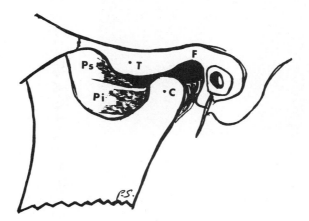

Figure 9–21. A diagram showing the relationships described in the text and in the preceding figures. The articular disc is shown in solid black, completely filling the space between the tuberculum (T) and the capitulum (C). The fossa (F) is filled with the posterior bulbous portion of the articular disc and the bilaminar zone of the disc. Note the superior (Ps) and the inferior (Pi) bellies of the external pterygoid muscles and the interval that separates them. This is usually a clearly-demarcated fascial zone. This diagram may be used to orient the succeeding anatomical dissections.

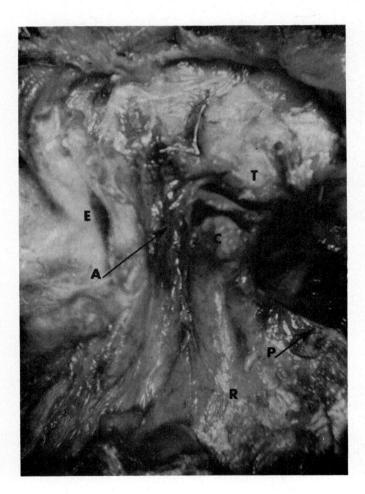

Figure 9–22. A dissection of the temporomandibular articulation in a fresh autopsy specimen shows the capitulum (C) and the tuberculum (T) as two bulbous elements in a biconvex joint with an interposed biconcave articular disc (meniscus). To orient the view please note the external auditory meatus (E) and the superficial temporal vessels (A). The articular disc (unlabeled here) divides the joint cavity into an upper and lower synovial cavity. The coronoid process (P) has been cut off the ramus (R) in order to apply pressure to distract the joint, thus exposing the synovial cavities, which ordinarily are only potential spaces.

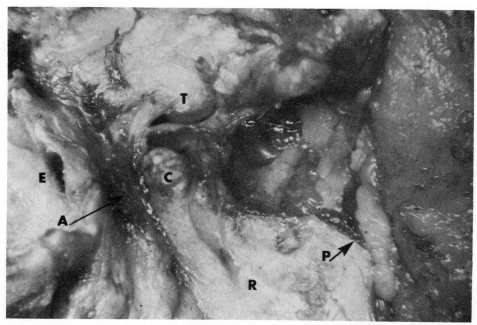

Figure 9–23. The same dissection of a fresh autospy specimen is seen from a different angle. Here the view is looking up onto the under- or condylar surface of the disc (unlabeled). One also sees part of the undersurface of the tuberculum (T). Note how much it resembles its counterpart, the capitulum (C). Here one can clearly see the conformity of the concavity of the articular disc to the capitulum (C) and similarly its concave adaptation to the convexity of the tuberculum (T). Again for orientation, (E) is the external auditory meatus, (A, arrow) points to the superficial temporal artery and vein, (R) is the ramus, and (P, arrow) is the cut coronid process that permits pressure to open up the joint spaces.

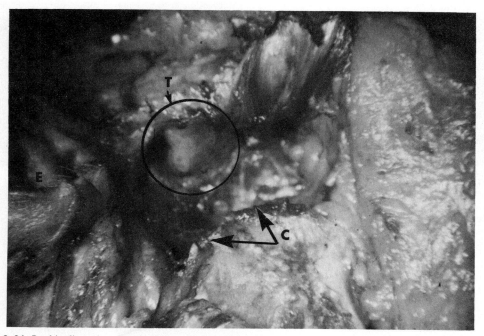

Figure 9–24. In this dissection of a fresh autopsy specimen, both the coronoid process and the condyle have been removed (C, double arrows). This inferiorly angled photograph shows the articular portion of the temporomandibular joint supplied by the cranial part. The tuberculum (T, encircled) shows a configuration of this articular surface that closely resembles the envelope of motion that has been generated by instruments attached to the mandible. Note also that, in spite of this shape in its essential geometry, it is a cylindrical structure. The external auditory meatus is labeled (E).

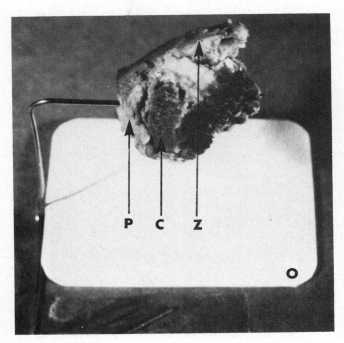

Figure 9–25. This photograph shows an intact block taken from a fresh autopsy specimen via the intracranial approach previously described (Fig. 9–14). The block is mounted so that it may be rotated around the pin and radiographed through a 360° range, thus duplicating all of the possible angles for TMJ radiography and some of the clinically impossible ones. These latter nevertheless provide interesting and useful information. (P) is the posterior edge of the block, (C) is the capitulum, and (Z) is the zygoma. (O) is the occlusal film which completes the experimental set-up.

Figure 9–26. These radiographs were produced by the method illustrated in Figure 9–25. In view (A) we see the capitulum and the adjacent tuberculum in close relationship. Note the dark space behind the capitulum. This is the unoccupied fossa that is filled with the posterior portion of the articular disc. In view (B) the capitulum lies beneath the tuberculum and the glenoid fossa is seen as a radiolucent space. In view (C) the capitulum and tuberculum are viewed as if seen in a PA view, which this in fact is. Note the precision with which the contours of these joint elements are harmony. The interval between them is a very good representation of part of the joint space. It is the only view that is closest to actual anatomical fact. View (D) completes the rotation and demonstrates how it is possible to prove that the capitulum lies in the glenoid fossa. Note that view (A) represents an anatomically correct position, as can be seen by the proper orientation of the zygoma. In all these views the zygoma may be used to orient the radiographs.

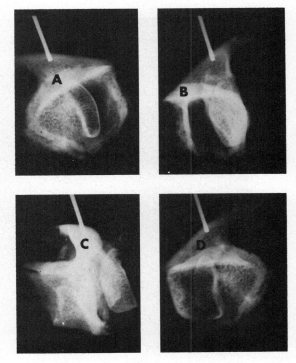

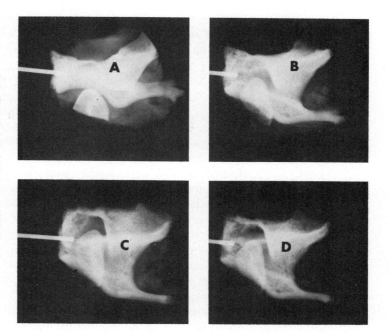

Figure 9–27. These radiographs demonstrate the results obtained from rotations using an incident ray which is directed laterally to the block. In (A) there appears to be a clear relationship of the capitulum to the tuberculum, while in views (B), (C), and (D) the "condyle-fossa" relationship varies from the conventional view in (B) to exaggerated ones in (C) and (D). It is important to note that these two-dimensional views can only be understood when the anatomy of the joint is thoroughly understood and the radiograph correctly interpreted. The radiograph has no independent validity outside of this synthesis.

BASICS IN TMJ RADIOGRAPHY

There are many who feel that any description of what appears in TMJ radiographs is only a description of what no one but the describer sees. A return to x-ray basics may be the beginning of an answer.

Some of the problems in interpreting radiographs of the TMJ are the result of a lack or lapse of understanding of the fact that x-rays of these and other joints produce an image in one plane which is really a projected translucency of all the calcified elements of the joint. The basic rules governing the apparent x-ray shapes and dimensions are as follows:

1. The part nearest the film appears smaller (or more nearly its actual size), while the part farthest from the film will appear enlarged.

2. Our appreciation of the actual three-dimensional appearance of a structure will be based upon our prior knowledge of the structure. Hence, correct and precise anatomical preknowledge is a critical factor. Consider the optical exercise in Figure 9–28. Note that the smaller face of the cube

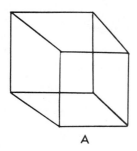
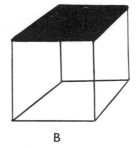
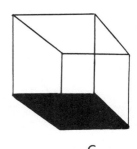

A   B   C

Figure 9–28. *A,* This is a diagram of the radiograph of a cube. The smaller face is closest to the film. In *B* we are free to interpret this as a cube seen from above or, in *C,* as a cube seen from below. Both *B* and *C* could be a valid interpretation of *A.* The distinction can only be made by the preknowledge that this is a cube; hence, the smaller face would be closer to the film.

(A) is closest to the film, but this can be interpreted as a cube seen from above B or as a cube seen from below C. Either B or C could be a valid interpretation of A. We would of course have to know the angulation of the incident ray in order to interpret the x-ray image. Knowing the general anatomical shape of the object in advance would permit us to develop a plastic three-dimensional visualization by a process of mental synthesis. As our experience increases, we learn to distinguish the dimension of depth in radiographic images and to note deviations from normal. The condyle is a three-dimensional object, and by first following the denser cortical outline of the articular facet on the anterior face of the condyle, we can then visualize its medial and lateral poles as well as the neck. We can also reconstruct the articular eminence by means of its known relationship, even though it is less distinct. Stereoscopy is helpful in this regard, although it is not usually employed. Consider the stylized shapes resembling the geometrical configurations of a condyle shown in Figure 9–29.

The following exercise will illustrate the principle under consideration. Stare at these two drawings; by relaxing your accommodation (i.e., staring through the page) you will be able to fuse the two images and produce a three-dimensional image of this "condyle." There will appear to be three images, but stare at the middle one. You will then see a three-dimensional figure and be able to distinguish the parts that lie nearer to you and those that are farthest from you. If you knew the angle from which an x-ray of such an object was taken, you would be able to determine the actual inclination of the object and its actual shape, provided that no distortion had been introduced other than the one dictated by the distance of surfaces from the film. Some of these would be caused by incident rays markedly divergent from the source (non-parallel, i.e., the result of a short cone technique), angulations other than those along the long axis of the object, or unknown angulations making interpretation difficult and often impossible. Other factors such as under-penetration (low voltage), over-penetration (high voltage), and fogging caused by excessive scatter will also reduce the diagnostic and interpretive quality of the radiograph. These are mentioned not to exhaust the knowledge on this subject but to indicate some of the

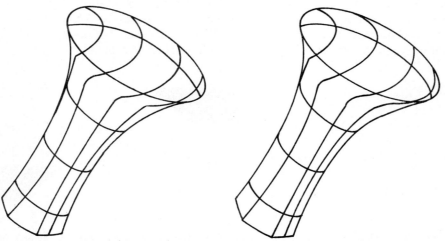

Figure 9–29. A stereoscopic pair of conventionalized "condyles." Consult the text for the technique of visualizing a three-dimensional effect.

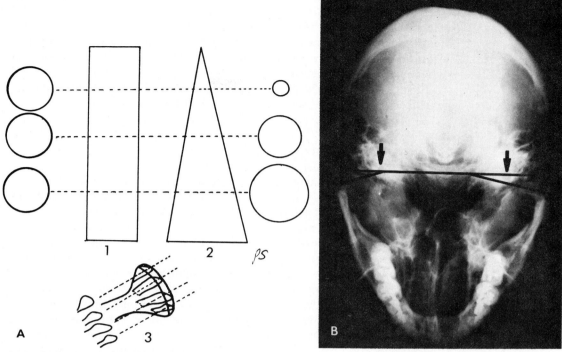

Figure 9–30. *A,* These diagrams illustrate the basic concepts of radiographic interpretation and of tomography. 1, 2, and 3 are, respectively, radiographs of a cylinder, a cone, and a condyle. We can tell from the sections of each what they are in three dimensions, provided we can preselect the correct axis. Sections, actual or radiographic by means of tomography, must be perpendicular to this axis. For example, other sections at other than right angles to these objects would not produce sections from which the true solid could be deduced. The cylinder would produce ellipses, the cone, conic sections including parabola and hyperbola and ellipses. *B,* In order to produce an image of the capitulum that will represent a true cross-section of the capitulum the following technique is suggested. A preliminary vertex projection is taken. The carotid canals are joined by a straight line, as illustrated. Lines intersecting this base line are drawn through the long axes of the condyles. The angle thus formed is the angle of correction of the tomograph. A vertical angle of fifteen degrees will overcome superimposition of structures. This corrected tomograph will permit a more reliable interpretation of the bony surfaces of the capitulum.

problems which limit the accuracy and reliability of TMJ radiographic interpretation.

Another way of dealing with the problem of interpreting a one-plane image as a three-dimensional structure is to radiograph one selected plane at a time, as in tomography. The synthesis of the structure is achieved by reassembling the separate sections. In this system the focal point chosen is the center of rotation of an axis which joins the point of origin of the x-ray and the film. Consider the geometric figures shown in Figure 9–30*A*; represented on a plane they are a triangle and a rectangle. Tomography would enable us to visualize the triangle, because of its array of diminishing circles, as actually being a cone, while the rectangle with sections of the same-sized circles would be visualized as a cylinder. Similarly, sections of the condyle would be seen as a series of irregular contours which together make up the complex three-dimensional head of the mandible (capitulum). These sections, combined with the usual "flat film," would complete our visualization of a capitulum. The tuberculum is more difficult to visualize, mainly because it is a less dense bone. In exposures which provide correct penetration for the capitulum, only its denser cortical margins appear.

Nevertheless, with practice it too may be visualized and its contours traced. Attempts at three-dimensional visualization in the interpretation of TMJ radiographs have been conspicuously absent in the literature. It has been totally replaced by a single-plane concept relating the condyle to the fossa, and this has resulted in measurements of an artefact as a real joint space, as we have already demonstrated.

Figures 9–31 to 9–36 illustrate radiographic and tomographic views of the TMJ; gross anatomy is shown in Figures 9–37 and 9–38.

THE PRINCIPLE OF TOMOGRAPHY

Tomography, or planigraphy, is a method of producing a radiograph in which a selected plane is in focus on the film while those above and below it are blurred. This is accomplished by linking the source of the x-ray and the film and rotating them around a center of rotation. The center of rotation is selected to coincide with the depth of the plane to be kept in focus. By adjusting the center of rotation, the plane in focus may be varied in depth. To accomplish this, the x-ray tube and the film carrier are yoked together by a rigid bar or C-frame so that their motion is synchronous; the center of rotation of the entire assembly is therefore identical with the depth of the selected plane. This simple arrangement has many variations involving complex cycloidal movements, but the principle involved in all tomography is the preselection of a focal plane and the synchronous movement of source and film. This is a result of the fact that when the x-ray source and the film

Text continued on page 219

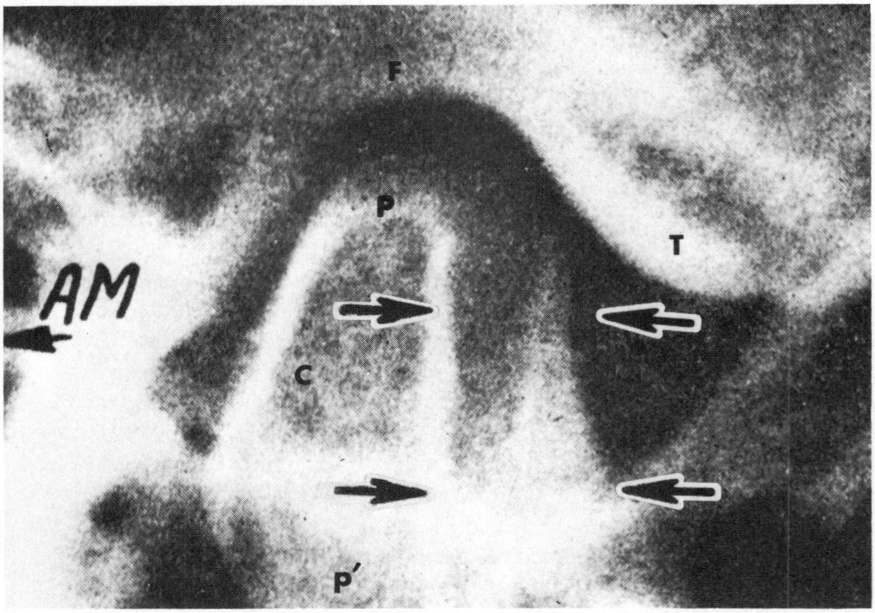

Figure 9–31. A TMJ radiograph which appears to show the relationship of the capitulum (P) to the glenoid fossa (F); actually, (P) and (P′) are poles of the capitulum (condyle) seen from above. However, (P′), the lower pole in this radiograph, is not included in the film. The actual areas of the functioning articulation lie between two parallel planes standing perpendicular to the arrows. (AM) is the auditory meatus, as labeled in the original radiograph. (From Weinberg, L. A.: Temporomandibular joint function and its effect on centric relation. J. Prosthet. Dent., *30*:176, 1973. Reprinted by permission)

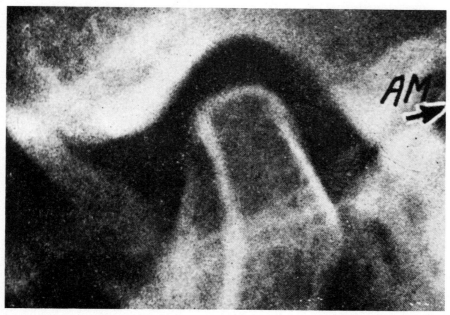

Figure 9–32. An otherwise excellent radiograph of the TMJ, which clearly shows the condyle with its lower pole missing and demonstrates that this is a projection of three-dimensional structures whose relationship on a flat plane cannot be taken on its own merit. (From Weinberg, L. A.: Temporomandibular joint function and its effect on centric relation. J. Prosthet. Dent., *30*:176, 1973. Reprinted by permission.)

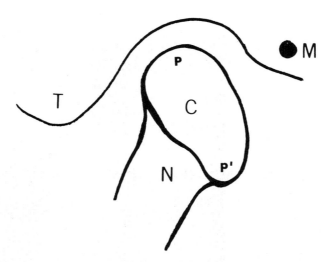

Figure 9–33. Diagram which may be used to orient Figures 9–31 and 9–32. Here the two poles (P) and (P′) of the condyle (C) as well as the neck (N) are drawn. (C) represents the articular facet which articulates with a similar and congruent facet on the articular tubercle (T), which is not drawn here for clarity.

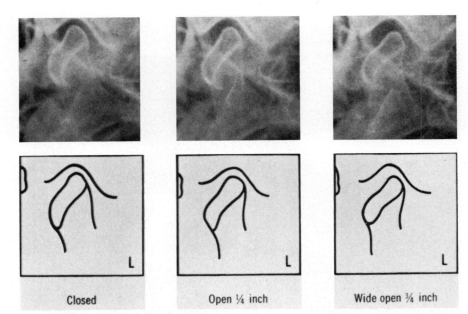

Closed   Open ¼ inch   Wide open ¾ inch

Figure 9–34. These radiographs and the accompanying diagrams illustrate what is seen when the conventional TMJ radiographs are taken so that the entire condyle, tuberculum, and fossa area are included. Notice the radiographic appearance of slight movement as the frames from L to R are compared. This is because the movement is taking place in a plane roughly parallel to the viewer; hence it is minimized. There is obviously no relation between the degree of opening, one-quarter inch and three-quarters inch, and the incremental change in the so-called joint space, which should appear as a ratio of 2 to 1. (From Morgan, D. H.: Mandibular joint pathology. Dent. Radiogr. Photogr., *43*:1, 1970. Reprinted by permission.)

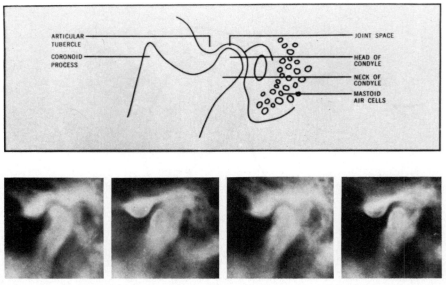

Figure 9–35. Tomography illustrates the changing shape of the condyle and its relationship to the articular eminence (tuberculum). Note the marked differences in the so-called "condyle-fossa" relationship. Tomography corrected for the horizontal angle of the capitulum (condyle) would have produced more valid cross-sections of the capitulum-tuberculum relationships. (From Coin, C. G.: Tomography of the temporomandibular joint. Dent. Radiogr. Photogr., *47*:2, 1974. Reprinted by permission.)

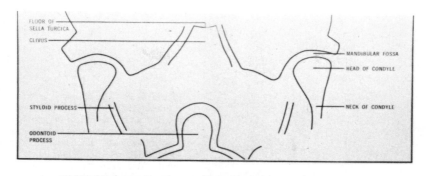

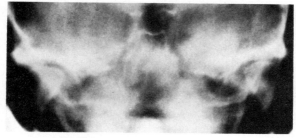

Figure 9–36. Such a posteroanterior view is most useful in visualizing the joint space. See the diagram above in which it is incorrectly labeled "mandibular fossa." Actually the glenoid fossa would lie above these structures and in this radiograph would be masked by the tuberculum. Note, however, the congruence of the convexity of the capitulum and the tuberculum. (From Coin, C. G.: Tomography of the temporomandibular joint. Dent. Radiogr. Photogr., *47*:2, 1974. Reprinted by permission.)

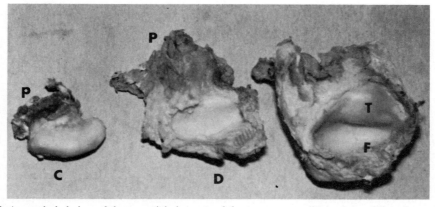

Figure 9–37. An exploded view of the essential elements of the temporomandibular joint. (C) is the capitulum with its attached pterygoid muscle (P). Note the articular face of the condyle which exactly fits the lower compartment of the disc (meniscus) (D). Note the attachment of the inferior belly of the external pterygoid (P). The surface beneath the meniscus in the middle structure in this photograph is shaped concavo-convex. The convex portion fits into and occludes with the glenoid fossa while the concave portion fits the convexity of the tuberculum. The functional relationship thus achieved through the interposed biconcave disc is to stabilize and permit complex movements of a biconvex joint.

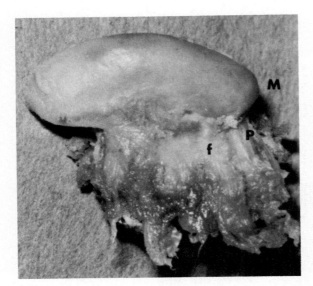

Figure 9–38. The anterior articular facet of the capitulum (condyle). Note the medial extension of the inferior belly of the pterygoid muscle (P), which permits the execution of complex lateral and rotatory movements. The meniscus (disc), as can be seen in the previous figure, has a similar attachment. Also note (f), the clear fascial separation between the inferior belly and the superior belly, thus providing independent movement of condlye and meniscus.

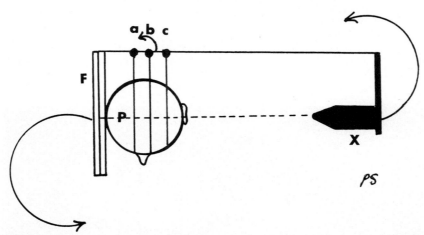

Figure 9–39. This diagram illustrates the basic principle of tomographic radiography. Two familiar elements are present, the film plate (F) and the x-ray source (X). The indispensable patient is labeled (P). The x-ray source and film plate are yoked together so that they can rotate as a unit. As the curved arrows indicte they rotate reciprocally. The various centers of rotation are indicated by the small letters (a, b, and c). Where these intersect the dotted line of the incident ray in this diagram there is no movement with respect to the incident ray and the film. All other planes are blurred; hence, by selecting the point of rotation of the linked x-ray source and film plate we can select the sectional plane to be radiographed. In TMJ radiography this would consist of several exposures, starting with a plane just below the skin and ending with a plane approximately 3 cm. below the skin. Depending on the amount of information desired consistent with safe exposures, one can reconstruct a three-dimensional record of the joint radiographically. The absence of superimposition enhances the diagnostic qualities of the radiograph for the purpose of visualizing changes in the surface of the bony structures as well as radiopaque or radiolucent changes in the bodies of the bone.

are rotated around the object radiographed only the center of rotation will be stationary with respect to the source and the film. Any plane above or below it will be in relative motion and hence cause blurring (Fig. 9–39).

It is also possible to arrange the film in a multiple stack array and simultaneously obtain a range of views. Many do not realize that the various devices for producing a panoramic view of the dentition of the mandible and maxillar are tomographic devices and reproduce a preselected section through these structures, not a flat film (i.e., superimposition of all planes of the solid structures).

References

1. Woodburne, R. T.: Essentials of Human Anatomy, 2nd ed. New York, Oxford University Press, 1961, p. 221.
2. Romanes, G. J.: Cunningham's Textbook of Anatomy, 10th ed. London, Oxford University Press, 1964, p. 226.
3. Grant, B. J. C.: A Method of Anatomy, 5th ed. Baltimore, The Williams and Wilkins Co., 1952, p. 704.
4. Gray, H., and Goss, C. M.: Anatomy of the Human Body, 28th ed. Philadelphia, Lea and Febiger, 1968, p. 300.
5. Nagle, R. J., and Sears, V. H.: Denture Prostheses. St. Louis, The C V. Mosby Co., 1962, p. 47.
6. Merrill, V.: Atlas of Roentgenographic Positions, 3rd ed. St. Louis, The C. V. Mosby Co., 1967, p. 326.
7. Jacobi, C. A.: Textbook of Anatomy and Physiology in Radiologic Technology. St. Louis, The C. V. Mosby Co., 1968, p. 148.
8. Hjortsjo, C. H.: Studies on the Mechanics of the Temporomandibular Joint. Lunds Universitets Arsskrift, *51*:2, 1954.
9. Sarnat, B. G.: The Temporomandibular Joint, 2nd ed. Springfield, Ill., Charles C Thomas, 1964, p. 31.
10. Moss, M. L.: Functional Anatomy of the Temporomandibular Joint. In Schwarz, L.: Disorders of the Temporomandibular Joint. Philadelphia, W. B. Saunders Co., 1966, p. 87.
11. Pillmore, G. U.: Clinical Radiology. Philadelphia, F. A. Davis Co., 1946, p. 222.
12. Bailey, H.: Physical Signs in Clinical Surgery. Baltimore, The Williams and Wilkins Co., 1960, p. 91.
13. Sullivan, W. E.: The function of articular discs. Anat. Rec., *24*:49, 1922.
14. Scheman, P.: Anthropoid comparisons of the anatomy of the external pterygoid muscles of the fetal and adult domestic pig. J. Dent. Res., *46*:1337, 1967.
15. Nørgaard, F.: Arthrography of mandibular joint. Acta Radiol., *25*:679, 1944.
16. Jacobsen, H. H.: On the normal arthrogram of the mandibular joint. Acta Radiol., *27*:93, 1946.
17. Gillis, R. R.: Roentgen-ray study of the temporomandibular articulation. JADA, *2*:1321, 1935.
18. Upedegrave, W. J.: Temporomandibular articulation x-ray examination. Dent. Radiogr. Photogr., *26*:41, 1953.
19. Petrilli, A., and Girley, J. F.: Tomography of the temporomandibular joint. JADA, *26*:218, 1939.
20. Ricketts, R. M.: Various conditions of the TMJ as revealed by cephalometric laminography. Angle Ortho., *22*:98, 1952.
21. Fukuda, E., and Yasuda, I.: On the piezoelectric effects in bone. J. Appl. Physics, *3*:117, 1964.
22. Frost, H. M.: Bone Dynamics in Osteoporosis. Springfield, Ill., Charles C Thomas, 1966.
23. Farrar, W. B., and McCarty, W. L.: Anterior dislocation of the disc (abstract). American Academy of Craniomandibular Orthopedics, 2nd Annual Meeting, New Orleans, 1976.
24. Weinberg, L. A.: Temporomandibular joint function and its effect on centric relation. J. Prosthet. Dent., *30*:176, 1973.
25. Weinberg, L. A.: Technique for temporomandibular joint radiographs, J. Prosthet. Dent. *28*:284, 1972.

PART II: RADIOLOGY OF THE TEMPOROMANDIBULAR JOINT

Arnold Berrett, M.D.

Whenever the clinician is faced with a suspected temporomandibular joint problem, an x-ray examination must be included as part of the total evaluation of the patient. Some of the x-ray methods employed will be described as follows.

RADIOLOGIC INVESTIGATION OF THE TMJ

CONVENTIONAL RADIOGRAPHY: TRANSCRANIAL OR TRANSFACIAL

The TMJ is usually evaluated by means of conventional films. Unfortunately, this method is of limited value and should be utilized with a great deal of caution. From a technical point of view, the TMJ is one of the most difficult parts of the body to visualize clearly by means of x-ray films. Clear demonstration of the TMJ is very hard to accomplish because superimposed structures interfere with visualization. This important fact is not appreciated by most dentists. In addition to the problem of superimposition with conventional x-ray techniques (transcranial or transfacial), some anatomical structures are distorted while others are elongated. Also, the clinician must keep in mind that normal variations in different invididuals compound the problem. Even with special head-holding devices for immobilization, comparable x-ray films are difficult to obtain. Because of the numerous difficulties encountered, some dentists omit any type of x-ray examination. Furthermore, the newer and more sophisticated x-ray methods are frequently not readily available to most practicing dentists. From a practical point of view, however, it is essential to obtain transcranial radiographs. This should form an integral part of the patient's record. Despite the various technical difficulties previously mentioned, it is essential to make every effort to obtain satisfactory radiographs of some diagnostic value.

TOMOGRAPHY (NONCOMPUTED)

Linear Tomography

In 1930, in an effort to overcome some of the problems enumerated, linear tomography was incorporated as an additional x-ray method. In this technique, a special attachment is added to a standard x-ray machine. With tomography, it is possible to isolate a selected section for study and mechanically obscure interfering anatomical structures both above and below the level of interest. Linear tomography was found, however, to be too crude a method for evaluating the complex anatomical structures of the head and neck. Thus, it has been largely abandoned by diagnostic radiologists in the study of the TMJ.

It should be pointed out that some dentists employ cephalometric linear tomography for evaluation of the TMJ in patients undergoing orthodontic and other treatments. This method enables them to detect TMJ abnormalities or to ensure their absence prior to the initiation of treatment.[19]

Panoramic Tomography

The panoramic (Panorex) method is comfortable for the patient because with one projection condyles, rami, and body are visualized. It is therefore a convenient method for screening patients for suspected fractures and deformities. Since distortion is inherent in this method, it is not suitable for detailed visualization of the temporomandibular joint. Despite this, the panoramic method is frequently employed for the examination of the TMJ (Fig. 9–40).

Pluridirectional Tomography

In the past 15 years, I have employed a new type of tomography using a pluridirectional medical x-ray unit, designed specifically for modern tomography.[2] Most of the early work undertaken with this machine involved the visualization of the fine structures of the ears, such as the ossicles, semicircular canals, and internal auditory canals. As a result of this work, it became apparent that here at last was a method capable of visualizing the fine structures with a great deal of clarity. This device was therefore employed to study the TMJ. With this unit, it is now possible to detect subtle abnormalities of the condylar articular surface, the joint space, and the fossa. We are now able to detect minor changes impossible to see with any other method, with the possible exception of the new computed tomography units.

Recent technical advances employing special tomographic x-ray units, such as the polytome, have radically altered the way we view the TMJ. We

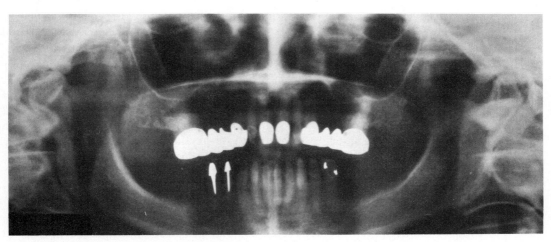

Figure 9–40. This shows the entire mandible as demonstrated by panoramic radiography. Here the temporomandibular joints are visualized at the periphery and are thus not sharply delineated.

are now in a position to demonstrate the TMJ with a great deal of clarity, so that even minor and subtle osteoarthritic or degenerative changes can be detected.

The value of this method has been stressed in a publication from the Mayo Clinic by Stanson and Baker.[20] They state that "soon after routine lateral tomography was begun in July, 1973, our overall quality improved greatly and our diagnostic detection rate and accuracy increased." These findings are confirmed in a recent publication by Rosenberg and Silha.[15] Even with this new form of tomography, limitations exist. The clinician must constantly be aware that certain structures, such as the muscles, ligaments, joint capsule, and cartilage, are not visualized by tomography unless they are calcified or ossified or unless some opaque material is added, as in arthrography.

The following points should be stressed concerning the value of pluri-directional tomography in the evaluation of TMJ problems:

1. This technique provides a good deal of detail about intrinsic bony structures of the condyle, fossa, and surrounding region.

2. The relationship of the condyle to the fossa may be studied in order to evaluate the joint space. Narrowing of this space may indicate disc damage and may be the first radiological sign of an underlying osteoarthritic process.

3. The mobility of the condyle may be evaluated by comparing x-ray films taken with the mouth closed, in resting position, with those taken with the mouth open. It is essential to compare the two sides.

4. The presence of suspected tumors and fractures may be ruled out before a final diagnosis is made and treatment instituted.

5. Tomography is extremely valuable for the patient presenting with an atypical clinical picture and for the patient who is not responding to treatment in the usual manner. It is also useful when a prompt relapse takes place during a period of observation.

6. Tomography is especially important for patients who have pain that is not related to occlusal muscle syndrome but is likely to be caused by an intrinsic joint disease, such as osteoarthritic or degenerative joint disease.

7. Tomography is of particular value in examination of infants and children because fractures and other diseases are often overlooked. In these circumstances, adequate treatment may not be instituted. Thus, the diagnosis may only be made years later, when the patients present with marked asymmetry or deformity of the mandible or face. In order to avoid this, TMJ problems in infants and children should be very carefully evaluated by means of tomography.

8. Tomography is of value in the postoperative changes in the TMJ that are difficult to evaluate. Some surgical procedures involve the placement of a partial or complete prosthesis in one or both joints. Following such procedures, a baseline study should be obtained in order to determine the exact location of the prosthesis. If any problems arise in the postoperative period, this information should prove of great value.

9. Tomography may be used in evaluating the efficacy of mandibular occlusal splints (Fig. 9–41).

10. Before planning extensive dental rehabilitation, clinical evaluation of the TMJ is advisable, even if the patient is free of symptoms. In cases of doubt, a tomographic examination is suggested. This may avoid problems at a later date. Latent or subclinical TMJ disease may be activated into a painful problem by extensive dental work.

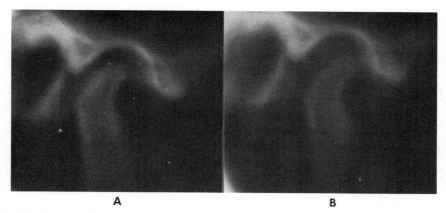

A   B

Figure 9–41. This illustrates the value of tomography in determining the efficiency of mandibular occlusal splints. *A,* Without the splint, slight superior as well as posterior joint space narrowing is seen. *B,* With the splint, the head and fossa assume a normal relationship.

11. In some patients, tomography may be the only source of needed information (see Fig. 9–58).

12. Finally, we have employed tomography to study the changes in the TMJ following treatment.

Corrected or Selected Tomography

To improve the diagnostic quality of the TMJ tomogram, I employ corrected or selected tomography.[16] This is done because the long axis of the condyle in the horizontal plane usually runs obliquely. The medial pole generally points medially and posteriorly. It is essential to determine the degree of obliquity so that the necessary correction is made prior to the tomographic examination. The objective is to rotate the head so that the long axis of the condyle is either parallel to or at right angles to the film. The obliquity of the two condyles is determined by obtaining a conventional film taken in the full base or submentovertical projection. Straight lines are then drawn through the middle of the long axes of the two condyles. These lines are projected posteriorly to intersect the midsagittal plane. The resultant angles are measured on the two sides (Fig. 9–42). These angles determine the degree of rotation that is required for the head. Again, the aim is to align the long axis of the condyle parallel to the film for the frontal projection and at right angles to the film for the lateral projection. In the lateral projection, the tomographic cuts are therefore perpendicular to the long axis (profile). It is important to stress that the degree of obliquity on the two sides may be different. Thus, every examination is "tailor-made." When the long axis of the condyle does not run obliquely, rotation of the head is unnecessary (Figs. 9–43, 9–44). It is essential to examine both sides for comparison. Also, the examination should be undertaken in both lateral and frontal projections. The lateral tomographic examination is undertaken in both the mouth-closed and mouth-opened positions. The normal opening pattern is regarded as being at least 45 mm. There is, however, a great deal of variation from person to person (Figs. 9–45 to 9–47).

It is advisable to include the entire ramus of the mandible when lateral sets of radiographs are obtained. In infancy and childhood, numerous

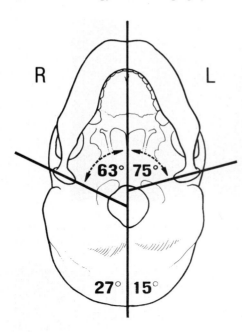

Figure 9–42. The obliquity of the two condyles is different. On the right side, the angle is 63°. Therefore, the head on this side has to be turned 27° (90° − 63° = 27°). On the left side, however, less rotation of the head is necessary, requiring only 15° (90° − 75° = 15°).

Figure 9–43. On the left side, only slight rotation of the head is needed, because the long axis is almost at right angles to the midsagittal plane. On the right side, a greater degree of rotation of the head is required.

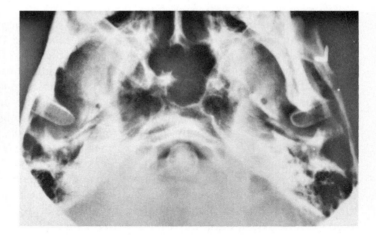

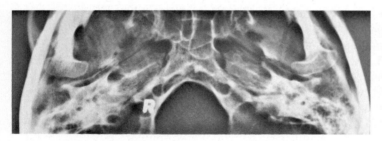

Figure 9–44. On the left side, very slight rotation of the head is necessary, because the long axis is almost at right angles to the midsagittal plane. On the right side, however, no rotation is needed, because the long axis is at right angles to the midsagittal plane.

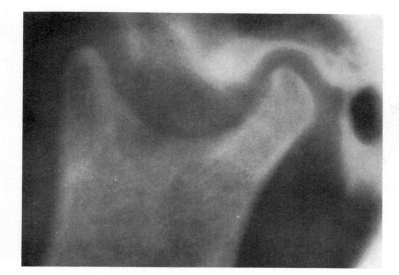

Figure 9–45. Demonstration of normal anatomical structures in the region of the superior ramus of the mandible.

Figure 9–46. Normal temporomandibular joint (lateral tomogram).

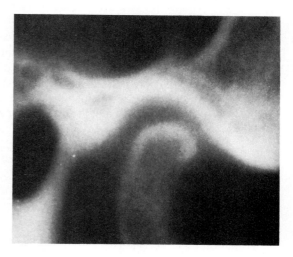

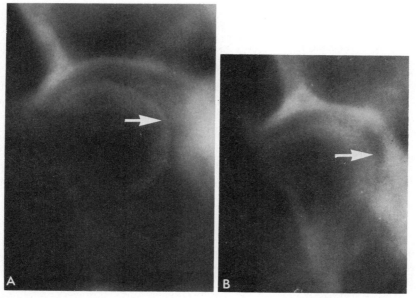

Figure 9–47. Right temporomandibular joint as seen in *A*, the oblique tomogram; *B*, frontal tomogram. These projections are particularly valuable for the visualization of the medial aspect of the head (arrows).

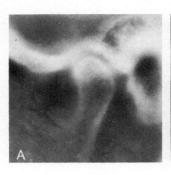 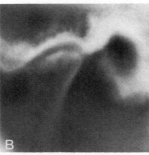

Figure 9–48. In this patient, the joints are very different on the two sides. *A,* Right; *B,* left. On the left side, there is marked flattening of the superior aspect of the condyle. This is associated with shortening of the neck and as a result of this, the ramus on this side is reduced in height. The fossa is also a little shadow, resulting in further bony shortening. Because of this, on opening, the jaw deviates to the left.

abnormalities may affect the TMJ region, which at a later stage may lead to stunting of growth and shortening of the ramus on that side. The same situation may also be found in adults. Advanced osteoarthritis may be responsible for flattening of the condyle as well as shortening of the ramus on the involved side. This may be associated with deviation of the jaw toward the short side (Fig. 9–48).

In the lateral projection with the mouth closed, the condyle is seen to occupy the anterior portion of the cavity of the fossa. The joint space is occupied primarily by the disc, which acts as a cushion or shock absorber, separating the bony structures. The joint space, superiorly and posteriorly, should measure at least 2.5 mm. When the joint space measures 2 mm. or less, narrowing of the joint space has occurred and disc damage should be suspected.

The following radiological features should be carefully observed and the two joints compared:[4] shape of the condylar head (round, flattened, irregular); surface of the anterior and superior aspects of the head (smooth, irregular, notched); contour of the cortex (intact, interrupted, condensed); structure of the medulla; inclination and length of the ramus of the mandible; abnormalities of the articular eminence; mobility of the head in relation to the articular eminence; depth of the fossa; position of the head in the fossa; width of the joint space; and associated abnormalities (tumor, unilateral hyperplasia or hypoplasia).

ARTHROGRAPHY

Temporomandibular joint arthrography was first described in 1947 by Norgaard,[13] who injected a radiopaque solution into the joint cavities. The procedure was seldom performed because of various technical difficulties. Recently, arthrography has enjoyed a revival, largely because of greater interest in the temporomandibular joint; it is now undertaken frequently in many centers. The main indication for this procedure is to determine the location of the disc in "internal derangement" of the joint. Because of space limitations, arthrography will not be described here, and the reader is referred to the standard works on the subject.

COMPUTED TOMOGRAPHY (CT)

Some preliminary examinations for the TMJ have been undertaken with CT in an attempt to determine anterior displacement of the disc. This new modality appears to have value in replacing TMJ arthrography in selected patients. Further work in this area is awaited with eager anticipation.

CINEFLUOROSCOPY OR CINERADIOGRAPHY

This method affords an opportunity to view jaw movements during continuous functions, such as speech, mastication, and deglutition. It is of value when performing arthrography. For the most part, such studies are limited to special diagnostic problems and research purposes.

DIAGNOSING TMJ DISORDERS

Disorders involving the TMJ may be approached in the following manner. Pain and discomfort in the TMJ region may be due to (1) diseases in one of the nearby structures, or (2) diseases in the region of the TMJ that are either part of some generalized process or localized to the TMJ.

It is important to determine first whether the problem involves the TMJ itself or perhaps is due to some local disease in one of the surrounding structures. Many conditions are found in this group. They range from minor neuralgias and dental diseases to malignant tumors of the parotid gland as well as the intracranial cavity. The actual site of the primary disease may be clinically completely silent. These patients, however, present with well-defined pain and discomfort, which is localized to the temporomandibular joint. The clinical features may be so well defined and localized to the TMJ that the patients find it difficult to believe that the actual intrinsic abnormalities is located not in the joint itself but in a nearby structure. Thus, if a patient has a TMJ problem, and thorough investigation, including tomography, reveals no obvious abnormality of the joint, a careful search should be made in the surrounding structures for a possible cause of the clinical findings. It should also be stressed that in pursuing an underlying cause, a thorough radiological examination is indicated, including the conventional routine radiographs of the skull, paranasal sinuses, cervical spine, and chest. Tomography, too, plays an important role. This method is particularly valuable in the region of the head and neck, where structures are small and the anatomical relationships complex. The styloid process, for example, is difficult to demonstrate by conventional x-rays. It is, however, easily visualized with modern tomography. The styloid process may be fractured by trauma to the neck.[8] Also, occasionally, the tip of the styloid process is injured during tonsillectomy. Trauma to the styloid process may be responsible for pain in the TMJ (Fig. 9–49).

In pursuing a diagnosis involving structures other than the TMJ, the collaboration of various other medical specialists is often necessary. The cause of the symptoms may be in the ear, nose, sinus, throat, cervical spine, or temporal and carotid arteries. In these instances, the primary disease—for example, infection or neoplasm in the maxillary sinus—is sometimes clinically silent. It may, however, be responsible for referred pain to the side of the face, and may therefore present as a TMJ problem. Other conditions that should be included in this group are enlarged lymph glands, cysts, or tumors of the nasopharynx. Adenopathy of the parotid gland, too, may cause symptoms in the TMJ. Finally, it should be stressed that various facial pains in the TMJ region may be secondary to intracranial disease as well as some disorders of the nervous system, involving one or more cranial nerves. These problems may require angiography, computed tomography, and various other neuroradiological examinations (Figs. 9–50 to 9–53).

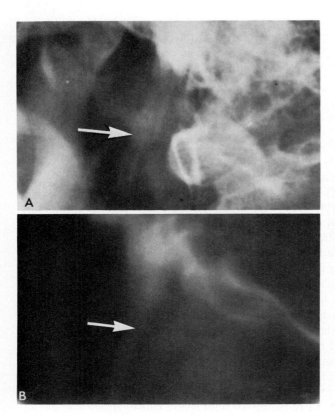

Figure 9–49. *A,* The styloid process as seen on a conventional radiograph. Visualization is to some extent obscured by overlying structures. *B,* With tomography, however, the styloid process is isolated and thus is more clearly seen.

Figure 9–50. The patient is a 68-year-old male who presented with severe pain in the right temporomandibular joint. The pain was referred from a carcinoma of the right antrum, which is opaque and shows breakdown of the lateral wall.

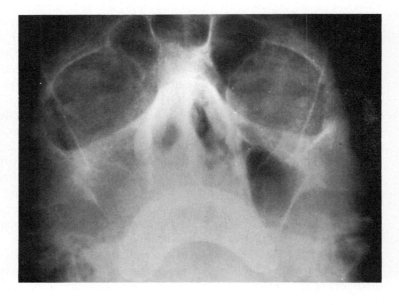

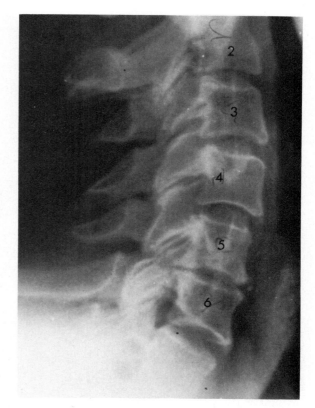

Figure 9–51. Intervertebral disc space narrowing is noted at the C5-6 level. Prominent osteophytes are present and these encroach upon the spinal canal.

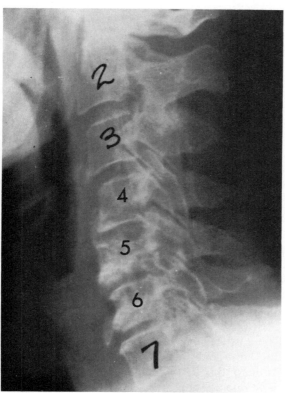

Figure 9–52. This radiograph shows marked irregularity of the body of C5 due to a metastatic deposit from a known primary carcinoma of the breast.

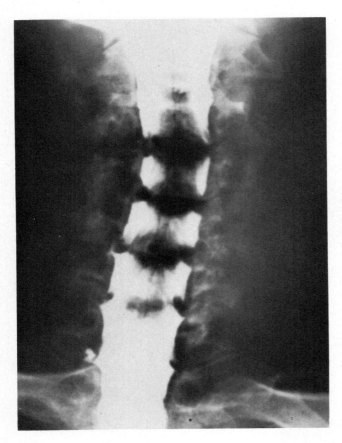

Figure 9–53. The cervical region is seen in the frontal projection during myelography. The opaque column shows a stepladder type of appearance secondary to protrusions at the level of the intervertebral disc spaces.

TMJ DISEASES: GENERALIZED OR LOCALIZED

Diseases of the TMJ itself may be subdivided into two large categories: generalized systemic disease and disease localized to the TMJ.

In generalized systemic disease, TMJ involvement is part of a generalized process. This may be found in rheumatoid arthritis, acromegaly, and various other conditions. Also, pain in the TMJ region may be secondary to a known primary malignancy. Primary carcinoma of the breast frequently metastasizes to bones. Occasionally, a metastatic deposit may be found in the ramus of the mandible.

A common condition localized to the TMJ is "TMJ dysfunction syndrome."[9] This has many other names, such as "pain-dysfunction syndrome." For convenience, the term "dysfunction" will be employed here. This is a common condition that is usually unilateral. It has been described extensively in both the medical and dental literature in the past 40 years. Despite the fact that this is a common condition, it is frequently undiagnosed or misdiagnosed because it mimics many different diseases and produces a wide variety of symptoms. These will be considered in brief as local and peripheral symptoms.

TMJ dysfunction should be suspected if any of these local symptoms are present: a clicking, cracking noise and crepitation on movement of the jaw,[17] tenderness and pain around the TMJ, and occasionally trismus. Limitation of jaw movement is frequently noted.

Peripheral pain is frequently referred to areas in the head, neck, and face. Stiffness of the neck muscles is not an uncommon finding. The pain that is encountered may resemble migraine, trigeminal neuralgia, or various other facial pains, or the pain typical of sinus problems or temporal arteritis. Occasionally, there is no pain, but dizziness, tinnitus, and hearing loss are present. These symptoms are mentioned to emphasize the complexity and diversity of the problem.

A few important aspects of dysfunction should be stressed. It must be kept in mind that the problem primarily involves the muscles of mastication and generally is an acute condition of short duration. Although in a small percentage of patients the condition resolves without any treatment, the vast majority generally respond to various forms of treatment. However, in some patients, the condition becomes chronic and eventually leads to degenerative joint disease. It is important to be aware that features of dysfunction may be encountered in the chronic phase. The clinician must, however, keep in mind that the dysfunction is no longer a primary muscle condition but is now secondary to an underlying arthritic process. Although resultant symptoms may be troublesome and painful, the changes in the joints are frequently subtle and difficult to detect by conventional x-ray methods (transcranial). Therefore, it is not surprising that the diagnostic yield is less than satisfactory. Because of this, intrinsic diseases of the joint, such as osteoarthritis or degenerative joint disease, have frequently been overlooked, and many patients have sought out numerous physicians and dentists in an aimless search to obtain relief from their symptoms. A few patients have been referred for prolonged psychiatric treatment. From a patient's point of view, this is often a long, expensive, painful, and ultimately unsuccessful undertaking.

The studies of McCarty[18] and others have provided further evidence that some patients considered to have "functional" disorders of the TMJ actually have intrinsic abnormalities involving the disc and other structures. This group of conditions is usually labeled "internal derangements of the TMJ." In many respects, this resembles "internal derangements of the knee joint," a very common orthopedic problem.

OSTEOARTHRITIS OR DEGENERATIVE JOINT DISEASE[3]

Osteoarthritis or degenerative joint disease is generally subdivided into two broad categories: primary and secondary.

The secondary variety is usually the result of trauma or some other intrinsic disease of the joint. A good example is the skier who fractures an ankle. During the period of healing, secondary osteoarthritis frequently develops. This is more likely to occur if the fracture line runs into the articular surface of the joint.

Under similar circumstances, comparable changes will occur in the TMJ. Chronic trauma may produce such changes as well. Secondary osteoarthritis may also occur in the chronic phase of numerous other intrinsic arthritic conditions.

The primary variety is generally described as a condition of "wear and tear" and is more common with increasing age. Some consider this an inevitable process of aging; however, recent evidence indicates that this is not completely true. Some of these views have recently been postulated by

Kelley and co-workers,[11] who state "[osteoarthritis] is not an inevitable part of aging, nor is it a simple wear and tear process." In fact, the condition may also be found fairly frequently in younger individuals (below 40 years of age). Primary osteoarthritis is a common affliction, and therefore it is not surprising that it is often found in the TMJ when this is carefully examined with modern x-ray techniques. There is one aspect of the management of patients with degenerative joint disease that is very undesirable. Since many health professionals are of the opinion that little can be done for an osteoarthritic process, it is not surprising that the patients are frequently told to just live with it. They are given a prescription for a tranquilizer and are told to go home and forget about it. Again, this concept is questioned by Kelley and associates,[11] who state that "the pessimistic and hopeless attitude that [osteoarthritis] always proceeds inextricably downhill to a joint destruction is no longer warranted. The pathogenic steps are not mysterious and pathological changes may be reversible."

Primary osteoarthritis is perhaps best subdivided into two clinical groups: (1) osteoarthritis of aging, which is common and frequently asymptomatic; and (2) osteoarthritis that occurs in younger individuals. This tends to be more active and is frequently responsible for chronic facial pain and other related problems.

CLINICAL CLASSIFICATION OF OSTEOARTHRITIS

Primary osteoarthritis is a slow process that develops over a period of months or years. Boering has subdivided the condition into the following three stages: initial stage, intermediate stage, and late (chronic) stage.[4]

Initial Stage

In the initial phase, we find biochemical changes in the joint. It should be stressed that at this stage the process is easily reversed. Should the condition continue to progress, the intermediate stage will result.

Intermediate Stage

In the intermediate phase, microscopical changes are found in the joint, but there are no significant x-ray film changes. With further progression, the late or chronic phase will result.

Chronic (Late) Stage

In the chronic stage, anatomical changes occur in the joints that can usually be easily detected by modern x-ray techniques. Exactly when symptoms arise is sometimes difficult to determine. In the early phase of the disease, the symptoms may be severe. On the other hand, in the chronic or late phase, the condition may be quiescent or "burnt out." Thus, very few symptoms may be encountered. An acute flare-up may, however, take place at any time during the course of the disease. If this should occur during the chronic phase, an acute dysfunction will result, which will still be secondary to the underlying degenerative process.

If we are to achieve good results, it is essential to make the diagnosis in the early phase of the condition. The more advanced the condition, the greater the difficulty in management.

It should be remembered that in the early stage, or biochemical phase, the process is easily reversed with treatment. When the microscopical changes are evident, reversing the process becomes more difficult. Finally, in the chronic stage, in which we encounter anatomical changes, the complete reversal becomes even more difficult. Even here, however, we often find some healing or remodeling.

RADIOLOGICAL CHANGES IN OSTEOARTHRITIS

As stated previously, the normal joint space, as seen in the lateral projection, is occupied by the disc and other soft tissue structures (Fig. 9–46). The disc acts as a cushion or shock absorber that separates the bony condyle from the fossa. In the early phase of osteoarthritis, because of damage to the disc, it becomes thinned, fragmented, and sometimes perforated. As a result, narrowing of the joint space takes place, and the spatial relationship between the condyle and fossa is disturbed. Frequently the condyle will be retruded, and this is associated with a loss in the vertical dimension. The resultant narrowing of the joint space is clearly demonstrated with modern x-ray techniques (Figs. 9–54 to 9–56). It is of the utmost importance for health professionals managing TMJ problems to be aware of this. It is essential to try to facilitate the healing process at this early stage and not wait for the more advanced changes to take place. When the disc is damaged, bone-to-bone contact tends to take place, and thus it is not surprising that bony changes will occur in both the condyle and the eminence.

If the condition is not treated in its early phase, it usually continues to progress, and further changes will be seen in the bony structures themselves. Flattening of the mandibular condyle in the anterior half of the superior aspect is a common finding. The flattening is frequently associated with bony

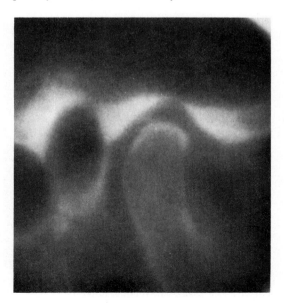

Figure 9–54. This radiograph shows very slight narrowing of the joint space posteriorly. This was confirmed clinically. The vertical height is well maintained. More advanced changes are seen in Figure 9–55.

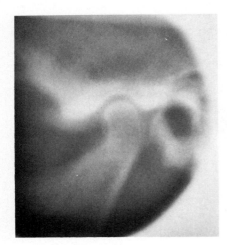

Figure 9–55. Narrowing of the joint space, which is generally secondary to disc damage. In addition, the superior aspect of the condyle shows subchondral sclerosis.

condensation or subchondral sclerosis. Periosteal bone apposition takes place at the junction of the head and neck, resulting in thickening of this region. Another characteristic feature is the formation of osteophytes or bony spurs (Fig. 9–57).

Osteophytes occur most commonly on the anterior aspect of the condyle but may also occur in other regions (Fig. 9–58). Sometimes fractures may occur through the base of an osteophyte. This is one form of loose body within the joint. It is not surprising that some cases of chronic degenerative joint disease are complicated by fractures involving other parts—for example, the condyle itself. The additional fracture will usually cause an exacerbation of the patient's symptoms, with the pain becoming more severe.

As the condition advances, further flattening of the superior aspect of the condyle takes place. This is sometimes associated with the appearance of translucent, more or less round pseudocysts. In the advanced stage, the condyle is frequently considerably decreased in size. The shortening may also involve the neck, with the result that the ascending ramus on one side

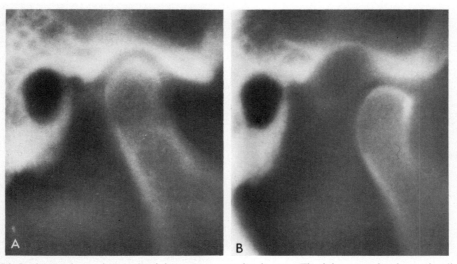

Figure 9–56. Both superior and posterior joint space narrowing is seen. The joint space has been visualized in *A*, mouth closed, and *B*, mouth opened positions. More advanced changes are seen in Figure 9–57.

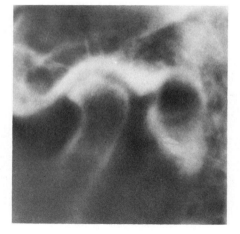

Figure 9–57. In addition to narrowing of the joint space, the anterior half of the superior aspect of the condyle is flat. Also, an osteophyte appears to be forming anteriorly.

is shorter than the one on the opposite side (see Fig. 9–48). Under these circumstances, the mandible will frequently deviate toward the shorter side.

With further progression, bony changes are seen in the eminence, which becomes flat so that the fossa enlarges. Normally, the eminence is rounded. Also, an osteophyte is sometimes seen in the anterior aspect of the eminence. Another finding that may be encountered is subluxation. A flat eminence facilitates subluxation. This is more likely to occur if the condyle and neck are also flat and short. Under these circumstance, the patient may complain of very little pain or discomfort but may indicate that the jaw subluxates when an attempt is made to eat something hard, like an apple. The jaw will slide forward and the patient may experience difficulty in getting it back into position (Fig. 9–59).

In severe bilateral osteoarthritis with loss of bone, one may also find

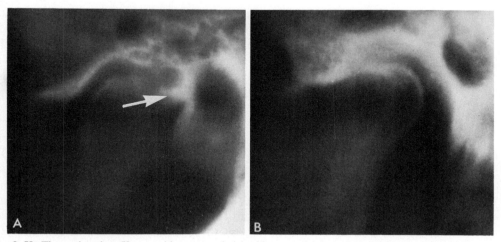

Figure 9–58. The patient is a 59-year-old woman who, besides complaining of discomfort in the left temporomandibular joint, also experienced severe headaches that were confined primarily to the left side. *A*, A tomographic examination revealed a tiny osteophyte, which was seen to arise from the posterior aspect of the fossa (arrow). It should be stressed that it is impossible to demonstrate a tiny osteophyte of this type by any other method. The patient then underwent a long period of conservative treatment. *B*, A follow-up examination undertaken three years later no longer shows the osteophyte. This is an example of self-healing. There was a corresponding alleviation of the patient's symptoms.

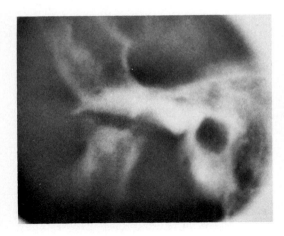

Figure 9–59. Advanced changes of degenerative joint disease. Obvious erosion of the condyle and neck is noted, which is responsible for bony shortening. The fossa is large and flat, with the eminence eroded. In this situation, subluxation can easily take place.

that only the posterior teeth touch. This may cause an anterior open bite. If the condition continues for a long time, the degenerative changes result in a deforming arthritis. It is regrettable that most publications on the subject stress the advanced changes, and little or no attention has been devoted to the early diagnosis of the condition. Many of us wait for the so-called classic features of the disease, which generally represent the late phase, to appear before we institute treatment.

It should be stressed that there is no simple correlation between what is occurring inside the joint and the symptoms experienced by the patient. There is a great deal of variation from patient to patient and at different times in the same individual. This was stressed by Osler, who stated, "It is more important to know the patient who has the disease, than to know the disease which has the patient."

Some dentists view osteoarthritic changes in the TMJ as an awesome and perplexing problem shrouded in mystery. This is probably due to lack of familiarity. Comparable osteoarthritic changes are found in the joints of the fingers as well as in some of the larger joints, such as the knee and hip. These are described in standard textbooks of orthopedic surgery and rheumatology.

Symptoms of degenerative joint disease in the TMJ are (1) local symptoms, (2) peripheral symptoms, (3) ear symptoms, and (4) any combination of these. These symptoms are commonly encountered in patients with osteoarthritis of the TMJ. It is very important to recognize that similar symptoms may be seen in the dysfunctions described in some detail earlier. It is important to note carefully the total duration of the symptoms. They are usually of short duration in the dysfunctions and tend to be rather protracted in osteoarthritis.

The next group of patients is fairly commonly encountered by clinicians treating osteoarthritis and therefore deserves special attention: those patients with few or no symptoms (occult or subclinical). This is a very important group that has received very little attention in the literature. Under certain circumstances, a patient without symptoms may suddenly develop symptoms. There are a number of conditions that may be responsible for this. Trauma in general is the most common cause; automobile accidents are the great offender. Other conditions are iatrogenic, sometimes occurring with extensive dental work. Prolonged opening of the mouth may be traumatic to the

TMJ. This is something that individuals in the healing profession should constantly keep in mind so that they will handle the TMJ at all times with extreme care. If this is not done by anesthesiologists and the various other health professionals during intubation or while undertaking various endoscopic examinations, damage to the TMJ may take place. This is more likely to occur if the patient is under general anesthesia and is unable to communicate with the dentist or physician.

There are numerous other causes that may convert a patient with asymptomatic disease to a patient with acute pain and other related symptoms. These include the "classic stroke." Here, in addition to paralysis of half the body, the jaw is deflected to the side of paralysis and the tongue is deviated to the same side. This is really a form of subluxation; therefore, it is not surprising that this too may traumatize the TMJ.

When evaluating the current status of a patient with suspected osteoarthritis of the TMJ, certain guidelines must be followed. It is of the utmost importance to take into consideration the total picture. This must include the history, physical examination, x-ray films, and any other pertinent information. As stated previously, the TMJ is demonstrated with a great deal of clarity by modern tomographic x-ray techniques. This, however, provides only part of the total evidence. *It is indeed unfortunate that some medical and dental consultants for insurance companies and other health groups base their criteria for eligibility on the evidence provided only by the x-ray films, without taking into consideration other important data.* Another source of error is the fact that the total duration of the patient's symptoms is not given enough consideration. This is shown in patients with a clinical history lasting many months or years, associated with definite x-ray changes, who are misdiagnosed as having myofascial pain–dysfunction syndrome. The fact that this is an acute process of short duration involving primarily muscles of mastication and other related soft tissues is overlooked. When presented with a patient with a long history of TMJ discomfort, it is essential to consider an intrinsic organic process of the joint.

It should be emphasized that osteoarthritis or degenerative joint disease is a condition frequently found in the TMJ examined with modern tomographic techniques. It occurs in individuals of all ages. Osteoarthritis of the TMJ is basically a medical or orthopedic condition similar to that found in other joints of the body affected by this primary joint disease. For this reason osteoarthritis, when it occurs in the TMJ, cannot be considered purely a dental condition. However, because of the close proximity, both anatomically and physiologically, to the teeth and related structures, these conditions are frequently labeled dental. They can be managed very effectively by dentists knowledgeable in diseases of the TMJ. They can, of course, be treated equally well by physicians with special training in this area. There are situations when the patient is best managed by the combined talents of both a dentist and a physician.

OTHER CONDITIONS INVOLVING THE TMJ

There are many other conditions which involve the temporomandibular joint. They frequently present with pain and discomfort and thus should be included in the differential diagnosis of the TMJ dysfunction syndrome.

TRAUMA

Most fractures and dislocations following acute trauma are diagnosed and treated in emergency rooms of hospitals and for the most part do not present much difficulty. Sometimes, however, fractures and dislocations present in an unusual manner and escape attention. At a later stage they may thus present clinically as a temporomandibular joint dysfunction syndrome. If one is confronted with a patient with temporomandibular joint dysfunction syndrome who is not responding to treatment, a previous undetected fracture should be considered.

Besides direct extrinsic trauma to the jaw and face, the TMJ may be traumatized by abnormal sleeping positions or manipulations during general anesthesia and prolonged dental procedures. These factors are responsible for intrinsic trauma of a chronic nature. Other forms of trauma include chronic or recurrent dislocation as well as minor degrees of subluxation which may be self-reducing. Any injury may be responsible for joint effusion, strained ligaments, and perhaps anterior dislocation of the disc. If untreated, these conditions may lead to remodeling deformities of both the condyle and eminence. Finally, a traumatic arthritis may result with subsequent fibrosis and limitation of movement. Sometimes degenerative changes may take place.

It is important to stress that in cases of trauma in childhood involving the TMJ area, a very careful evaluation, including tomography, is essential. In children, unreduced fractures tend to be clinically insidious and escape detection until obvious deformity of the mandible becomes apparent in later years. This may or may not be associated with ankylosis. Also, condylar fractures should be considered when evaluating a victim of child abuse (Fig. 9–60).

One should keep in mind that spontaneous dislocation or chronic recurrent dislocation occasionally may be encountered which is unrelated to trauma. It is usually regarded as being caused by lack of muscle coordination.[1] This condition has been mistaken for a parotid gland tumor.

INFECTION

Because of antibiotics, pyogenic arthritis is rare in many parts of the world. This condition is occasionally found as an aftermath of infection of childhood. Usually, however, infection spreads from the middle ear or mastoid region to the TMJ. Infection may also follow trauma or an operative procedure. In the acute phase infection produces an acute inflammatory arthritis with exudation and restriction of movement. If the condition persists joint ankylosis will result in the chronic phase. In childhood, destruction of the growth center may take place, leading to impaired mandibular growth.

CONGENITAL AND DEVELOPMENTAL ANOMALIES

There are a number of conditions which interfere with normal growth, development, and function of the TMJ. These may predispose to or aggravate TMJ diseases. Only a few of these conditions will be considered. In agenesis

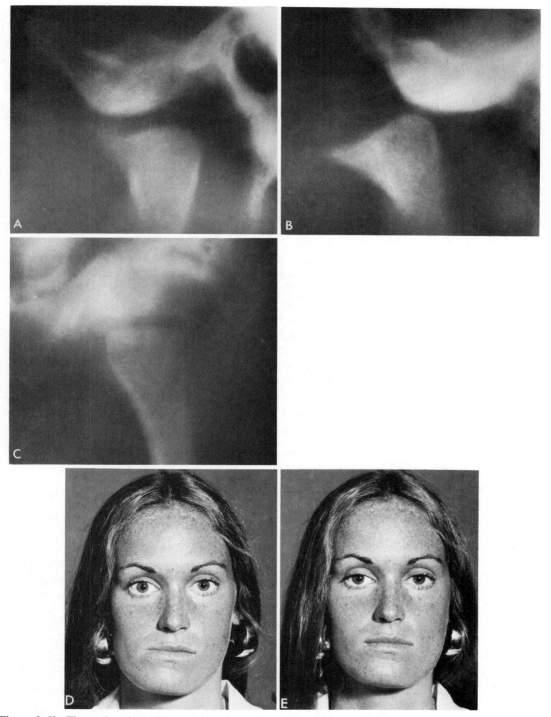

Figure 9–60. The patient is a 19-year-old woman. A number of abnormalities were demonstrated in the left temporomandibular joint. The head of the condyle was flattened and appeared to articulate with the eminence. A spur is seen to arise from the anterior aspect of the condylar head. The fossa is small. These features were clearly demonstrated in both *A* (mouth closed) and *B* (mouth opened) positions, as well as *C* (frontal projection). The changes noted were considered to be due to trauma occurring early in life. It is interesting to note that the patient did not present with any temporomandibular joint discomfort but mainly had referred ear symptoms, such as tinnitus and dizziness. *D,* Deviation of the mandible to the right. *E,* Following treatment, the mandible is seen to be in the midline.

of the condyle, one of the condyles fails to develop. This is usually associated with underdevelopment of the side of the mandible, with a tendency of the jaw to deviate toward the affected side. Similarly, such conditions as infection and trauma in infancy or early childhood may also stunt growth.

It should be stressed that congenital anomalies, such as agenesis or hypoplasia of the condyle, are invariably associated with equivalent malformations in the temporal bone, particularly the middle ear and ossicles. This association is of the utmost importance in the differential diagnosis. It helps to distinguish congenital from acquired deformities due to trauma or infection.[14]

ANKYLOSIS

Another condition which should be mentioned is ankylosis accompanied by limitation of movement, a common finding. Ankylosis may be fibrous or bony. Fibrous ankylosis is usually caused by external trauma. Bony ankylosis is frequently due to infection or suppurative disease. When ankylosis is the end result of trauma or infection occurring in childhood, condylar growth may be arrested, and as a result an antegonial notch develops on the affected side. The notch is found on the inferior aspect of the body of the mandible in the region of the insertion of the masseter muscle. Its depth and striking appearance are often accentuated by the formation of a large blunt bony spur, which projects downward and backward from the angle of the mandible. The earlier the insult, the greater the deformity.

Painless restriction of jaw movement is found in a condition called chronic mandibular hypomobility.[1] This may be caused by ankylosis (intracapsular), capsular fibrosis, or muscular contracture (extracapsular). The underlying cause is usually old trauma or infection (Fig. 9–60).

RHEUMATOID ARTHRITIS

Rheumatoid arthritis affects many joints of the body including the TMJ. Comroe[6] states that acute involvement of the TMJ occurs in 20 per cent of the cases of rheumatoid arthritis. Other publications[5,7] on the subject, in which tomography was employed, report a higher incidence of involvement because, with tomography, we are now able to detect subtle changes and small erosions. During the acute phase, swelling and tenderness may be noted with restricted movement.

Radiological examination at this stage may demonstrate limited mobility as well as demineralization. As the condition advances, cartilage may be destroyed, and this will lead to joint space narrowing. This is frequently associated with cortical erosions and later with flattening of the joint surfaces. Sometimes a decrease in the depth of the fossa secondary to erosion of the eminence is noted. In the chronic phase, osteoarthritic lipping of the condyle or spur formation and marginal proliferation are seen. Fibrosis and ankylosis tend to be rare.

In Still's disease, or juvenile rheumatoid arthritis, the TMJ may also be involved. When this takes place in early childhood serious interference with mandibular growth and facial asymmetry may be the end result. At this late stage the condition may be mistaken for agenesis of the mandibular condyle.

It is perhaps worth mentioning that in ankylosing spondylitis approximately one third of the patients will show temporomandibular joint involvement, similar to the incidence in rheumatoid arthritis. Psoriasis is another condition which may be responsible for similar changes in the temporomandibular joint.

TUMORS AND TUMOR-LIKE CONDITIONS

True neoplasms of the TMJ, which may be benign or malignant, are rare. In young people chondromas or osteochondromas may be found. On rare occasions these undergo malignant degeneration. When growth has ceased, osteomas are found. Here the condylar head is enlarged and shows an unusual trabecular pattern (Fig. 9–61).

Malignant lesions may be primary or secondary. Examples of primary lesions are chondrosarcomas of the mandible and synovial sarcomas, as well as fibrosarcomas of the joint capsule. These are rare. Malignant lesions are usually metastatic. They may arise from a distant site, such as carcinoma of the bladder, or extend from a malignant neoplastic process in a nearby structure, such as the parotid gland or nasopharynx. Such patients usually present with a tender swollen joint, which does not respond to conservative treatment (Fig. 9–62).

There are a number of non-neoplastic conditions that cause enlargement of the condyle and should thus be considered in the differential diagnosis:

1. Osteoarthritis may cause enlargement of the condyle. This is due to a reactive type of change, as well as osteophyte formation.

2. Chronic bilateral unreduced anterior dislocation sometimes leads to gross enlargement of the condyle.

3. Fibrous dysplasia may cause bony thickening. Sometimes in this condition, cystlike expansion of the condyle is found. This has been described by Miles.[12] There are a few other conditions which should be included, such as acromegaly and Paget's disease.

4. Condylar hyperplasia is an uncommon condition of unknown etiology. It is usually found in young people. The condition is generally unilateral and more frequent in women. There are two forms: (a) In the more common variety the mandible is deviated to the unaffected side. Here the increase in growth appears to be taken up by the body of the mandible. Secondary remodeling of the fossa takes place in order to accommodate the enlarged condyle. It is obviously essential to differentiate this condition from the numerous other causes of facial and mandibular asymmetry. (b) In the rarer form, the head is large and the neck becomes elongated and may even assume a spiral shape. There is little deviation of the mandible. It is perhaps important to stress that this condition is usually found in young people and growth of the jaw terminates with maturity, in contrast to the enlargement of the condyle secondary to a true neoplasm.

CONCLUSIONS

The radiology of the temporomandibular joint is a much neglected subject. It is hoped that recent developments in tomography will play a

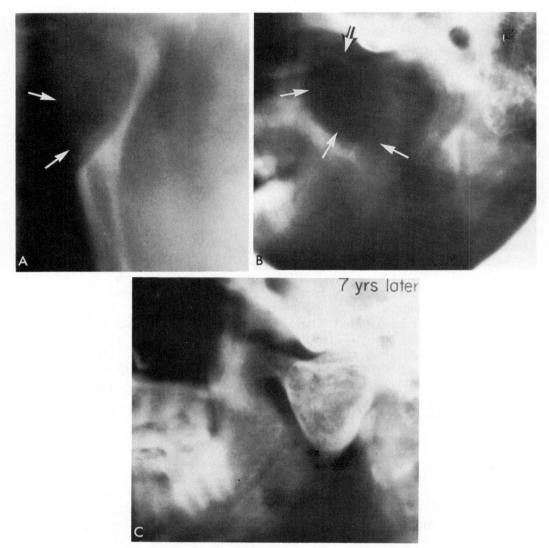

Figure 9–61. *A*, Frontal tomogram; *B*, lateral tomogram; *C*, lateral tomogram following treatment. The patient is a 27-year-old male with a large destructive lesion caused by an aneurysmal bone cyst (outlined by arrows). This is well seen in the frontal and lateral tomograms. The lesion was treated by curettage and radiation therapy. Very good healing is noted in the follow-up examination taken seven years later, as is seen in the lateral tomogram, *C*. (The author is indebted to Julius Smith, M.D., of New York City, for permission to publish this case).

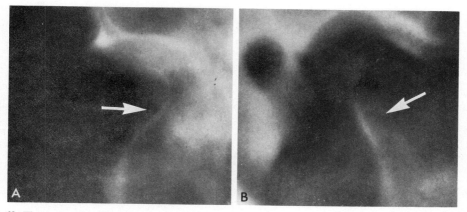

Figure 9–62. The patient is a 69-year-old male who complained of very severe pain in the right temporomandibular joint of about six weeks duration. Numerous transcranial radiographs of the right temporomandibular joint were taken by several dentists. No abnormality was demonstrated. Tomographic examination in frontal, *A*, and lateral, *B*, projections shows an obvious extensive destructive process. This was regarded as being a metastatic deposit from a known primary carcinoma of the bladder.

significant role in clarifying many of the complex problems which exist in this area. This method is extremely valuable in the evaluation of the temporomandibular joint and its surrounding structures.

References

1. Bell, W. L.: Orofacial Pains: Differential Diagnosis. Dallas, Texas, Denedco of Dallas, 1973.
2. Berrett, A., Brunner, S., and Valvassori, G. E.: Modern Thin-Section Tomography. Springfield, Ill., Charles C Thomas, 1973.
3. Blackwood, H. J. J.: Arthritis of the mandibular joint. Br. Dent. J., *115*:317, 1963.
4. Boering, G.: Arthrosis Deformans Van Het Kaakgewricht. Groningen, Drukkerij Van Denderen, 1966.
5. Chalmers, I. M., and Blair, G. B.: Rheumatoid arthritis of the temporomandibular joint. Q. J. Med., *42*:369, 1973.
6. Comroe, B. I.: Arthritis and Allied Conditions, 5th ed. Philadelphia, Lea & Febiger, 1953.
7. Ericson, S., and Lundberg, M.: Alterations in the temporomandibular joint at various stages of rheumatoid arthritis. Acta Rheum. Scand., *13*:257, 1967.
8. Freese, A. S., and Scheman, P.: The Postgraduate Dental Lecture Series: Management of Temporomandibular Joint Problems. St. Louis, C. V. Mosby Co., 1962.
9. Gelb, H., and Tarte, J.: A two-year clinical dental evaluation of chronic headache: The craniocervical-mandibular syndrome. JADA, *91*:1230, 1975.
10. Helms, C. A.: Personal communication, 1982.
11. Kelley, W. N., Harris, E. D., Ruddy, S., Sledge, C. B.: Textbook of Rheumatology. Philadelphia, W. B. Saunders Co., 1981.
12. Miles, A. E. W.: Chondrosarcoma of the maxilla. Br. Dent. J., *88*:257, 1950.
13. Nørgaard, F.: Temporomandibular Arthrography. Copenhagen, Ejnar Munksgaards Forlag, 1947.
14. Pruzansky, S.: The Temporomandibular Joint. Otolaryngol. Clin. North Am., *6*:523, 1973.
15. Rosenberg, H. M., and Silha, R. E.: Dental Radiography and Photography, Vol. 55. Rochester, N.Y., Eastman Kodak Co., 1982.
16. Rozencweig, D. R., and Martin, G.: J. Prosthet. Dent., *40*:67, 1978.
17. Shore, N. A.: TMJ dysfunction. N.Y. State Dent. J., *34*:5, 1968.
18. Solberg, W. K., and Clark, G. T.: Temporomandibular Joint Problems. Chicago, Quintessence Publishing Co., 1980.
19. Stack, B. C., and Funt, L. A.: Personal communication, 1976.
20. Stanson, A. W., and Baker, H. L., Jr.: Routine tomography of the TMJ. Radiol. Clin. North Am., *14*:105, 1976.

10

Functional Considerations in Early Limited Orthodontic Procedures

H. T. PERRY, D.D.S., Ph.D.
E. W. MARSH, D.M.D.

The correction of malposed teeth in the growing child and the modification of maloccluded maxillary and mandibular arches offer a positive means for the prevention of craniocervical mandibular syndrome symptoms. The endeavors of a dentist not only encompass esthetics and improved dental health but also must, of primary necessity, provide a functioning oral environment for the dynamics of the stomatognathic system. The usual day-to-day functions of occlusion, articulation, respiration, mastication, and deglutition should be the foremost concerns. By applying their skills, practitioners are acting in a true preventive fashion to correct early childhood and adolescent dysfunction patterns, which, if left uncorrected, may significantly contribute in early adulthood to symptoms of functional inadequacy, pain, and accelerated tissue breakdown and disrepair. Dental practitioners must strive to provide the child's developing dentition and total masticatory apparatus with a stable, healthy, and correctly functioning environment. Thus they may prevent the many sequelae of craniocervical mandibular disturbances attributed to adult malocclusion and/or occlusal imbalances.

In over 30 years of teaching dental students and graduate students, as well as lecturing to dentists and physicians in this country and other nations, one salient fact has emerged: the dental (and medical) knowledge of the functioning stomatognathic system is woefully inadequate. We believe that the fault lies with our dental cirriculum committees. Too often, students learn the facts of each system and tissue, but their interrelation and coordination in function and dysfunction are not stressed, and in some dental departments the dynamics of the system are not even mentioned. This is not intended, however, as a blanket condemnation of all schools. In the past few years, we have seen the emergence of departmental and even interdepartmental efforts to correlate the health science foundations of our profession with our responsibility to achieve a healthy, stable, and acceptably articulating dentition. It seems logical to us that this correlation can best be achieved by combining the basic and clinical sciences in a mutually receptive and respective fashion.

In a book such as this, and particularly in this chapter, the relationship of the neuromuscular system to normal and abnormal jaw function cannot be stressed too greatly. Normal function leading to health and stability is our ideal goal. The consequences of abnormal function and the sequelae of dysfunction and pathology must be avoided. Space, and perhaps clinical interest, does not permit an extensive review of all the basic science information so important to proper diagnosis and treatment planning. It is imperative, however, to cite some of the more salient works that are directly related to the concept which we are presenting: namely, that early intervention by the dentist to correct malocclusion and improper centric jaw relations permits the child or adolescent patient to achieve an "altered centric"[1] with simple treatment procedures. This altered or corrected centric then provides an optimal functional environment for the natural forces of growth and development and coordinated neuromuscular activity.

NEUROMUSCULAR PHYSIOLOGY OF JAW MOVEMENT

Extensive literature concerning the physiology of jaw movement is available to the interested clinician. Noteworthy are the works of Ahlgren,[2] Ballard,[3] Brill et al.,[4] Corbin and Harrison,[5] Dellow,[6] Kawamura,[7] Hickey et al.,[8] Lammie,[9] Jerge,[10] McNamara,[11] Moyers,[12] Perry,[13] Schaerer et al.,[14] Walsh,[15] Woelfel et al.,[16] and others.

It has been shown that mandibular movement is initiated in utero even before the development of the temporomandibular joints is complete.[17, 18] The infant's stomatognathic function is intimately associated with nutrition, respiration, and primitive vocalization.[19] Thus, long before the eruption of the teeth, the neuromuscular circuits are developing. The neural elements of the temporomandibular joints, a topic summarized by Clark and Wyke,[20] are initiating their future role in mandibular movement. The musculature, with its Golgi tendon end organs and muscle spindle systems, is also functioning but not with its future capacity or efficiency. From prenatal mandibular movements to early neonatal function, the increase of neural activity is apparent.

With the eruption of the teeth, a new element of reflex jaw movement emerges. The periodontal ligament possesses a discrete and extensive network of touch, tactile, and proprioceptive endings. The proprioceptive (proprius, self; ception, awareness) endings send centripetal signals to the mesencephalic nucleus of the trigeminal (fifth cranial) nerve. It is this nucleus that eventually plays an important role in the functional and parafunctional movement of the mandible. It is the only sensory nucleus that is located within the central nervous system, and in addition to proprioceptive fibers for the fifth cranial nerve, it also may carry fibers for the seventh and ninth cranial nerves. Collaterals from the cell bodies of this nucleus have a synapse with the motor cells for the muscles of mastication in the masticator nucleus. Thus, the monosynaptic reflex for mandibular movement receives further reinforcement with the eruption of the teeth.

As the child's jaw grows in concert with the craniofacial components, the neuromuscular system receives a constant torrent of reinforcing signals. The various functions of the body that are associated with movement of the mandible bring into action cerebral level activity and other cranial nerve systems. Different patterns of neuromuscular activity are apparent for mastication, vocalization, respiration, deglutition, and even emotion.

One of the principal functions of the oral cavity is mastication. As dentists, our efforts are directed at optimal tooth contact during masticatory movements. Of particular interest in this chapter is the jaw–tooth relation (occlusion and articulation) and muscle function or dysfunction.

The components of mandibular function and their interrelations are illustrated in Figure 10–1. Here we have presented some of the areas and actions of the many dependent units.

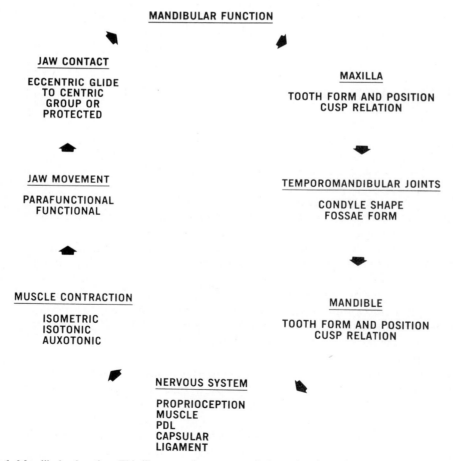

Figure 10–1. Mandibular function. This illustrates the numerous independent but related parts of the stomatognathic system. Dysfunction or disease in any area will affect the entire system.

Some of the peripheral sense organs of the trigeminal touch–tactile system are illustrated in Figure 10–2. Sensory cell bodies are located in the bilateral gasserian ganglia. Figure 10–3 shows the pain and temperature sensing system of the fifth cranial nerve. Central sensory projections make a primary synapse in the chief sensory nucleus. From this nucleus, secondary neurons ascend the brain stem on either the ipsilateral or contralateral side to make reflex connections with other cranial nerves, or they ascend to the cerebral cortex for conscious recognition.

The Trigeminal Brainstem System (Diagrammatic)

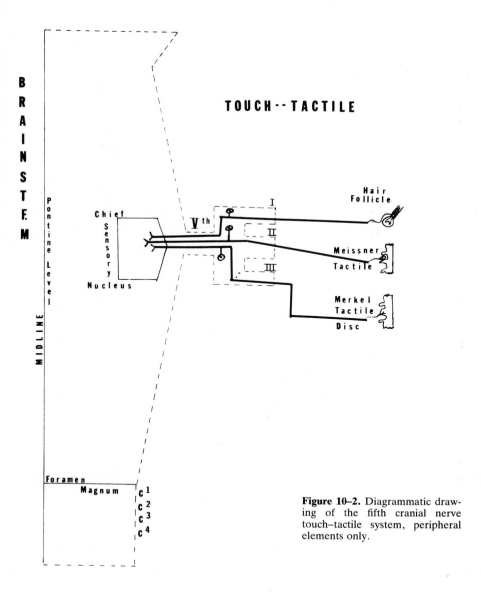

Figure 10–2. Diagrammatic drawing of the fifth cranial nerve touch–tactile system, peripheral elements only.

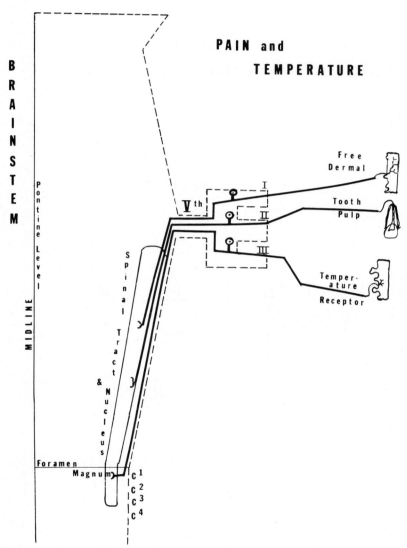

Figure 10–3. Diagrammatic drawing of the fifth cranial nerve, pain and temperature system, peripheral elements only.

The principal areas of proprioceptive sensory endings for the trigeminal nerve are illustrated in Figure 10–4. These sensory receptors project their central fiber toward and through the gasserian ganglion without the deposition of the sensory cell body in that ganglion. Rather the cell bodies are located in a concentrated area of the brainstem, the mesencephalon; thus the name mesencephalic nucleus, which is the only evidence of sensory cell bodies located within the central nervous system. A collateral projection

The Trigeminal Brainstem System (Diagrammatic)

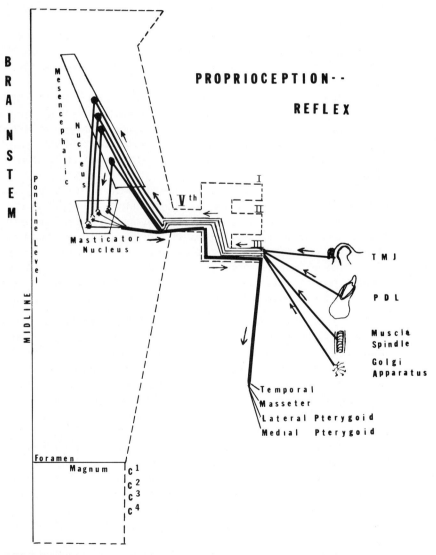

Figure 10–4. Diagrammatic drawing of the fifth cranial nerve, proprioception and jaw reflex system.

from the cell bodies in the mesencephalon to the masticator (motor) nucleus of the trigeminal system is seen. A synapse, the first, is made here with the anterior horn cells of the trigeminal system. These are the motor cells for the masticatory musculature. Thus we have a monosynaptic arc for the "jaw jerk" and for the reflex jaw movements of mastication, deglutition, and so forth.

Although not illustrated, the masticator nucleus also receives fibers from the pyramidal cells of Betz (the outer cortical mantle), which are responsible for volitional movements of the mandible.

The correction of malocclusion potentially can improve the masticatory muscle function pattern. An electromyographic investigation showed that gross incoordination of the various mandibular muscles exists in the presence of severe tooth–jaw malocclusions.[21] Several salient observations are relevant to the concept of improved function with early orthodontic procedures. Prior to citing these, however, a brief description of the study is warranted.

The subjects' ages varied from 11 to 26 years. Thus, there were very few mixed dentitions and no deciduous dentitions, but it may be assumed that the patterns of function had already developed in the subjects at younger ages.

Young persons, all possessing neutrocclusion (Class I, Angle), participated as the control group. They were a nonorthodontically treated sample, without disorders of the stomatognathic system and possessing all of their permanent teeth with the exception of third molars. Their dentitions were judged sufficiently acceptable, and no orthodontic correction was recommended or required.

The test subjects were young persons with severe Class II, Division 1 (Angle) malocclusions. Prior to the initiation of orthodontic treatment, these children were examined electromyographically. The movements of the bilateral temporal and masseter muscles were recorded with surface electrodes as a homogeneous bolus (gum) was chewed. Throughout orthodontic therapy whenever major treatment procedures changed, electromyographic records were taken. The most striking records for each subject were those from which these significant conclusions were drawn:

1. Individuals in the control group exhibited a high degree of synergy in the peak contraction times of the four muscles studied. Coordination of contraction cycles on both the bolus and nonbolus sides reflected a harmonious occlusal table. In those control subjects with known occlusal interferences, there was an asynchronous pattern of peak contraction of the four muscles. This in no way compared with the asynchrony seen in the test group, but it was evidence of incoordination.

2. In the control group, it appeared that peak contraction achievement was concomitant with centric occlusion, at which point the muscles relaxed to initiate another chewing cycle.

3. The test subjects with malocclusions exhibited an entirely different sequence of muscle activity, with gross asynchrony in the achievement of peak muscle contraction times. The four muscles appeared to be "searching" for the occlusal table of maximum contact in each chewing cycle.

4. Orthodontic treatment achieved a more synchronous pattern of

the four muscles. Even at retention, however, the coordination of the four muscles never reached the efficiency seen in the control group. After a period of tooth stabilization and selective occlusal grinding, another degree of improved synchrony and coordination became apparent.

The study conclusively illustrated the intimate association between tooth–jaw and jaw-to-jaw functional relation and the activity of the neuromuscular system. In other words, the musculature accurately mirrors the functional capacity of the dentition. Cuspal interferences (e.g., malposed teeth) were of greater importance in creating muscle asynchrony and disharmony (function) than was the anteroposterior relation of the jaws (esthetic).

SYMPTOMS OF MAXILLARY–MANDIBULAR DYSFUNCTION

In our efforts to relieve symptoms of dysfunction, we have found it valuable to use differential diagnostic procedures. Using these procedures, we have noted a simple triad of symptoms: joint sounds, irregular patterns of mandibular movement, and craniocervical mandibular pain that we believe is indicative of past or present maxillary–mandibular dysfunction.

Joint Sounds

"Clicking" or "Popping"

The exact cause of this sound symptom seems to be less understood than that of crepitus. Various causes have been cited.[22, 23, 24] It does seem logical from histologic and anatomic studies that there are separation and incoordination of the superior surface of the condyle and the inferior dense fibrous surface of the meniscus. This could be related to microtrauma of the temporomandibular ligament, which would decrease its supportive role in maintaining condyle-disk relation in translatory movement, or it may even be attributable to an incoordination of contractions of the inferior and superior heads of the lateral pterygoid muscle. Still another, though unproven, possibility is the presence of a "gabled" superior condyle surface which, in translation of the mandible into the eminence, passes the anterior lip of the meniscus and gives the rude "snap" or "pop." In our experience, we consider the "click" of the joint to be a functional rather than pathologic sequela, although it may be pathognomonic.

We have clinically examined a child, aged 4 years, 8 months, with a "click" of the right temporomandibular joint. This sound was associated with a right buccal crossbite of the deciduous teeth distal to the canine. One author has reported the presence of a "click" in a newborn child.[25]

It is quite common for a patient to complain of "clicking" in the joint without the dentist's being able to palpate or to hear the sound. In these instances, a stethoscopic examination may confirm the "click." Usually it is possible to confirm this sound by the rapid jerklike movement of the mandible as the patient opens his mouth; the sound may be loud enough to be heard 3 feet or more from the patient.

In our experience, the "click" has usually been associated with occlusal imbalances or arch relation discrepancies. In certain instances, however, its first occurrence is subsequent to jaw trauma in a person with a malocclusion.

Crepitus

We believe these joint sounds are more indicative of pathosis than "clicking." The sound may be compared to that created by crushing a piece of heavy bond or parchment paper in a clenched fist. It is a grating sound, without the sharp, acute delineation of the "click." We have noted crepitus in children with rheumatoid arthritis, in patients having high condylar fractures, and in those who have sustained a heavy blow to the chin. Others also have confirmed its presence in frank joint pathosis.[26, 27] Its occurrence is less common in patients in the age range referred to in this chapter (5 to 15 years).

THE TEMPOROMANDIBULAR JOINT AND LIGAMENT. The temporomandibular joint is a complex functioning unit. In an effort to amplify its importance to our subject matter, we have included a few illustrations to emphasize intrajoint relations and components.

The temporomandibular ligament extends from the inferior border of the zygomatic arch to the lateral condylar pole and is one of the primary supporting ligaments of the temporomandibular joint. A lateral dissection of the temporomandibular joint is illustrated in Figure 10–5. The features of the area are labeled and further detailed in Figures 10–6, 10–7, and 10–8.

PERFORATION OF THE MENISCUS AND CONDYLE. Perforations are most often seen to occur first in the lateral-superior region of the disk. This is the thinnest area of the disk and would be interposed between the condyle and eminence (Fig. 10–9).

Both condyles shown in Figures 10–9 and 10–10 were from persons with absence of one or more teeth posterior to the mandibular first premolars. No bridges or dentures were present (Fig. 10–10). Figure 10–11 is a diagrammatic explanation of a "click." As the condyle moves down and out of the fossa, it moves at a greater rate than the meniscus. The superior surface of the condyle passes over the anterior margin of the disk. As this occurs, the "click" is heard. Later, as the subject closes, the condyle remains anterior to the disk, and the subject complains of a "pinching" sensation or fullness in the ears. If the mandible is depressed voluntarily, as would occur in a suppressed yawn, the condyle and disk assume their proper relation only to be disassociated at the next protrusive or opening movement.

Figure 10–12 is a diagrammatic interpretation of crepitus. The roughened surface of an osteoarthritic condyle, perforated disk, or articular remodeled fossa gives the grating sound with movement.

Irregular Patterns of Mandibular Movement

Opening from Occlusion

Deviation of the mandible from a smooth pattern in the transition from occlusion to maximal opening may be indicative of pathologic or functional

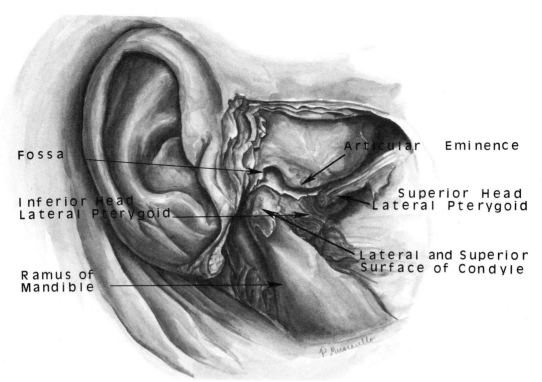

Fossa

Inferior Head
Lateral Pterygoid

Ramus of
Mandible

Articular Eminence

Superior Head
Lateral Pterygoid

Lateral and Superior
Surface of Condyle

Figure 10–5. Lateral dissection of temporomandibular joint.

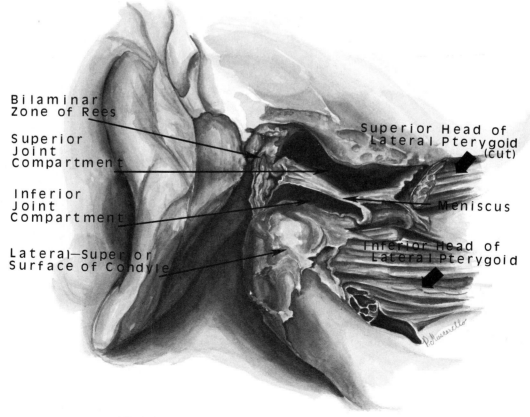

Bilaminar
Zone of Rees

Superior
Joint
Compartment

Inferior
Joint
Compartment

Lateral–Superior
Surface of Condyle

Superior Head of
Lateral Pterygoid
(Cut)

Meniscus

Inferior Head of
Lateral Pterygoid

Figure 10–6. Lateral dissection of temporomandibular joint.

253

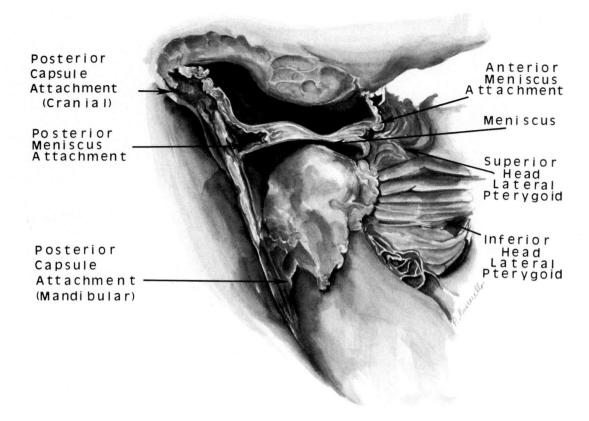

Posterior Capsule Attachment (Cranial)

Posterior Meniscus Attachment

Posterior Capsule Attachment (Mandibular)

Anterior Meniscus Attachment

Meniscus

Superior Head Lateral Pterygoid

Inferior Head Lateral Pterygoid

Figure 10–7. Lateral dissection of temporomandibular joint.

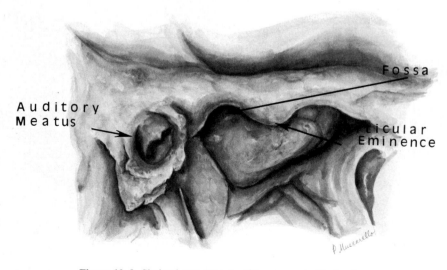

Fossa

Auditory Meatus

Articular Eminence

Figure 10–8. Skeletal components of temporomandibular fossa.

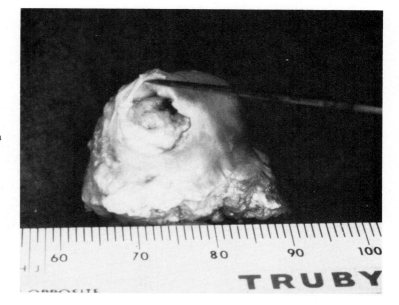

Figure 10–9. A perforation of a meniscus found in autopsy.

disturbance. The usual anterior aspect of opening should not exhibit jerking or midline shift nor should it be apparent that the subject is exerting excessive voluntary effort to achieve maximal opening. Several factors may contribute to an unusual or deviate opening pattern:

1. Myospasm (splinting) of certain muscles to inhibit painful pressures on joint structures associated with condyle movement.

2. Asymmetrical fossa and eminence forms that anatomically would create irregular movement patterns.

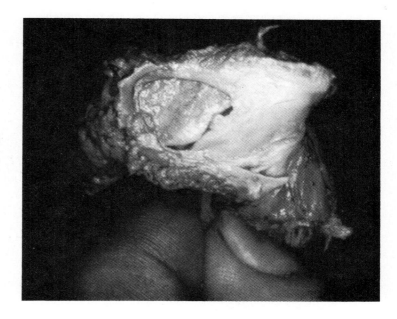

Figure 10–10. A larger meniscus perforation with definite osteoarthritic remodeling of the superior and anterior condyle surfaces.

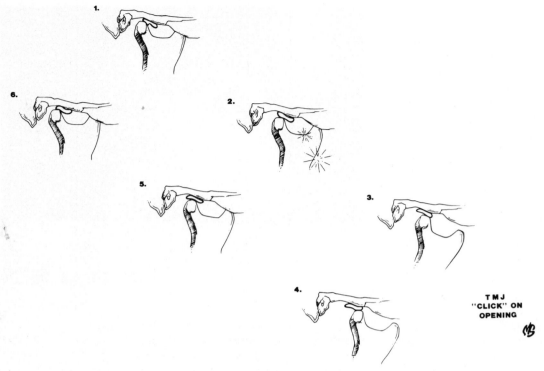

Figure 10–11. Diagrammatic illustration of a temporomandibular joint "click."

3. Asymmetrical condyle forms that, on opening, also create irregular movement patterns.

4. Unilateral meniscus pathosis that creates an uneven translatory path.

5. Unilateral and even bilateral condylar pathosis that also creates irregular mandibular translatory patterns because of differential condylar volumes in the fossae and on the eminences.

We are able to correct and alter disturbances caused by myospasm that may be related to irregular occlusal table relations in occlusion and ar-

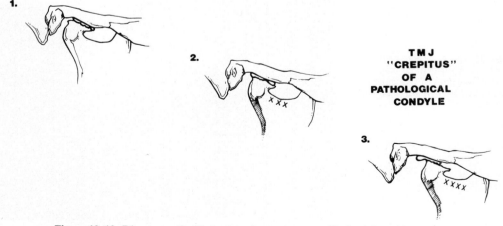

Figure 10–12. Diagrammatic illustration of a temporomandibular joint with crepitus.

ticulation. We may be able to compensate with oral reconstruction for those disturbances that are related to asymmetrical fossae, eminence, and condyle forms. However, we are grossly misinforming our patients and grossly misinformed ourselves if we believe we can reverse disturbances caused by meniscus or condylar pathosis. The best we may do in the latter is to arrest or slow the pathosis if it is indeed caused by occlusal table irregularities.

Closure from "Rest" Position to "Full Occlusion"

The free-way space is the most fertile area for our preventive and health maintenance efforts. As the mandible closes from a phonetically established vertical dimension to full occlusion, the presence of interfering cusps can adversely affect the smoothness of the movement. The closure pattern is not a true mechanical alteration, but more likely a proprioceptively guided reflex path. The mandible may deviate in maximum occlusion, which may be eccentric because of the lack of occlusal table balance. The interruption of the smooth closure may be attributable to a single tooth in supraocclusion or to an arch quadrant in crossbite. In a few instances, it may even be caused by complete arch interference wherein the maxillary arch is excessively expanded to inhibit any occlusal table contact with a constricted mandibular arch occlusal table.

Thus, the deviation of mandibular movement in closure is most frequently caused by factors that can be corrected. Indeed, we are obligated to correct them because their continued presence could well lead to future pathosis of the condyles, menisci, capsules, and fossae.

Craniocervical Mandibular Pain

This final symptom of the differential triad we utilize is the most common cause for patient concern and consultation. Pain is a peculiar sensory modality, an individual experience that is not physiologically oriented, as are all other sensory stimuli, but is indicative of pathosis or impending damage to the body.

We have previously divided the pain types into the following three gross categories:[28] (1) "dull aching" pain, characteristic of deep, poorly localized skeletal muscle spasm; (2) "sharp shooting" pain, related to facial, ligamentous, or capsular irritation; and (3) a "tight drawing" pain, which is most likely to be caused by tension and which is more uncomfortable and noxious than truly painful.

Certainly, the features of craniocervical mandibular syndrome pain are covered in excellent and extensive detail in other chapters of this text. However, we recommend a superior source of reference, the work of Wyke and his associates of the Neurological Unit of the Royal College of Surgeons of England.

DIAGNOSIS AND TREATMENT

Figure 10–13 shows a differential diagnosis flow chart. On the left top half we must be able to recognize those patients whose problems are self-correcting or so minor that treatment is not indicated. If we are certain that no treatment will lead to the lower section, we must intercede. Our basic science background permits us to select and treat these with the correct clinical procedures, thus moving the patient into the top right section of the chart.

Many times, if we lack the diagnostic or clinical ability to treat their problems properly, our treatment iatrogenically sends them to the lower section of the illustration. Thus this diagram reaffirms the importance and interrelation of our basic and clinical sciences, not only in diagnosis but also in treatment.

The correction of severe structural malocclusions or complicated functional malocclusions requires a complete armamentarium of diagnostic tools and equipment, usually found only in the specialist's office. It was, therefore, decided to present only those cases that would respond favorably to a simpler corrective procedure. The diagnostic aids for the cases that follow include apical or panoramic radiographs, the study casts of the dentition, and a total patient dental history. In some instances the causative factor of the functional malocclusion may be obtained in the patient history information. However, in each of the following cases, the focus of our presentation is in the corrective procedures and not in the causative agent or agents. It is germane to emphasize that if the buccal crossbite is caused by a pernicious digital habit, correction may be doomed to relapse if the

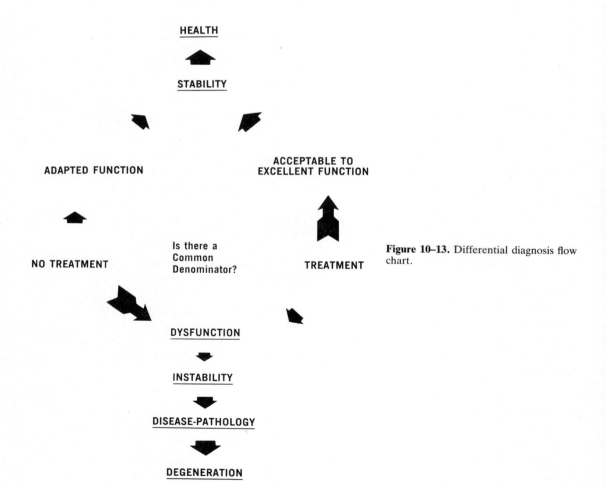

Figure 10–13. Differential diagnosis flow chart.

habit is not corrected. In this matter a good deal of common sense and diagnostic skill on the dentist's part is necessary for success.

DECIDUOUS DENTITION CROSSBITES

Deciduous Unilateral Buccal Crossbite

Quite often we elect to ignore a deciduous crossbite if only the maxillary and mandibular canines are involved. It is true that the usual labial eruption of the maxillary permanent canines will correct the crossbite with loss of the deciduous teeth. If, however, a radiograph reveals a palatally positioned permanent canine, we prefer to correct the deciduous crossbite. Similar logic is used in evaluation of crossbites of the first deciduous molars if they are the only teeth in crossbite, since eruption of the permanent tooth may be self-corrective.

Our concern is directed toward those patients whose deciduous canines or deciduous first and second molars are in lingual crossbite. This full buccal crossbite occlusion predisposes to a unilateral shift of the mandible to the side of crossbite. The musculature presents an irregular contraction pattern and, with continued vertical growth of the face and dentition, an imbalance occurs that may be reflected in slight facial asymmetry and cant to the occlusal plane.[29] It is, therefore, a matter of consequence if we do not treat these malocclusions at this age.

We have many mechanical methods at our disposal for correction of the deciduous unilateral crossbite. We may prefer a fixed appliance. Certainly, its advantage is control: we place it and the patient wears it. The removable appliance is patient-controlled, and without his cooperation our efforts are useless. We have chosen to illustrate the correction of the deciduous dentition crossbite with a removable appliance, although other types of removable or fixed appliances would suffice (Fig. 10–14).

Crozat Appliance

The Crozat is an extremely useful appliance for correctly diagnosed cases.[30] Its principal function is to tip the teeth, and such is the need in the majority of these unilateral crossbite problems (Fig. 10–15 *A, B*).

The fabrication and construction of the Crozat appliance is well described and illustrated by Taylor.[31] His articles and manual are recommended for any dentist who would consider the use of the Crozat. (Also, reputable dental laboratories will construct the appliance for the dentist once suitable prescription orders are made.) If the dentist or assistant does wish to construct his own appliances in the laboratory, we recommend a short course on the subject.

Deciduous Anterior Crossbite

It must be assumed that in this instance we are not dealing with the true Class III (Angle) growth pattern. Rather, we have the pseudo-Class III so often seen with the deciduous maxillary central incisors in linguover-

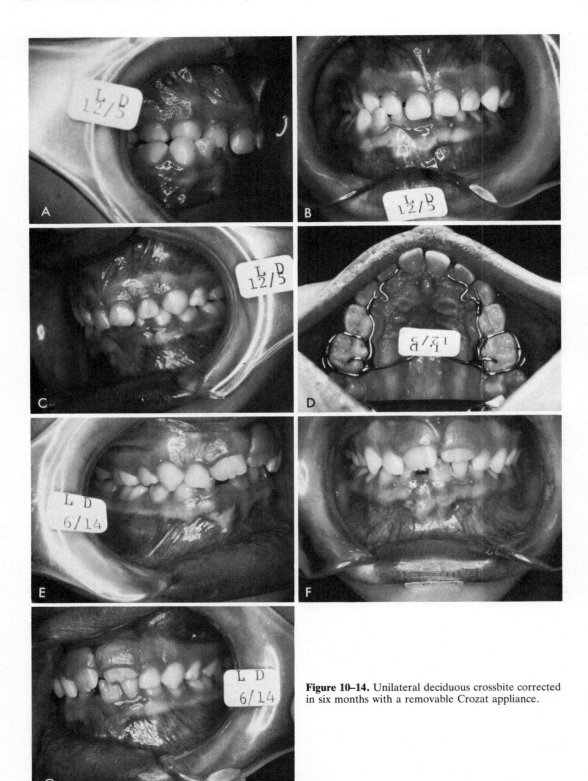

Figure 10–14. Unilateral deciduous crossbite corrected in six months with a removable Crozat appliance.

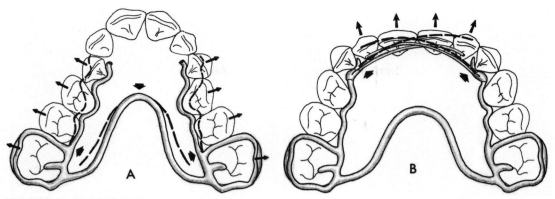

Figure 10–15. *A,* Maxillary Crozat designed for unilateral or bilateral expansion. *B,* Maxillary Crozat designed for anterior tooth advancement.

sion to the mandibular incisors. In these patients we advance the deciduous maxillary incisors over the deciduous mandibular incisors to give a better functional (and developmental) pattern. Quite often, if the arch length is adequate and the anteroposterior jaw relation is acceptable, our early intervention insures that future orthodontic therapy will not be needed (Fig. 10–16).

Fixed Lingual Appliance With Anterior Reversed Finger Springs

This is a simple appliance to construct. Molar bands or stainless steel-chrome deciduous tooth crowns are fitted on the deciduous maxillary second molars. A maxillary impression is taken with the bands or crowns in place. After the impression is withdrawn from the mouth, the bands or crowns are removed and placed in the impression in their proper position. The impression is poured in dental stone. After separation of the impression and cast, the base of the cast is trimmed for ease of work. A gold* or Truchrome** .040 diameter wire is closely adapted to the lingual aspect of the bands or crowns and then properly contoured to the lingual–gingival area of the buccal surfaces of the maxillary anterior teeth. The space between the lingual base wire and the lingual surfaces of the maxillary deciduous incisors is from 4 to 5 mm. If the lingual arch is too close to the incisors, the lingual recurved finger springs do not have sufficient space for action. The lingual base wire is adapted in the same fashion on the contralateral side of the arch.

At this point, the clinician solders one point of the wire to the molar band or crown, then checks that the lingual arch is in passive contact with the contralateral molar. If he is satisfied that it is passive, the second solder joint is made. The work cast should now appear as though a lingual holding arch has been constructed, with no deciduous maxillary incisor contact.

The recurved or reversed finger spring must be made of a resilient wire

---

*J. Aderer, Inc., Long Island City, N. Y.
**Rocky Mountain Dental Supply Co., Denver, Colorado.

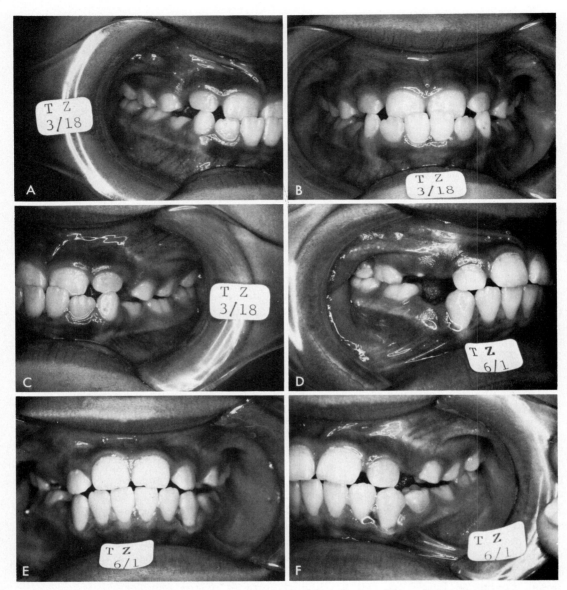

Figure 10–16. Maxillary anterior tooth advancement with fixed lingual recurved finger springs. Total treatment time was four months.

of .026 or .024 diameter. We have found that gold wire is the most effective.* This wire has a great deal of workability, and the long spring arm has a very superior force delivery system to the lingually positioned incisors.

The bands, lingual arch, and soldered finger springs are removed from the cast. The springs are adapted as illustrated, and then the appliance is polished and cemented in place.

The patient is carefully instructed concerning foods that will damage

*J. Aderer, Inc., .026 inch No. 4 gold wire.

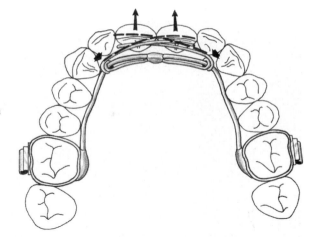

Figure 10–17. Fixed maxillary lingual arch with recurved anterior finger springs.

or break the appliance. Usually we do not activate the appliance at the time of cementation; our first adjustment may be done one or two weeks after placement. It is quite simple to press the thumb on the occlusal aspect of the second deciduous molar and, with the opposite hand, bend the lingual arch wire down a quarter of an inch with a Howe plier. This is done bilaterally, and the thumb pressure on the tooth supports the band and tooth from undue force. With the appliance held away from the lingual surface, the finger springs are easily advanced a few millimeters for initiation of lingual-to-labial force. Now the lingual arch is rebent to its original position.

The activation described is adequate for a period of four to six weeks, provided the patient does not deliberately or accidentally displace the finger springs. Subsequent activation is done as described. One common problem with this, and all finger spring appliances, is the possibility that the springs may over-ride the tooth's incisal or occlusal surface. To avoid this, it is wise to place a slight gingival bend in each finger spring at the time they are activated (Fig. 10–17).

Unilateral and Bilateral Buccal Deciduous Tooth Crossbites

The essential factor in correction of this type of malocclusion is a bilateral force delivery system; most often the forces directed bilaterally are equal, but this is not always necessary. In these cases, an excellent mode of treatment is the fixed Barnes appliance. It may consist of bands on the deciduous second molars alone or on the deciduous second molars or first permanent molars and deciduous canines or permanent canines. The appliance consists of a recurved lingual–palatal arch, which, with proper adjustment, provides equal or unequal lateral forces.

The Barnes appliance is indirectly fabricated in much the same manner as the previously described appliance. A very heavy gauge (.036 to .040) wire should be used; our preference is for Truchrome or gold (Figs. 10–18 and 10–19).

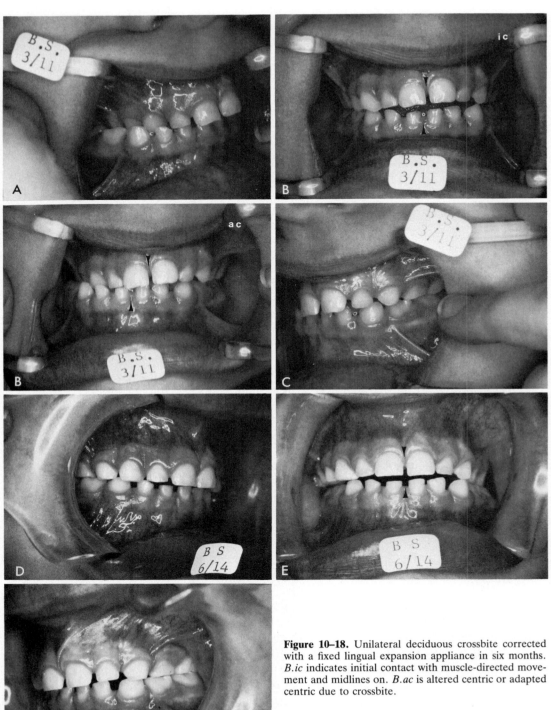

Figure 10–18. Unilateral deciduous crossbite corrected with a fixed lingual expansion appliance in six months. *B.ic* indicates initial contact with muscle-directed movement and midlines on. *B.ac* is altered centric or adapted centric due to crossbite.

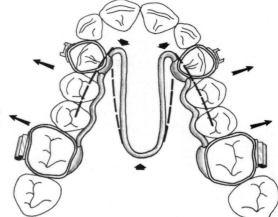

Figure 10–19. Fixed maxillary expansion appliance as used to correct crossbite (altered centric) of patient in Figure 10–18.

TRANSITIONAL DENTITION

The opportunity for the correction of a functional malocclusion often may not present itself in the deciduous dentition stage. On other occasions the practitioner may postpone early treatment in the hope that the permanent first molars will erupt in proper buccal–lingual relation. In the latter situation, it is quite possible that normal tongue function, facial growth, or just an end-to-end deciduous buccal occlusion may permit normal permanent first molar occlusion. However, if the deciduous maxillary molars' buccal cusps are in the occlusal fossae of the mandibular deciduous molars, the maxillary and mandibular first molars will rarely erupt correctly. The constricted maxillary arch form extends posteriorly and includes the partially unerupted first molars.

In these patients with transitional dentition crossbite, we prefer to await the complete eruption of the permanent maxillary first molars.

Preformed maxillary first molar bands with .045 inch buccal tubes are firmly seated on those teeth. A maxillary impression is made with the bands in place. The impression is removed and checked to be certain that the buccal tubes of the bands did not "pull" the impression from the side of the tray. If the impression is inaccurate, the constructed appliance will not fit or, if it does, it may exert abnormal or undesired forces.

The lingual aspect of the inner surface of the bands is waxed to provide a space between the band and the plaster that is soon to be poured. When this wax is melted during soldering, it provides a "heat space" to enhance the soldering procedure.

The impression is then poured in either plaster or stone. After the final plaster set, the cast is separated from the impression. The nonanatomical portion of the cast is trimmed.

We use a simple dental surveyor to hold the working cast as we solder.

The appliance we prefer to use for the transitional dentition is a modification of the lingual arch with a labial arch and Oliver loops or tie back stops. Gold* lingual extensions are soldered to the lingual aspect of each

---

*J. Aderer, Inc., Long Island City, N. Y.

molar band. These are closely adapted to the lingual surface of the maxillary teeth anterior to the deciduous canine or permanent lateral incisor, depending on the extent of the crossbite.

The bands and their attached lingual extensions are removed and polished. The bands are then cemented to the patient's permanent first molars after their fit and the contact of the lingual extensions have been checked.

After the excess cement has been removed, we adapt a .045 inch gold* wire from one buccal tube to the other. This wire is adapted to fit into the buccal tubes passively and to "stand away" from the teeth approximately 5 mm. This is especially important in the anterior portion of the arch, where contact with the incisors could cause unnecessary tooth movement or, in rare instances, tooth devitalization.

After this heavy buccal wire has been passively adapted, two Oliver loops or tie back stops are soldered, one on each side, anterior to the molar–buccal tubes. These will provide a means of tying the buccal arch in, and will also allow a means of arch advancement as the crossbite is corrected. Prior to tying the buccal arch, an expansion of one-half inch to each side is placed in the wire. The wire is then seated and tied for its first period of activation.

The patient is checked at three or four week intervals and additional expansion is achieved. The total treatment time depends on the extent of the crossbite, the density of the bone, the number of teeth in crossbite, and the occlusal cuspal locking. For example, cases involving deep fossae and long cusps require more time than those involving flat cusps and shallow fossae. On an average, our treatment times may extend from four to six months.

It may be necessary, with extensive tooth movements, to make additional buccal arches as the length of the arch increases with expansion. These arches are directly constructed in the same fashion as the original.

After the crossbite has been corrected, it is often advisable to hold the arches in position with the passive expanding appliance. This pre-retention procedure permits the teeth and alveolar bone to stabilize. We often follow this procedure for two or three months. Upon removing the appliance, we place a Hawley maxillary retainer to insure our treatment result. The patient wears the retainer both night and day for six months; then, over the next six months, the use of the retainer at night is gradually decreased (Figs. 10–20, 10–21, and 10–22).

PERMANENT DENTITION

Bilateral Expansion With Palatal Expansion Appliance

Extensive papers on this appliance by Wirtz[32] and Haas[33] have appeared in the literature. They have documented most appropriately the indications, contraindications, and application of this procedure. We illustrate our position and preferred appliance with one case.

---

*J. Aderer, Inc., Long Island City, N. Y.

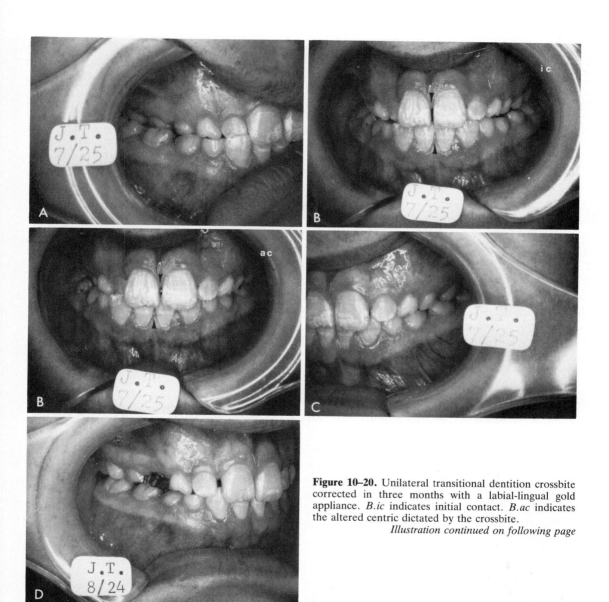

Figure 10–20. Unilateral transitional dentition crossbite corrected in three months with a labial-lingual gold appliance. *B.ic* indicates initial contact. *B.ac* indicates the altered centric dictated by the crossbite.

Illustration continued on following page

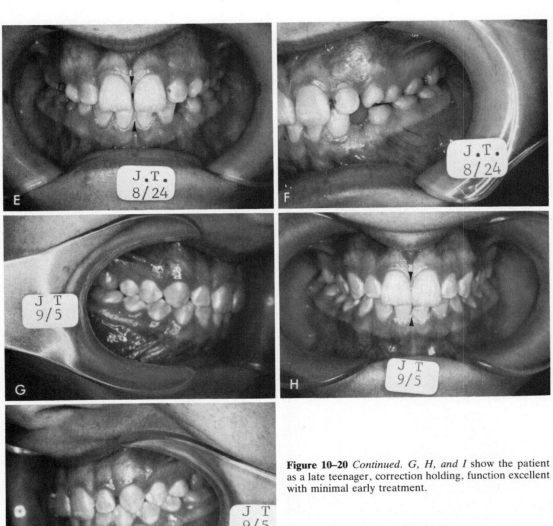

Figure 10–20 *Continued. G, H, and I* show the patient as a late teenager, correction holding, function excellent with minimal early treatment.

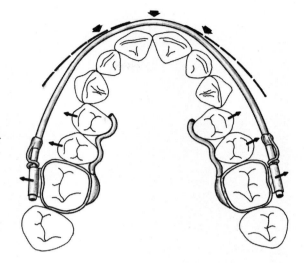

Figure 10–21. Fixed labial-lingual expansion appliance.

Most frequently these patients have bilaterally collapsed, Omega-shaped maxillary arches. The palatal vault is high, the nares are often narrowed, and evidence of mouth breathing may be present in the form of dry anterior mucosa, fissured angles of the lips, and as cephalometric evidence of adenoid and tonsillar tissue enlargement. The mandibular arch is often well formed and oval-shaped, with adequate arch length. The tongue with a low posture has maintained a nearly ideal mandibular arch form.

Our preferred procedure utilizes a high-tension spring,* which is soldered to the bands. We seat preformed bands on the permanent first molars and the first premolars. An impression is taken with the bands in place. The impression is removed and the laboratory procedure of waxing, pouring, and trimming is identical to that for the previously described appliance.

The lingual extensions of the appliance are adapted to the lingual arch form from molar to premolar. If the second maxillary molars are in crossbite, lingual extensions are made from the first molar to the second molar to sweep them buccally with the expansion.

The spring appliance is soldered to the lingual aspects of the four preformed bands. Since the appliance is patient activated, it is important that the wrench insert hole is in a position that the patient can find and activate. One should check the direction of activation, since it must be expansive, and also check the working of the wrench and screw and the expansion distance available before soldering.

After all solder joints have been completed, the appliance is removed, polished, and checked again for workability. The appliance is seated to check its fit and, if satisfactory, cemented into position.

The patient is instructed in oral hygiene and activation. He is also advised of possible pain in the teeth, the maxillary arch, and the area lateral to the orbit from the maxillary zygomatic to the frontal zygomatic suture area.

We instruct our patients to start with a quarter turn in the morning and

---

*Minne-Expander, Ormco Orthodontic Supply Co., Glendora, California.

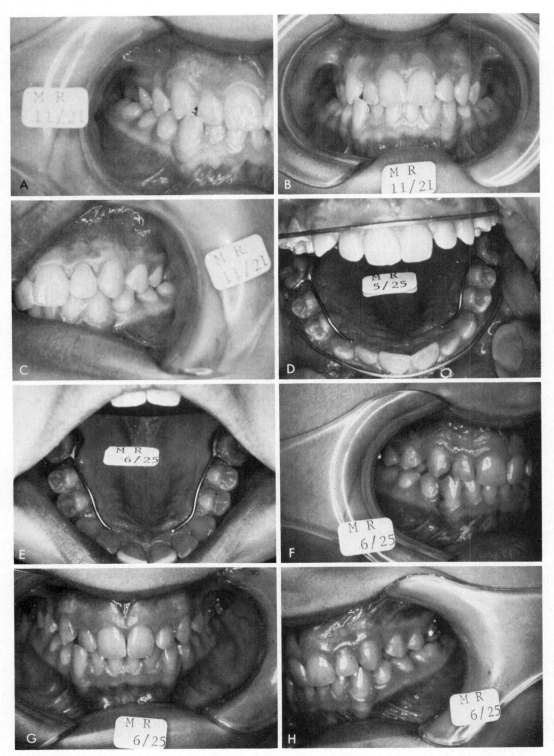

Figure 10–22. Permanent dentition crossbite corrected with fixed labial-lingual appliance. *D* Illustrates overcorrection. *E, F, G,* and *H* show settling. Further treatment will be required later to align maxillary anterior teeth.

a quarter turn in the evening. We check the patients on a ten-day schedule.

As expansion occurs, the bilateral space-gaining often opens the bite mechanically and creates a midline diastema. The former often does not close without full orthodontic treatment, and the latter closes as the teeth align themselves in the arch. Thus, to the astute diagnostician, these patients are often candidates for full orthodontic treatment after arch expansion. Some may even require orthodontic–surgical procedures. It is therefore imperative that accurate pretreatment records are obtained and that both patient and parent are apprised of the possible need for comprehensive treatment at a future date (Fig. 10–23).

Here again we use the expansion appliance as an early retention appliance. Once the expansion has been achieved, the appliance remains in the mouth for two to four months. In this time, some of the midline diastema and open bite features close. Teeth that are not fixed in the appliance do stabilize. Following this period of stabilization, a regular Hawley retainer is fabricated and placed. The usual retention pattern is then followed.

We quite often find that the bilateral permanent dentition expansion cases, such as those described, require a full fixed orthodontic appliance to take suitable advantage of the expansion. Thus it is advisable in these situations to have the mechanical armamentarium available for total correction.

With the exception of the last case, we have purposely avoided those instances wherein a full fixed orthodontic appliance is indicated. Our intention has been to illustrate simple fixed and removable appliances which are capable of correcting early any minor tooth interferences that alter maxillary and mandibular relation. The human jaw, jaw joints, and neuromuscular system are especially adaptive in the young child and adolescent; however, with latent pubertal and early adult development, the noxious functional aberrations cited earlier may introduce irreversible changes within the stomatognathic system. It thus behooves the dental diagnostician to review accurately those many simple and complex tooth positions in young patients that are responsible for altered centric. The early correction of those situations, which are not self-corrective, insures that the patient will experience acceptable and satisfactory jaw function.

If we are not able to correct these jaw relation problems at an early age, their continued existence may introduce the pain-dysfunction syndrome in conjunction with bruxism habits, myospasm, and associated symptoms.[34]

It may seem judicious to the clinician to introduce limited therapy in these young adult and adult patients rather than orthodontically correcting the malocclusion. Such procedures could involve bite plate therapy, diagnostic splints, occlusal rehabilitation, or occlusal equilibration. The latter two procedures are irreversible and certainly should only be pursued in a few instances. The work of Laskin and colleagues on occlusal equilibration stresses the importance of the dentist in properly diagnosing and treating with occlusal equilibration.[35] It would seem logical in treating these adult patients to seek the combined diagnostic and treatment recommendations of several specialty areas involved, and then, if all the therapeutic avenues are blocked, to resort to the compromise of occlusal rehabilitation and/or occlusal equilibration.

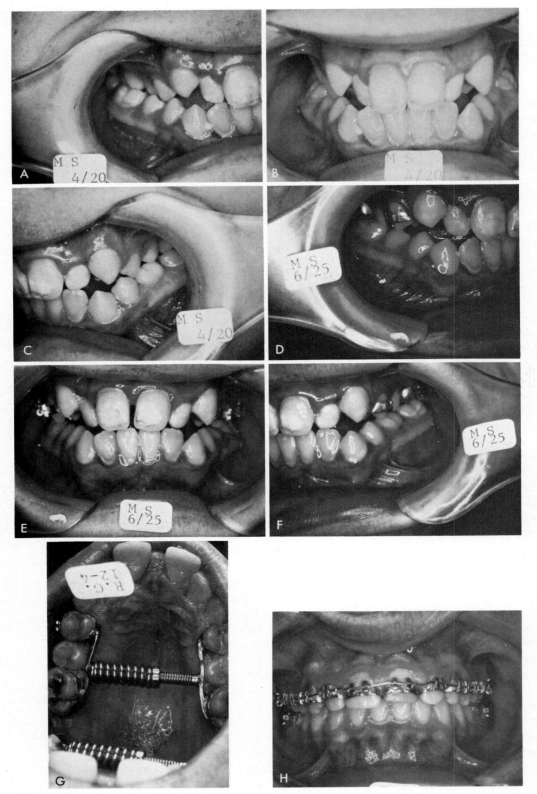

Figure 10–23. Bilateral permanent dentition crossbite. *D, E,* and *F* show patient after three weeks of initial expansion. *G* is a photograph of the fixed palatal screw appliance in another patient. *H* is of the same patient as in *G* after placement of a full edgewise maxillary arch to consolidate and coordinate arch form.

CONCLUSION

Today's deep concern for preventative dental procedures endorsed by third party plans, combined with a dental-health–oriented population, should encourage all dental practitioners to avoid the damaging sequelae and possibly painful symptoms of craniocervical mandibular dysfunction. We have endeavored to present our views by emphasizing the neuromuscular system of jaw movement, the anatomical and pathological basis of function and/or dysfunction, and the relatively simple, but multiple, mechanical means at the clinician's disposal for early treatment of improper mandibular–maxillary relations which are due to tooth positions.

Figure 10–13 illustrated our interest and concern for an increased

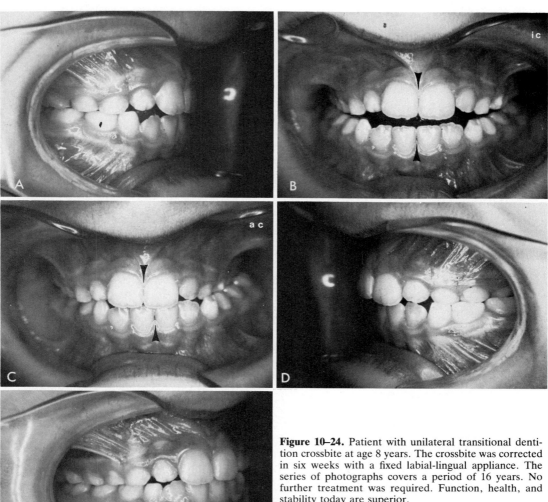

Figure 10–24. Patient with unilateral transitional dentition crossbite at age 8 years. The crossbite was corrected in six weeks with a fixed labial-lingual appliance. The series of photographs covers a period of 16 years. No further treatment was required. Function, health, and stability today are superior.

Illustration continued on following page

diagnostic base for all of dentistry. In that illustration we placed our diagnostic skill at the center and asked if there was a "common denominator" to assure us that we have made the proper diagnosis and treatment or no-treatment decision. To date, we do not believe we have found such a factor; but we believe it exists, and we continue to search for it.

In this schematic cycle, we must be able to assess those cases which are self-corrective to their initial dysfunction symptoms. In those instances, they will adapt and go on to health and stability. However, if our past clinical experience and diagnostic knowledge informs us that we must treat to avoid dysfunction, instability, disease, or pathology to the point of degeneration, we must institute early and proper treatment procedures to correct the problem. Still one other aspect of our dilemma in treatment is

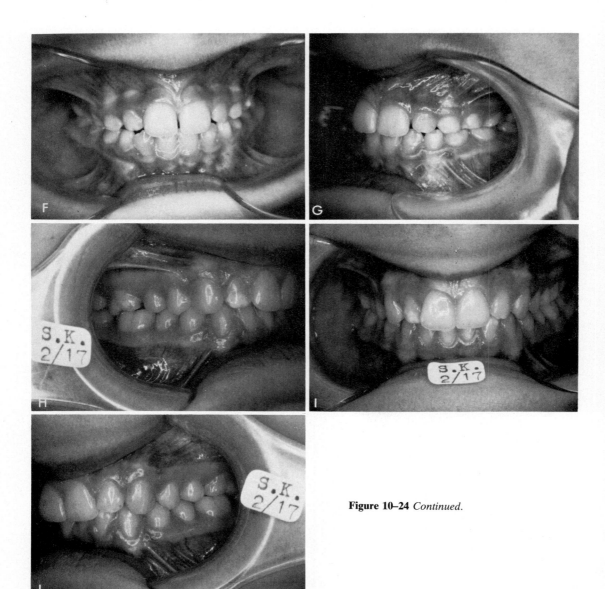

Figure 10–24 *Continued.*

the iatrogenic insults we inadvertently impose on our patients and their dentitions. This is emphasized with the arrow on the right of Figure 10–13, below "treatment." We must forever be alert to avoid this path in treatment. Too often, we ignore this vector until we are at the irreversible level of "degeneration."

Thus, we would stress, it is not only necessary to know "when" and "how" to treat these jaw dysfunction and altered centric problems, but it is just as important to know when not to treat.

Dentistry today has entered a most comprehensive and challenging period. All of us are called upon daily to make decisions that may easily affect the lifetime dental and physical health of our patients. It is, therefore, most imperative that our basic science knowledge, treatment procedures, and mechanical armamentarium be extensive and complete. Our patients deserve our very best, and we as dentists are obligated to assure that they are provided with nothing less.

Figure 10–24 emphasizes the potential that we all possess. This illustrates a unilateral buccal crossbite of the transitional dentition. Mechanical treatment consisted of six weeks with a fixed removable maxillary expansion appliance. The sequence of illustrations covers a period of 16 years to age 24. The dental health, function, and stability are superior and the effort on our part was minimal.

It is not too difficult to imagine the dysfunction sequelae, facial asymmetry, and impaired oral health that could have resulted if no treatment had been instituted. It is also possible to imagine the difficulty and prolonged treatment that later adolescent orthodontic appliances would have entailed.

Therefore we emphasize again the importance of early treatment and preventive procedures which are within the province of all of us with common sense, sound diagnosis, and simple appliances.

References

1. Levy, P. H.: Clinical implications of mandibular repositioning and the concept of an alterable centric relation. Dent. Clin. North Am., *19*:543, 1975.
2. Ahlgren, J.: Kinesiology of the mandible: an EMG study. Acta Odont. Scand., *25*:593, 1967.
3. Ballard, C. F.: A consideration of the physiologic background of mandibular posture and movement. Dent. Pract., *6*:80, 1955.
4. Brill, N., Lammie, G., Osborne, J., and Perry, H. T.: Mandibular position and mandibular movements; a review. Br. Dent. J., *106*:391, 1959.
5. Corbin, K. B., and Harrison, F.: Function of the mesencephalic root of the fifth cranial nerve. J. Neurophysiol., *3*:423, 1940.
6. Dellow, P. G.: Control mechanisms of mastication. Ann. Aust. Coll. Dent. Surg., *2*:81, 1969.
7. Kawamura, Y.: Recent Concepts of the Physiology of Mastication. Advances in Oral Biology, Vol. 1. New York, Academic Press, 1964, pp. 77–109.
8. Hickey, J. C., Stacey, R. W., and Rinear, L.: Electromyographic studies of mandibular muscles in basic jaw movements. J. Prosthet. Dent., *7*:565, 1957.
9. Lammie, G. A.: Dental Orthopedics, Oxford, The Alden Press, 1966.
10. Jerge, C. R.: The neurologic mechanism underlying cyclic jaw movements. J. Prosthet. Dent., *14*:667, 1964.
11. McNamara, J. A.: Neuromuscular and skeletal adaptations to altered orofacial function. Center for Human Growth and Development. The University of Michigan, Ann Arbor, Michigan, 1972.

12. Moyers, R. E.: Some physiologic considerations of centric and other jaw relations. J. Prosthet. Dent., *6*:183, 1956.
13. Perry, H. T.: Kinesiology of the Temporal and Masseter Muscles in Chewing a Homogenous Bolus. An unpublished Ph.D. thesis, Northwestern University, Evanston, Illinos. 1961.
14. Schaerer, P., Stallard, R. E., and Zander, N. A.: Occlusal interferences and mastication: an electromyographic study. J. Prosthet. Dent., *17*:438, 1967.
15. Walsh, J. P.: Neurophysiological aspects of mastication. Dent. J. Austral., *23*:49, 1951.
16. Woelfel, J. B., Hickey, J. C., Stacy, R. W., and Rinear, L. L.: Electromyographic analysis of mandibular movements. J. Prosthet. Dent., *10*:688, 1960.
17. Humphrey, T.: Development of mouth opening and related reflexes involving the oral area of human fetuses. Alabama J. Med. Sciences, *5*:126, 1968.
18. Castelein, P. T.: The Histological, Anatomical and Roentgenographic Investigation of the Temporomandibular Joint Region in the Eight to Thirty Week Human Fetus, Unpublished M.S. Thesis, Northwestern University, Chicago, Illinois, 1972.
19. Bosma, J. F.: Human Infant Oral Function. In: J. F. Bosma, Ed.: Symposium on Oral Sensation and Proprioception. Springfield, Illinois, Charles C Thomas Co., 1967.
20. Clark, R. K. F., and Wyke, B. D.: Arthrokinetic reflexogenic system in the temporomandibular joint. J. Anat., *117*:216, 1974.
21. Perry, op. cit.
22. Sicher, H.: Oral Anatomy, 4th ed. St. Louis, The C. V. Mosby Company, 1965.
23. Rees, L. A.: Structure and function of the mandibular joint. Br. Dent. J., *96*:125, 1954.
24. Perry, H. T.: Relation of occlusion of temporomandibular joint dysfunction; the orthodontic viewpoint. JADA, *79*:137, 1969.
25. Berry, D. C.: Clicking of temporomandibular joints in the newly born. Br. Dent. J., *124*:3, 1968.
26. Moffett, B. C., Johnson, L. C., McCabe, J. B., and Askew, H. C.: Articular remodeling in the adult human temporomandibular joint. Am. J. Anat., *115*:119, 1964.
27. Blackwood, H. J. J.: Pathology of the temporomandibular joint. JADA., *79*:118, 1969.
28. Perry, H. T.: The symptomology of temporomandibular joint disturbance. J. Prosthet. Dent., *19*:288, 1968.
29. McNamara, op. cit.
30. Smythe, R. B.: The Crozat removable appliance. Am. J. Orthod., *55*:739, 1969.
31. Taylor, W. H.: Adjustment and Design Technique of the Crozat Appliance. A laboratory manual privately published by the author, 1970. Personal communication, 1970.
32. Wirtz, R. A.: Skeletal and dental changes accompanying rapid midpalatal suture opening. Am. J. Orthod., *58*:41, 1970.
33. Haas, A. J.: The treatment of maxillary deficiency by opening the midpalatal suture. Angle Orthod., *35*:200, 1965.
34. Perry, H. T. et al.: Occlusion in a stress situation. JADA, *60*:78, 1960.
35. Goodman, P., Greene, C. S., and Laskin, D. M.: Response of patients with myofacial pain-dysfunction syndrome to mock equilibration. JADA, *92*:755, 1976.

11

Effective Management and Treatment of the Craniomandibular Syndrome

HAROLD GELB, D.M.D.

OVERVIEW

The syndrome with which we are dealing has alternately been referred to as the TMJ syndrome, myofascial pain–dysfunction syndrome, TMJ arthrosis, and dysfunctional temporomandibular joint arthritis. The distinction between these various entities was discussed in Chapter 3. It is evident that the significant differentiation lies in the degree of exposure of the joint and musculature to microtraumata, "wear and tear," and dysfunction.

The symptom complex is diverse and seemingly unrelated clinically. It may include head, ear, neck, and facial pain; vertigo without nystagmus; tinnitus (subjective ear noise); clicking and crepitation within the joint on opening or closing; burning and pricking sensations of the side of the tongue and the roof of the mouth; fatigue; difficulty in swallowing; spontaneous subluxation of the mandible; chronic sore throat; forgetfulness; changes in hearing ability and clogged ears; and diverse muscle spasm throughout the body.

Far and away the most frequently reported symptom is pain. The muscle groups most frequently involved are listed in Tables 11–1, 11–2, and 11–3, representing patients referred from three different sources. The types of dentitions observed in these two medical studies plus a purely dental one are listed in Tables 11–4, 11–5, and 11–6. It should be noted that patients from the headache study evidenced pain on palpation of the condylar heads through the external auditory meatuses in 179 of 200 cases and in 152 of 200 cases in the private TMJ practice group. This is one of the chief methods of ruling out the myofascial pain–dysfunction syndrome diagnostically. Our

TABLE 11–1. Symptoms of 742 Patients With Temporomandibular Joint Syndrome*

AGE GROUP	10–20	21–30	31–40	41–50	51–60	61–70	71–80	TOTAL
Males	15	31	47	20	36	30	12	191
Females	35	81	115	125	123	50	22	551
Muscles in spasm								
Internal pterygoids	43	109	137	109	115	53	36	602
External pterygoids	30	87	96	101	83	52	22	471
Masseters	20	45	76	49	49	13	14	266
Temporalis	8	27	58	39	38	16	11	197
Sternomastoids	20	40	81	47	46	26	14	274
Posterior cervicals	5	12	33	40	33	20	8	151
Mylohyoids	—	13	9	14	2	2	2	42
Trapezius	4	2	16	12	4	6	3	47
Others	1	6	3	5	3	7	1	26
Ear symptoms								
Tinnitus	11	51	70	83	58	28	10	311
Hearing loss	—	19	40	17	25	5	1	107
Pre-auricular pain	12	19	25	33	17	2	1	109
Post-auricular pain	14	7	5	17	24	10	2	79
Auricular	19	25	43	52	71	41	12	263
Temporomandibular joint								
Clicking	6	28	22	38	31	3	4	132
Crepitation	2	12	14	30	17	7	4	86
Pain	28	61	75	67	55	23	11	320
Limited motion	6	4	6	4	5	1	3	29
Bruxism	12	24	42	30	23	13	3	147
Head pain								
Facial	8	11	15	16	22	6	1	79
Occipital	—	8	3	9	19	3	2	44
Cervical	—	5	8	11	5	3	1	33
Headaches	4	24	43	33	32	14	2	152
Dizziness	9	27	25	31	23	16	2	133

*The types of dentition observed in this study are given in Table 11–4.
From Gelb, H., et al.: The role of the dentist and the otolaryngologist in evaluating temporomandibular joint syndromes. J. Prosthet. Dent., *18*:500, 1967.

TABLE 11–2. Symptoms of 200 Patients With Temporomandibular Joint Dysfunction*

Age Group	1–10	11–20	21–30	31–40	41–50	51–60	61–70	71–80	Total
Males	1	6	10	19	11	9	1	0	57
Females	0	14	31	32	32	24	8	2	143
Muscles in muscle spasm									
Internal pterygoids	1	20	38	44	38	30	7	0	178
External pterygoids	1	20	41	50	41	32	8	2	195
Masseter	0	13	30	39	36	30	9	1	158
Temporalis	1	16	29	35	35	27	6	2	151
Sternomastoid	1	12	34	28	33	25	3	2	138
Posterior cervical	1	9	31	41	37	27	5	2	153
Mylohyoid	0	4	16	23	32	27	3	1	106
Trapezius	1	6	18	33	26	16	9	2	111
Others	0	12	31	31	23	17	2	0	116
Ear symptoms									
Tinnitus	0	0	6	26	27	25	7	1	92
Hearing loss	0	0	1	0	4	5	8	2	20
Preauricular pain	1	10	35	22	25	28	3	2	103
Auricular pain	0	3	10	2	6	7	4	0	32
TMJ symptoms									
Clicking	1	15	24	21	38	8	16	1	124
Crepitation	0	0	0	4	7	5	8	2	26
Pain	0	11	10	14	12	9	5	2	63
Bruxism	0	8	17	13	4	6	3	0	51
Head pain									
Facial	0	0	5	4	2	1	2	0	14
Occipital	0	0	3	6	3	4	2	0	16
Cervical	1	14	20	30	11	8	4	2	90
Temporal	1	8	27	47	32	14	4	1	134
Vertigo	0	4	2	6	3	3	4	1	23

*The types of dentition observed in this study are given in Table 11–5.

From Gelb, H., and Tarte, J.: A two-year clinical evaluation of 200 cases of chronic headaches: the cranicervical-mandibular syndrome. JADA, *91*:1230, 1975.

TABLE 11–3. Symptoms of 200 Patients with Temporomandibular Joint Syndrome from a Dental Study*†

Age Group	10–21	21–30	30–41	41–50	51–60	61–70	71–80	Total
Males	3	20	14	6	8	1	2	54
Females	15	34	37	28	16	12	4	146
Muscles in spasm								
Internal pterygoids	15	41	41	28	16	11	4	156
External pterygoids	17	44	46	31	19	12	5	174
Masseters	16	50	44	28	22	11	5	176
Temporalis	15	44	42	25	16	10	5	167
Sternocleidomastoid	16	46	45	29	18	10	4	168
Posterior cervicals	15	45	43	27	17	10	3	160
Mylohyoids	12	34	35	27	16	9	4	137
Trapezius	16	44	45	29	16	10	4	164
Others	17	52	50	33	21	12	6	191
Ear symptoms								
Tinnitus	3	15	24	10	9	6	4	71
Hearing loss	2	9	19	5	5	5	4	49
Stuffiness	6	20	28	17	13	6	5	95
Popping or whooshing noise on opening or closing	10	43	43	22	14	5	5	142
Temporomandibular joint								
Clicking	6	30	36	23	7	8	3	113
Pain	16	54	51	33	21	13	6	194
Bruxism	9	29	35	19	12	10	2	116
Head pain								
Facial	5	14	19	9	9	6	1	63
Occipital	13	1	9	6	7	2	2	40
Cervical	1	10	9	9	5	5	1	40
Temporal	2	12	29	17	8	5	4	77
Vertigo	3	13	30	12	11	6	4	79

*The types of dentition observed in this study are given in Table 11–6.

†From Gelb, H., and Bernstein, I.: Clinical evaluation of two hundred patients with temporomandibular joint syndrome. J. Prosthet. Dent., *49*:237, 1983.

TABLE 11–4. Distribution of Patients

	No. Patients	% of Total
Full complement of teeth	148	20
Complete upper and lower dentures	74	10
Complete upper and partial lower dentures	60	8
Fixed partial dentures	14	2
Partially edentulous; no replacement	363	49
Removable partial dentures	83	11

From Gelb, H., et al.: The role of the dentist and otolaryngologist in evaluating temporomandibular joint syndromes. J. Prosthet. Dent., *18*:501, 1967.

TABLE 11–5. Rehabilitation Instituted in 97 Patients After Treatment for Temporomandibular Joint Dysfunction

METHOD OF TREATMENT	NO. PATIENTS
Selective occlusal adjustment	25
Orthodontics	37
Fixed partial prostheses	17
Cast gold occlusal overlay	14
Complete maxillary and mandibular dentures	4

Distribution of 200 Patients by Dental Status

DENTAL STATUS	NO.	%
Full complement of teeth	50	25
Complete maxillary and mandibular dentures	7	3.5
Removable partial prostheses	29	14.5
Complete maxillary partial mandibular dentures	4	2
Fixed partial prostheses	34	17
Partially edentulous—no replacements	76	38

From Gelb, H., and Tarte, J.: A two-year clinical evaluation of 200 cases of chronic headache: the craniocervical-mandibular syndrome, JADA, *91*:1230, 1975.

TABLE 11–6. Distribution of 200 Patients from a Dental Study*

Fully complemented	110	148
With fixed bridgework	38	
Partially edentulous with no replacement	25	30
With some fixed bridgework	5	
Full upper and full lower dentures	6	
Partial dentures	10	
Full upper and partial lower dentures	6	

*From Gelb, H., and Bernstein, I.: Clinical evaluation of two hundred patients with temporomandibular joint syndrome. J. Prosthet. Dent., *49*:239, 1983.

TABLE 11–7. FINDINGS

CHIEF COMPLAINTS

TMJ Pain NO. %	Head-ache NO. %	Facial Pain NO. %	Ear Pain NO. %	Neck Pain NO. %	Click NO. %	Tinittus NO. %	Other NO. %
57 28.5	83 41.5	18 9	9 4.5	22 11	6 3	2 1	3 1.5

REFERRALS

Dentist NO. %	Physician NO. %	Other Health Professionals NO. %	Other Patients NO. %	Media NO. %
123 61.5	24 12	16 8	28 14	9 4.5

ILIAC CREST

Right Only	Left Only	Both
12	123	19

GASTROCNEMIUS

Right Only	Left Only	Both
102	16	16

PREVIOUS TMJ THERAPY

Drugs	Surgery	Equilibra-tion	Appliance	Restorations or Prosthesis	Chiropractor	Other	Combo.
106	12	14	38	18	12	38	69

CHRONIC ILLNESS

Endocrine Hyst. Thyroid	Surgery	Psychologic	E.N.T.	Orthopedist	Combo.
1 38	126	69	81	105	134

TABLE 11–8.

		Total
Deviant Swallowing Pattern		144
Clicks		
Click on Opening and Closing		49
Unilateral Click on Opening		20
Unilateral Click on Closing		28
Bilateral Opening Click		2
Bilateral Closing Click		7
Anterior Wall Tenderness		
	— Both Ears	38
	— Right	82
	— Left	108
	— One side only	114
High Eye & Low Hip on Same Side		
	— Right	147
	— Left	3
Previous Orthodontic Therapy		43
Orthodontia with Extractions (Bicuspid)		15
Previous History of Trauma		
Within Past Five years		46
Five Years or Longer		99
Had Both		24
Midline Deviation on Same Side as High Eye		
	Closed—Right and Left	65
	Open— Right and Left	82
High Eye and Anterior Wall Tenderness on Same Side		
	— Yes	86
	— No	62

experience indicates the most prevalent disorder may be either temporomandibular joint arthrosis or temporomandibular joint osteoarthritis.

As previously mentioned, because the symptoms are of multifactorial origins to which the other chapters in this book address themselves, the treatment is of necessity multiprofessional. Consequently, medical consultation and treatment often take place before or concomitantly with oral orthopedic procedures (Fig. 11–1).

The problem then is one of treating *acute* pain or *chronic* pain. "Acute" pain is usually transient and the result of infection, injury, or internal disease. If the cause is diagnosed correctly, and then treated or removed, the pain generally disappears. Suppose, for example, that the cause cannot be

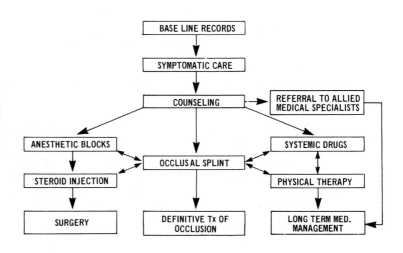

Figure 11–1. University of California TMJ Clinic Diagnostic and Treatment Tree. (Reprinted, with permission, from McNeill, C.: Modern oral preventive techniques. J. Prosthet. Dent., *30*: 571, 1973.)

discovered or removed and that the pain continues for a prolonged period of time; it is then categorized as "chronic." These cases are more bothersome and much more difficult to handle.

I would say that the myofascial pain–dysfunction syndrome falls into the acute classification, whereas dysfunctional temporomandibular joint arthritis is in the chronic class. It is simply a matter of location, duration, time of occurrence, radiation, and referral (see Fig. 3–1 in Chapter 3).

As we all know, chronic pain is our most serious disabling disease. Its cost in human suffering is incalculable; its cost in medical expense dollars was estimated in 1974 at 25 billion dollars a year.[1]

Dr. John Bonica[2] states that there are myriad examples of pain that is the disease itself, not a symptom: migraine, low back pain, phantom pain, and psychogenic pain. Dr. Bonica points out three requirements that must be met: (1) a detailed history must be done and a complete work-up made, including neurologic, psychologic, and sociologic evaluation; (2) the mechanism of the pain must be determined; and (3) treatment must be planned that takes into account the patient's age, life-expectancy, and obligations. "Meeting these requirements is a time-consuming process, for which a multidisciplinary team approach is ideal," Dr. Bonica has stated. "However, the physican (or dentist or other health professional) who is willing and able to devote the necessary time to the problem can achieve good results."

It is unfortunate that the various pain clinics throughout the country mainly specialize in low back pain. A few clinics treat only headaches exclusively. The TMJ clinics as well as TMJ specialists also treat only one facet of the chronic pain problem. For the benefit of mankind, and not to just give lip-service to the "holistic" approach to chronic pain, it would be wonderful to combine the knowledge, skill, and judgment of all three of these aspects under one roof. Only in this way can the patient really resolve his or her problem. The psychogenic problems as a result of this diagnostic and treatment deficiency, which are reported in Chapter 8, would not be as numerous as the literature would lead us to believe. Often this type of patient may present with the following physiologic symptoms that may also be considered to pinpoint depression: sleep disturbance, lack of appetite, alteration of taste, dry mouth, burning tongue, constipation or diarrhea, low back pain, fatigue, easily brought to tears, unhappy with their lot in life, oral mucosal inflammations, and ulcerations.[3]

ORAL ORTHOPEDIC MANAGEMENT

Orthopedists and osteopaths have long been aware of the importance of bilateral balance and its relationship to optimal function. The orthopedist uses numerous appliances to help establish functional balance and harmony of the lower extremities, and he or she also institutes measures to prevent growth divergencies. Furthermore, he or she prescribes therapeutic exercises that will produce optimal physical conditioning for a given patient at a given time. Realizing that the potential of each patient varies with sex, age, physical and mental health, environmental factors, and socioeconomic status, the physician encourages activities and exercises that will promote the highest degree of synchronized neuromuscular joint balance. Thus, it is hoped that both a healthy functioning mind and body will result.

The dentist who practices orthopedically (namely, jaw-to-jaw, which also includes that relationship to the face, head, neck, and back) in a truly holistic fashion will institute measures for optimal craniomandibular positioning. In essence, neuromuscular joint balance with proper activity and exercise will be restored before actual fabrication of the final prosthesis. If the anatomic structures that will act in conjunction with the contemplated prosthesis are conditioned with training appliances in an orthopedic manner, optimal maxillo-mandibular relations can be recorded with confidence.[4] This supersedes past as well as present endeavors which focus their attention primarily on tooth-to-tooth relationships. In order to have a better understanding of this total concept, the postural considerations involved in treatment will now be explored.

POSTURAL CONSIDERATIONS INVOLVING THE HEAD, NECK, AND BACK

The types of treatment for back pain vary widely, depending upon whether the patient sees a medical physician or osteopath. Some patients are just told to stay in bed. Others may have surgery, massages, body manipulation, or heat treatment prescribed. They may be fitted with corsets, braces, or pelvic pulling traction devices with weights strung over the foot of the bed.

Approximately 50 per cent of the population has some inborn skeletal defect, such as one leg that is shorter than the other, outgrowths of bone from the sides of the spine, or a so-called "extra" vertebra in the lower back. However, many people live nicely with such anomalies, provided they have good supporting muscles and are not subject to unusual trauma or infection.

Whatever the causes of backaches—physical, emotional, or both—most doctors agree that man's spinal equipment got short-changed when he evolved from his four-legged status to that of an upright biped, and that this made his back vulnerable to miseries.

Irvin M. Korr, a research physiologist at Kirksville College of Osteopathy, once said: "We've taken the magnificent cantilever bridge, the arched spinal apparatus and four supporting limbs of the quadruped and turned it into a sky-scraper. . . . Whereas the four-legged creature has a low center of gravity on a very broad base, upright man has a high center of gravity supported on a very small base—his two legs—and so we are constantly challenged to keep the center of gravity in line with that base. Moreover, we have put a brain on top of the sky-scraper—and this presents us with additional problems."[5] Furthermore, Sicher and DuBrul[6] have stated: "The final and decisive changes in the skull of man are related to the acquisition of the upright posture which necessitated a strong curvature around an axis passing through the two acoustic organs." Gregory[7] adds: "The upright posture is not entirely an unmixed blessing, since it has made civilized man liable to fallen arches, to assorted hernias, and to all the unpleasant visceral prolapses and similar ills that flesh is heir to."

Research at the Chicago College of Osteopathic Medicine[8] demonstrated electromyographically the effect of a short leg on dental occlusion. Absence of the heel lift (only three eighths of an inch) to compensate for the shortened lowered extremity markedly altered the firing sequences observed during chewing, but when the lift was replaced the muscles once again showed the normal firing pattern for proper occlusion. Once again, the unity of the body mechanism becomes apparent, with the stress of posture extending all the way up to the masticatory muscles, not down as we usually see it from the dental viewpoint.

Travell[9] reported that, if one leg is only a quarter of an inch shorter than the other, the entire body can be tilted enough to cause pain throughout the skeletal system. So slight a difference can distort the entire skeleton, causing a "see-saw" condition that pulls one shoulder down a full inch. This may never be recognized until, for example, the person is hurt in a fall or accident. Then the muscles on the short side may go into spasm, exaggerating the original tilt and reversing it as the "long" leg is pulled up by the tightened muscle mass.

The goal of the physician or osteopath then is to restore normal muscle function, freeing muscles of the extra workload that was placed on them. However, by that time, the body may have adjusted to a life-long abnormal tilt, and simply adding on a piece of extra heel will not correct things.

Therefore, it is reasonable to conclude that some of the developmental and dysfunctional problems encountered in the craniomandibular syndrome are in some way related to the adaptations necessary for maintenance of body posture.

According to Mohl[10] two important planes should receive attention when considering head posture. The *first*, the "Frankfort plane" (orbitomeatal plane), passes through the upper margins of the external auditory meatus (porion) and the lower margin of the left orbit (orbitale). It should correspond to a natural horizontal plane when a subject is in the anatomical position and the gaze is directed toward a vertical mirror on which he fixes the pupils of his eyes or when he looks ahead into the far distance. The *second* is the plane that passes through the horizontal semicircular canals of the inner ear (Fig. 11–2). Several different experiments have shown that the position of the horizontal semicircular canals in the cranium is functionally related to the spatial orientation of the head.

It was noted that in humans the horizontal semicircular canals are horizontal only when the head is flexed at about a 30° angle from the erect position, as one would measure by the Frankfort plane. This 30° flexion may possibly be related to the feeding position of the head either to fulfill a functional need or because of some phylogenetic imperative. Cineradiographic movies of the masticatory act show head position to be extremely dynamic.

Whereas the anterior parameter of the postural variation is approximately 30° at flexion, the posterior extreme of head extension at the end of the drinking act is in the neighborhood of 45°. It can therefore be assumed that, during a typical meal, if one were to measure the variable head position, as it relates to the Frankfort plane, a range of at least 75° would be seen.[10]

Posselt[11] was one of the first to demonstrate changes in the postural rest position when the Frankfort plane of the head was altered. Brill and his associates,[12] all physiologists, stated that changes in a relaxed patient's head posture will alter rest position of the mandible, namely, with the head inclined backwards the mandible moves away from the maxilla and the free-way space is increased.

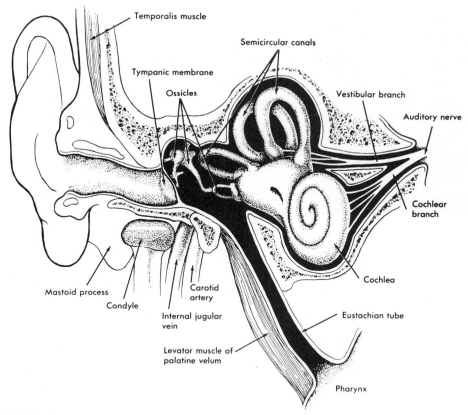

Figure 11–2. Note the superior, posterior, and horizontal semicircular canals. The horizontal canals are parallel to the ground or floor in the alert state. They are almost parallel to the hard palate. The head is usually tipped at a 30° angle while eating to keep these semicircular canals parallel to the ground. (Reprinted with permission from Grieder, A., and Cinotti, W. R.: Periodontal Prosthesis. St. Louis, C. V. Mosby Co., 1968, Vol. I, p. 246.)

It was over 50 years ago that Schwarz[13] observed these very same happenings and hypothesized that the normal and abnormal development of the occlusion may be related to chronic head posture. For argument's sake, children with enlarged tonsillar and adenoidal tissue, unable to breathe properly, will keep their mouths open, carrying the head into an extended position, especially during sleep, thereby causing a change in the final eruption pattern of the teeth as a result of the change in mandibular posture.

Now, it is fairly obvious that any action or condition that affects a related muscle group will consequently alter postural rest position of the mandible. It has recently been demonstrated on rats[14] that masticatory muscle activity is altered in response to rotation, tilting, and flexion of the head. Tonic neck reflex definitely has an influence on the masticatory muscles. With all this evidence at hand, it can logically be assumed that changing the head-to-thorax relation will strongly affect mandibular posture.

Posselt has remarked that rest position can be said to be a position on the path of a habitual closing movement (Fig. 11–3). If this statement is accepted, one can logically conclude that, since rest position is altered by a change in head position, the habitual path of closure is also altered by such a change. Posselt concludes: "The positions obtained by means of habitual closing movements are moved farther posteriorly when the head and/or the

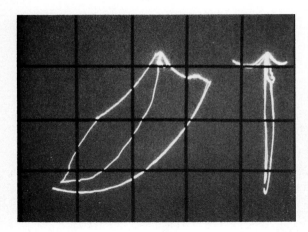

Figure 11–3. Posselt's envelope of motion obtained on Jankelson kinesiograph. (From Gelb, H.: Evaluation of static centric relation in the T.M.J. dysfunction syndrome. Dent. Clin. North Am., 19:3, 1975, pp. 519–530.)

trunk are reclined, though they do not then become maximally retruded positions."[11]

McLean has demonstrated that as patients on a tilt table are raised from a completely supine position (0°) to 30°, then to 60°, and finally to an upright position (90°), the lower teeth make contact with the upper teeth in an increasing mesial direction.

McLean and co-workers analyzed occlusograms along with electromyographically recorded masseteric silent periods, which normally occur immediately after tooth contact. They found that silent period durations decreased as the subject was raised on the tilt table to the erect position. The occlusograms also changed as body position was altered. The most abnormal occlusograms and the longest masseteric silent periods were recorded in the supine position. The occlusograms and electromyographic records improved as the tilt table was raised.[15, 16]

The concept of the presence of an optimal, muscularly determined mandibular position is most appealing, but it has been thought to be difficult to register, especially in the presence of a neuromuscular or temporomandibular joint problem or when the dentition is missing or mutilated. The time has come for this muscularly determined optimal mandibular position to be produced with relative ease and confidence.

TREATMENT PROCEDURES

In instituting therapeutic procedures, the practitioner should aim at two main goals: (1) keep them simple, and (2) allow them to be reversible if possible. As was noted in Chapter 3, treatment depends on an accurate and attentive history and examination.

There are five main avenues of treatment:[17]

   I. Physiologic and physiotherapeutic treatment to eliminate muscle tension and pain, the logical first step in treatment.

  II. Elimination of occlusal and jaw imbalance through the use of an orthopedic repositioning appliance, which will permit the muscles to close the mandible in the muscular position without the teeth directing the closure into a different position (with elimination of the trigger areas and spasm, the occlusion should be corrected).[18, 19]

III. Control of oral habits and associated exercise therapy.
IV. Assisting the patients in the control of their tension and stress.
 V. Medication and systemic therapy.

CRANIOMANDIBULAR REHABILITATION

I. Physiologic and Physiotherapeutic Modalities

A. Heat application. Heat has varied effects on the area being treated: it increases local circulation, acts as a sedative, and lowers muscle tension. In addition, it increases permeability of membranes, metabolic activities, transudation, and, depending on the source of the heat, increases the extensibility of collagen and muscle structures. Heat modalities may be either superficial or deep.[20] The most commonly used modalities are heating lamps, moist and dry heating pads and packs, moist application with towels and wash cloths, and canvas-covered packs of silica gel placed in a cabinet with water heated to approximately 170° Fahrenheit and then wrapped in toweling. Usually 15- to 20-minute applications four times a day are effective.

B. Ultrasound. This increases the heat to deep structures. Application of ultrasound to human joints has demonstrated the highest elevation of temperature to be in the bone and menisci, with the next highest temperature in the capsules.[21] Favorable therapeutic results have been reported in cases of arthritis, as well as in other conditions of the TMJ.[22-24]

C. Cryotherapy. Many of the low back pain clinics have found the use of cold to be more effective than heat in certain instances. The use of ice pack application to the base of the skull or the suboccipital area at the very beginning of a tension headache will often help patients control their headaches if applied repeatedly. Therapac (Fig. 11–4) is more rigid than other forms of cold compresses and delivers a measured amount of cold, since it is completely melted within 20 minutes and the patient's skin is never burned by it. For continued use by the patient at home, it is the most effective way of applying ice, and it can be recommended for use about four times a day, but not to exceed eight times.[29] Some of the reasons for the effectiveness of cold are as follows: (1) sensory impulses arising at end organs in the skin have been shown to be proportional to the thermal gradient expressed in milligram calories per second per square centimeter, with defined correlation of pain sensitivity in various body parts with concentration of histamine in the skin, so that deep cold penetration lowers the thermal gradient, interrupting massive concentration of pain threshold–lowering histamines in the skin; (2) the spread of pain can be interrupted by a sudden cold stimulus to an area into which pain spread would normally occur, thereby raising cutaneous pain threshold in the area of the original pain site by counter-irritation; and (3) topical cold application under light pressure offers controlled tactile/thermal stimuli at a point below discomfort-producing pain, serving to modify pain intensity.

D. Local anesthetics. These are helpful in the relief of pain and limitation associated with this syndrome. Basically, anesthetics act by interrupting the pain-spasm cycle, permitting a pain-free period for exercise where their effectiveness is most noted. This is discussed in greater detail in Chapter 4 and elsewhere in the medical and dental literature.[25-28]

It is necessary to differentiate between those trigger areas which will

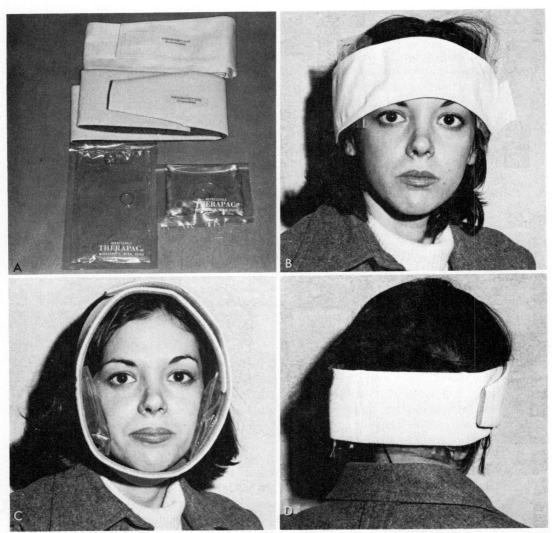

Figure 11–4. *A*, Therapac Product Line: Therapac Refreezable R × 2 flat and folded, Theraband/A Autoclavable Bandeau, and Theraband/D Disposable Bandeau. *B*, Freeze folded Therapac R × 2 applied to both temporal areas using Theraband/A Bandeau. *C*, Freeze folded Therapac R × 2 applied to both masseter muscles using Theraband/D Bandeau. *D*, Flat R × 2 Therapac applied to posterior cervical musculature using Theraband/D Bandeau.

respond to surface anesthetics such as ethyl chloride, Fluori-Methane, and novocaine iontophoresis, and those trigger points that are palpable in the muscles and require injection of the local anesthetic directly into these painful areas. Injection of normal saline and dry needling will be equally effective.

Methods of Administering Local Anesthetics

1. On the surface of the skin overlying the painful muscles. With the patient sitting upright in the dental chair, have him place the thumb of his hand on the side to be sprayed under the body of the mandible, and the other four fingers held together so as to shield the eyes. The dentist places his index finger in the patient's ear and then sprays the area of the temporomandibular joint, masseter and temporalis muscles. The stream of Fluori-Methane or ethyl chloride spray should cover an area of skin about one and one-half inches in width, and is applied at about a 45° angle using a medium nozzle at a distance of one and one-half feet from the face. Sweeping movements which are deliberate and slow are used, being certain not to frost the skin. Begin slow exercise of the jaw by opening and closing as soon as possible. Continually check the degree of opening, the amount of residual pain, and the muscle areas that are still tender before spraying again. Treatment should last not longer than five minutes. In case of sensitive skin, Borofax ointment may be used. Surface anesthetics have been found to enhance reduction in dislocation and relief of postoperative trismus (Fig. 11–5).

2. Infiltration of a local anesthetic directly into painful muscle trigger areas. To be most effective, the local anesthetic must be injected directly

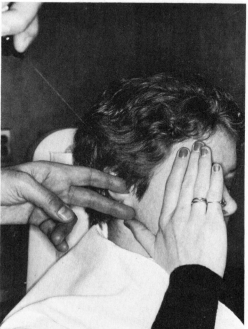

Figure 11–5. Spraying ethyl chloride or Fluori-Methane over the temporomandibular joint and masseter area. Note that the patient protects eye as dentist protects patient's ear. The patient gently opens and closes as the area is sprayed.

into the painful areas of the particular muscle involved. When a painful area is located it is infiltrated with the anesthetic, and by further probing additional areas are sought until no others can be located (Fig. 11–6). Frequently, painful areas in other muscles are also relieved, with the infiltration of the most painful one. This is especially true of the internal pterygoid muscle; when it is injected, pain leaves most of the other muscles on that side of the face and neck. Injections are usually made with a 25 gauge needle attached to an aspirating syringe using either lidocaine hydrochloride, 1 per cent without epinephrine, or procaine, 0.5 per cent without epinephrine. This procedure is described in greater detail in Chapter 4.

E. Tetanizing and sinusoidal currents. Tetanizing current is applied to the area in muscle spasm, fatiguing the muscle, and sinusoidal current then helps to recover gradual rhythmic movement. The exact method of use is described in greater detail in Chapter 4.

F. Electrogalvanic stimulation. The Electro Galvanic Stimulator is used to deliver a wide range of intensity (voltage) to activate the most refractory injured muscle through its nerve point or directly over the muscle. This instrument not only provides higher voltage but also delivers increasingly rapid pulses achieving extended excitability and conductivity ranges without the usual painful heating or unpleasant side reactions of similar galvanic devices.

This form of therapy has a marked effect on the trophism of tissues by stimulating local circulation. Patients have reported a painless increase in

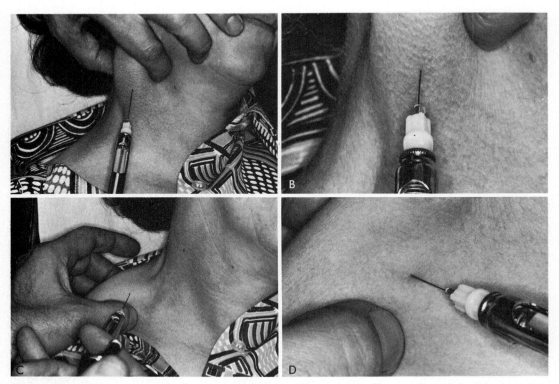

Figure 11–6. *A,* Trigger point injection of sternocleidomastoid muscle. *B,* Close-up view of the injection of the trigger point of the sternocleidomastoid muscle. *C,* Trigger point injection of trapezius muscle. *D,* Close-up view of the injection of the trigger point of the trapezius muscle.

Illustration continued on opposite page

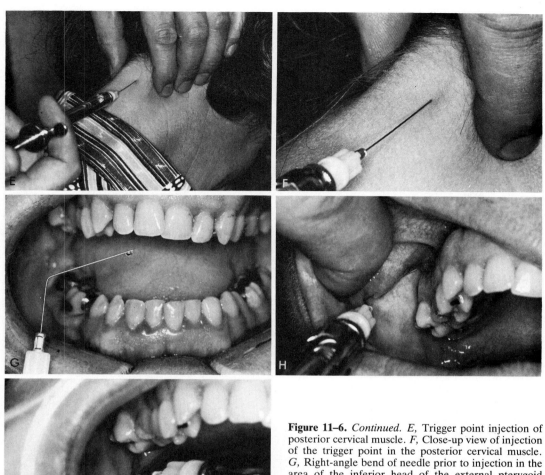

Figure 11–6. *Continued. E,* Trigger point injection of posterior cervical muscle. *F,* Close-up view of injection of the trigger point in the posterior cervical muscle. *G,* Right-angle bend of needle prior to injection in the area of the inferior head of the external pterygoid muscle. *H,* Close-up view of injection into the area of the inferior head of the external pterygoid muscle. *I,* Trigger point injection of internal pterygoid muscle.

mobility of joints afflicted by acute or chronic conditions such as rheumatism or arthritis. An important advantage in the application of this modality of treatment is its ability to be well tolerated, no matter how painful the condition which is being treated. We generally pulse at 80 cycles per second for ten minutes while treating the spastic muscles, and then exercise the muscle for five minutes at 4 to 5 cycles per second (Fig. 11–7). Its use and action are discussed in Chapter 5.

    G. Transcutaneous nerve stimulation. In 1967 Shealy[30] reported the successful control of chronic benign pain through an electrical device: the dorsal column stimulator implanted over the painful area. He discovered that chronic pain could be controlled with a battery device alone. The device was called "Electreat." It was improved and was named the Transcutaneous Neuro-Stimulator.[30] Since that time many new TNS instruments have been brought to the market. Our instrument of choice is the Pain Suppressor,

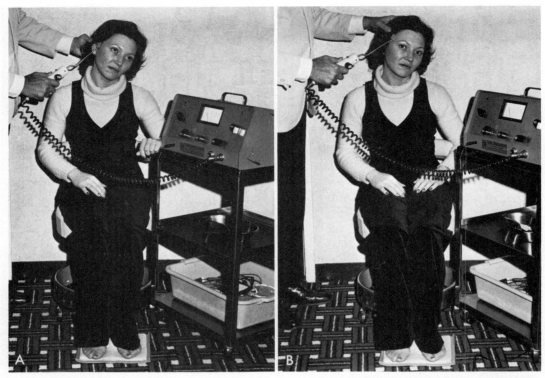

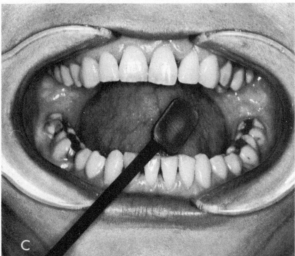

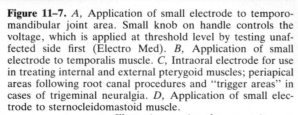

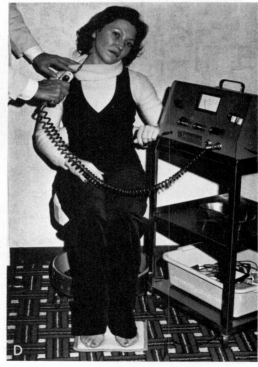

Figure 11–7. *A,* Application of small electrode to temporomandibular joint area. Small knob on handle controls the voltage, which is applied at threshold level by testing unaffected side first (Electro Med). *B,* Application of small electrode to temporalis muscle. *C,* Intraoral electrode for use in treating internal and external pterygoid muscles; periapical areas following root canal procedures and "trigger areas" in cases of trigeminal neuralgia. *D,* Application of small electrode to sternocleidomastoid muscle.

Illustration continued on opposite page

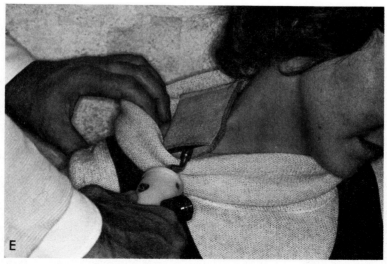

Figure 11–7 *Continued. E,* Application of large electrode to trapezius muscle.

which we have been using for the past eight years with excellent results. Its operation is based on the following theory: (1) interference with the sensation of pain in the brain, and (2) increase in blood flow between the electrode positions with bilateral effect. These benefits are provided while operating below the level of sensation. The Pain Suppressor is a subsensation (threshold) device which most people are able to detect (when the instrument intensity is adjusted to high) in the form of one of the following sensations: itching, pins and needles, warmth, bite (like mosquito), and an optical flicker (when used in or around the head). The operator should turn up the intensity until one of the above sensations is felt and then reduce the intensity until no sensation is detected. Should the patient again feel the sensation after several minutes, the intensity should be reduced again. Optimal treatment is 9 to 12 minutes at a time, which can be repeated several times a day as prescribed by the dentist or physician (Fig. 11–8). The recommended locations for the placement of the electrodes correspond to motor points, trigger points, or points that lie across the superficial branches of motor or sensory peripheral and cranial nerves (Fig. 11–9). For more information on the Pain Suppressor, see Chapter 5.

H. Alpha Stim 2000. A new instrument that has proved to be quite effective is the Alpha Stim 2000. It is a TNS unit designed to selectively stimulate the large afferent A beta neurons. It is a multimodality instrument, actually two instruments in one, effecting maximum patient comfort during therapy and affording continuous relief afterward. Modality A is an alternating current microampere stimulator with hand-held probes or remote electrodes. It is pretimed for 6, 8, or 12 seconds, 2, 5, or 10 minutes, or for continuous stimulation. The frequency is adjustable from 0.5 to 320 hertz (cycles per second) and the current may be set from 25 to 500 μA. Modality B is an alternating or direct current milliampere stimulator with two separate outputs each varying the intensity of two electrode pads. The pulse width is continuously adjustable from 0.75 to 200 microseconds and the frequency ranges from 3 to 80 Hz.

I. Light massage. Massage of the structures of the face should be applied

Text continued on page 301

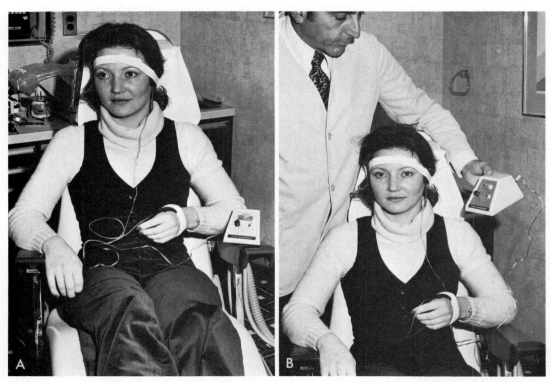

Figure 11–8. *A,* Patient using transcutaneous nerve stimulator to treat TMJ pain. The active electrode (the red one on a machine) is held in place over left TMJ with adhesive strap. The dispersive electrode (black) is placed at a lower point on the body (Hoku area–webbed area between thumb and forefinger). (Pain Suppression Labs Inc., 1200 Route 46, Clifton, New Jersey 07013.) *B,* Doctor monitoring use of pain suppressor TENS while treating painful TMJ.

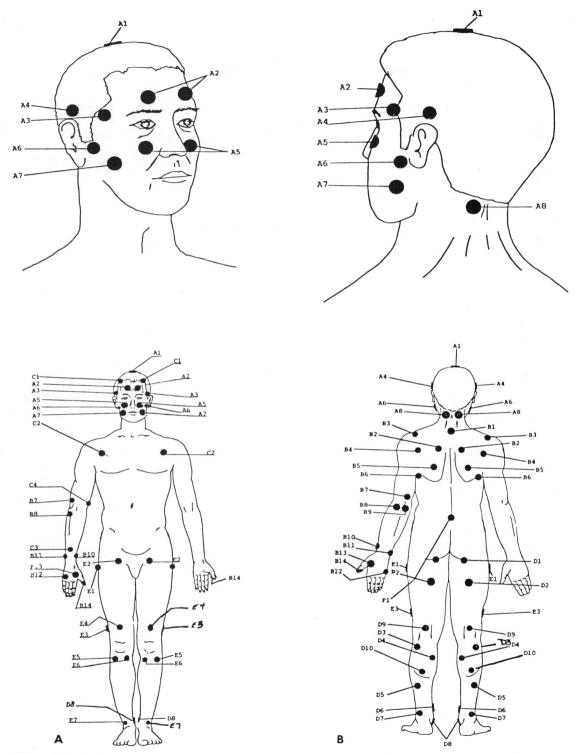

Figure 11–9. *A,* Recommended locations for placement of active (red) electrodes. *B,* Recommended location for placement of dispersive (block) electrodes. The active (red) electrode is usually placed higher up on the body than is the dispersive (black) electrode. (Supplied by Jeffrey Mannheimer, M.A., R.P.T.) *C–E,* Identification of codes for positions of electrodes.

Illustration continued on following pages

PHYSICAL POSITION OF ELECTRODE LOCATIONS

Trigger Points, Motor Points, and points that lie across superficial branches of motor or sensory peripheral and cranial nerves.

CODE	POSITION	Peripheral Nerve Innervation
A1	At vertex of head, center point of line connecting the two apexes of the ears and the mid-sagittal line.	Greater occipital and supraorbital nerves.
A2	Above eyebrow one finger-breadth over center of eye. Motor point of frontalis muscle.	Supraorbital branch of ophthalmic division of trigeminal nerve.
A3	In depression or fossa directly lateral to eyebrow.	Lacrimal and upper zygomatic branches of the trigeminal and facial nerves.
A4	About one inch above the apex of the ear.	Greater occipital nerve and auriculotemporal branch of the trigeminal nerve.
A5	Infraorbital, below center of eye. Motor point of Orbicularis Oculi.	Infratrochlear and infraorbital nerves and a branch from temporal portion of facial nerve.
A6	Anterior to tragus of the ear in depression formed when the mouth is open. Over temporal-mandibular joints.	Greater auricular and auriculotemporal nerves.
A7	Motor point and trigger point of Masseter muscle. Can palpate muscle by biting down hard. Anterior and superior to angle of jaw.	Greater auricular and sensory and motor branches from facial and trigeminal nerves respectively.
A8	Trigger point of splenius capitus. Just below occiput in depression formed by upper trapezius and sternocleidomastoid muscles.	Greater and lesser Occipital Nerves.
B1	Cervical - Thoracic junction, between spinous processes of C7 and T1.	Posterior primary rami of C8 and T1.

C

Figure 11–9 *Continued.*

Illustration continued on opposite page

CODE	POSITION	PERIPHERAL NERVE INNERVATION
B2	Motor Point of Middle Trapezius. Just lateral to upper thoracic spinous processes.	Spinal accessory nerve.
B3	Posterior between acromion and greater tubercle of humerus.	Axillary and Supraclavicular nerves.
B4	Trigger point and motor point of Infraspinatus muscle. In center of infrascapular fossa.	Suprascapular nerve
B5	Trigger point and motor point of lower trapezius muscle.	Spinal accessory nerve.
B6	Motor point of Teres Major in Posterior axillary fold.	Subscapular nerve. Also lies near or over the axillary and radial nerves.
B7	One inch above the olecranon of the ulna in depression formed when the elbow is bent.	Overlies branches of radial nerve and its posterior brachial cutaneous nerve.
B8	Motor points of brachioradialis and/or extensor carpi radialis longus just below elbow on posterolateral side.	Superficial radial nerve, and dorsal antebrachial cutaneous nerve.
B9	Posterior aspect of the elbow in depression between olecranon of ulna and tip of medial epicondyle of the humerus.	Overlies the ulnar nerve.
B10	About 1½" above the styloid process of the radius between the brachioradialis and abductor pollicis longus tendons.	Overlies the superficial radial nerve and lateral antebrachial cutaneous nerve.
B11	Between bony cleft of radial aspect of the styloid process of the ulna and the tendon of the flexor carpi ulnaris.	Overlies the superficial dorsal and palmar branches of the ulnar nerve.

D

Figure 11–9 *Continued.*

Illustration continued on following page

CODE	POSITION	PERIPHERAL NERVE INNERVATION
B12	On ulnar border of the hand at end of transverse crease proximal to the fifth metacarpal joint when a fist is formed. Motor point of abductor digiti quinti muscle.	Volar and dorsal cutaneous branches of the ulnar nerve.
B13	Motor point of first dorsal interosseous muscle. Dorsal surface of the hand between the first and second metacarpals at midpoint of radial side of second metacarpal.	Superficial branches of the radial and musculocutaneous nerves and volar proprius branch of the median nerve deeply.
B14	On radial and volar aspect of the tip of the thumb.	Distal superficial cutaneous branches of the radial and median nerves.
C1	In the corner of the forehead just within the anterior hairline. The distance between the right and left locations is equal to that between the two greater occipital tuberosities.	Overlies branches of the trigeminal and facial nerves.
C2	Trigger and motor point of pectoralis major.	Medial and lateral anterior thoracic nerves.
C3	Motor point of extensor pollicis longus. Between radius and ulna.	Overlies dorsal and lateral cutaneous branches of radial nerve and lateral cutaneous nerve of the forearm - a branch of the musculo=cutaneous nerve.
C4	1½" above the elbow in groove medial to biceps tendon.	Lateral antebrachial cutaneous nerve - anterior branch from musculo=cutaneous nerve.
C5	On dorsal surface of hand between fourth and fifth metacarpals. In depression superior to MCP joint.	Superficial cutaneous branches of the radial and ulnar nerves.
D1	Gluteal fold, midway between ischial tuberosity and greater trochanter of femur.	Overlies the sciatic nerve and posterior cutaneous nerve of the thigh.
D2	Upper hamstring area, in midline of leg.	Posterior cutaneous nerve of thigh.

E

Figure 11–9 *Continued.*

with care so as not to traumatize any soft tissue by too active pressure against the bones of the skull. It is possible to apply a bit more pressure in massaging the stronger muscles of the neck and upper back. Massage over the joint and masseter region in the morning and evening with a small quantity of counter-irritant unguent containing methyl salicylate is comforting. Vibrators may be used for the temporary relief of muscle spasm.

II. Elimination of Occlusal and Jaw Imbalance

We are now ready to treat jaw-to-jaw as well as tooth-to-tooth malrelationships. The two most important factors to be considered at this time are (1) the status of head posture and (2) balancing the occlusion in all parafunctional ranges.

As stated before, our major goal at this time is to create the optimal orthopedic program for each of our patients, which will best enable them to cope with any future stressful situations. This is done by using the clinical criteria mentioned in Chapter 3 (Fig. 11–10). Using these criteria we can

CRITERIA FOR STARTING A CASE

I **VISUALIZATION**

    A. FACE
    B. MID-LINE DEVIATION
       I. CLOSED
       2. ON OPENING
    C. LEVEL OF SHOULDERS,
       HIPS, BREASTS, KNEES

II **PALPATION**

GREATEST LOSS OF
V.D. GENERALLY ON
SIDE OF SHORT LEG

    A. MUSCLES OF:
       I. MASTICATION
       2. NECK
       3. BACK
       4. LEGS (CALVES)
    B. CONDYLES THROUGH EXTERNAL
       AUDITORY MEATUSES

III **TMJ X-RAYS**

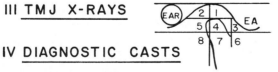

IV **DIAGNOSTIC CASTS**

V **PHONETICS**

    CLOSEST SPEAKING SPACE - S, SH, CH,
                        J, Z, ZH
    FREE-WAY SPACE IS USUALLY BETWEEN
    3.07 - 3.67 mm. BUT HAS BEEN SHOWN
    TO VARY FROM 0-10 mm.

VI **APPLIED KINESIOLOGY TESTING PROCEDURES**

                              (SEE CHAPTER 16)

Figure 11–10. Criteria for starting a case.

CRITERIA FOR FINISHING

I HEAD POSTURE
II BALANCE FOR PARAFUNCTION
   A. MAXIMUM INTERCUSPATION
      AT C.O. AT PROPER VERTICAL D.
   B. RIGHT AND LEFT LATERAL
      EXCURSIONS - MAY BE GROUP
      FUNCTION BUT GENERALLY
      CUSPID PROTECTION
   C. NO BALANCING SIDE INTER-
      FERENCES
   D. OPTIMUM CONTACT IN PROTRUSIVE,
      DISOCCLUDE POSTERIORLY
   E. NO CENTRIC
      RELATION PREMATURITIES

Figure 11–11.

now differentiate between those cases which can be treated simply by occlusal equilibration and those that need orthopedic repositioning of the jaws.

If it is now determined that the patient is at the correct level of vertical dimension (Steps II, III, and V) and that he has a normal free-way space, we can then proceed to recontour tooth inclines according to the criteria for finishing a case (Fig. 11–11). It should be stated that there are many methods[31–40] and concepts for equlibration or balance of natural dentitions (Fig. 11–12), but our clinical experience and the research reported in the literature have led us to follow the procedures as outlined in Figures 11–12 and 11–13. *Any method may be utilized provided the end result meets these criteria.* For many years, I have used the technique of Jankelson[38] very successfully, but I believe the procedures introduced by Ross[32] greatly simplify this aspect of therapy. It should be emphasized that a truly stable occlusion cannot be obtained if the patient has a deviant swallowing problem. This is discussed in greater detail in Chapter 15.

CLINICIAN	DIRECT OCCLUSAL FORCES IN LONG AXIS	DISTRIBUTE FORCES ONTO AS MANY TEETH AS POSSIBLE	ADJUST OCCLUSION TO A HINGE AXIS POINT	ADJUST OCCLUSION TO A LINE (LONG CENTRIC)	ADJUST TO ELIMINATE CENTRIC PATHWAY PREMATUR-ITIES	ADJUST TO ATTAIN GROUP FUNCTION IN LATERAL MOVEMENTS	ELIMINATE BALANCING SIDE PRE-MATURITIES	CUSPID PROTECTED OCCLUSION IN LATERAL MOVEMENTS	ADJUST OCCLUSION PROPHYLAC-TICALLY
D'AMICO	YES	YES	YES	NO	YES	NO	YES	YES	?
GLICKMAN	YES	YES	NO	NO	YES	NO	YES	NO	NO
JANKELSON	YES	YES	NO	NO	YES	NO	YES	NO	NO
RAMFJORD	YES	YES	NO	YES	YES	YES/NO**	YES	NO/YES**	NO
SCMIDT	YES	YES	YES*	NO*	YES	NO	YES	NO	YES
SCHUYER	YES	YES	NO	YES	YES	YES/NO**	YES	NO/YES**	NO
STUART & STALLARD	YES	YES	YES	NO	YES	NO	YES	YES	NO
GELB	YES	YES	NO	NO	YES	YES/NO**	YES	NO/YES**	NO

  * ADJUSTMENT TECHNIQUE ALLOWS LINE MOVEMENT
** IF OCCLUSION IS CUSPID PROTECTED AND CUSPID IS ABLE TO WITHSTAND FORCES --- GROUP
      FUNCTION IS NOT SOUGHT
     IF THERE IS GROUP FUNCTION AND THE TEETH ARE ABLE TO WITHSTAND FORCES --- CUSPID
        PROTECTED OCCLUSION IS NOT SOUGHT

DIAGRAM COURTESY OF DR. ARTHUR GOLD, DEPARTMENT OF PERIODONTOLOGY, TUFTS UNIVERSITY COLLEGE OF DENTAL MEDICINE

Figure 11–12.

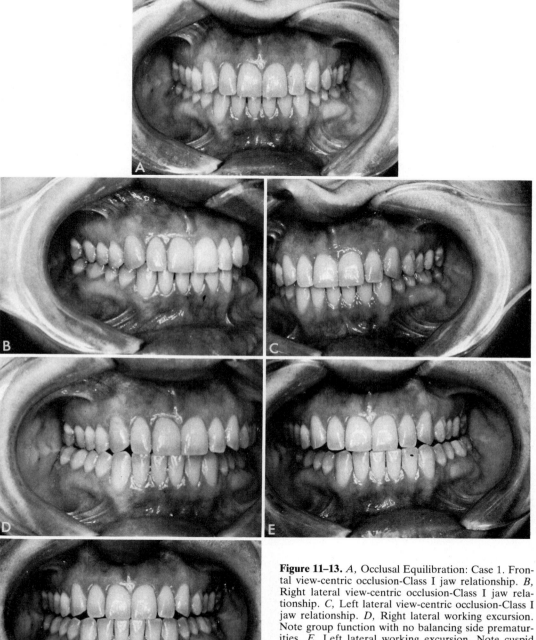

Figure 11–13. *A,* Occlusal Equilibration: Case 1. Frontal view-centric occlusion-Class I jaw relationship. *B,* Right lateral view-centric occlusion-Class I jaw relationship. *C,* Left lateral view-centric occlusion-Class I jaw relationship. *D,* Right lateral working excursion. Note group function with no balancing side prematurities. *E,* Left lateral working excursion. Note cuspid protection with no balancing side prematurities. *F,* Optimum protrusive contact with disocclusion posteriorly.

Illustration continued on following page

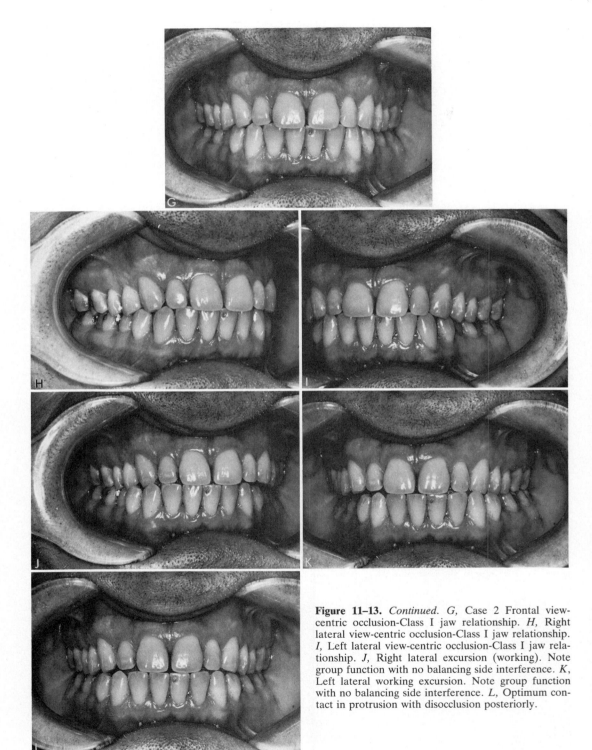

Figure 11–13. *Continued. G,* Case 2 Frontal view-centric occlusion-Class I jaw relationship. *H,* Right lateral view-centric occlusion-Class I jaw relationship. *I,* Left lateral view-centric occlusion-Class I jaw relationship. *J,* Right lateral excursion (working). Note group function with no balancing side interference. *K,* Left lateral working excursion. Note group function with no balancing side interference. *L,* Optimum contact in protrusion with disocclusion posteriorly.

OBJECTIVES FOR CORONAL RESHAPING*

Temporomandibular joint pain and dysfunction are frequently related to stress situations, such as anxiety, anger, fear, and frustration. Stress may initiate clenching and grinding or it may perpetuate and even increase the intensity and frequency of the habits if they are already present. In addition, stress may affect the manner in which the patient responds during treatment of pain or dysfunction, or both. It may prolong or exacerbate an existing condition.

Frequently an individual has difficulty in moving the mandible easily if there is little or no overjet between the maxillary and mandibular anterior teeth or if the bicuspids and molars have steep interlocking cusps. The difficulty occurs because the maxillary teeth lock the mandibular teeth in intercuspal contact position and inhibit anterior and lateral movements. If an individual with steep interlocking teeth clenches or grinds the teeth considerable muscle spasm and pain may develop.

The initial objective of treatment should be to relieve the pain and muscle spasm by unlocking this tight relationship and permitting the mandibular teeth to move more easily. The unlocking is done initially with relaxing techniques and a removable occlusal appliance. If the condition does not respond or if it regresses after initial response, coronal reshaping should be considered. The objectives should be to increase anterior overjet and to reduce steep maxillary molar and bicuspid cusps.

The following outline describes in detail the specific objectives to be achieved with coronal reshaping of anterior and posterior teeth.

CORONAL RESHAPING

General Rules for All Teeth

1. Convert lateral forces to vertical forces.
2. Confine vertical forces within that part of the crown supported by the root.
3. Reduce size of contacts.
4. Establish a series of small symmetrical contacts.
5. Reduce mobility from wedging and rocking forces.
6. Increase overjet and overbite of all anterior and posterior teeth.
7. Eliminate plunger cusp mechanisms.

Rules for Anterior Teeth: Improve Anterior Guidance

A. Reshaping to be done in intercuspal contact position (centric occlusion).
1. Correct incisal level of mandibular and maxillary teeth.
2. Correct labiolingual curve of mandibular teeth.
3. Correct labial curve of maxillary teeth.
4. Produce a series of incisal edge markings on mandibular teeth.
5. If it is not possible to produce incisal edge markings on mandibular teeth because of long labial contacts, produce a series of labial markings as close to the incisal edge as possible.

---

*The objectives and general rules for coronal reshaping were written by Ira Franklin Ross, D.D.S.

B. Reshaping to be done in protrusive and lateral protrusive positions and excursions.

    6. Produce optimum (not always the most) contact in protrusive and lateral protrusive positions and excursions on maxillary and mandibular teeth.

C. Reshaping of maxillary lateral incisors in all positions and excursions.

    7. Reduce or eliminate, if possible, contact on maxillary lateral incisors in protrusive, lateral protrusive, and lateral positions and excursions.

D. Reshaping to treat mobility.

    8. Reduce or eliminate, if possible, mobility of maxillary and mandibular anterior teeth during vertical mandibular movements.

    9. Reduce or eliminate, if possible, mobility of maxillary and mandibular anterior teeth during protrusive and lateral protrusive positions and excursions.

    10. Reduce or eliminate, if possible, contact and/or mobility of maxillary central and lateral incisors during lateral positions and excursions.

Considerations for Cuspids

1. Cuspids function with all teeth during vertical mandibular movements; with anterior teeth during protrusive and lateral protrusive positions and excursions; and with posterior teeth during lateral position and excursion. Therefore, the cuspid must be considered both an anterior and a posterior tooth.

2. Harmonize those surfaces of the cuspid that contact in protrusive and lateral protrusive positions and in excursions with similar contacting surfaces of other anterior teeth.

3. Harmonize those surfaces of the cuspid that contact in lateral position and excursion with similar contacting surfaces of other posterior teeth.

4. An important question is whether contact should be on the cuspid alone (cuspid protected occlusion) during excursive movements, or whether contact should be shared with neighboring teeth (partial or full group function). The decision varies from one individual to another and depends upon the length and shape of teeth, their periodontal support, and occlusal forces directed against them. If the cuspids are long, with steep inclines, most lateral contact will probably be on cuspids alone. If cuspids are flat, there will probaby be group function.

Rules for Posterior Teeth: Improve Posterior Guidance

A. Reshaping to be done in intercuspal contact position (centric occlusion).

    1. Correct modifying factors of posterior guidance as much as is possible and practical. These factors include occlusal curve, marginal ridges, buccolingual diameters, plunger cusps, tooth-to-ridge relations, and relation of mandibular teeth to maxillary teeth.

    2. Produce buccal peak contact on mandibular bicuspids.

    3. Produce buccal peak and inner lingual contact on mandibular molars.

    4. Produce optimal (not the most) contact on maxillary bicuspids. Ideal contact is in the central section, but this is not always possible and practical because of the shape and position of teeth.

    5. Produce optimal contact on maxillary molars. Ideal contact is in the

central section and on the outer lingual, but this is not always possible and practical because of the shape and position of teeth.

6. Reshape contact area of maxillary bicuspids and molars to permit entrance of opposing buccal peaks.

B. Reshaping to be done in lateral excursions (working and balancing cusps).

7. Produce shallow cuspal inclines of maxillary posterior teeth.

8. Shorten and round cusps of maxillary posterior teeth.

9. Eliminate balancing cusp contacts on maxillary and mandibular bicuspids and molars.

10. Produce optimal (not always the most) contact on posterior teeth during lateral excursions. There may be cuspid contact only (cuspid protected occlusion), or two or more teeth may be in contact (partial or total group function). The amount of contact that should be produced during lateral excursions depends upon the length and shape of teeth, their periodontal support, and occlusal forces directed against them.

11. Reduce or eliminate, if possible, mobility of maxillary posterior teeth during vertical and lateral positions and movements.

Comment

These objectives have been prepared with the treatment of neutro-occlusion in mind because neutro-occlusion represents the classic concept of occlusion. Obviously, not all individuals have neutro-occlusion. Therefore, these objectives must be modified for individuals who do not have neutro-occlusion and for whom this relation is not practical. Even though the ideal may not be achieved in all cases, the dentist can reduce destructive occlusal forces by adapting these objectives to meet the specific needs of patients.

Orthopedic Repositioning of the Mandible

The next step in therapy is the repositioning of the mandible with its condyles to produce an optimal neuromuscular balance as well as bilateral condyle-fossae and jaw relationships. This diagnostic decision was the result of assessing the information obtained at the first visit. The corrected wax bite was tried at the second visit, and the patient is not only able to see the facial change (approximates a nonsurgical face-lift) but feels the difference on palpation through the external auditory meatuses as well as a diminution in tenderness in some of the masticatory, neck, and back muscles. The back muscles were found to be the most involved group of muscles in our most recent study.[42] A click on closing also disappears with this diagnostic wax bite. Symptoms reappear with the removal of the wax bite, which convinces the patient of its efficacy. If the patient is in extreme pain and the loss of vertical dimension is considered to be a prime cause, a soft rubber night guard is prepared on the Omnivac, which is to be worn until the third visit (Fig. 11–14).

At the third visit, we insert the *mandibular orthopedic repositioning appliance,* which is constructed to cover the lower posterior teeth only. The reasons for using this type of appliance are as follows:

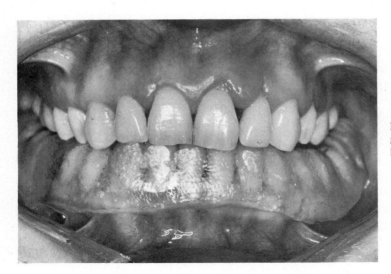

Figure 11–14. Soft rubber night guard fabricated on Omnivac using patient's lower diagnostic cast.

1. They can be constructed quickly and are easy to correct or adjust.

2. They provide the patient with functional comfort in the shortest period of time.

3. The clinician has an opportunity to familiarize himself with the case and effect any changes that he deems advisable.

4. The procedure is *reversible*; the appliances can be discarded, if not effective, without damaging the teeth or changing the jaw position during the first three to four months of therapy.

5. They are hygienic, comfortable, and inconspicuous.

6. The dentist has an opportunity to discover if psychogenic factors are more deep-seated, requiring the patient to seek psychiatric consultation and therapy.

7. Phonetically they can be checked to see that they do not invade the free-way space.

8. If myofunctional therapy has to be instituted, the tongue can contact the palate without a layer of acrylic in its way during deglutition.

9. If the patient should go into a lateral excursion, these appliances can contact the natural cuspids. With an upper appliance acrylic generally covers the linguals of the upper cuspids, altering the mechanics of the joint structures when the appliance is removed prior to reconstruction of the dentition.

10. The patient can make optimal contact in protrusion, and still disocclude posteriorly.

11. From the standpoint of conservation, the dentist truly has a functional architectural rendition of the correct jaw relationship in all planes of space. Since the habitual jaw relationship was a factor in the production of symptom, time is required to decondition this neuromusculature reflex and recondition the structures to a more harmonious muscle, jaw, and tooth relationship. At this time it is important to restate that, in most instances, if properly diagnosed, the optimal interarch relationships must be *produced* and not just *obtained*.

Some members of the profession have said that such appliances "intrude the posterior teeth" or enhance supereruption of the lower anterior teeth. What is observed as intrusion of the lower posterior teeth is actually the spatial change occurring as a result of an orthopedically corrected jaw imbalance. Furthermore, if optimal contact of the maxillary and mandibular incisors is made during protrusion and at incision, then supereruption should not occur.[43] In cases of severe bruxing and clenching, some intrusion of the posterior teeth will be noticed. However, since a large percentage of our cases will be finished orthodontically using functional appliances, with passive eruption of the posterior segments, this is not considered an insurmountable problem.

It is now that we insert the appliance, and balance for parafunctional excursions. In the order outlined in Figure 11–11, we proceed to balance the appliance in centric occlusion, with the patient constantly looking in the mirror (Fig. 11–15). This is necessary, since the patient has never functioned at this position before, and time will have to elapse for the corrected jaw relationship to be conditioned (Fig. 11–16). After centric stops have been definitively incorporated into the occlusal topography of the acrylic appliance, we guide the patient into right lateral (Fig. 11–17) and then left lateral excursions, holding our hands distal to the ramus so that the patient will give us a pure right and left lateral excursion. If this is not done, you will find the patient going into lateral retrusion on excursion (Fig. 11–18). We then have the patient move into a protrusive relationship with optimal contact (Fig. 11–19), and finally we retrude the mandible to the terminal hinge position to remove centric relation prematurities (Fig. 11–20). We are satisfied to make contact simultaneously on the last molars only. It is our contention, and that of other investigators,[44-46] that the true locus of the retruded contact position is recorded inferior to the intercuspal position, rather than posterior to it, indicating that centric relation position is essentially an open one.

This appliance is adjusted on a continuing basis over the course of therapy (three to six months), as the neuromuscular system is brought to homeostasis through the use of exercise, local anesthetics, physiotherapy, biofeedback, myofunctional therapy, medication, and systemic therapy. At the conclusion of TMJ therapy, the required prosthetic and restorative efforts will be able to be completed with confidence, since the possibility of future TMJ dysfunction will be minimal. Each patient is given instructions for wearing the orthopedic repositioning appliance (Fig. 11–21).

Text continued on page 315

Figure 11–15. Patient constantly looking into hand mirror as orthopedic appliance is being balanced into corrected jaw relationship.

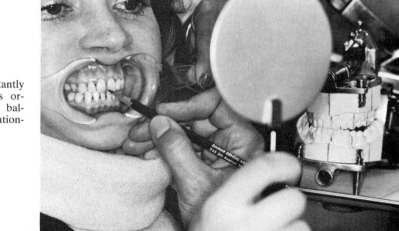

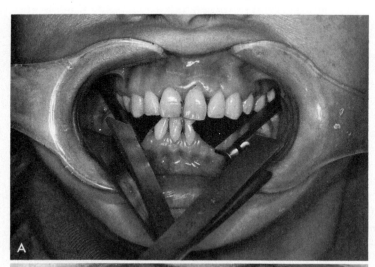

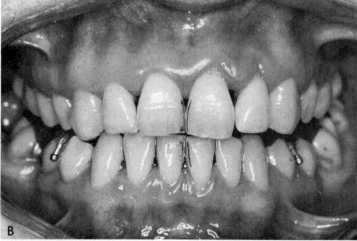

Figure 11–16. *A*, Articulating paper held in holders used bilaterally to establish occlusal stops at centric occlusion. *B*, Orthopedic repositioning appliance occlusally balanced in centric occlusion at corrected interarch relationship. A normal free-way space exists.

Figure 11–17. *A*, Appliance being balanced in right lateral excursion with cuspid protection. No balancing side interferences on the left. *B*, After right lateral excursion with cuspid protection has been accomplished.

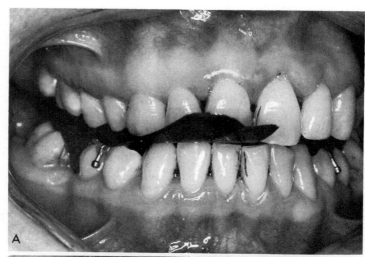

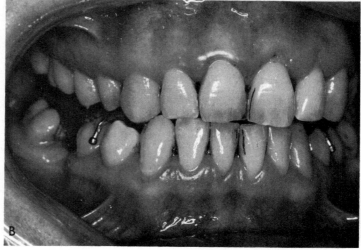

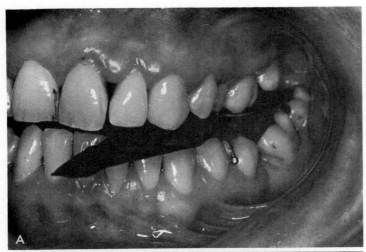

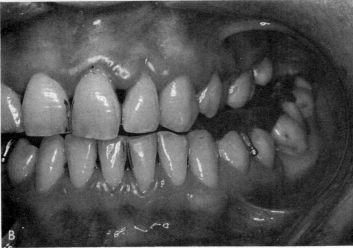

Figure 11–18. *A*, Appliance being balanced in left lateral excursion with group function on bicuspids and first molar. *B*, After left lateral excursion with group function has been accomplished. Note the amount of enamel worn off the incisal surface of the lower cuspid as a result of previous pathologic occlusion. There are no balancing side prematurities on the right.

Figure 11–19. *A,* Balancing appliance so that optimum contact will be established on the central incisors. Posterior teeth disocclude posteriorly. *B,* After balancing appliance so that optimum contact is made on maxillary and mandibular central incisors. Posteriors disocclude posteriorly.

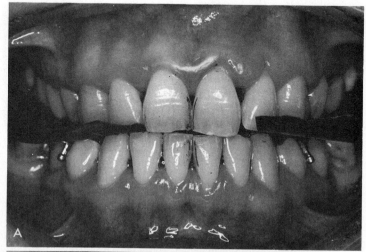

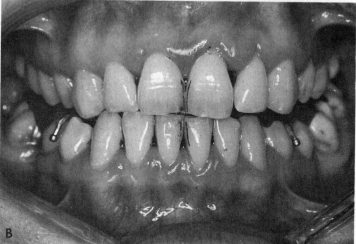

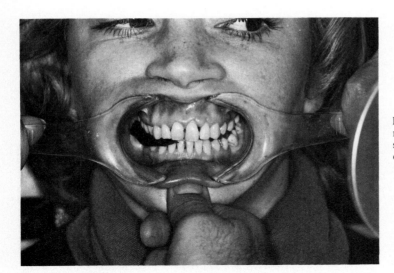

Figure 11–20. Patient being forcibly retruded to the terminal hinge position by the clinician to remove centric relation prematurities.

Since the treatment you are to receive is mainly orthopedic in nature we have fabricated an orthopedic jaw repositioning appliance for you. This appliance will help muscles which are in spasm to relax and will reduce pain. It is not a cure in and of itself.

During the first week wear it for short periods of time. Increase the time that it is kept in the second week. I prefer that you wear it all the time, but if you are uncomfortable while eating, you may remove it.

I believe you should restrict yourself to a soft diet, i.e., eggs, hamburger, chicken, fish, soft cheeses, yogurt, soups, various breakfast cereals, salads, souffles, and certain desserts. Avoid steak, raw vegetable, hard crusted bread, lobster, apples and other foods difficult to chew.

While you are under treatment, I suggest that you do not yell or yawn or open too widely. Do not move your jaw side to side to see if it clicks or grates or hurts. Do not chew gum, do not grit or clench your teeth. Repeat to yourself over and over again during the day, "lips together, teeth apart."

Remove your appliance after each meal and wash it out under the tap in the bathroom. Also rinse out your mouth so no food collects around the teeth. Whenever you brush your teeth, brush your appliance at the same time out of the mouth.

In order not to aggravate muscles of the neck, jaws, and back, avoid carrying, pushing, or lifting heavy objects (groceries, sewing machines, laundry, windows, stalled cars, etc.).

Obeying these rules will hasten your recovery.

Figure 11–21. Patient instructions for wearing the orthopedic repositioning appliance.

Fabrication of Mandibular Orthopedic Repositioning Appliance

1. We remove the diagnostic wax bite and make sure the set screw is tightened at the proper vertical dimension (Fig. 11–22).

2. With the case mounted on the Galetti articulator, which is one of very few articulators capable of registering three-dimensional mandibular changes, the lower model is first coated with liquid foil (Fig. 11–22 A, B). Then we box out the undercuts with carding wax, and finally, we wax down on the cast a prefabricated wrought lingual bar (Fig. 11–22 C, D, E, F).

3. We then bend two ball clasps with reverse bends on the lingual, to fit between the second bicuspids and first molars on the right and left sides (Fig. 11–23). We connect them to the bar with fast-setting acrylic.

4. With powder and liquid mixed to the manufacturer's specification, we make a roll of the acrylic and add it lingually and occlusally, leaving the buccal area free (Fig. 11–24).

5. The upper posterior teeth are coated with petrolatum and then closed into the soft acrylic overlying the lower posterior teeth at the pre-set level of vertical dimension (Fig. 11–25).

6. The lower model is removed from the articulator after the acrylic sets. It is then placed in a pressure cooker to further cure the acrylic at 120°F for 15 minutes (Fig. 11–26).

7. The case is removed from the pressure cooker, returned to the articulator, balanced, and then polished (Fig. 11–27).

After balancing the appliance in the patient's mouth, as described previously, we can add additional acrylic to the appliance in the mouth if it wears down or if more vertical dimension is desired. This is done by applying petrolatum to the upper teeth, adding fast-setting acrylic to the lower teeth, and having the patient close to the desired jaw relationship, which is indicated by using a hand mirror and pencil together with placement of the small fingers in the external auditory meatuses (Fig. 11–28).

If the patient is wearing a lower removable partial denture we can add fast-setting acrylic right over the denture teeth and the abutment teeth, coat the upper teeth with petrolatum, and have the patient close to the desired position, as mentioned above. If the edentulous areas become sore during function, *tissue treatment* material can be added to the edentulous areas for comfort.

Should the patient be wearing full upper and lower dentures, we can first make them stable by using tissue treatment material, then overlay all the lower teeth with fast-setting acrylic, and then have the patient close to the desired relationship (as described above) after applying petrolatum to all the upper teeth. Another method would be to mount the models on the Galetti articulator, reposition the jaws, and take a wax registration of the correction. Try the diagnostic bite in the mouth, check it as outlined previously, then cut the wax in half and add the acrylic to one side at a time.

A patient usually has marked reduction in symptoms or complete remission within 90 to 120 days. After waiting to see if the patient maintains this state of well-being for at least two months, we are now ready to permanently restore the occlusal relationship.

Text continued on page 325

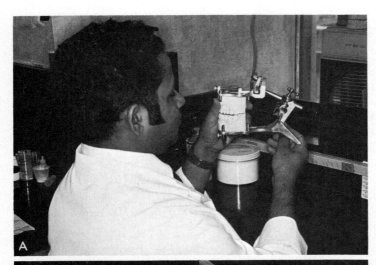

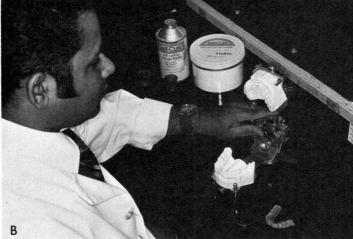

Figure 11–22. *A,* Set-screw secured on Galetti articulator. *B,* Diagnostic wax bite removed prior to bending wrought lingual bar.
Illustration continued on opposite page

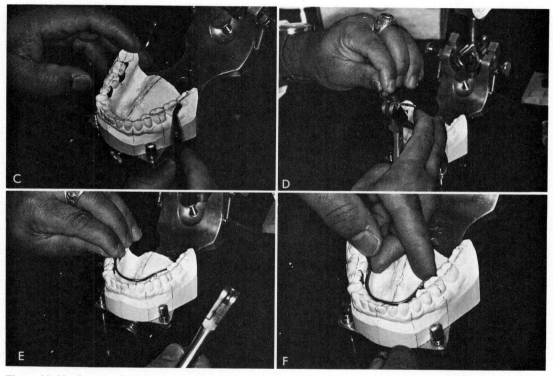

Figure 11–22. *Continued. C,* Undercuts are boxed out on the lingual aspects of the posterior teeth before painting the surfaces of these teeth with a separating medium. *D,* Starting to bend wrought lingual bar with bar-bending pliers. *E,* Trying wrought lingual bar inside lower model to see if contour fits lingual surfaces of the mandible. *F,* Final fitting of wrought lingual bar inside mandibular arch.

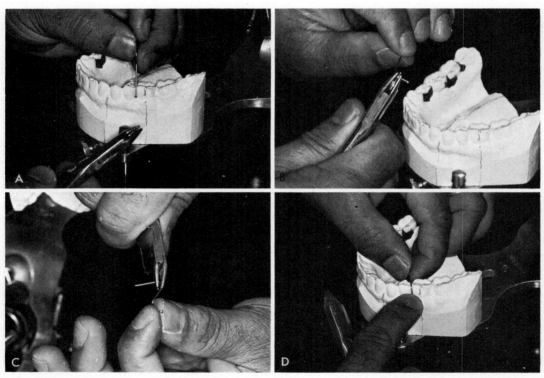

Figure 11–23. *A,* Fitting the ball clasp between the second bicuspid and first molar. *B,* Making occlusal bend of clasp with three-pronged plier. *C,* Making lingual bend of clasp with three-pronged plier. *D,* Trying clasp on model.

Illustration continued on following page

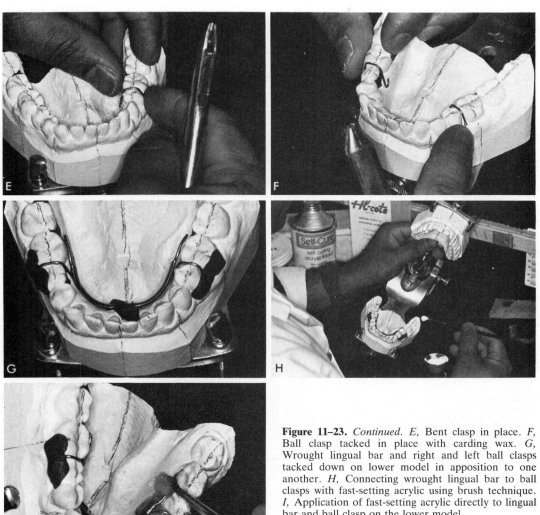

Figure 11–23. *Continued. E,* Bent clasp in place. *F,* Ball clasp tacked in place with carding wax. *G,* Wrought lingual bar and right and left ball clasps tacked down on lower model in apposition to one another. *H,* Connecting wrought lingual bar to ball clasps with fast-setting acrylic using brush technique. *I,* Application of fast-setting acrylic directly to lingual bar and ball clasp on the lower model.

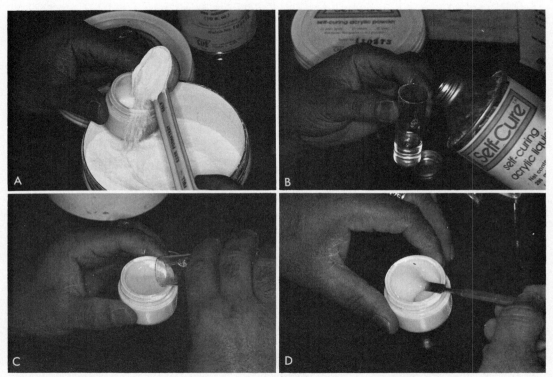

Figure 11–24. *A*, Measuring out acrylic powder as specified by manufacturer for the lingual and occlusal portions of the orthopedic repositioning appliance. *B*, Measuring out liquid monomer in glass vial according to manufacturer's specification. *C*, Mixing acrylic powder and monomer together in glass jar. *D*, Mixing ingredients with a spatula to disperse contents and get a more uniform mix.

Illustration continued on opposite page

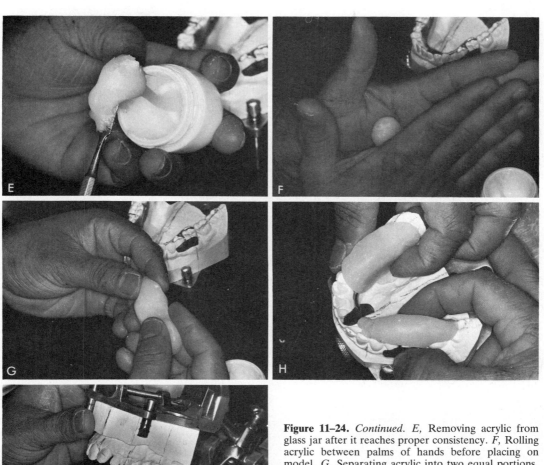

Figure 11–24. *Continued. E,* Removing acrylic from glass jar after it reaches proper consistency. *F,* Rolling acrylic between palms of hands before placing on model. *G,* Separating acrylic into two equal portions. *H,* Placing the acrylic over bicuspids and molars in both lower posterior quadrants. *I,* With the set-screw at the proper vertical dimension, getting set to close the articulator.

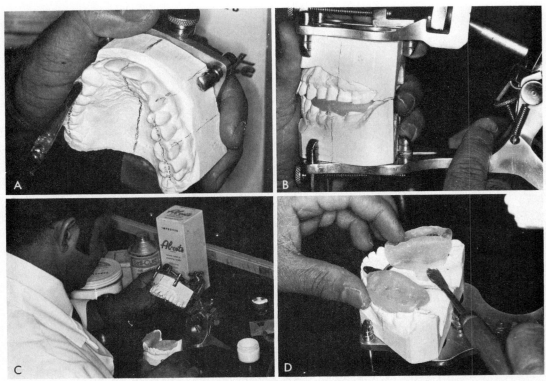

Figure 11–25. *A*, Separating medium or petrolatum applied to maxillary posterior teeth. *B*, Articulator closed, making sure set-screw is fixed and then closing into the soft acrylic. *C*, The articulator is opened as the acrylic begins to polymerize. *D*, The processed appliance is removed from the lower model.

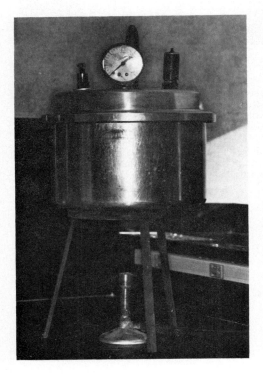

Figure 11–26. The processed orthopedic appliance is placed in the pressure cooker for heat treatment, which will make it stronger.

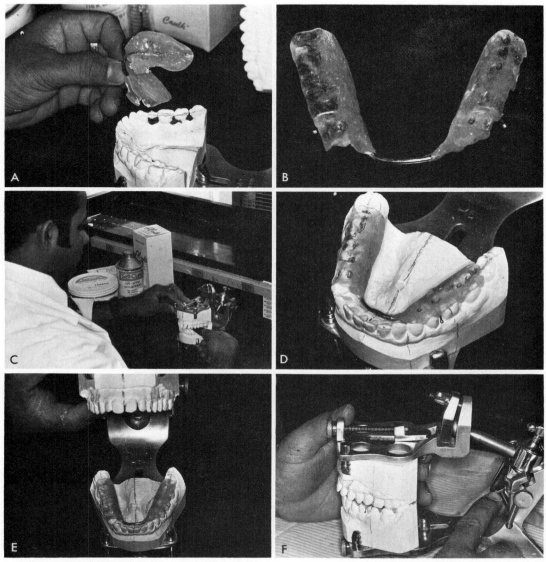

Figure 11–27. *A*, Orthopedic repositioning appliance removed from mandibular model after being in pressure cooker. *B*, Excess acrylic removed from the appliance. *C*, Repositioning appliance placed back on lower model on Galetti articulator and balanced in centric occlusion. *D*, Centric occlusion vertical stops established on occlusal surface of mandibular orthopedic appliance. *E*, Mandibular appliance polished and ready for insertion into patient's mouth on third visit. *F*, Occlusal vertical dimenson maintained throughout all procedures.

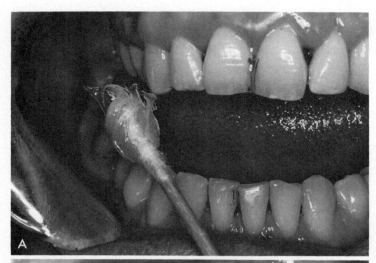

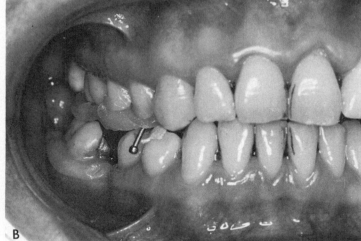

Figure 11–28. *A,* Placing petrolatum on the upper posterior teeth prior to adding fast-setting acrylic to the mandibular repositioning appliance. *B,* Adding fast-setting acrylic to the mandibular repositioning appliance to increase vertical dimension, correct wear patterns, and repair fractures.

RESTORATION OF OCCLUSAL RELATIONSHIP

This may be done in the following ways:

1. Orthodontics. Removable appliances such as Crozat lend themselves well to this type of completion therapy. Acrylic added to the inside of cribs on the molars can maintain the corrected jaw relationship as teeth are moved (Fig. 11–29). If the degree of vertical correction posteriorly is not too great, we can remove the acrylic over the second molars (on the mandibular appliance) and allow them to supererupt. This usually takes four to six months (Fig. 11–30). Then remove the acrylic over the first bicuspids and break the contact mesially and distally with a Mizzy hand separator or lightning strips. These teeth usually erupt into occlusion in six to nine months. Other types of appliances that may be used can be seen in Figure 11–31. If we look at our original models carefully, we will notice that so-called *dual bites* are nothing more than lack of eruption of these posterior teeth to their full growth potential. This is usually caused by faulty eruption patterns, deviant swallowing problems, oral habits such as clenching and bruxing, and iatrogenic factors such as orthodontics with two and four bicuspid extractions. Most cases present as Angle Class II, Division I. As a matter of fact, the most prevalent condition is overclosure, with loss of vertical dimension.

2. Overlay partials. These can be cast preferably in gold, but may be cast in chrome-cobalt alloy (Fig. 11–32). The final study casts are poured and mounted on an articulator, using the patient's final appliance to make the transfer accurate. This can be simplified by placing a small amount of soft acrylic between the anterior teeth with the orthopedic repositioning appliance still in position over the posterior teeth. Once this anterior jig has polymerized, wax check bites of the relationship of the posterior segments can be made with the appliance removed.

3. Partial dentures can be constructed very easily, since the final jaw relationship has already been established over a period of months, and the final case can be planned with greater detail.

4. Full upper and lower dentures, similarly, can be reproduced with relative ease, since the patient's final jaw relationship has already been established.

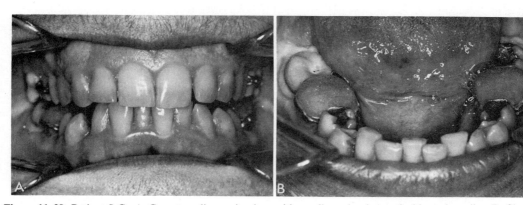

Figure 11–29. Patient S.G. *A,* Crozat appliances in place with acrylic occlusal stops inside molar cribs. *B,* Close-up view of acrylic stops inside molar cribs.

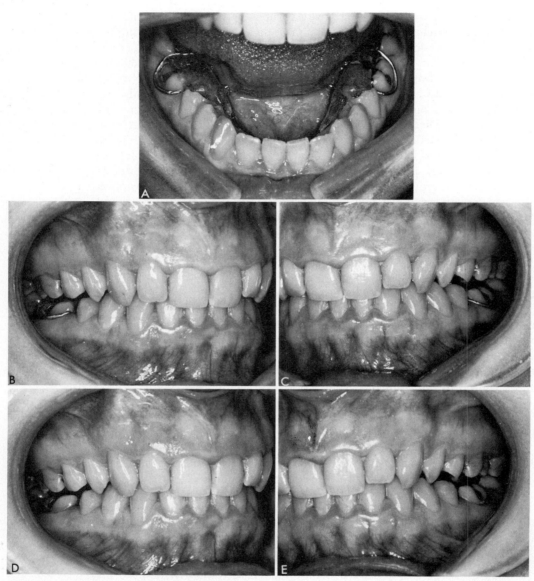

Figure 11–30. Patient H.L. *A*, Mandibular orthopedic appliance in place with acrylic removed over second molars and first bicuspids. *B*, Right lateral view with mandibular orthopedic appliance in place. *C*, Left lateral view with mandibular othopedic appliance in place. *D*, Right lateral view of mandible in corrected jaw relationship with second molar and first biscuspid supererupted to maintain vertical dimansion. The second biscuspid and first molar will gradually erupt on their own or with orthodontic intervention. *E*, Left lateral view of mandible in corrected jaw relationship with second molar and first bicuspid supererupted to maintain vertical dimension.

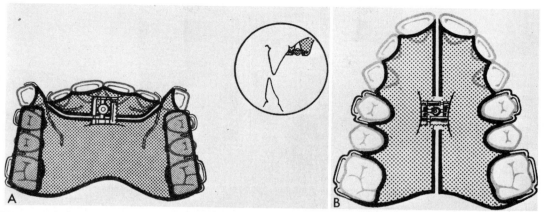

Figure 11–31. Other types of orthodontic appliances. *A,* Upper appliance with screw to move anterior segment labially. *B,* Upper appliance used to expand posterior segment. (From Dickson, G.C., Wheatly, A. E.: An Atlas of Removable Orthodontic Appliances. Kent, England, Pitman Medical Publishing Co., Ltd., 1965.)

5. Fixed prosthesis also becomes easier to accomplish, since, prior to the preparation of any teeth, the final jaw relationship has already been established with all excursive functional movements included. It is simply a matter of working lower right posterior quadrant against upper right posterior quadrant. With the appliance in place on the left side to act as a stop, the acrylic is removed on the right side and the teeth prepared. This is then repeated on the left side. Facetiously, the case can be mounted on a barn door hinge with an anterior stop, and then balanced in the mouth, and a successful result will be obtained. This is true because, prior to the preparation of teeth, the patient was brought, neuromuscularly, well within his or her adaptive limits. Since all physiological processes of the body have a range of normal, even if some human error is incorporated into transferring a case from the mouth to the articulator and back again, we still remain well within the patient's adaptive range (Fig. 11–33).

If only the lower two posterior quadrants need to be reconstructed, then the final appliance can be placed over the original model, taken to the laboratory, and a resin overlay can be punched out using the Omnivac Precision Vacuum Adapter (Fig. 11–34). Vertical dimension is measured with markings on the chin and nose, the posterior teeth are prepared, fast-setting acrylic is placed into the resin mould and placed over the prepared teeth, and the patient is asked to close gently. The vertical dimension is checked with a caliper on the nose and chin markings; condylar position is checked through external auditory meatal palpation. The temporary acrylic

Text continued on page 332

Figure 11–32. Various designs of overlay partials. Preferably cast in gold, but can be chrome-cobalt alloy or in combination with acrylic occlusal surfaces.

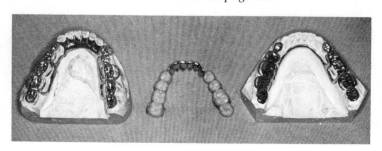

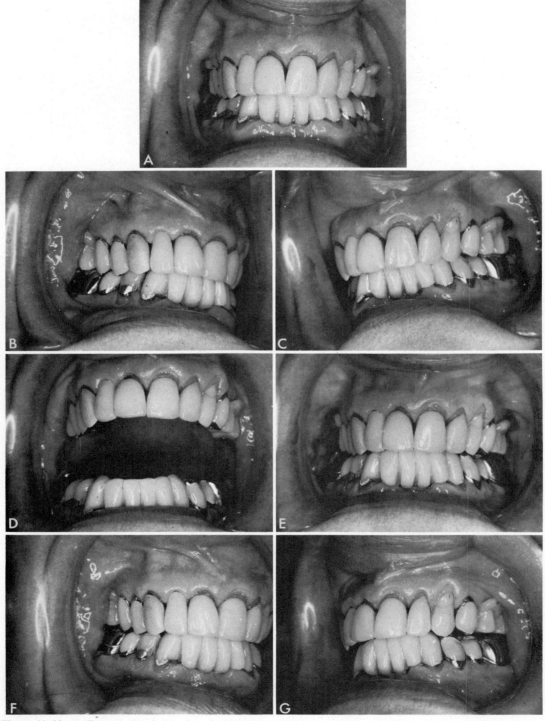

Figure 11–33. *A*, Frontal view–habitual occlusion. Note recession at gingiva of old restorations. *B*, Right lateral view–habitual occlusion. *C*, Left lateral view–habitual occlusion. *D*, Mouth open–limited movement–mandible deviating to right. *E*, Frontal view–orthopedically corrected jaw relationship. *F*, Right lateral view–orthopedically corrected jaw relationship. *G*, Left lateral view–orthopedically corrected jaw relationship.

Illustration continued on opposite page

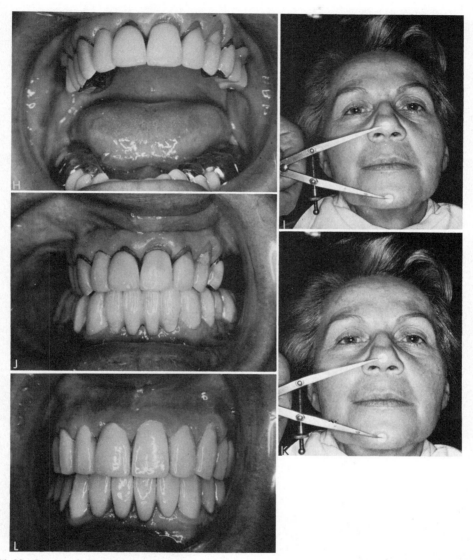

Figure 11–33. *Continued. H,* Mouth open–movement no longer limited but slightly deviated to right. *I,* Placement of nose and chin markers to check vertical dimension before and after preparation of teeth and placement of acrylic temporary bridgework. *J,* Lower acrylic temporary bridge cemented after teeth preparation. *K,* Rechecking vertical dimension after cementation of lower temporary acrylic bridge. Further confirmation can be made with palpation of external auditory meatuses (condylar position), TMJ x-rays, and phonetics. *L,* Ceramco bridges temporarily cemented after several weeks.

Illustration continued on following page

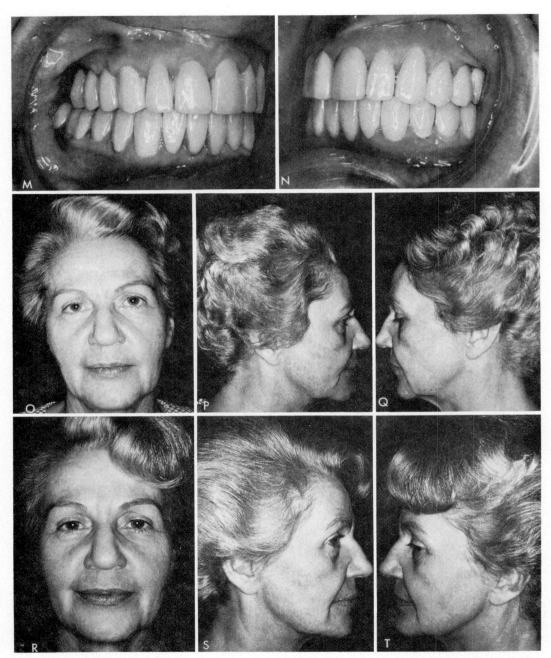

Figure 11–33. *Continued. M,* Right lateral view of temporarily cemented ceramco bridges. *N,* Left lateral view of temporarily cemented ceramco bridges. *O,* Frontal view–habitual occlusion. *P,* Right lateral view–habitual occlusion. *Q,* Left lateral view–habitual occlusion. *R,* Frontal view–orthopedically corrected jaw relationship. *S,* Right lateral view–orthopedically corrected jaw relationship. *T,* Left lateral view–orthopedically corrected jaw relationship.

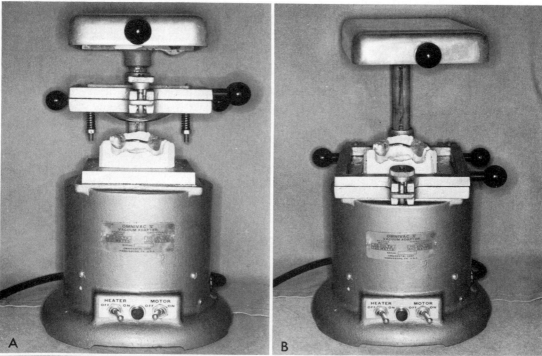

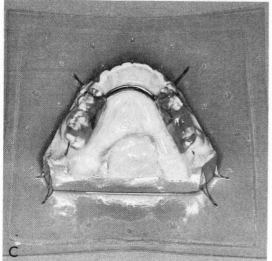

Figure 11–34. Omnivac Precision Vacuum Adapter. *A,* Patient's model with mandibular orthopedic repositioning appliance in place while resin is being heated. *B,* Heated resin being vacuum-formed over model and appliance. *C,* Vacuum-formed resin overlay after removal from Omnivac before being cut away from mode.

bridges are then balanced in all excursions and cemented in place. The cases can be finished simply by mounting the upper model on the horizontal platform of either a Gysi Symplex or Shofu Handy II articulator (Fig. 11–35), with the central incisors mounted against the anterior coronal line, and the mid-sagittal plane of the upper cast continuous with the midline of the mounting platform. Wax bites of the relationship previously established now permit the lower model with prepared teeth to be mounted to the upper cast with either stone or plaster. Upper and lower denture cases can be mounted in a similar fashion (Fig. 11–36).

Should the operator wish to complete his restorations on an arcon-type instrument, he can use the Whip-Mix articulator. The Quick Mount face bow works especially well, since ear positioners are used to locate the condylar axis (Fig. 11–37). The upper cast is mounted and then the lower with the appliance in place is articulated with the upper case using a wax, Dura-lay, or a zinc oxide eugenol paste registration. The condylar readings are set accordingly. After the teeth are prepared we can now replace the old model with the newly poured model by using wax check bites, which are duplications of the previously recorded centric occlusion and vertical dimension. Gnathologically carved occlusions can thus be produced.

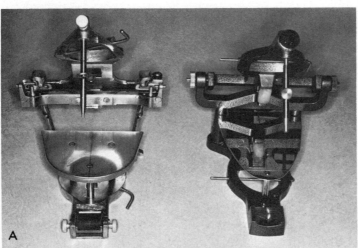

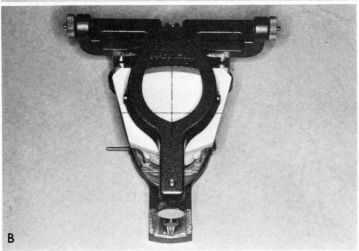

Figure 11–35. *A*, Gysi Symplex articulator on left and Shofu Handy II on the right. Note mounting platforms with mid-sagittal and frontal coronal markings. *B*, Upper model mounted on horizontal platform with mid-sagittal plane of upper cast lined up with mid-sagittal plane of mounting platform. Incisal edges of maxillary central incisors are set against frontal coronal line.

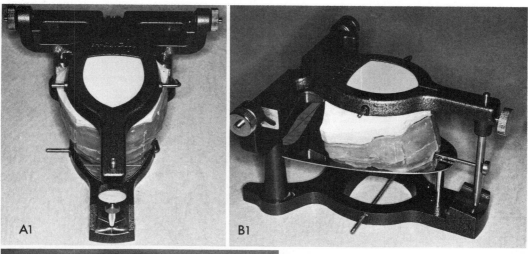

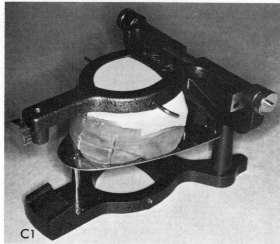

Figure 11–36. Mounting of upper and lower denture cases.

Those operators following the Pankey-Mann-Schuyler philosophy or the myocentric concept should be able to adapt their technique to these procedures with relative ease. In essence, the final jaw relations, which are registered after several months of usage, are neuromuscularly the most physiologic pantographic tracing or functionally generated paths that can be obtained.

III. Controlling Oral Habits and Associated Exercise Therapy

Making a patient aware of an oral habit, and then helping him or her to rebuild a new jaw behavior through the repetitive actions, is constructive. Just having them repeat the phrase "lips together and teeth apart" over and over again, reduces bruxing and clenching habits, since many people actually believe their teeth should be together at all times. Generally speaking, therapeutic exercises in the treatment of the craniomandibular syndrome should assist in restoring normal mandibular movement by improving the properties of power, elasticity, and coordination (see Chapters 4 and 15) that are required for normal function of the head, neck, and masticatory muscles.

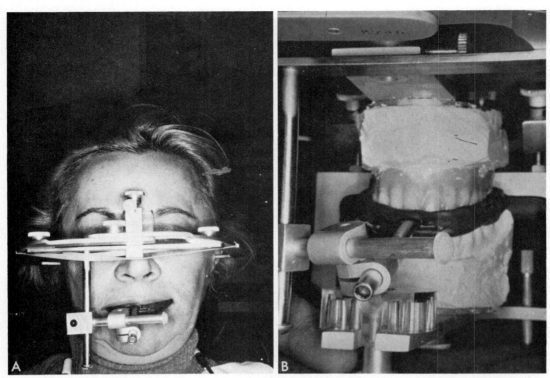

Figure 11–37. *A,* Use of Quick Mount face bow to mount maxillary cast on Whip-Mix articulator. *B,* Upper cast mounted on Whip-Mix articulator using Quick Mount face bow with ear positioners.

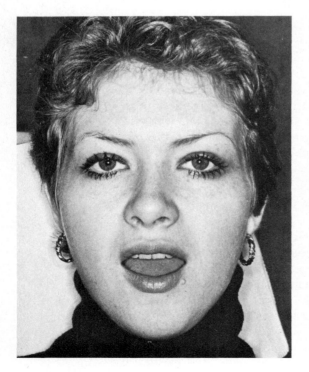

Figure 11–38. Active stretch. Patient is asked to open and close gently ten times as a warm-up, and then as widely as possible several times slowly.

Treatment of Limitation (Spasm and Contracture)[47]

ACTIVE STRETCH. This exercise consists of simply asking the patient to open his mouth as widely as possible. With the patient in a relaxed position on an examining table or in a dental chair, he or she is asked to open and close gently, using rhythmic hinge-like movements. These are repeated approximately ten times as a warm-up with the aid of a hand mirror. This is followed by having them open as widely as possible several times slowly. This exercise can be repeated a half dozen times. When vapor coolant surface sprays are used we employ active stretch exercises to gain greater opening and restore painless function (Fig. 11–38).

The external pterygoids always seem to be injured to some degree as a result of joint trauma. A midline opening exercise to correct disharmonies of the external pterygoid action is described in detail in Chapter 12. It is especially beneficial in the treatment of "clicking" upon opening. A protrusive exercise is used in conjunction with it.

REFLEX RELAXATION OR STRETCH AGAINST RESISTANCE. The physiological basis of the use of reflex relaxation is reciprocal inhibition. By providing resistance during symmetrical opening, reflex relaxation of the jaw-closing muscles is enhanced. In opening the jaw, the depressor group of muscles contracts arising from inhibition of the contraction of the elevators, their antagonists. Consequently, contraction of the jaw-opening muscles against force causes inhibition of the tension in the jaw-closing muscles. This relaxation is accomplished by placing a hand under the patient's chin and asking him to exercise against resistance, followed by relaxed rhythmic movements of active stretch of the masticatory muscles, as described previously (Fig. 11–39). The patient can also exercise by placing his hand under his chin on a table top and then opening against resistance (Fig. 11–40).

In conjunction with this exercise a retrusive exercise can also be utilized; both are effective in arresting opening clicks as a result of forced protrusive opening. Simply have the patient curl the tongue upward, place the tip of the tongue as far back in the roof of the mouth as possible (or on a torus palatinus if it is present), and then ask the patient to open and close the mouth gently so as to reactivate the retrusive muscles (suprahyoid, posterior temporalis, and posterior digastric). This exercise automatically limits mouth opening as well (Fig. 11–41). We reinforce this exercise by advising the patient to masticate with the jaw in a retruded position, and to never attempt to bite off a piece of hard or brittle food with the anterior teeth.

ASSISTIVE STRETCH. Passive stretch movement is accomplished by the efforts of the therapist, in active stretch by the patient, and by both parties in assistive stretch. Three methods have been used for assisting the patient in actively stretching the elevator muscles: (1) In the mechanical method, a mouth prop is generally used with spring and rachet removed. We have long since abandoned this form of assistive stretch, since the amount of force required is critical and many operators have been known to use too vigorous an application, causing injury to the muscles and joint structures. (2) Another method can be used directly, in the office, using only one hand, with resistance provided by the patient or an assistant (Fig. 11–42). The patient is instructed to use one hand or both for home treatment (Fig. 11–42).

These exercises are simple enough to perform, do not confuse the patients, and, coupled with other modalities of therapy, aid materially in resolving residual subclinical symptoms. They also act as deterrents to the

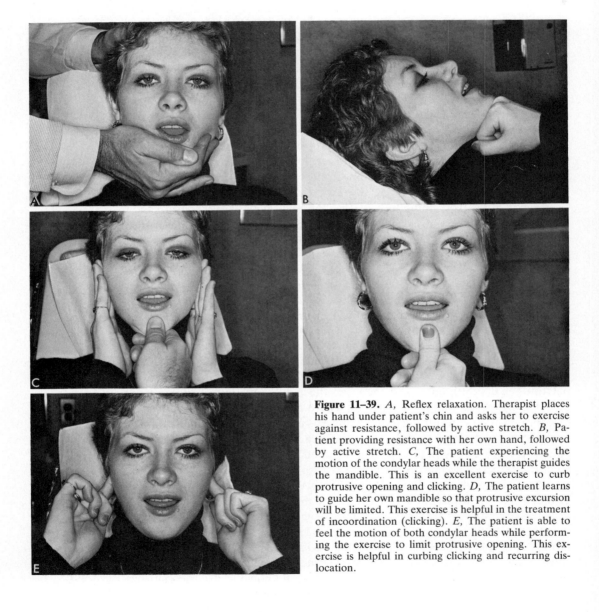

Figure 11–39. *A,* Reflex relaxation. Therapist places his hand under patient's chin and asks her to exercise against resistance, followed by active stretch. *B,* Patient providing resistance with her own hand, followed by active stretch. *C,* The patient experiencing the motion of the condylar heads while the therapist guides the mandible. This is an excellent exercise to curb protrusive opening and clicking. *D,* The patient learns to guide her own mandible so that protrusive excursion will be limited. This exercise is helpful in the treatment of incoordination (clicking). *E,* The patient is able to feel the motion of both condylar heads while performing the exercise to limit protrusive opening. This exercise is helpful in curbing clicking and recurring dislocation.

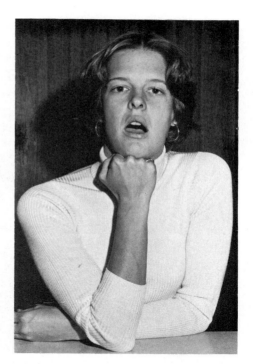

Figure 11–40. Patient making fist and placing it under the chin on a table top, then opening slowly against resistance.

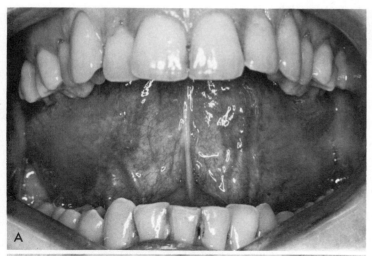

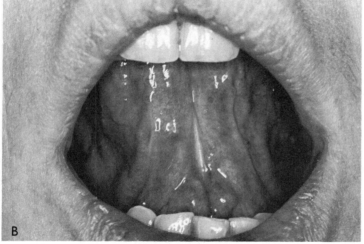

Figure 11–41. *A,* Patient curling tongue up, placing it as far back on palate as possible, and slowly opening and closing mandible in retrusion position. *B,* Same exercise at slightly wider opening. Note midline deviation to affected side.

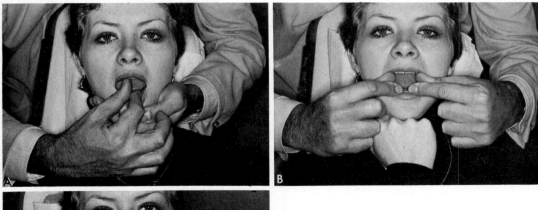

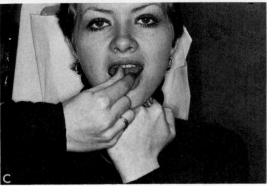

Figure 11–42. *A,*, With the therapist providing resistance, assistive stretch is performed using a single hand. *B,* Assistive stretch using both hands for more vigorous application. *C,* Assistive stretch as prescribed for home use, using one hand.

1. Place your fist under your chin and open slowly five times against pressure. Then, looking in the mirror, open five times without hand pressure, making sure your lower jaw does not come forward so that your lower teeth come out beyond your upper teeth. Do this 25 times in the morning and 25 times in the afternoon.

2. Place one half of a round toothpick between your upper teeth and the other half between your lower teeth. Now, looking into a mirror, open and close your mouth, keeping the toothpicks in alignment. Repeat this exercise 25 to 50 times in the morning and 25 to 50 times in the afternoon.

3. Curl your tongue upward and place the tip as far back in the roof of your mouth as you can. Now, holding it in place, open and close your mouth. You will notice that the lower jaw cannot come forward when you do this. Whenever you have spare time while reading, driving, or watching TV, practice this exercise.

4. Place your thumb against your upper front teeth and your index finger against your lower teeth. With a scissor-like motion, gently separate the upper and lower jaws. Do this several times, but stop if you experience pain. Repeat this exercise from time to time when you are reading or watching television.

Figure 11–43. Patient instructions for corrective temporomandibular joint exercises.

recurrence of painful symptoms. Each patient receives a sheet of instructions which lists several simple exercises. The ones that are beneficial for him are checked off (Fig. 11–43).

IV. Assisting the Patients in the Control of Their Tension and Stress

One of the best methods for limiting stress-induced muscle activity is biofeedback training. The basic aim of biofeedback training is to enable the individual to achieve a physiological state of complete relaxation and tension reduction through voluntary Alpha wave control. It is believed that this type of training can help most people reach and maintain this highly pleasant state of relaxed consciousness at will. It has been amply demonstrated that the physical state of deep relaxation achieved is substantially the same as that achieved by experienced Zen and Yoga masters and by persons well trained and experienced in Transcendental Meditation techniques. This entire subject is discussed in great detail in Chapter 14. Other techniques, such as hypnosis, are discussed in Chapter 13.

V. Medication and Systemic Therapy

"The usual reaction to pain," Halpern has written, "is to look for something to swallow to make it go away." Frequently enough if you swallow the right pill and the pain is uncomplicated and transient, it works well enough. It is so simple, easy, and cheap. But there is room for error—the wrong drug, the wrong dosage, or too much of a good thing—overuse.

"One of the things we've learned," he continues, "is that after about six weeks on opiates, or good strong analgesics, you don't buy anything by continuing to medicate the patient. In fact, you're probably buying more problems than you started with. Problems in terms of side effects, in terms of the emotional changes in the patient in terms of the fact that you do not cover the patient's pain with opiate/analgesic drugs after about six weeks."[48]

Dr. Halpern has outlined a useful guide which divides analgesics into three main categories: nonaddictive, moderately addictive, and strongly addictive.[49]

Nonaddictive Analgesics

1. Plain aspirin, for mild pain such as ordinary headaches, neuralgia, joint and muscle pain, and reduction of fever, is usually sufficient. One or two tablets (0.3 to 0.6 g.) every four hours has been shown to produce maximum results.

2. Aspirin combinations such as APC, which contain aspirin, phenacetin, and caffeine, are not superior to aspirin alone.

3. Sodium salicylamide is more soluble than aspirin and should act more rapidly, but it appears to be less effective than aspirin.

4. Phenacetin, which is used extensively in headache remedies, is equal to aspirin in reducing pain, but it is not as effective in reducing fever or inflammation, so it is not as effective in treating arthritis.

5. Acetaminophen is a substitute for phenacetin. It reduces the risk of methemoglobinemia, and is recommended for long-term use when aspirin is contraindicated. For reduction of pain and fever it is equal to aspirin, but not in its anti-inflammatory effect, and is thereby less effective in treating rheumatoid arthritis.

6. Phenylbutazone is used for acute flare-ups in short-term therapy, generally a week for gout, bursitis, or tendinitis. The short-term restriction is placed on it because of its toxicity, which carries the risk of agranulocytosis.

7. Indocin (indomethacin) is a specialized anti-inflammatory agent, specific for osteoarthritis of the hip, although it is also useful for gout and ankylosing spondylitis.

8. Tegretol (carbamazepine) is effective against the pain of tic douloureux (trigeminal neuralgia) but is quite toxic, causing agranulocytosis or aplastic anemia if not monitored carefully.

Moderately Addictive Drugs

1. Codeine can be given regularly for several months with little danger of dependence, but tolerance does develop. Side effects, similar to those occurring with other narcotics, are constipation, nausea, and vomiting.

2. Darvon (propoxyphene) is structurally related to methadone, and it is claimed to be in the potency range of codeine, with less chance of dependence.

3. Percodan (oxycodone) resembles codeine with similar or slightly better analgesic effect. Habit-forming potential is less than that of morphine but greater than codeine. Similar precautions should be observed as with other opiates.

4. Talwin (pentazocine) is a narcotic-like drug that is stronger than codeine. The manufacturer claims that 50 mg. of Talwin is equivalent to 60 mg. of codeine. It has an erratic effect on patients, and side effects include increased blood pressure, dizziness, nausea, and respiratory depression.

Strongly Addictive Drugs

1. Demerol (meperidine) is a synthetic narcotic that is similar in many regards to morphine. It is strongly analgesic but requires a 50 to 100 mg. dose to equal 50 mg. of morphine. Like morphine, Demerol changes the patient's perception of pain; he feels pain, but he is less anxious, calmer, and more comfortable. Both Demerol and morphine may cause constipation, nausea, and vomiting. They are usually not prescribed for our patients.

2. Methadone is a synthetic opiate with about the same potency as morphine, although it is not as good an all-around drug as morphine. Methadone is an excellent drug to use with chronic pain patients who have tolerance, but we do not recommend its use for the craniomandibular patient.

Besides many of the pain killers listed above, many chronic pain and craniomandibular syndrome patients have had numerous tranquilizers and muscular relaxants prescribed for them before arriving in our office. Among these are the following:

1. Meprobamate: 200 or 400 mg., three to four times a day.
2. Valium (diazepam): 2.5 or 10 mg., two to three times a day.

3. Librium (chlordiazepoxide): 5, 10, or 15 mg., two or three times a day.

4. Serax (oxazepam): 10 mg., three times a day.

5. Norflex (orphenadrine citrate): one tablet twice a day.

6. Robaxin (methocarbamol): 500 or 750 mg., two tablets three times a day.

7. Parafon Forte (chlorzoxazone and acetaminophen): two tablets four times a day.

8. Equagesic (meprobamate and ethoheptazine citrate with aspirin): one tablet four times a day.

The Physician's Desk Reference, with its supplements, should continually be consulted for dosage and contraindications.[50]

It is truly a paradox that painful suffering leads to the taking of drugs, which leads to increasing the dosage, which eventually leads to more pain and behavior problems. When the drug is systematically withdrawn, the patient often improves as he comes out of his confusion and depression. Since many of these patients are depressed when they first present for therapy, a combination of an antidepressant such as amitriptyline hydrochloride (10–25 mg. before bedtime) and Equagesic (three times a day) is very beneficial until the patient is detoxified.

Amitriptyline hydrochloride in conjunction with Equagesic can also be prescribed during the early phases of treatment in the following dosages:

1. During the first week: amitriptyline hydrochloride, one tablet three times a day in conjunction with Equagesic tablets three times a day. The dosage is reduced if improvement is noted.

2. During the second week: amitriptyline hydrochloride, one tablet twice a day in conjunction with Equagesic tablets twice a day. If additional improvement is noted, then the dosage is further reduced.

3. For the next month the dosage would be reduced to one tablet daily of each of the above drugs as a maintenance dosage.

It is desirable simply to detoxify chronic pain patients for whom no apparent reason is seen for continuing medication. Frequently the pain subsides as the patient is detoxified, while other more effective modalities, previously mentioned, are being instituted. It should suffice to have patients on simple aspirin or aspirin-like medication (10 g. four times a day).

THE PLACEBO EFFECT

Dorland defines a placebo as follows: "An inactive substance or preparation, formerly given to please or gratify a patient, now also used in controlled studies to determine the efficacy of medicinal substances."[51] Freese[52] has written "Powerful, omnipresent, magical, unique, and mysterious, potent—this is the picture of the mighty placebo, as old as recorded history, never fully understood nor adequately studied, it still stands in the shadow of scientific medical care, a powerful addition to the physician's grab bag of drugs, instruments, and knowledge. He has always used it, as did his ancestors the witch doctor, the priestess, and the medicine man—and they all still do. As recently as 1952 a study of some 17,000 prescriptions revealed that a third were placebos."

The placebo effect seems to be derived from a combination of factors that involve the patient, the doctor, and the relationship between the two. A meaningful doctor-patient interaction is most significant, allowing the patient to transfer his concern to an acknowledged scientist and healer.

The psychological state of the patient affects his or her response to both active and nonactive drugs, and relief from a placebo will be obtained if the level of concern and discomfort is high, and if the patient is convinced of the efficacy of the treatment. The environmental factor of receiving the therapist's attention also may influence receptivity to treatment.

The length of time that the dentist or physician spends with the patient and his ability to communicate the expectation that treatment will be efficacious are permanent factors. The placebo derives its power from the emotional relationships between therapist and patient, allowing the patient to express his emotions freely, especially during the history taking. The doctor can better understand the important developmental and situational highlights of the patient's life, thus establishing a satisfying and beneficial doctor-patient relationship. The placebo effect in most instances enhances the patient's well-being and thus is an essential aspect of modern medicine. More emphasis should be placed on the potency of the placebo and its positive effects.[53] This to a large measure may explain the term, "laying on of the hands."

Once we learn how to harness the placebo effectively, it may prove to be one of the most powerful tools at our disposal for treating pain. It may be the common ingredient which is essential for all effective pain therapies, without which each therapy is substantially weakened.

INJECTION OF CORTICOSTEROIDS

Intra-articular injection of corticosteroids into the temporomandibular joint has been advocated by several clinicians.[33, 54, 55] Deterioration was observed radiographically in 13 of 25 knee joints treated with steroid injections along with symptomatic improvement.[56] It was demonstrated that articular surfaces of the mandibular condyle in healthy monkeys develop degenerative histologic changes after six injections of hydrocortisone.[51]

We have never resorted to injection of corticosteroids into the TMJ, although we are presently experimenting with using the Pain Suppressor and the principle of iontophoresis to drive a 10 per cent micronized hydrocortisone ointment into the temporomandibular joint. This should enhance the possibility of remodeling of the articulating surfaces, once normal function has been restored orthopedically (objective evidence of patient feeling better). More about these injections is mentioned in Chapter 12.

DIET AND NUTRITION

A soft diet is recommended so as to reduce stress and strain to the long traumatized muscles and joints. Soft textured foods, such as fish, eggs, chicken, and hamburger, and those that do not require wide opening or excessive jaw movements are recommended. In severe cases, a liquid diet may be required.

Every patient who has undergone trauma or who is suffering from the craniomandibular syndrome should be treated for stress syndrome. The degree of stress varies with the previous stress reserve of the individual and his reacion to injury. Treatment includes administration of vitamin C (ascorbic acid) along with bioflavonoid and rutin for a total of 1 gram or more per day in divided doses. In this connection it may be significant that the tissue in the body that has the highest concentration of ascorbic acid is the adrenal cortex, and that a measure of adrenal cortical function in experimental animals subjected to stress is the quantitative determination of the gland's vitamin C context.[56] The patient should be encouraged to keep his diet low in carbohydrate, excluding all white flour and refined sugar products as well as the synthetic sweeteners, hard alcohol, and caffeine. Ostogen tablets, which contain fresh, raw veal bone and nucleoprotein extract, and which are cold processed to conserve natural enzymes and heat labile amino acids, are prescribed at a rate of one a day for six weeks. This supplement is believed to be of nutritional benefit in degenerative conditions of bone and teeth and aids in the amelioration of abnormal calcium deposits. At least 400 international units of vitamin E daily should be ingested, along with trace elements such as magnesium, zinc, and potassium. In addition, the vitamin B complex serves as a catalyst in the production of energy, so all the B vitamins are vital for a patient who is under stress.

Several new products directed at bone and tissue levels have been used in our TMJ/nutrition treatment program and are being marketed and distributed by Gnatho Nutrients.* They are as follows:

Gnatho Nutrients–GN Bone: This product has been formulated to help improve the nutritional environment of bones, teeth, ligaments, and tendons.
Dosage: 2 tablets daily after meals or as directed.

Gnatho Nutrients–GN Muscle: This product has been formulated to improve the nutritional environment to relieve muscle spasms and other neuromuscular involvement.
Dosage: 1 to 3 tablets three times a day after meals.
Maintenance: 1 to 2 tablets per day after meals.

Gnatho Nutrients–GN Connective Tissue: This product has been formulated to help improve the nutritional environment for aiding ligaments, tendons, and cartilage, and building of collagen.
Dosage: 2 to 3 tablets per day following meals.

A simplified low-stress diet is recommended for patients undergoing treatment for the craniomandibular syndrome (Fig. 11–44).

One other very important aspect of systemic therapy is the control of endocrine imbalance, described thoroughly in Chapter 6.

It should now be evident that the etiologic factors are numerous, and treatment of necessity is multiprofessional. A "holistic" approach must be incorporated into every health professional's treatment regimen.

In order to follow the patient's progress chronologically, a chart listing all the patient's symptoms and the effect that various therapeutic modalities have upon them should be kept (Fig. 11–45).

---

*Gnatho Nutrients, 3021 Darnell Road, Philadelphia, PA 19154–3293.

The following is only a suggested schedule, since there is a considerable variety available.

Breakfast: Poach, boil or fry (in natural oils) 1 to 2 eggs
                 Rice or oatmeal for cereal with a small amount of milk
                 and honey
                 Tomatoes (juice or canned)

Mid-Morning: A whole apple, orange, or a celery or cabbage based salad

Lunch: Cole slaw, fish, tomato juice, a potato, some vegetable

Mid-Afternoon: Fruit, banana, gelatine dessert

Supper: Broiled steak, veal, roast (or other muscle meat), raw
                 salad, baked potato, vegetable

Mid-Evening: Dessert

SUMMARY

A. The Low Stress Diet is a method of eating, not a "List of Foods."

B. We judge foods by four properties: Quantity, Quality, Concentration and Digestibility.

C. We eliminate excesses with the principle of moderation.

D. Excesses cause the following possibilities:

1. Systemic overload
2. Digestive overload
3. Foreign substances ingested

E. We rate foods according to basic Classifications and eat accordingly:

1. Vegetables: The "Golden Food"
2. Animal meat: Use in moderation, never with sugar
3. Carbohydrates: Use between meals, if at all
4. Fats and Oils: High quality is emphasized
5. Cereals and Grains: No processed grains
6. Inorganic Minerals: An individual problem

F. General Rules:

1. Eat only when hungry
2. Eat whole foods
3. Never eat sweets with meals
4. Animal food in moderation
5. Eat some raw food with every meal
6. Eat small meals

G. We list Special Rules as follows:

1. Tomatoes with meat
2. Vegetable juices are excellent
3. Cabbage instead of lettuce
4. Honey, vinegar, yogurt and molasses for salad dressings
5. No hydrogenated fats
6. Vegetables for between meal snacks

OBJECTIVES

The Low Stress Diet aids the detoxification mechanism by taking the stress off of the metabolic systems. You may notice the difference by increased energy, improved nerves and fewer digestion symptoms. Bowel movement should also be improved where there has been constipation.

Figure 11–44. Low-stress diet–simplified. (Standard Process Laboratoies, Inc., Milwaukee, Wisconsin.)

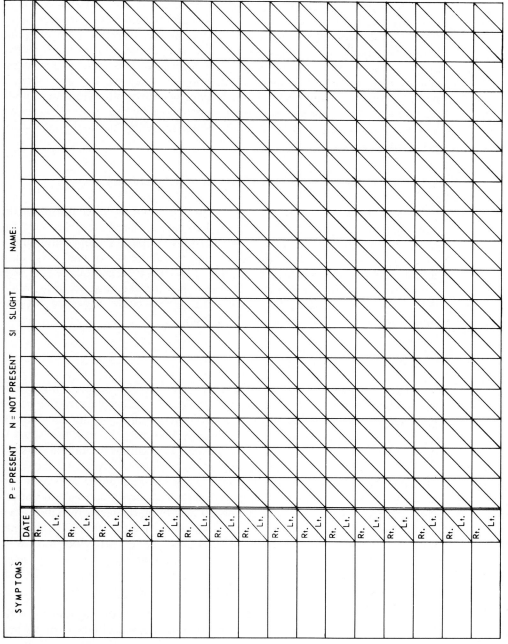

Figure 11-45. Symptom checklist. (Reprinted with permission from Shore, N. A.: Temporomandibular Joint Dysfunction and Occlusal Equilibration, 2nd ed. Philadelphia, J.B. Lippincott Co., 1976.)

ASSOCIATED PATHOLOGICAL CONDITIONS

PAROTID-MASSETER HYPERTROPHY–TRAUMATIC OCCLUSION SYNDROME

This syndrome has been explained by Blatt.[57] The patients examined not only had evidence of traumatic occlusion coupled with masseter hypertrophy, but they also had sialodochitis of the affected parotid gland. Sialograms indicated that the parotid duct was obstructed by the hypertrophied masseter when the teeth were in occlusion. This type of obstruction caused inflammation of Stensen's duct, with associated swelling and increased pain. Correction of the occlusal interference was most efficacious in relieving parotid symtoms. The sialodochitis was managed by rise of sialogogues and increased water intake by the patient. Bougienage and lacrimal dilators were sometimes required.[58]

ARTHRALGIA RELATED TO ORAL CONTRACEPTIVE DRUG USE

Cases have been reported of arthralgia related to the use of oral contraceptive drugs.[59, 60] The patients had latent rheumatoid arthritis that was precipitated by the ingestion of the drugs. When a patient complains of preauricular pain, the clinician should inquire if the onset of pain was related to the use of oral contraceptive pills. The onset of arthralgia can begin anywhere from three months to a year following the start of drug intake. Withdrawal of the drug for a six-week period could prove to be most significant, if no other cause has been found.

OROFACIAL DYSKINESIA

This is a movement disorder characterized by severe, involuntary dystonic movements of the facial, oral, and cervical musculature. It is usually believed to be either the result of an extrapyramidal disorder or a complication of phenothiazine and L-dopa therapy.[61] During the past few years we have noticed certain edentulous and partially edentulous dental patients with involuntary dystonic movements similar to, but not as severe as, those with orofacial dyskinesia (Fig. 11–46). The symptoms responded well to a combination of oral orthopedic therapy coupled with myofunctional therapy. It is possible that other patients diagnosed as having orofacial dyskinesia with symptoms strongly resembling it may be aided by correction of craniomandibular imbalance. Evidently the disruption of dental proprioception was a major factor in the etiology of orofacial dyskinesia. It generally affects persons more than 60 years of age, and it may be associated with torticollis or generalized dystonia. The following findings were of interest:

1. All attempts to establish an occlusion at the terminal hinge position failed, and the most comfortable and therapeutically effective mandibular position was several millimeters anterior to the terminal hinge position.

2. An apparently excessive vertical dimension of the occlusal prosthesis for these patients was most beneficial.

3. Most of the patients with orofacial dyskinesia also had symptoms of the craniomandibular syndrome.[62]

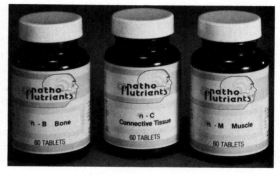

Figure 11–46. Gnatho Nutrients, helpful in improving nutrition for bone, connective tissue, and muscle, respectively.

TRIGEMINAL NEURALGIA

This is the most common facial neuralgia, responsible for one of the most excruciating pains known to man. In approximately 95 per cent of the cases seen, the second or third division of the trigeminal nerve is affected, with the ophthalmic branch of the fifth cranial nerve being involved in less than 3 per cent of the cases.[63] The patient describes a stabbing or electric shock sensation, lasting usually less than a minute. Initially the attacks are quite mild, and remissions lasting several months are common. With time, remissions become shorter and the pain becomes more severe, until finally attacks occur daily for many months. The pain is unilateral; in rare instances it may be bilateral involving one or more branches of the fifth cranial nerve. The pain never crosses the midline, and even in bilateral cases pain originating on one side does not cross to the other.

Pain is precipitated or "triggered" by various stimuli, including eating, talking, tongue and lip movements, yawning, touching the skin of the face, draft, sudden head movements, and, on occasion, walking, loud noise, or bright light; the onset is usually after the forty-fifth year.[64] No attacks occur during sleep at night. Attacks occur more often on the right side than on the left and are more common in females than in males.

The etiology of typical trigeminal neuralgia is unknown. It is questionable whether it is central or peripheral. Mechanical compression of nerve fibers has been considered a possible cause. It is currently suspected that a combination of degenerative changes in the gasserian ganglion, mechanical compression by a prominent petrous ridge, or an aberrant branch of the superior cerebellar artery may be involved in producing this pain.[65] Gardner was of the opinion that these factors produce demyelination, which in turn causes a short-circuiting of efferent fibers with afferent pain fibers, so that innocuous tactile stimuli to the face may cause abnormal discharges of the pain fibers, producing an attack.[66]

The classic treatment of trigeminal neuralgia has been alcohol injection of the gasserian ganglion and its branches or operative section of the preganglionic root of the fifth cranial nerve. Recently, carbamazine (Tegretol) and phenoliophendylate injections have been prescribed. Injection or operation can be complicated by painful numbness, while prolonged carbamazepine therapy can have serious side effects.

Several other methods of treatment have been reported successful but have not been used extensively. Disturbed physiology of the dural membrane enveloping the gasserian ganglion as a result of articular strain between the petrous portion of the temporal bone and the sphenoid bone has been supported by observation of structural imbalance between the right and left temporal bones where the nerve passes over the petrous apex. Releasing the dural stresses, due to strains on the cranial articulations and elsewhere in the body, is benefical, especially if diagnosed early.[67] Manual retraction of the mandible for 10 minutes three times a day has freed patients of trigeminal neuralgia in periods ranging from one week to one month. This treatment was based on the theory that tractions and displacement against bony and dural landmarks caused the degenerative changes in the trigeminal nerve.[68]

Our findings and those of other investigators[17, 64, 69] showed not only that mandibular dysfunction occurred on the same side as the neuralgic pain but also that rehabilitation of normal mandibular function according to physiologic orthopedic principles eliminated the paroxysmal painful attacks of trigeminal neuralgia. However, we found that complete remission did not always result until the tactile pressure on a tooth, triggering the paroxysmal pain, was eliminated. This generally was a single upper or lower posterior tooth. Although this tooth appeared normal on x-ray examination or pulp-tested vital, the tooth was referred for root canal therapy; following this therapy, all pain was eliminated. Occasionally the final triggering mechanism was found to be the sensitive exposed cemento-enamel junction on a clasped tooth. Desensitization or root canal therapy[70] removed this factor.

A recent study[71] highlighted the possibility that dental and oral diseases may be major and important contributing factors in the onset of not only so-called idiopathic trigeminal neuralgia but the atypical facial neuralgias as well. Thirty-eight patients with idiopathic trigeminal neuralgia and 23 subjects with atypical facial neuralgia showed in almost all the cases a close relationship between the pain they were experiencing and the existence of cavities in the alveolar bone and in the jaw bone itself. These cavities were at the sites of previously extracted teeth and although some were more than 1 cm. in diameter, they were usually not detectable by x-rays. They were detected and localized empirically based on the observation that peripheral infiltration of local anesthesia into or very close to the bone cavity rapidly abolished trigger and pain perception while the patient was under anesthesia. Histopathological examination of the bone removed from these cavities revealed a pattern characterized by a highly vascular abnormal healing response to bone removal. Preliminary microbiological studies of material taken from the walls of the cavity showed the existence within the walls of a complex, mixed polymicrobial aerobic and anaerobic flora. Treatment consisted of vigorous curettage of the cavities, repeated when indicated, plus administration of antibiotics to induce healing and filling-in of the cavities by new bone. The patients' responses to this therapy were marked to complete pain remissions. It was then noted that complete healing led to complete and persistent pain remissions.

In summary, it must be stated that present-day therapy of trigeminal neuralgia, or the craniomandibular syndrome, or both, recognizes no single method of treatment for all patients. After a thorough diagnostic evaluation each patient should be treated in an orderly sequence, starting with the most conservative methods, and proceeding to surgical procedures only after all other methods have failed.

HERPES SIMPLEX VIRUS AND TMJ DISORDERS

Recently, Adour and his co-workers[72, 73] established a causal relationship between the herpes simplex virus type I (HSV-I), Bell's palsy, and certain acute and chronic clinical manifestations of the temporomandibular joint syndrome.

The bases of Adour's hypothesis[74] are the following: (1) herpes simplex type I involvement in the trigeminal ganglion and the facial, glossopharyngeal, and other cranial nerves and ganglia is already well established;[74–75] (2) HSV-I resides in the various cranial ganglia and during exacerbations causes a cranial polyneuritis;[76, 77] (3) as HSV-I proliferates downward from a particular cranial ganglion or from a single neuron, demyelination of the affected nerve fiber or fibers takes place as an autoimmune reaction;[76] (4) a demyelinated nerve can have its ability to transmit neural impulses stopped so that a motor nerve so affected will produce neuropraxia or denervation (if the axon is destroyed) of the supplied muscle tissue;[74, 76, 77] (5) denervated skeletal muscles no longer function normally and exhibit such pathologic functions as fibrillation, contracture, fasciculation, and high tissue irritability along with local areas of muscle inflammation (myositis) with atrophy, often in discrete areas of the muscles.[76, 78]

In a recent study,[79] 25 patients with clinical symptoms of TMJ underwent electromyographic (EMG) and electronic mandibular motion analysis examinations. Twenty-three of the 25 subjects had clear clinical histories of herpetic viral infections (HSV-I). EMG testing revealed that in all the patients with history of herpetic infection, the masticatory muscles had dysfunction typical of permanent motor neuron damage. Pathologic states such as fibrillations, contracture, and fasciculation were frequently seen. This study supported published medical findings relating herpes simplex viral infection to the neuromuscular dysfunction of the temporomandibular joint.

HEADACHES RELATED TO A CONNECTIVE TISSUE DISORDER—A "NEW SYNDROME"[80]

The most common headaches that plague man are neurovascular in nature, but little if anything has been done to research the cause of this type of pain.

It has been reported in the literature that individuals who have a mitral valve prolapse syndrome (MVP) complain regularly of headaches that appear to be nonorganic in origin. In this group of patients, pathologic examination of the valve leaflets demonstrates specific types of degenerative changes (myxomatous in nature) in the connective tissue components of the valve.

In gross specimen studies of the temporomandibular meniscus, it has been reported that a defect in the integrity of the disc may be unrelated to the configuration of the bony structures. Since perforations that have been observed in the fibroelastic discs do not originate directly from inflammatory or degenerative bone disorder, they must be considered congenital, or attributable to some type of systemic disease process.

In a clinical study involving 50 patients with chronic head and neck pain originating from a nontraumatically induced TMJ dysfunction, it was found that over 90 per cent exhibited an MVP after a complete cardiovascular evaluation.

In correlating these findings, it was hypothesized that the fibroelastin component of the TMJ meniscus and the fibroelastin tissue of the mitral valve undergo similar degenerative changes. This joint damage causes a splinting reaction, trigger points, and pain from the craniofacial myofascial components independent of the dental occlusion.

Although conventional TMJ occlusal therapy did not relieve the head and neck pain in these patients because of a constant joint irritation from the disc degeneration, a treatment plan for associated connective tissue damage and valvular defects was successful in over 95 per cent of the subjects in the particular study group.

Case History 1

Patient H. G. is a 44-year-old Caucasian hosewife with three children. Her chief complaint was severe headaches for a period of 16 years when she first presented herself on February 4, 1974. They were diagnosed at one time as tension headaches and at another time as migraine. They occurred with the greatest intensity on the left side but occasionally were felt on the right side as well.

The pattern of pain radiated from the inner side of the right or left eye, to the temporomandibular joint on the affected side, then to the mastoid area, and from there down to the occiput and shoulder. The pain was lancinating and deep. She generally awakened with a headache every morning. If she took Demerol (25 to 100 mg.) before retiring she would not awaken with a headache. Her past medications included Valium, Anacin, Fiorinal, Cafergot and Sansert.

Secondary complaints included popping or whooshing noises on opening and closing on the left side. She also complained of pain between the upper left first and second bicuspids. She was aware of clenching or grinding her teeth during sleep and also during the day. Muscle fatigue was experienced as the day wore on.

She had a hysterectomy performed in 1964, and the headaches were more severe since that time. One would have suspected hormonal imbalance, since she reported that her skin was dry, her nails broke easily, she tired easily, and had numerous trigger points throughout her body. Referral to her family physician, who took SMA-12 and other tests, revealed nothing unusual.

Clinical examination revealed spasms and tenderness on palpation of the anterior, middle, and posterior fibers of the left temporalis; the zygomatic, body, and mandibular angle of the left masseter; the body and mandibular angle of the right masseter; right and left internal and external pterygoid muscles; right and left sternocleidomastoid muscles; left trapezius muscle; right and left mylohyoid muscles; right and left posterior cervicals; right and left deltoids; the middle and lower back muscles on the right; and lower back muscles on the left side. The temporomandibular joint was tender to palpation on the left as well as both coronoid processes (the left more so). On palpation of the condylar heads through the external auditory meatuses the left was tender.

The mandible was deviated to the right in the closed position, and on opening deviated more to the left and then back toward the right. The maximal interincisal opening was 46 millimeters. Examination of the face revealed the right eye to be higher, with the right hip and shoulder lower. The patient exhibited a deviant swallowing problem. She reported the occurrence of polio in the right leg at the age of 15.

Radiographic as well as clinical examination revealed no caries and an excellent periodontal condition. There was a narrowing of the joint space on both sides in closed position. The opening position found the condyles in good relation to the eminentia bilaterally. The patient was missing the lower right and left first molars, and the upper right cuspid was in lingual version (Fig. 11–47).

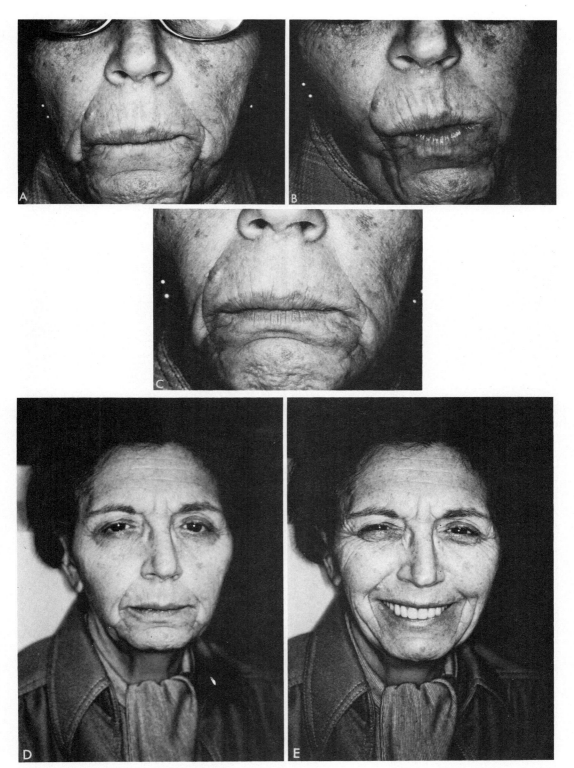

Figure 11–47. *A,* Patient exhibiting dystonic involuntary movements of the orofacial muscles. This view shows patient before treatment, wearing full upper denture and partial lower denture. *B,* Patient exhibiting almost continual involuntary movements of the orofacial muscles. Shown before treatment. *C,* Close-up view of orofacial muscles after orthopedic correction of jaw imbalance. *D,* Frontal view of patient after orthopedic correction of jaw imbalance. Notice cessation of involuntary dystonic movements. *E,* Frontal view of patient smiling, showing new full upper prosthesis.

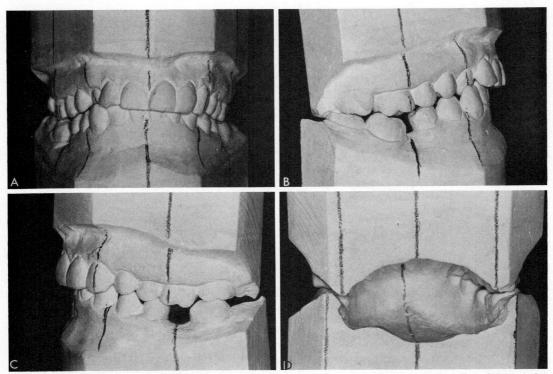

Figure 11–48. *A*, Frontal view of habitual occlusion. *B*, Right lateral view of habitual occlusion. *C*, Left lateral view of habitual occlusion. *D*, Posterior view of habitual occlusion.

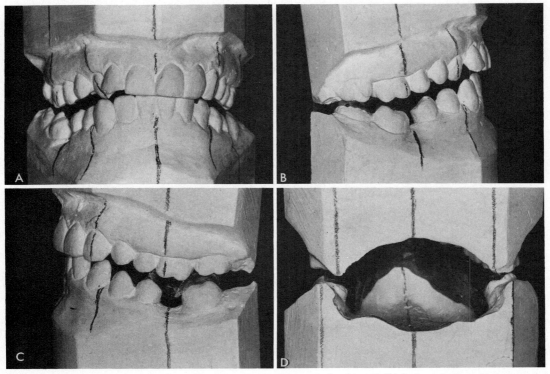

Figure 11–49. *A*, Frontal view of orthopedically corrected jaw relationship. *B*, Right lateral view. *C*, Left lateral view. *D*, Posterior view.

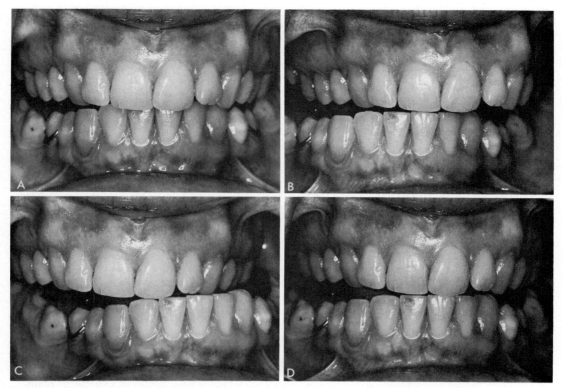

Figure 11–50. *A,* Centric occlusion produced with mandibular orthopedic repositioning appliance. *B,* Right lateral excursion with mandibular orthopedic repositioning appliance in place. *C,* Left lateral excursion with mandibular orthopedic repositioning appliance in place. *D,* Protrusive contact with mandibular orthopedic repositioning appliance in place.

Diagnosis of dysfunctional temporomandibular joint syndrome was established and treatment initiated.

We inserted a mandibular orthopedic repositioning appliance on February 12, 1974, to correct the jaw imbalance (Figs. 11–48 and 11–49). The trigger areas in the affected muscles were treated by injection of Xylocaine (2 per cent) with no epinephrine, as well as with high-voltage electrogalvanic stimulation and ethyl chloride spray with exercise. The patient was symptom free within three months. Orthodontic therapy using the Crozat appliance was instituted in August, 1974, to correct the cuspid on the right side. After this was completed, fixed bridges were placed in the lower right and left posterior quadrants (Fig. 11–50).

The patient is symptom free to this date.

Case History 2

Patient M. L. is a 43-year-old Caucasian housewife with three children. She presented herself to our office on March 17, 1975, complaining of head pain over the right eye and pain in the right temporomandibular joint, of nine months' duration. She was unable to perform her duties as wife and mother. Three years prior to the onset of symptoms she was involved in an automobile accident in which she was hit on the driver's side while driving. Her right lung collapsed as a result of that accident. In October, 1974, she fell and hit the right side of her face.

The pain of which she complained was dull, aching, and deep. Its onset could be abrupt or gradual, but it left abruptly. It was triggered by eating, yawning, and speaking but could be relieved by analgesics such as Darvon.

She was not aware of clenching or bruxing. She experienced popping or whooshing noises on opening and closing on the right side.

Clinical examination revealed spasm and tenderness on palpation of the anterior fibers of the right temporalis; the body and mandibular angle of the right masseter; the right and left internal and external pterygoids; the right sternocleidomastoid; the right and left trapezius muscles; the right and left posterior cervicals; and the middle back muscles on the right side. The right and left temporomandibular joints were tender to palpation, as were both coronoid processes. On palpation of the condylar heads through the external auditory meatuses both were tender.

The mandible was deviated to the right in the closed position but deviated to the left on opening. There was a click in the right TMJ on full opening and a click on terminal closure on the left side. The widest interincisal opening was 29 millimeters.

Examination of the face revealed the right eye to be higher. The patient exhibited a deviant swallowing habit.

Radiographs and clinical examination revealed no caries and a mouth that was periodontally sound. Temporomandibular joint x-rays revealed greater narrowing of the joint space on the left side than on the right side. It was also noted that there was very limited excursion of the condyles in their fossae upon opening widely, owing to limitation of movement of the mandible. The radiographs were negative for any evidence of fracture. The patient had a full complement of teeth with the upper right first and second bicuspids and the first molar in a crossbite relationship (Fig. 11–51).

A diagnosis of dysfunctional temporomandibular joint arthrosis was made, and treatment was initiated. A mandibular orthopedic repositioning appliance was inserted on April 17, 1975, to correct the maxillo-mandibular imbalance (Fig. 11–52). The trigger areas in the masticatory and neck musculature were treated by injection of Xylocaine (2 per cent) with no epinephrine, as well as with high-voltage electrogalvanic stimulation. The patient was rendered symp-

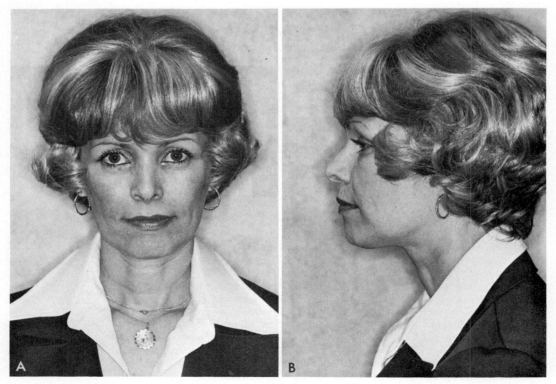

Figure 11–51. *A*, Frontal view of corrected jaw relationship. *B*, Profile view of corrected jaw relationship.

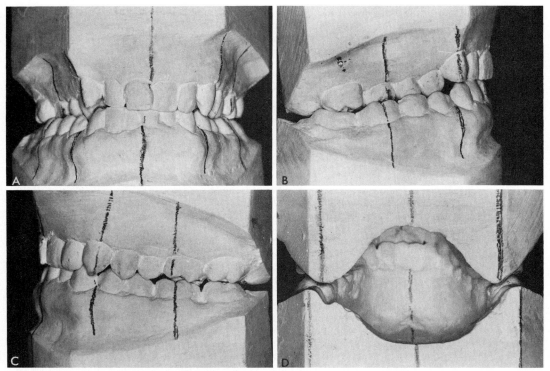

Figure 11–52. *A*, Frontal view of habitual occlusion. *B*, Right lateral view of habitual occlusion. *C*, Left lateral view of habitual occlusion. *D*, Posterior view of habitual occlusion.

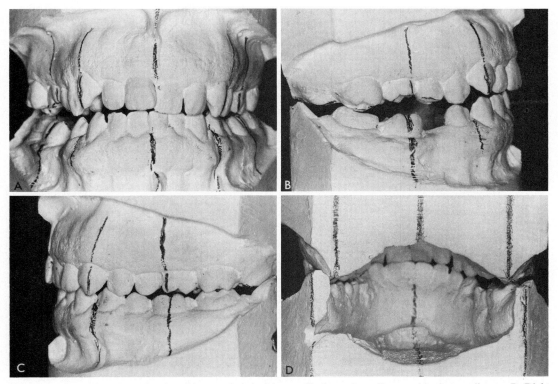

Figure 11–53. *A*, Centric occlusal position produced with mandibular orthopedic repositioning appliance. *B*, Right lateral view of corrected maxillo-mandibular relationship. *C*, Left lateral view of corrected maxillo-mandibular relationship. *D*, Posterior view of corrected maxillo-mandibular relationship.

tom free in five weeks. However, she sustained additional trauma as the result of another automobile accident on October 18, 1975. Symptoms reappeared for a short period of time, but were relieved quickly by treating the affected musculature. She would have had more severe symptoms had she not been wearing her oral device. As a consequence of this accident she had to have the lower right second bicuspid removed. In April, 1976, she was fitted with Crozat appliances to correct the crossbite relationship on the right side and to even out the arch form in the anterior segments (Fig. 11–53). Upon completion of orthodontic therapy, fixed bridgework was necessary in the upper and lower right posterior quadrants.

Case History 3

Patient J. T. is a 22-year-old single Caucasian schoolteacher at a state school for the mentally retarded. Her chief complaint was headache above her eyes on her forehead occurring several times a week for the past year. She first presented herself for examination on February 26, 1976.

The pain was most severe on the left side. The area of onset was the temporomandibular joint. The pain was of an aching quality and deep seated. It would come on and leave abruptly, generally being precipitated by chewing tough meat or when she was extremely tired. Restricted mandibular movement would relieve her discomfort. She was aware of clenching her teeth not only while awake, but also during the night. Secondary complaints included popping or whooshing noises on opening and closing her mouth.

Clinical examination revealed spasm and tenderness on palpation of the anterior and middle fibers of the left temporalis muscle; the zygomatic, body, and mandibular angle of the right masseter muscle; the left mylohyoid muscle; the right and left external pterygoid muscles; the right and left trapezius muscles; the left intercostal muscles; and the supraspinatus and infraspinatus muscles on the left side. The left temporomandibular joint and coronoid process were tender to palpation, and crepitation, as well as a sagittal closing click, was heard on auscultation. The maximal interincisal opening was 48.5 millimeters, and there was no deviation on opening. The patient revealed a deviant swallowing habit. Examination of the face revealed that the left eye was higher, and the lip line was lower on the right and higher on the left.

Periapical radiographs as well as clinical examination showed no evidence of caries and an excellent periodontal condition. The patient had undergone orthodontic therapy between the ages of 12 and 16, with four bicuspid extractions. Temporomandibular joint radiographs demonstrated superior displacement of the condyle on the right side (position 1–2) and posterior displacement on the left side (position 2–5). In the open position both condyles were in good relation to the eminentia articularis. A noticeable discrepancy in

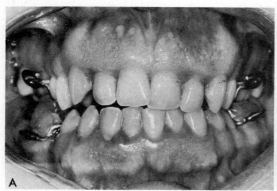
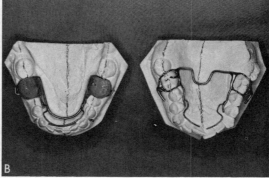

Figure 11–54. *A,* Upper and lower Crozat appliances in place. Note acrylic placed within cribs of lower first molars to maintain vertical stops in the corrected jaw relationship. *B,* Lingual view of upper and lower Crozat appliances.

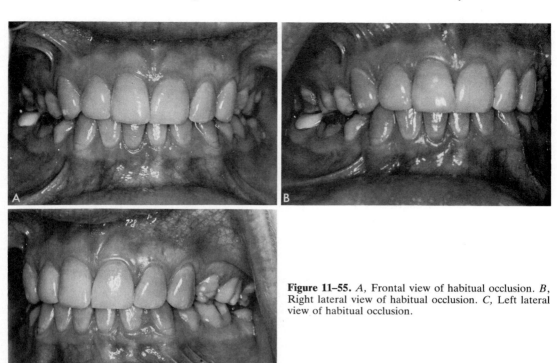

Figure 11–55. *A*, Frontal view of habitual occlusion. *B*, Right lateral view of habitual occlusion. *C*, Left lateral view of habitual occlusion.

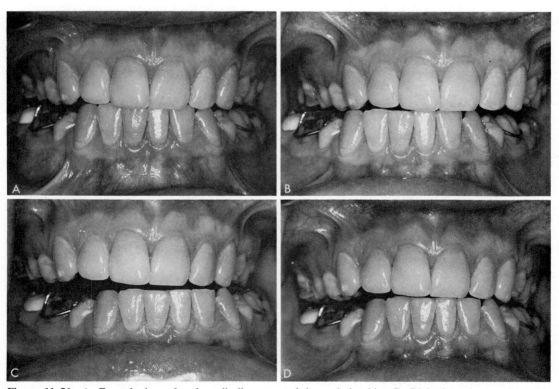

Figure 11–56. *A*, Frontal view of orthopedically corrected jaw relationship. *B*, Right lateral excursion with mandibular orthopedic repositioning appliance in place. *C*, Left lateral excursion with mandibular orthopedic repositioning appliance in place. *D*, Protrusive excursion with mandibular repositioning appliance in place. Note that all the upper teeth on the right side are off the plane of occlusion.

size and shape between the upper and lower six anterior teeth and the lower posteriors was evident (Fig. 11–54).

Diagnosis of dysfunctional temporomandibular joint syndrome was made, and treatment was initiated.

A mandibular orthopedic repositioning appliance was inserted on March 17, 1976 (Fig. 11–55). The trigger areas in the affected muscles were treated by injection of Xylocaine (2 per cent) with no epinephrine, and high-voltage electrogalvanic stimulation was used. Exercises for protrusive opening were also instituted. The patient was symptom free within three and one-half months (Fig. 11–56). Orthodontic therapy was then started to super-erupt the lower posterior teeth, which obviously had not reached their full growth potential into their physiologic vertical position.

Case History 4

Patient R. C. is an 18-year-old single Caucasian dental assistant. Her chief complaint was pain in the right and left sides of her face with a marked deviation of the mandible on the right side. The only means by which she could be relieved of the pain or prevent deviation of the mandible was to have her jaws wired by an oral surgeon (Fig. 11–57). At one point she was fitted with an upper Hawley appliance at a local temporomandibular joint clinic after the wires were removed (Fig. 11–58A, B, C, D).

On March 2, 1976, she presented at the Temporomandibular Joint Clinic at the French and Polyclinic Hospital Health Center and Medical School (Fig. 11–59A, B). At this time, her pain was deep, aching, and continuous. It was at its worst at bedtime. The usual pain-killers did not relieve her pain.

Clinical examination revealed spasm and tenderness in the middle posterior fibers of the right temporalis; the posterior fibers of the left temporalis; the body and mandibular angle of the right and left masseters; the right and left internal and external pterygoid muscles; the right and left sternocleidomastoid muscles; the right and left trapezius muscles; the right and left posterior cervical muscles; the right and left supraspinatus muscles; the right and left infraspinatus muscles; and the right intercostal muscles. Both temporomandibular joints were tender to palpation. There was swelling in the neck area.

The mandible was deviated to the right in an approximated closed position and on opening. The interincisal opening was restricted. In order to take study casts, it was necessary to inject the trigger points in the right and left internal pterygoids and right masseter. The right temporomandibular joint was sprayed with ethyl chloride as the patient gently opened and closed her mouth. The patient's facial appearance returned to normal in a very short period of time (Fig. 11–60A, B).

Radiographs as well as clinical examination revealed no caries and sound periodontal structures. There was some narrowing of the joint space on both sides in the closed position. The opening position found the condyles to be in good relation to the eminentia following the trigger point injections. The patient was missing the lower left first molar. The upper left bicuspid was lingually displaced, and there were diastemas mesial and distal to the lower left cuspid. The patient exhibited a deviant swallowing habit.

A diagnosis of dysfunctional temporomandibular joint syndrome was made and treatment initiated.

A mandibular orthopedic repositioning appliance was inserted on April 13, 1976, and balanced in various excursions. Further treatment of the affected muscles was carried out by means of trigger point injections, ethyl chloride spray, exercise, and electrogalvanic stimulation. The patient was taught to correct her midline opening pattern with toothpicks placed between the upper and lower central incisors. She was also taught how to limit her opening into protrusion. She improved greatly within three months, and a fixed bridge was recommended for the lower left quadrant in addition to occlusal equilibrium (Fig. 11–61). She returned to her own dentist for treatment.

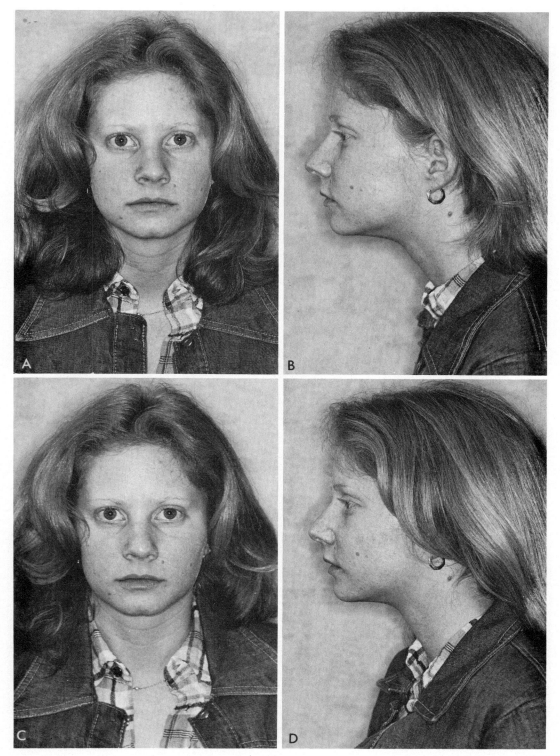

Figure 11–57. *A*, Frontal view before treatment. *B*, Profile view before treatment. *C*, Frontal view of corrected jaw position. *D*, Profile view of corrected jaw position.

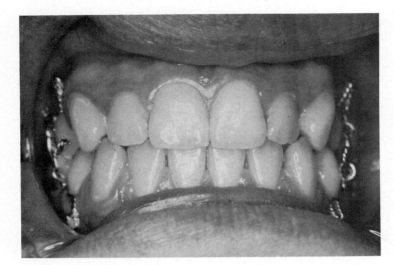

Figure 11–58. Patient with interarch wires in place.

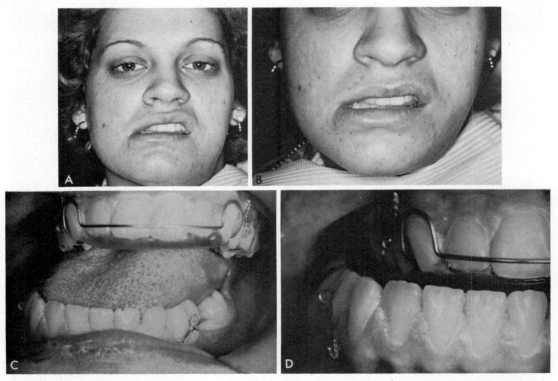

Figure 11–59. *A,* Frontal view of patient with wires removed, wearing upper Hawley appliance. *B,* Close-up frontal view of patient with wires removed, wearing upper Hawley appliance. *C,* Patient with mouth open, wearing upper Hawley appliance. *D,* Patient trying to close mouth with upper Hawley appliance in place. (Courtesy of Dr. Robert A. Saporito.)

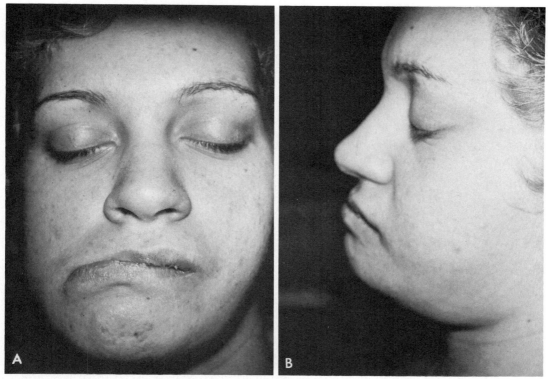

Figure 11–60. *A*, Frontal view of patient with interarch wiring removed. *B*, Profile view of patient with interarch wiring removed. (Courtesy of Dr. Robert A. Saporito.)

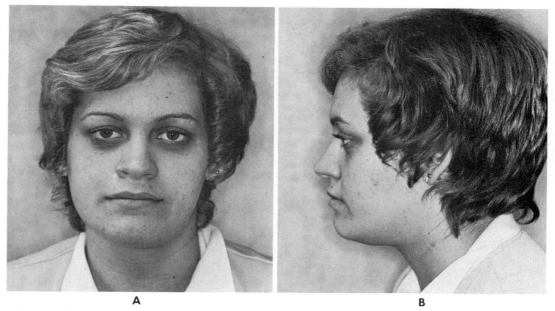

Figure 11–61. *A*, Frontal view of patient with muscles relaxed. *B*, Profile view of patient with muscles relaxed.

Case History 5

Patient E. C. is a 45-year-old Caucasian housewife with two children. Her chief complaint was constant pain for the past 16 months in her temples, ears, neck, shoulder, and arms when she first appeared in our office on January 6, 1976. The pain was deep, aching, and constant. She also complained of frequent vertigo and nausea. There were secondary complaints, such as stuffiness in both ears, tinnitus, numbness of her face and arms, and even difficulty with breathing on occasion. Clinical examination revealed spasm and tenderness in the anterior, middle, and posterior fibers of the left temporalis muscle; the middle and posterior fibers of the right temporalis muscle; the zygomatic, body, and mandibular angle of the left masseter muscle; the body and mandibular angle of the right masseter muscle; the right and left internal and external pterygoid muscles; the right and left sternocleidomastoid muscles; the right and left trapezius muscles; the left mylohyoid; the left posterior cervical; the right and left infraspinatus muscles; and the right and left sacrospinal muscles. There was tenderness on palpation of the right temporomandibular joint and both coronoid processes.

The mandible was deviated to the left in the closed position, but it deviated to the right on opening. The interincisal opening was restricted to 34.5 millimeters. There was tenderness of the left condylar head when palpated through the external auditory meatus on opening and closing.

Examination of the face showed the left eye to be higher and the left shoulder and hip lower. The patient had a deviant swallowing habit (Fig. 11–62).

Radiographic and clinical examination revealed no caries but many amalgam restorations. There were teeth missing in the lower right and left posterior quadrants and the upper left posterior quadrant. There was minimal periodontal involvement. Temporomandibular joint radiographs demonstrated narrowing of the joint space on both sides in the closed position and restricted movement in the opening position. The patient was wearing an upper appliance to treat her TMJ problem when she first arrived in our office (Fig. 11–63).

A diagnosis of dysfunctional temporomandibular joint arthritis was made and treatment initiated.

On January 21, 1976, a mandibular orthopedic repositioning appliance was inserted and balanced in all excursions (Fig. 11–64). The trigger areas in the affected muscles were treated by injection of Xylocaine (2 per cent), with no epinephrine, in conjunction with high-voltage electrogalvanic stimulation, ethyl chloride spray, and exercise. The patient was referred for endocrine consultation in May and was found to be deficient in estrogen. Following the use of Premarin, the patient was much better at the end of the summer. She was recently fitted for a lower overlay partial denture. The patient still has residual symptoms and is in need of long-term medical management.

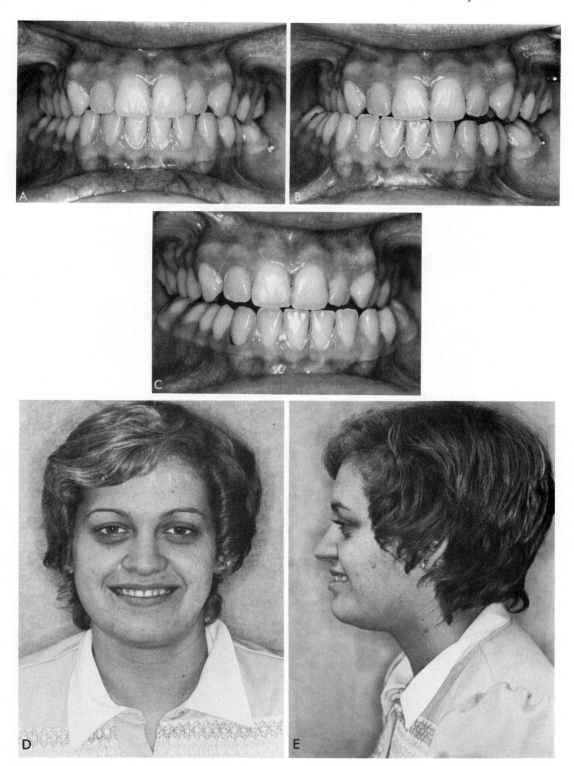

Figure 11–62. *A,* Frontal view of dentition after elimination of pain and dysfunction. *B,* Right lateral excursive movement after elimination of pain and dysfunction. *C,* Left lateral excursive movement after elimination of pain and dysfunction. *D,* Frontal view of patient at completion of TMJ treatment. *E,* Profile view of patient at completion of TMJ treatment.

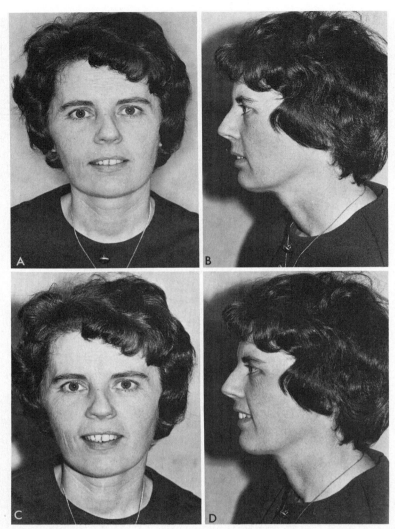

Figure 11–63. *A*, Frontal view of patient before treatment. *B*, Profile view of patient before treatment. *C*, Frontal view of patient after orthopedic jaw correction. *D*, Profile view of patient after orthopedic jaw correction.

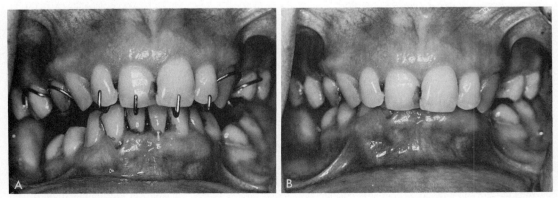

Figure 11–64. *A*, Frontal view of patient wearing an upper appliance to treat TMJ dysfunction. *B*, Frontal view of habitual occlusion showing noticeable loss of vertical dimension.

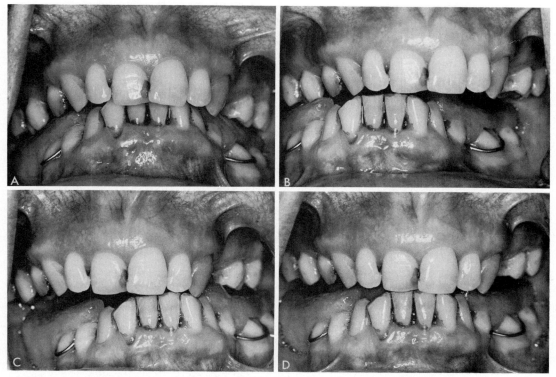

Figure 11–65. *A,* Frontal view of centric occlusion produced with mandibular orthopedic repositioning appliance. *B,* Right lateral excursion with mandibular repositioning appliance in place. *C,* Left lateral excursion with mandibular repositioning appliance in place. *D,* Protrusive excursion with mandibular repositioning appliance in place.

References

1. Mines, S.: The Conquest of Pain. New York, Grosset and Dunlap, 1974.
2. Bonica, J. J.: The Management of Pain. Philadelphia, Lea and Febiger, 1974.
3. Alling, C. C., and Burton, H. N.: Diagnosis of chronic maxillofacial pain. Alabama J. Med. Sci., *10*:75, 1973.
4. Wood, G. N.: Centric occlusion, centric relation and the mandibular posture. J. Prosthet. Dent., *20*:292, 1968.
5. Carey, F.: Your Aching Back. New York Post, July 15, 1970, p. 39.
6. Sicher, H., and DuBrul, E. L.: Oral Anatomy, 5th ed. St. Louis, C. V. Mosby Co., 1970.
7. Gregory, W. K.: The upright posture of man: a review of its origin and evolution. Proc. Am. Philos. Soc., *67*:339, 1928.
8. Strachan, F., and Robinson, M. J.: Short leg linked to malocclusion. Osteopath. News, April, 1965.
9. Travell, J.: Lecture presented to Florida Dental Association Annual Meeting, May, 1974.
10. Mohl, N. D.: Head posture and its role in occlusion. N.Y. J. Dent., *42*:17, 1976.
11. Posselt, U.: Studies on the mobility of the human mandible. Acta Odont. Scand., *10*:1, 1972.
12. Brill, N., Lammie, G. A., Osborne, J., and Perry, H. T.: Mandibular positions and mandibular movements. Br. Dent. J., *106*:391, 1959.
13. Schwarz, A. M.: Positions of the head and malrelations of the jaws. Int. J. Ortho. Oral Surg. Radiol., *14*:56, 1928.
14. Funakoski, M., and Amano, N.: Effects of the tonic neck reflex on the jaw muscles of the rat. J. Dent. Res., *52*:668, 1973.
15. McLean, L. F., Brenman, H. S., and Friedman, M. G. F.: Effects of changing body position on dental occlusion. J. Dent. Res., *52*:1041, 1973.
16. McLean, L. F.: Gravitational influences on the afferent and efferent components of mandibular reflexes. Ph.D. dissertation. Philadelphia, Thomas Jefferson University, 1973.

17. Moore, D. S., and Nally, F. F.: The diagnosis and management of paroxysmal trigeminal neuralgia in association with a temporomandibular joint dysfunction. Oral Surg., *38*:876, 1974.

18. Posselt, U.: Physiology of Occlusion and Rehabilitation. Oxford, Blackwell Scientific Publications, 1962.

19. Krogh-Paulson, W. G., and Olsen, A.: Occlusal disharmonies and dysfunction of the stomatognathic system. Dent. Clin. North Am., 1966, p. 627.

20. Alexander, R. E., Taylor, C. G., Cinquemani, N. F., and Kramer, H. S.: Use of physical therapy in oral surgical practice. Oral Surg., *28*:671, 1970.

21. Lehman, J. F., et al.: Heating of joint structures by ultrasound. Arch. Phys. Med. Rehabil., *49*:28, 1968.

22. Nash, D. F. E.: The clicking jaw. Practitioner, *161*:61, 1948.

23. Grieder, A., et al.: Evaluation of ultrasonic therapy for temporomandibular joint dysfunction. Oral Surg., *31*:25, 1971.

24. Erickson, R. I.: Ultrasound—a useful adjunct in temporomandibular joint therapy. Oral Surg., *18*:176, 1964.

25. Travell, J.: Rapid relief of acute "stiff neck" by ethyl chloride spray. J. Am. Med. Wom. Assoc., *4*:89, 1949.

26. Travell, J.: Ethyl chloride spray for painful muscle spasm. Arch Phys. Med. Rehabil., *33*:291, 1952.

27. Travell, J., and Rinzler, S. H.: The myofascial genesis of pain. Postgrad. Med., 425, 1952.

28. Schwartz, L. L.: Disorders of the Temporomandibular Joint. Philadelphia, W. B. Saunders Co., 1959, pp. 232–238.

29. Shealy, C. N.: The Pain Game. Millbrae, California, Celestial Arts, 1976, p. 95.

30. Shealy, C. N., et al.: Electrical inhibition of pain, experimental evaluation. Anesth. Analg. Curr. Res., *46*:299, 1967.

31. Ramfjord, S. P., and Ash, M. M.: Occlusion, 2nd ed. Philadelphia, W. B. Saunders Co., 1971.

32. Ross, I. F.: Occlusion. St. Louis, C. V. Mosby Co., 1970.

33. Shore, N. A.: Temporomandibular Joint Dysfunction and Occlusal Equilibration, 2nd ed. Philadelphia, J. B. Lippincott Co., 1976.

34. Lucia, V. O.: Modern Gnathological Concepts. St. Louis, C. V. Mosby Co., 1961.

35. Dawson, P. E.: Evaluation, Diagnosis and Treatment of Occlusal Problems. St. Louis, C. V. Mosby Co., 1974.

36. Guichet, N. F.: Principles of Occlusion. Anaheim, Denar Corp., 1970.

37. Krogh-Paulsen, W. G.: Management of the occlusion of the teeth. *In* Schwartz, L. L., and Chayes, C. M. (eds.): Facial Pain and Mandibular Dysfunction. Philadelphia, W. B. Saunders Co., 1968.

38. Jankelson, B.: Management of the Occlusion. A Postgraduate Seminar in Dentistry. University of Missouri at Kansas City, 1965.

39. Mann, A. W., and Pankey, L. D.: The P. M. philosophy of occlusal rehabilitation. Dent. Clin. North Am., Philadelphia, W. B. Saunders Co., Nov., 1963, pp. 621–636.

40. Glickman, I., Pameijer, J. H. N., Roeber, F. W., and Brion, M. A. M.: Functional occlusion as revealed by miniaturized radio transmitters. Dent. Clin. North Am., Philadelphia, W. B. Saunders Co., July, 1969, pp. 667–679.

41. Ross, I. F.: Personal communication, 1983.

42. Gelb, H., and Bernstein, I.: Clinical evaluation of two hundred patients with temporomandibular joint syndrome. J. Prosthet. Dent., *49*:234, 1983.

43. Gelb, H., and Tarte, J.: A two-year clinical dental evaluation of 200 cases of chronic headache: the craniocervical-mandibular syndrome. JADA, *91*:1230, 1975.

44. Knop, F. J., Richardson, B. L., and Bogstad, J.: Motions of the mandible related to modern gnathologic concepts. J. Prosthet. Dent., *24*:148, 1970.

45. Gelb, H.: Evaluation of static centric relation in the T.M.J. dysfunction syndrome. Dent. Clin. North Am., 1975, pp. 519–530.

46. Jankelson, B.: Reality vs. the inherited mythology of occlusion. Calif. Dent. Assoc. Meeting, San Francisco, Oct. 1–3, 1976.

47. Schwartz, L. L.: Disorders of the Temporomandibular Joint. Philadelphia, W. B. Saunders Co., 1959, p. 223.

48. Halpern, L. M.: Drugs against pain. *In* Mines, S. (ed.): The Conquest of Pain. New York, Grosset and Dunlap, 1974.

49. Halpern, L. M.: Analgesics and other drugs for the relief of pain. Postgrad. Med., *53*:91, 1973.

50. Physician's Desk Reference, 38th ed. Oradell, New Jersey, Medical Economics Co., 1984.

51. Dorland's Illustrated Medical Dictionary, 26th ed. Philadelphia, W. B. Saunders Co., 1981.

52. Freese, A. S.: Pain. New York, Penguin Books, 1975, p. 133.

53. Benson, H., and Epstein, M. D.: The placebo effect: a neglected asset in the care of patients. JAMA *232*:1225, 1975.

54. Horton, C. P.: Treatment of arthritic temporomandibular joints by intra-articular injection of hydrocortisone. Oral Surg., *6*:826, 1953.

55. Henny, F. A.: Intra-articular injection of hydrocortisone into the temporomandibular joint. J. Oral Surg., *12*:314, 1954.

56. Travell, J.: Mechanical headache. Headache, April, 1967, pp. 23–29.

57. Blatt, I.: The parotid-masseter hypertrophy traumatic occlusion syndrome. Laryngoscope, *79*:624, 1969.

58. Mahan, P. E.: Pathophysiology of facial and oral pain. *In* Goldman, H., et al. (eds.): Current Therapy in Dentistry. St. Louis, C. V. Mosby Co., 1974.

59. Bole, G. G., Jr., et al.: Rheumatic symptoms and serological abnormalities induced by oral contraceptives. Lancet, *1*:323, 1969.

60. Spiera, H., and Platz, C. M.: Rheumatic symptoms and oral contraceptives. Lancet, *1*:511, 1969.

61. Sutcher, H. D., Underwood, R. B., Beatty, R. A., and Sugar, O.: Orofacial dyskinesia. JAMA, *216*:1459, 1971.

62. Sutcher, H. D., Underwood, R. B., and Beatty, R. A.: Orofacial dyskinesia: Effective prosthetic therapy. J. Prosthet. Dent., *30*:252, 1973.

63. Kerr, F. W. L.: Mechanisms, Diagnosis and management of some cranial and facial pain syndromes. Surg. Clin. North Am., *43*:951, 1963.

64. Blair, G. A. S., and Gordan, D. S.: Trigeminal neuralgia and dental malocclusions. Br. Med. J., *4*:38, 1973.

65. Kruger, L.: Structural aspects of trigeminal neuralgia: A summary of current findings and concepts. J. Neurosurg., *26*:106, 1967.

66. Gardner, W. J.: Concerning the mechanism of trigeminal neuralgia and hemifacial spasm. J. Neurosurg., *19*:947, 1962.

67. Lay, E. M.: The osteopathic management of trigeminal neuralgia. J. Am. Osteopath. Assoc., *74*:373, 1975.

68. Carney, L. R.: Considerations on the cause and treatment of trigeminal neuralgia. Neurology, *17*:1143, 1967.

69. Nordh, A. F.: Trigeminal neuralgia and mandibular dysfunction. Sven. Tandlak. Tidskr., *67*:1, 1974.

70. Uppgaard, R. O.: Trigeminal neuralgia of dental origin. Northwest Dent., *46*:267, 1967.

71. Ratner, E. J., Person, P., et al.: Jawbone cavities and trigeminal and atypical facial neuralgias. Oral Surg., *48*:3, 1979.

72. Adour, K. K.: Bell's palsy, a complete expression of acute benign cranial polyneuritis. Primary Care, *2*:717, 1975.

73. Adour, K. K., Byl, F. M., Hilsinger, R. L., Jr., Kahn, Z. M., and Sheldon, M. I.: The true nature of Bell's palsy: Analysis of 1,000 consecutive patients. Laryngoscope, *88*:1017, 1978.

74. Adour, K. K.: Acute temporomandibular joint pain–dysfunction syndrome: Neurotologic and electromyographic study. Am. J. Otolaryngol., *2*:114, 1981.

75. Schear, M.: Neurologic disease and mandibular dysfunction. In Schwartz, L., and Chayes, C. M. (eds.): Pain and Mandibular Dysfunction. Philadelphia, W. B. Saunders Co., 1968, p. 116.

76. Adour, K. K.: Costen's syndrome revisited: Cranial polyganglionitis as a form of tempo-romandibular joint pain dysfunction syndrome. Paper delivered before Equilibration Society, February 1982.

77. Stien, R., and Tonning, R. M.: Acute peripheral facial palsy. Arch Otolaryngol., *98*:187, 1973.

78. Foged, J.: Temporomandibular arthrosis. Lancet, *2*:129, 1949.

79. Gordon, J. R., and Thomas, E.: Influence of herpes simplex virus on jaw muscle function: A preliminary study. J. Craniomandib. Pract., *2*:32–38, 1983/1984.

80. Bennish, A., and Tilds, B. M.: Headaches related to a connective tissue disorder—a "new syndrome." Paper delivered before The American Association for the Study of Headache meeting, June 1979.

12

Surgery of the Temporomandibular Articulation

PAUL SCHEMAN, D.D.S.

A decade and a half ago, a chapter such as this would have been an important and even a central chapter on TMJ problems. Today, with the recognition that most of the problems are functional, this subject has come to occupy a place of greatly decreased importance as a method of dealing with temporomandibular joint problems. As I and others have pointed out, intrinsic diseases of this joint are rare. While most of the problems in this region for which patients seek help are functional and are even "non-joint" problems, as in the myofascial pain–dysfunction syndrome (MPD), there are two conditions for which surgery is the modality of choice: ankylosis and condylar fracture in the young.

In the past, the following conditions were considered by many to be amenable to surgical solutions:

1. Chronic dislocation (subluxation).

2. Joint pain refractory to treatment with or without "clicking" and sometimes only for clicking.

3. Cephalic, facial pain, refractory to other treatment, i.e., surgery as a last resort.

4. Costen's syndrome which did not respond to "opening the bite" and for which the alternate diagnosis was "hypertrophy of the meniscus."

Except for chronic dislocation, surgery is not usually done or recommended. The basic rationale for the lessened choice of surgery is, primarily, its poor record of success and, second, the progressive development of a more precise understanding of the anatomy and physiology of this joint. Laskin's research into the clinical entity which he called myofascial pain–dysfunction syndrome illuminated the physiopsychosocial aspects of the disease. For this whole class of clinical problems surgery is irrational, and it is important for surgeons to understand that these patients will become willing subjects for irrational treatment. In spite of recorded success, surgery for conditions in which surgery is not the direct and rational remedy should not be employed. These patients have responded well to a multitude of nonsurgical therapies.

ANKYLOSIS

The chief condition for which surgery of the joint is indicated is ankylosis. As this is written, one must realize that when ankylosis occurs one cannot properly speak of "surgery of the joint," since the joint is obliterated. A more precise statement would be that we are concerned with restoring mobility to the mandible in the face of absence of joint function.

This condition results most often from an osteoma or ossification that is possibly idiopathic or the result of a birth injury. It may also result from untreated fracture at an early age in life, i.e., in infancy, before the age of 13, and more rarely in all ages as a result of pannus formation following severe rheumatoid arthritis or other inflammatory conditions resulting in calcification, dense fibrosis, or ossification. In children the form of rheumatoid arthritis known as Still's disease is a cause.

Specific infections, such as gonococcal infection, which has a predilection for the TMJ (as well as the sternoclavicular joint), have been responsible for ankylosis of the TMJ in the past. With the reappearance of gonorrhea among larger numbers of the population, it may in the future result in an increased incidence of ankylosis. From the point of view of the clinician the knowledge that this disease attacks the TMJ should lead to a preventive stance through venereal disease control, case finding, and early or at least prompt treatment following diagnosis. Birth injury and child abuse are other possible causes of ankylosis. Following such trauma, hemorrhage into the joint spaces and into the adjoining fascial planes may occur, which may explain the often massive ossification which extends beyond the limits of the anatomical structure of the joint. Perhaps in the early stages of life connective tissue is capable of undifferentiated activity, and hence exhibits one of its developmental options, the production of bone. An analogy may be made with the problem of removing all of a tumor to prevent recurrence. Therefore, gap arthroplasty to treat ankylosis may fail because of this osteogenic potential of young connective tissue. The use of inert materials such as silicone or methylmethacrylate is rational in this light. These may serve to prevent the bridging of the gap by interrupting the vascularity of the distal bone segment of the resected mandible. The nature of the material used or its shape is immaterial, as long as it has proven histocompatibility.

SURGICAL MANAGEMENT OF ANKYLOSIS

Surgery for the relief of ankylosis begins with a diagnostic radiological survey that must include conventional lateral projection (oblique lateral transcranial projections), a vertex projection, and tomography along the long axis of the condyle as established by the vertex projection (see Chapter 9). These views will establish the extent of the ankylosis and determine the surgical plan, which includes the selection of the initial incision. If careful

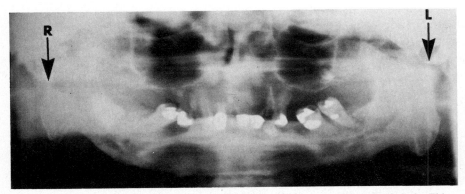

Figure 12–1. This is a panoramic tomographic x-ray of the mandible showing a bilateral ankylosis. This patient had been operated on in childhood but developed a recurrence. On the right there is more mobility as a result of bone resorption. On the left there is little motion in spite of the radiographic appearance of a pseudoarthrosis.

radiography determines that the ankylosis extends to the level of the coronoid notch of the mandible or beyond, the incision of choice is a submandibular one. This incision, made popular for vertical osteotomies for the correction of mandibular prognathism, has the advantage of being cosmetically safe and of avoiding injury to the facial nerve (Figs. 12–1 to 12–3).

TECHNIQUE

Assuming the lesion does not extend beyond the anatomical neck of the condyle, the surgical approach to this region is by way of a preauricular

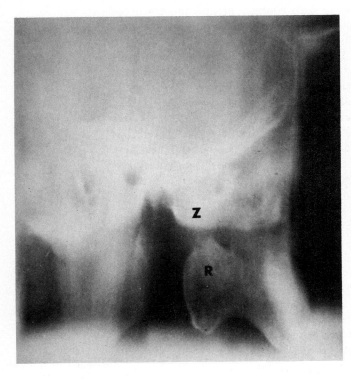

Figure 12–2. This is the left side of this case of bilateral ankylosis. Between the zygoma (Z) and the ramus (R) may be seen an atrophied mandible with resorption in the area of the condyle. This has resulted in some mobility on this side. Note the clarity and lack of superimposition of structures that is obtained by means of tomography.

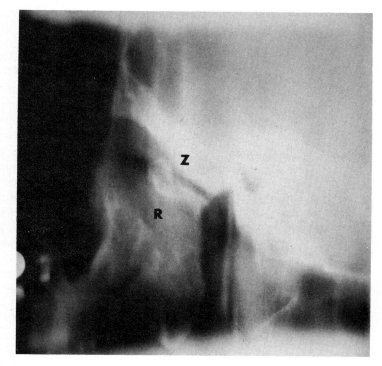

Figure 12–3. This is a tomographic radiograph through the right side of the mandible in the plane of the pseudoarthrosis. It may be seen between the zygoma (Z) and the ramus of the mandible (R). It illustrates the diagnostic quality of a tomograph. Note the "blurring out" of the deeper cranial structures in the top right portion of the radiograph as well as the clarity of the selected plane through the ramus and the pseudoarthrosis.

incision. The structures to be avoided are the auriculotemporal branch of the fifth nerve, the superficial temporal vein and artery, and, in extending the dissection forward, the temporal branch of the facial nerve. Ordinarily this nerve presents no problem in this surgical field, but there are variations in its arborization as it leaves the root of the facial nerve that may bring some of its branches closer to the capitulum. Careful blunt dissection in any area anterior to the capitulum as well as the avoidance of rough or excessive retraction of the ventral (anterior) edge of the flap will avoid injury to this nerve.

The skin and the superficial and deep fasciae are brought forward (ventrally) by means of blunt dissection. Superficial bleeding vessels rarely need to be clamped and tied. In this connection it has been my practice to inject lidocaine hydrochloride with 2 per cent epinephrine or other vasoconstrictors into the line of the incision and anterior to the capitulum into the insertions of the external pterygoid muscles, even when general anesthesia is employed, in order to provide a relatively bloodless field and permit the use of lighter planes of anesthesia.

The elevation of the flap will expose the lateral ligament of the joint, which, in the presence of a mass such as an osteoma, will appear as a dense and not easily detached structure. A vertical incision is made in the ligament. The use of *sharp* periosteal elevators will permit the elvation of this ligament. It may be necessary at this point in the procedure to extend the vertical incision until it is considerably longer than the mass. If this is done care must be taken to elevate the overlying tissues because the temporal branch of the facial nerve crosses the neck of the condyle in the region of the posterior (dorsal) end of the coronoid notch. Again, one must be gentle and cautious in dissection and retraction. In many instances elevation of the ligament is not required and it may be taken en bloc.

In all cases of ankylosis the joint cavities are obliterated and therefore the mass takes on a pyramidal shape, with the base of the pyramid along the root of the zygoma. This is used as a guide to the line of bone excision. Using an oscillating saw and a blade with a ribbed back in order to provide a stop, an initial cut is made parallel to the inferior (caudal) border of the zygoma. The attachments of the superior and inferior bellies of the external pterygoid muscles are detached by first clamping them and then carefully severing them with Metzenbaum scissors as close to the mass as possible. It is not advisable to complete the detachment of the external pterygoids at this time, since there is a medial extension of the muscle that cannot be brought into view at this point in the procedure. Blind dissection may sever branches of the internal maxillary artery (see Fig. 9–1). By stripping away the lateral ligament and the periosteum around the neck of the condyle, a small, flat or slightly curved retractor is worked around the anterior face of the neck of the condyle so that it will act as a stop for the subsequent use of the saw for sectioning the neck of the condyle below the mass.

The purpose for this caution is to avoid a pterygoid branch of the internal maxillary artery which often comes between the superior and inferior heads of the muscle and to preserve the sphenomandibular ligament, which, along with the stylomandibular ligament and the associated muscles (except the severed external pterygoid), will provide the functional support of the mandible after removal of the mass. With the retractor in place the oscillating saw is used to sever the neck of the condyle. Following this cut a bone-grasping forceps is placed on the neck of the condyle which is involved in the mass, and the mandible is depressed so that a gap is produced between the cut ends. The periosteal elevator is now employed to strip away the periosteum from the medial surface of the condyle as well as the anterior surface until it can be worked up behind the medial surface of the mass. It is then replaced by a broader retractor to act as a stop for the extension of the superior cut which was made at the base of the pyramidal mass. With this stop in place, a saw without a rib stop is placed in the oscillating head and the previous cut completed. It may be necessary at this point to use a rongeur to mobilize the segment. The bone-grasping forceps, however, will permit the rotation of the mass out of the tissue bed, and by means of blunt and judicious sharp dissection the remaining attachment of the external pterygoid and deep fascia may be freed.

All of the connective tissue, i.e., the capsule of the "joint," must be removed and included in the surgical specimen, since this tissue may have osteogenic potential and result in recurrence of a bony bridge. The clamp is removed from the ends of the external pterygoid and bleeders are tied off if they occur. The surgical cavity is debrided and a rongeur used to remove spicules and to smooth roughened surfaces. If there is oozing of blood a Gelfoam pack is placed in the cavity and the incision is closed with closely spaced, interrupted skin sutures. A small drain is sometimes placed in the most dependent portion of the incision if the mass removed resulted in a deep cavity, particularly in its medial extension. As noted above, covering the cut end of the mandible with an inert material may serve to prevent the re-formation of a bony bridge. Silastic caps, methylmethacrylate, and vitreous carbon (experimental) may be used. In the case of the latter, Klasson and I have shown that vitreous carbon will produce a pseudosynovium when implanted into the iliac crest of a dog. In our experiment, after the iliac crest was re-entered, we found that the vitreous carbon implant, in the shape of a cylinder, rotated in an almost frictionless way in its bony cavity. Histological section showed complete absence of inflammation or foreign body reaction and also the presence of a dense fibrous tissue capsule with a homogenous interface with the vitreous carbon. The possibility of thus producing a pseudoarthrosis needs to be investigated. The use of dexamethasone, 8 mg., in the operative infusion, as well as the administration of 4 mg. of the drug in the postoperative infusion for the first 24 postoperative hours, is recommended.

POSTOPERATIVE CARE

In older patients because of the frequency with which organisms are sequestered in adult bone, prophylactic antibiotics are recommended. A Barton bandage will provide stability and a sense of comfort postoperatively, but, since exercise is essential to success in restoring mobility, it should be removed on the third postoperative day. A liquid diet is given for four postoperative days, and on the fifth day the patient may be given a soft diet. The patient should be encouraged to chew as early in the recovery as possible. Rehabilitative exercises to avoid deviate mandibular movements will be described later in this chapter.

FRACTURE OF THE CONDYLE

Based upon the fact that the condyle is a growth center, fractures of the condyle in persons under the age of 16 in females and 18 in males should be corrected by open reduction of the displaced bony fragments. In adults, the incidence of complications following untreated condylar fractures is so low that one should be reluctant to undertake a procedure that is not without the risk of some morbidity.

In cases in which one elects to do an open reduction, the procedure recommended by Thoma is the best. One should follow his surgical procedure as well as his recommended instrumentation. Some condylar fractures are accompanied by such severe medial displacement of the condylar fragment that considerable time, as well as ingenuity, in locating the fragment is required. As in the previous discussion of the preoperative radiography that should precede all surgery of the TMJ, it is here reiterated that a vertex projection followed by standard and tomographic views along this predetermined condylar angle be obtained in order to determine the operative strategy before entering the operating room. If at all possible, the joint capsule should not be penetrated or the joint cavity entered. Hemorrhage into the joint space is an undesirable sequela of all joint surgery, as is hemorrhage into the joint cavity as a result of trauma, as I shall point out later.

Wiring of the condyle to the ramus of the mandible need not be rigid or precise; however, wire ends should be buried in the drill holes and bone fragments removed. Closure is the same as for the previously described operation for ankylosis, with one caution. It is obvious from the above that this operation will be performed upon young people, for whom appearance is extremely important. Attention must be paid to following accepted surgical principles which will result in exceptional cosmetic results. In all facial surgery, techniques of skin closure practiced by plastic and reconstructive surgeons should be studied and scrupulously applied. For this reason also, drains are not advised in open reduction of condylar fracture, since after reduction there should not be dead space. On the other hand, one should be careful to express all of the blood resulting from the surgery by means of a 4 × 4 in the shape of a cylinder that is rolled over the operative field from anterior to posterior (ventral–dorsal), thus expressing blood and fluid from the operative area.

The following surgical procedures have been performed by others, but to date, in my opinion, they are not conditions for which surgery is the only or even the primary method of treatment.

MENISCECTOMY

This procedure is employed in cases of pain and dysfunction or in the presence of these symptoms accompanied by joint sound and erratic or deviate mandibular movements. Some surgeons have described hypertrophied articular discs as the cause of the problem. There is as yet no convincing evidence that hypertrophy of the disc exists as an entity, and while degeneration is a condition that affects all tissues, histopathological evidence for disc degeneration independent of arthritis is likewise scanty. In view of the paucity of such evidence, and considering that many such operations have been performed yielding many surgical specimens, it cannot be considered an established procedure as far as histopathological evidence is concerned. Discs have undergone changes, as have the bony elements of the joint. These are mainly progressive thinning of the disc, often with perforations. Rheumatoid arthritis is rare in the TMJ, and osteoarthritis is not, but disc removal is not a treatment for osteoarthritis. On the other hand, many patients with the same or similar complaints have benefited from nonsurgical procedures. Since the ability of the temporomandibular articulation to remodel itself in response to changes in occlusion, as well as being a concomitant of age, loss of dentition, and habits, is well known and established, removal of a critical element of the joint may be described as an example of "therapeutic impatience" and is not recommended.

CHRONIC DISLOCATION

Many attempts have been made to deal with this entity as if one were correcting the tendency of the condyle to "leave its socket" and thus "to dislocate." If, on the other hand, this is understood as a disharmonious movement of the interarticular disc and the condyle secondary to nonsynchronous movement of the two bellies of the external pterygoid muscles, which is followed by spasm of the masseter and the temporal and internal pterygoid muscles, a different approach would suggest itself. The one exception is chronic dislocation in the elderly, which will be discussed later.

Three approaches have been used to deal with the problem of chronic recurrent subluxation or dislocation. The first has been to limit the arthrodial or translatory movement of the capitulum by means of fascia lata ties or wires. This method, plus the use of exercises, has had a limited success. The second approach has been to resect the zygoma proximal to the articular tubercle in order to increase its effective height, thus providing a stop to the movement of the capitulum. The third method has been the reduction in the tuberculum in order to provide for an unimpeded return of the capitulum, even though it is still capable of excursions into the infratemporal area. This last method does not have sufficient history for proper evaluation. One must, of course, realize that this last technique requires that the superior synovial cavity of the joint be entered. The possibility of hemorrhage into the space in the presence of a decorticated tuberculum runs the risk of obliteration and calcification of the space with undesirable sequelae, to say the least. In general, the joint per se should not be entered, since our present technology does not permit us to replace all or parts of it.

Functional Considerations in Dislocation

In careful studies of the physiology of the temporomandibular joint neuromuscular apparatus, one is struck by the fact that as long as the disc and the condyle move in harmony, the mandible is capable of extremes of movement which radiographically appear to place it in the infratemporal fossa, from which position it returns smoothly and painlessly. In some individuals, however, in anterior boundaries of this excursion the masseters, temporals, or internal pterygoids contract and prevent the return of the jaw. If caught early enough, injections of lidocaine hydrochloride into the muscles in spasm will result in the reduction of the "dislocation" (Fig. 12–4).

Curariform drugs will produce the same result, but a safer drug is ketamine, which will swiftly correct the problem without any jaw manipulation whatsoever. To return to the special case of the elderly who fall asleep with the jaw agape and awaken unable to close the jaw, intramuscular ketamine has proved efficacious. More important, however, is the nocturnal use of a jaw sling to prevent this distressing occurrence.

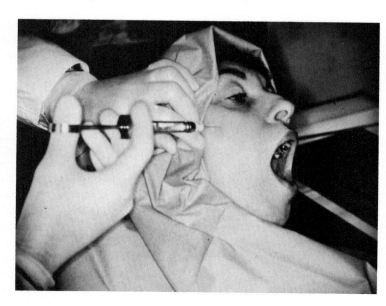

Figure 12–4. "Dislocation" of the mandible relieved by injection of lidocaine hydrochloride into the external pterygoid muscles. Note use of a sterile technique.

The author has observed that in patients with chronic dislocation problems the external pterygoid muscles are not as well developed as the other muscles of mastication. The main limit to anterior movement of the condyle is the bulk of well-developed external pterygoid muscles as the capitulum moves over the tuberculum. There is other evidence in these patients that they do not employ vigorous lateral masticatory movements, as noted in their occlusion, as evidenced by wear facets and by other indices of such movements, such as the ease and vigor with which they can execute them upon demand. In a discussion of surgical methods of treating dislocation, it is surely begging the question to introduce preventive concepts, but the point to be made here is that exercises designed to strengthen external pterygoid function may be worth trying before invasive techniques are employed.

CONDYLECTOMY

The use of this method to deal with functional disease of the joint is irrational. Condylotomy with the use of implants shares the irrationality of condylectomy, since it addresses itself to the abnormality (which it is designed to correct) of the capitulum without taking into account that this abnormality (irregularity in the surfaces of the joint components) is reflected in the surfaces of the disc and in the tuberculum. The implant made in whatever shape cannot correct this condition. What is needed is a prosthetic joint replacing all articulating surfaces. At present this awaits the arrival of future skills. For this reason, such attempts must fall far short of a proper biological solution.

ACUTE TRAUMA

MANAGEMENT

The chief causes of injury to the TMJ are falls, automobile accidents, boxing blows, or assaults with weapons which may cause either fracture or contusions with varying degrees of blood or fluid accumulations in the joint or joints. As stated before, most fractures of the condyles in adults do not require surgery, and since the fractures are almost always extracapsular, there is no injury to the joint complex per se. Contusions and sprains, particularly of the external pterygoid muscles, cause bleeding into the joint cavity. In the absence of radiographic evidence of fracture these conditions may be diagnosed clinically by noting severe tenderness or exquisite pain in the area of the joint with minimal backward pressure on the chin, and severe to complete limitation in mandibular opening. In the case of external pterygoid injury or sprain there is complete absence of protrusive movement if the injury is bilateral, and severe deviation to the injured side if it is unilateral. In cases in which there is considerable fluid or blood in one or both joint spaces, there will be protrusion of the mandible and in the presence of posterior dentition there will be posterior occlusal prematurities with a resultant anterior open bite.

The primary problem that must be dealt with is the removal or dispersal of the fluid or blood in the joint. This is done by the injection of hyaluronidase into the superior synovial cavity under very strict aseptic conditions. In the case of suspected sprain of the external pterygoid muscles with possible extravasation of blood into the infratemporal space, intravenous streptokinase-streptodormase (Varidase) should be considered in addition to the local instillation of hyaluronidase. It is presupposed that a careful medical history will precede any of these treatments, especially in order to elicit a history of past allergic reactions to these drugs.

Healing of joint injuries is extremely slow because of the avascularity of the disc. In some instances the disc is torn by the trauma and healing takes place by means of the formation of another lamina of the disc which covers or masks the injured area without actually producing a repair, as in other tissues. This is consistent with good and painless function, although it may be accompanied by joint sounds. Most important to the overall treatment of joint trauma is the proper prescription of rest for the first two months of the treatment and progressive exercise for the remainder of a period of several months.

THE PHYSIOTHERAPY OF TMJ TRAUMA

The Rest Phase of Treatment

It is obviously difficult to enforce complete rest in joint injuries. Even wiring the jaws does not afford rest, since it often results in clenching which not only aggravates the trauma to the joint structures but also is painful when the presence of even minimal amounts of fluid makes it impossible to retrude the mandible. Considering all the disadvantages, it is better to rely upon the patient's own tendency to splint the mandible when in pain and for the patient to select a jaw position that is free of pain and hence free of pressure from joint fluid. Some patients will receive relief from the external application of moist heat. A soft diet as tolerated is suggested. Analgesics are almost always required and aspirin is the drug of choice, except when bleeding is a part of the problem. Aspirin may be used later in these cases after all possibility of bleeding is considered to be past, usually after the first five days, with gradual subsidence of pain. In patients who cannot tolerate aspirin or who are sensitive to it nonsalicylate analgesics may be used. If drugs like meperidine or large doses of codeine are required, one should suspect fracture.

The Exercise Phase of Treatment (Figs. 12–5 to 12–20)

The Midline Exercise

The external pterygoid muscles are always injured to some degree as a sequela of joint trauma. After the initial period of rest the first objective is to prescribe an exercise that will correct the disharmonies of external pterygoid action. These may be classified as bilateral disharmonies resulting in deviation of the mandible to the side of greater injury and unilateral disharmonies between the upper and lower bellies of the external pterygoids unilaterally or in various combinations of unilateral and bilateral disparate movement. These are corrected by a midline exercise which, when accomplished successfully by the patient, results in all muscles moving harmoni-

Text continued on page 385

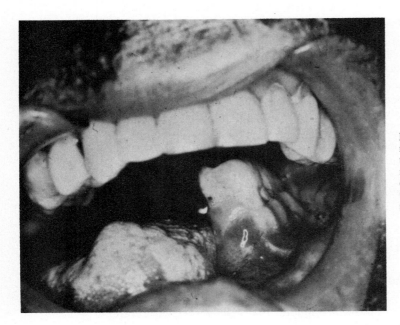

Figure 12–5. Following a hemi-mandibulectomy, this patient was unable to move the remaining mandibular segment into proper occlusion. Note the marked deviation of the mandible toward the surgical side.

Figure 12–6. Following the exercises, the patient achieves an excellent degree of control and muscle strength. Note the unassisted movement of the hemimandible into an acceptable relationship.

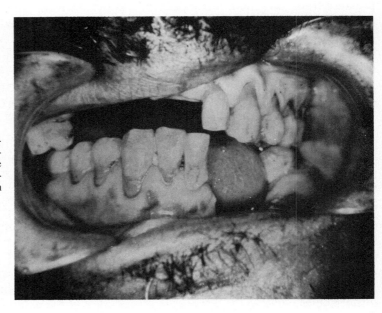

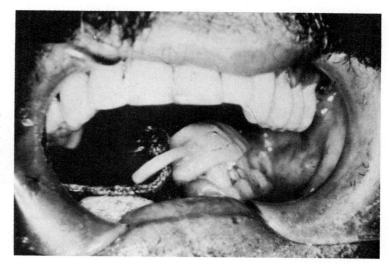

Figure 12–7. Apparatus for performing an exercise against resistance to improve the patient's control of a hemimandible. It consists of an acrylic overlay splint with provision for the attachment of a line to pulley to weight appliance.

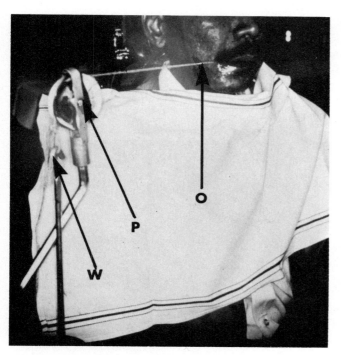

Figure 12–8. The patient is shown here using an exercise device to restore muscular control to his remaining mandibular segment. An intraoral appliance fitted over his teeth is attached to a line (O), which passes over a pulley (P) that supports a weight (W). The effect of the exercise is to develop control and strength in the muscles of the mandibular segment. This is possible in the same way as it is possible for us to move our fingers with one set of muscles in each digit.

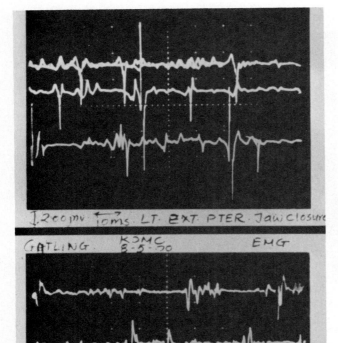

Figure 12–9. Electromyographic tracings of the potentials produced by the external pterygoid muscles before and after the exercises. Below are the relatively low potentials produced before the exercise, and above are the considerably enhanced potentials that resulted from the use of the exercises.

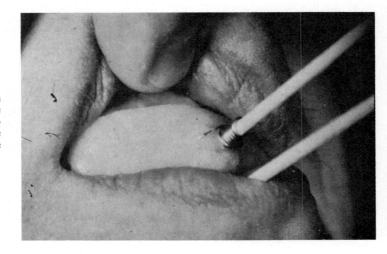

Figure 12–10. The device shown here will permit a patient whose dentition does not permit the insertion of a marker or whose midline is grossly off to perform the midline exercises (see text).

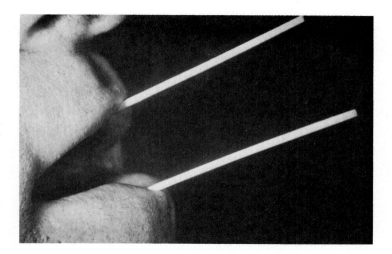

Figure 12–11. Midline exercises must be done with precision. In performing them, no deviation of the mandible should be tolerated. If it occurs, the patient must return to centric and begin again.

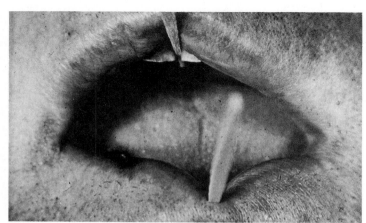

Figure 12–12. Deviation caused by jaw injury. Note disparity of midline markers placed between the mandibular and maxillary central incisors.

Figure 12–13. When the patient is asked to open her mouth the mandible is seen to deviate to one side (arrow), as can be clearly seen from the markers inserted between the maxillary and mandibular central incisors. The muscles on the patient's left side, particularly the pterygoids, are pulling harder than those on the right. Also note the limitation in opening due to lack of translatory (protrusive) movement.

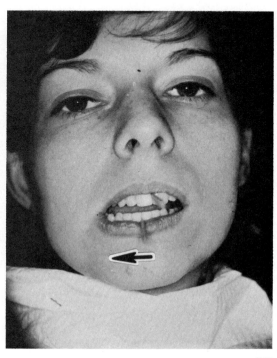

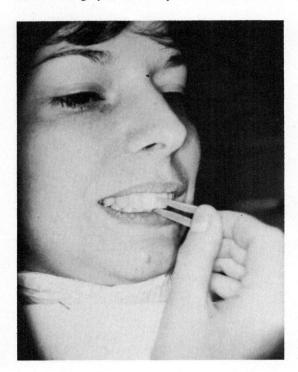

Figure 12–14. The patient is seen adjusting the midline markers, inserted between the maxillary and mandibular incisors, so that they coincide. Note that the mandible has been closed into the patient's convenient or habitual interdental relationship.

Figure 12–15. The patient checks on the accuracy of the exercise by observing the position of the midline markers when the mandible is moved. If the mandible deviates in opening, the patient is instructed to return the mandible to its starting position and begin the midline exercise again.

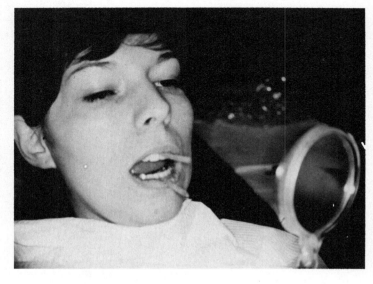

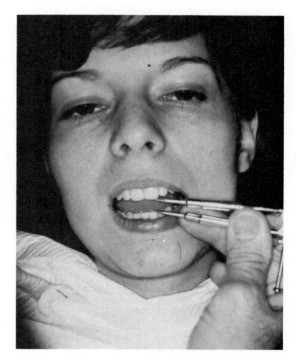

Figure 12–16. The divider measures the extent of the limitation in jaw opening. This is transferred as a line of this length to the patient's chart. It may also be expressed and recorded in millimeters.

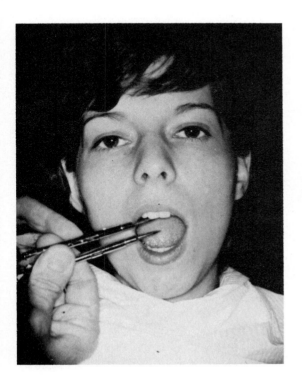

Figure 12–17. The divider here indicates the improvement in the degree of opening achieved by the midline exercise. The patient's chart will record these comparative changes.

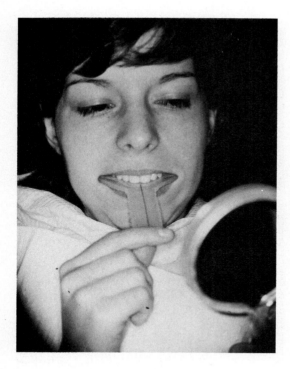

Figure 12–18. A protrusive exercise is performed by the patient. Here she is shown inserting a flat polyethylene device, shaped as an arch to conform to the arch of the mandible and maxilla. Note the midline marked as a black line. The mirror is again used as a means of checking on the accuracy with which the mandible slides forward, following the midline to insure even muscular effort.

Figure 12–19. A lateral view of the maneuver shown in Figure 12–18, showing protrusion of the mandible. Note that interdental biting pressure is maintained in this exercise so that it becomes an exercise under a load because of the resistance of the material used in the appliance. This hastens an increase in muscle bulk and strength of function.

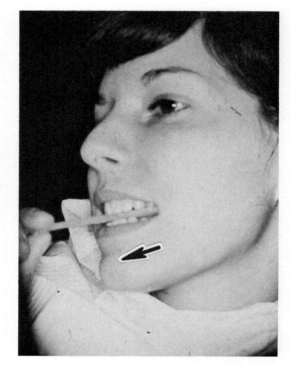

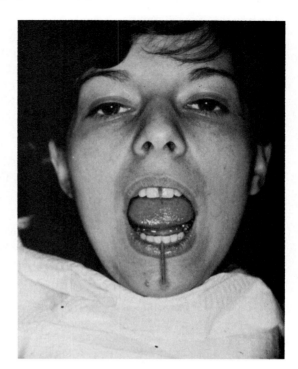

Figure 12–20. This demonstrates the degree of opening achieved by combining protrusion of the mandible with opening. The ginglymoid (hinge) and arthrodial (gliding) movements result in a maximized degree of opening.

ously. It is apparent that should any one of these muscles move out of harmony with the others the mandible would deviate to one side or another. This exercise, as I have previously described, is performed by the patient with the aid of two Stim-U-Dents or toothpicks placed between the central incisors of the maxilla and the mandible. While looking in a mirror, the patient *carefully* and *slowly* opens the mouth. Using the markers as a guide, the patient performs the exercise, returning to a starting position in centric *if any deviation occurs*. The patient performs the midline exercise until he can do it perfectly, or else returns to centric to begin again.

At the beginning, the patient may not be able to open very wide without deviation, but he should be asked to persist, since this will result in a corrective effort—i.e., the muscle pulling harder will have to slacken off while the muscle not putting forth the effort will have to increase its activity. Persistence will be rewarded by a re-establishment of harmonious muscle movement and the restoration of full opening without deviation.

The exercise is based upon some fundamental facts about muscle physiology. First, it must be understood and conveyed to the patient that these muscles, whose action is seen only in the resultant movement of the mandible, are voluntary muscles. They are muscles that are strongly habituated through long use, but they are voluntary nevertheless and hence can be retrained. Second, one does not normally see mandibular movement as one sees movement of the digits of the hands. One of the most important reasons the hands and fingers can be so exquisitely trained is by means of eye–hand coordination, e.g., piano playing, fine craftsmanship. This is absent for the mandible. The use of the mirror and the insistence upon exact and correct performance of this midline exercise provides this "eye–mandible" feedback or coordination. This use of the mirror in speech therapy is a well-established method of teaching the person who has not spoken from birth.

There has been a great deal of clinical proof for the efficacy of this exercise. For example, in the clicking joint which is due to failure of the disc to move in harmony with the capitulum, the correct performance of this exercise will eliminate the click. In hemimandibulectomy it is possible, using a marker and a mirror, to retrain the hemimandible to move in a path determined by the patient. Such a case is illustrated here in which this exercise was supplemented by an augmented version in which the patient worked against a weight. This resulted not only in restoring muscle control over the mandibular segment so that the occlusion of the dentition in the segment was restored, but also, as can be seen, there is electromyographic evidence of enhancement of the muscle potentials.

The Protrusive Exercise

When the patient has succeeded in performing the midline exercise to an acceptable degree of opening, as measured at the midline anteriorly, he should begin to perform a protrusive exercise.

Again, using the mirror and the midline markers, the patient proceeds as follows: The marker between the incisors of the maxilla is left at its manufactured length, while the marker to be placed between the mandibular incisors is shortened by approximately 5 mm. The patient is asked to protrude the mandible so that the ends of the markers are even. This will require both the internal and external pterygoids to move harmoniously. It is important that in the maneuver the patient observe the midline rule, that is, no deviation during the maneuver and a return to centric should this occur.

With the successful performance of this relatively passive exercise, the patient is graduated to a loaded protrusive exercise which is designed to require the muscles to perform more work. This is accomplished by means of a polyethylene device of the following type.

Using a model of the mandible, a sheet of polyethylene is cut to conform to the arch and is also provided with an integral handle. By means of a black suture, a midline is placed in the middle of the handle. In front of a mirror, the patient inserts the "bite plate" in the mouth and closes the teeth upon it. The same protrusive exercise is now performed against the resistance of the plate. This exercise will quickly strengthen the muscles and produce progressively more controlled protrusive movement as well as longer excursions.

When the patient can perform these exercises well and without discomfort, he may be instructed in combining both protrusive and mouth-opening exercises to achieve maximal control of muscle function.

When this objective is achieved, the problem becomes one for the practitioner who will undertake whatever restorative dentistry is required or whatever occlusion correction may be required. With restored control over the muscles the patient will be able to provide the clinician with a stable and reproducible, maxillo–mandibular relationship which at the time, or any time after the injury, he could not do.

In this connection, it is important to remember that centric relation or convenience relation is a position that the patient provides the dentist with. In many instances, and particularly after injury, the patient is unable to do so. Exercises to correct this situation are essential and, indeed, a precondition to any dental treatment which depends upon the restoration of occlusal and therefore muscle function (Figs. 12–21 to 12–34).

Text continued on page 394

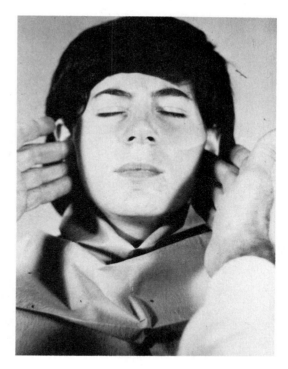

Figure 12–21. Visual inspection from in front of the patient to determine symmetry.

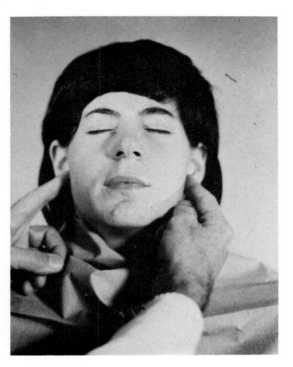

Figure 12–22. Palpation anterior to the joint.

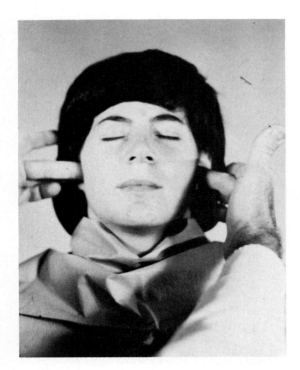

Figure 12–23. Palpation posterior to the joint and through pressure forward from the external ear canal.

Figure 12–24. Pull the ear back and out to differentiate pain caused by pathosis in the external ear.

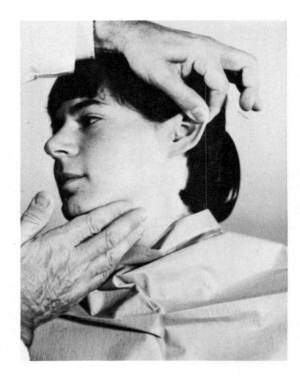

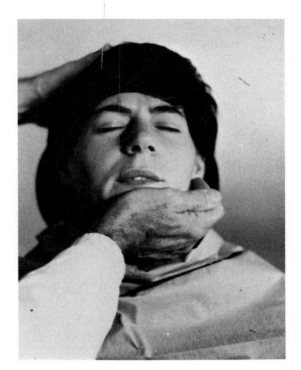

Figure 12–25. Push the mandible back with the heel of the hand to discover acute arthritis or presence of inflammatory exudate in the joint spaces.

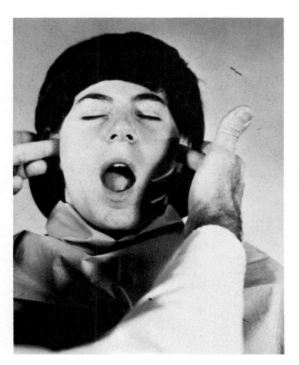

Figure 12–26. Firm palpation of the joint area during opening.

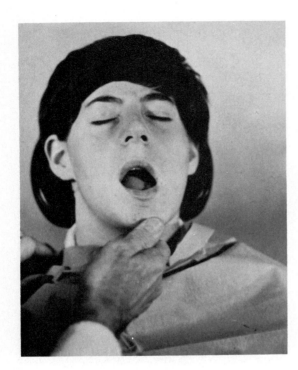

Figure 12–27. Patient is asked to open mouth. Note the deviation to one side indicating an imbalance in muscle function. See chart for diagnostic significance of partial or total trismus or inability to close mouth.

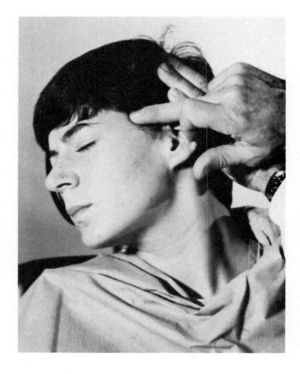

Figure 12–28. Palpation for tenderness in the temporal muscles.

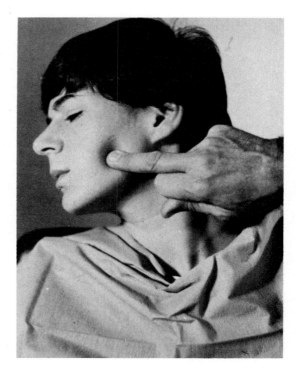

Figure 12–29. Palpation for tenderness in the masseter muscle.

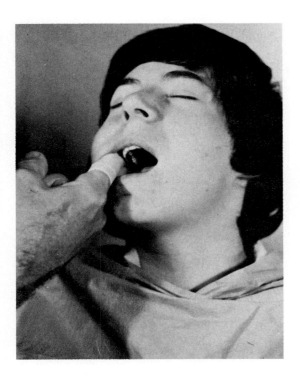

Figure 12–30. Palpation for tenderness in the external pterygoid muscle. The gloved finger is inserted behind the maxillary tuberosity as the patient is requested to close the mouth partially. The finger pressure is directed medially and superiorly.

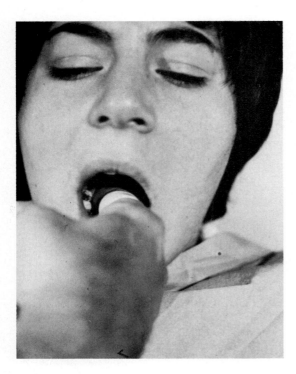

Figure 12–31. Palpation for tenderness of the internal pterygoid muscle. The gloved finger is inserted along the lingual surface of the mandible and advanced so it palpates the muscle in the area of the sublingual and pharyngeal surface of the mandible in the region of the muscle insertion.

Figure 12–32. Palpation for tenderness in the sternomastoid muscle.

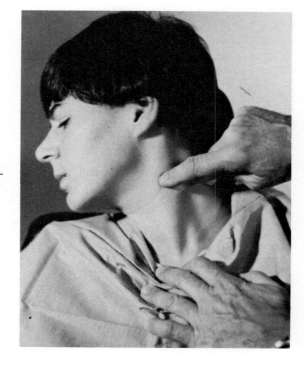

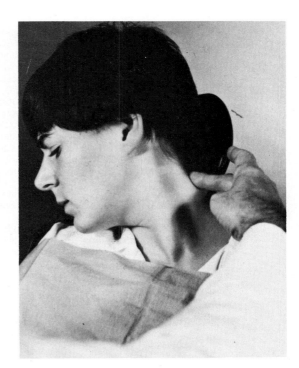

Figure 12–33. Palpation for tenderness in the trapezius muscle, upper part.

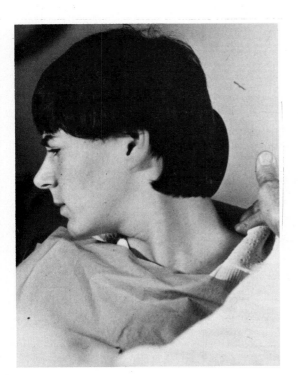

Figure 12–34. Palpation for tenderness of the trapezius, lower part.

References

Amer, A.: Approach to surgical diagnosis of the temporomandibular articulation through basic studies of the normal. JADA, *45*:668, 1952.

Boering, G.: Temporomandibular Joint Arthrosis. Doctoral Thesis, Drukkerij van Denderen, Groningen, Holland, 1966. Dutch with summary in English.

Boman, K.: Surgical treatment of recurrent dislocation of the jaw. Acta Chir. Scand., *136*:191, 1970. (Adv. Oral Surg., abstract 553, *3*:79, 1973.)

Carlsson, G. E. et al.: Remodeling of the TMJ. Oral Sci. Rev., *6*:53, 1974.

Clark, R. K. F., and Wyke, B. D.: Temporomandibular articular reflex control of the mandibular musculature. Int. Dent. J., *25*:289, 1975.

Costen, J. B.: Treatment of mandibular joint reactions. J. Med. Assoc. Alabama, *29*:45, 1959.

Dixon, A. D.: Structure and functional significance of the intra-articular disc of the human temporomandibular joint. Oral Surg., *15*:48, 1962.

Farrar, W. B.: Differentiation of temporomandibular joint dysfunction to simplify treatment. J. Prosthet. Dent., *28*:629, 1972.

Fountain, H. W.: The temporomandibular joints—a fulcrum. J. Prosthet. Dent., *25*:78, 1971.

Freese, A., and Scheman, P.: Management of Temporomandibular Joint Problems. St. Louis, The C. V. Mosby Co., 1962.

Goodman, P., Greene, C. S., Laskin, D. M.: Response of patients with myofascial pain-dysfunction syndrome to mock equilibration. JADA, *92*:755, 1976.

Greenfield, B. E., and Wyke, B.: Reflex innervation of the temporomandibular joint. Nature, *211*:940, 1960.

Hilloowala, R. A.: The temporomandibular joint: a diginglymus joint. J. Prosthet. Dent., *33*:328, 1975.

Hjortsjö, C. H.: Views on the general principles of joints and movements. Acta Ortho. Scand., *29*:134, 1959.

Hjortsjö, C. H.: The Mechanics of the Temporomandibular Joint (film). Archives of Scientific Films, No. 1, 1959. Dept. of Anatomy, University of Lund, Sweden.

Hjortsjö, C. H.: A new apparatus for demonstrating the mechanics of the temporomandibular joint. Odontol Revy, *8*:443, 1957.

Ingervall, B., Bratt, C. M., Carlsson, G. E., Helkimo, M., and Lantz, B.: Duration of swallowing with and without anesthesia of the temporomandibular joints. Scand. J. Dent. Res., *80*:189, 1972.

Kameros, J., and Himmelfarb, R.: Treatment of temporomandibular joint ankylosis with methyl methacrylate interpositional arthroplasty: Report of our cases. J. Oral Surg., *33*:282, 1975.

King, W. A.: A diagnostically significant crepitus in the temporomandibular joint. Am. J. Orthodont., *49*:741, 1963.

Klasson, D. H., and Scheman, P.: Purified carbon as a tissue replacement. Int. Surg., *62*:179, 1977.

Krogh-Poulsen, W. G.: Functional anatomy of the temporomandibular joint. Rev. Fr. Odontostomat., *18*:453, 1971.

Lorimier, A. A.: Arthropathies of the temporomandibular joint. Am. J. Surg., 616, May, 1953.

Mazaheri, M., and Biggerstaff, R. H.: Standardized sectional laminographs of the temporomandibular joint. J. Prosthet. Dent., *18*:489, 1967.

Mincey, D. L., Barnhart, G. W., and Olson, R. E.: A simplified exerciser for the temporomandibular joint following condylotomy. Oral Surg., *39*:844, 1975.

Moffett, B.: The morphogenesis of the temporomandibular joint. Am. J. Orthodont., *52*:401, 1966.

Morgan, D. H.: Temporomandibular joint surgery, correction of pain tinnitus and vertigo. Dent. Radiogr. Photogr., *46*:27, 1973.

Munro, R. R.: Coordination of activity of the two bellies of the digastric muscle in basic jaw movements. J. Dent. Res., *51*:1663, 1972.

Omnell, K. A., and Petersson, A.: Radiography of the temporomandibular joint utilizing oblique lateral transcranial projections. Odontol. Revy, *27*:77, 1976.

Oshrain, H. I.: Involvement of the temporomandibular joint in a case of rheumatoid arthritis. Oral Surg., *8*:1039, 1955.

Pomp, A. M.: Psychotherapy for the myofascial pain dysfunction syndrome: a study of factors coinciding with symptom remission. JADA, *89*:629, 1974.

Ramfjord, S. P., and Blankenship, J. R.: Interarticular disc in wide mandibular opening in rhesus monkeys. J. Prosthet. Dent., *26*:189, 1971.

Rönning. O. et al.: The involvement of the TMJ in juvenile rheumatoid arthritis. Scand. J. Rheumatol., *3*:89, 1974.

Sabin, M. Synchronized sonometric and cine-fluorographic analysis of the crepitant temporomandibular joint. University of Illinois College of Dentistry Lecture Series, Sept. 5–7, 1969 (from TMJ Research Center).

Sarnat, B. G.: The Temporomandibular Joint. Springfield, Ill., Charles C Thomas, 1964.

Sarnat, B. G., and Laskin, D. M.: Diagnosis and Surgical Management of Diseases of the Temporomandibular Joint. Springfield, Ill., Charles C Thomas, 1962.

Scheman, P.: The articulating surfaces of the human TMJ. N.Y. State Dent. J., *39*:294, 1973.

Scheman, P., Milstoc, M., and Scheman, P.: TMJ trabeculation as an expression of joint function. N.Y. State Dent. J., *40*:595, 1974.

Scheman, P.: An aspect of temporomandibular joint dysfunction—the unstable bite syndrome. N.Y. State Dent. J., *32*:12, 1966.

Schwartz, L.: Disorders of the Temporomandibular Joint. Philadelphia, W. B. Saunders Co., 1966.

Simon, S. D., Litchman, H. M., and Silver, C. M.: Orthopedic management of affections of the temporomandibular joint (meniscectomy advised). Presented at the 118th annual convention of the AMA, N.Y. Coliseum, N.Y.C., July 13–17, 1969.

Sonneson, B.: The temporomandibular joint during lateral involvement of the mandible (a tomographical investigation in the living person). Odontol. Revy, *7*:369, 1956.

Sullivan, W. E.: The function of articular discs. Anat. Rec., *24*:49, 1922.

Tsukamoto, S., Umeda, T., Tamari, Y., and Kawakatsu, K.: Electro-myographic activities of jaw muscles in ankylosis of the temporomandibular joint. Oral Surg., *25*:117, 1968.

Ulik, R., and Zenker, W.: On a new operative method for the elimination of habitual luxation of the temporomandibular joint. Wien. Klin. Wochenschr., *73*:892, 1961.

Ward, J. R.: Questions and answers, "clicking" jaw motions. JAMA, *195*:195, 1966.

Weinberg, L. A.: Technique for temporomandibular joint radiographs. J. Prosthet. Dent., *28*:284, 1972.

Weinberg, L. A.: Temporomandibular joint function and its effect on centric relation. J. Prosthet. Dent., *30*:176, 1973.

Weisengreen, H. H.: Observations of the articular disc. Oral Surg., *40*:113, 1975.

Yavelow, I., and Arnold, G. S.: Temporomandibular joint clicking. Oral Surg., *32*:708, 1971.

Zampelli, M., Salkin, L. M., Vandersall, D. C., and Denbo, J. A.: Rheumatoid arthritis of the temporomandibular joint: case report. J. Periodontol., *45*:26, 1974.

13

The Role of Hypnosis in the Treatment of Craniomandibular Dysfunction

JEFFREY S. TARTE, D.D.S.

It is the most highly organized bit of matter in the universe, this three-pound, electrochemical, double handful of cells that thrives on change, allows us to move, to see, to think, to create, to love, and to be conscious of our actions. Since man first became aware of its existence, he has struggled to comprehend its miracle and miseries, punching crude holes in the bones that protect it and arbitrarily assigning moral and intellectual values to the lumps and bumps in its outer surface.

The brain itself is an awesome mass of 10 billion cells that never sleep. Its electrochemical mass is so dense in some regions that 100 million cells fit into one cubic inch, and every one is connected to as many as 60,000 others. This gelatinous mass has evolved over a period of two billion years. Somewhere in this miracle of design and evolution the abstract concept of consciousness is defined, and by definition altered states of consciousness exist.

Webster defines consciousness as the knowledge of what is happening around one: the totality of one's thoughts, feelings, and impressions. Man probably was able to alter his awareness effectively as soon as the process of cerebration evolved. The caveman's fascination with a flickering flame probably made him the first human to experience the trance phenomenon. The earliest meditative religions may, in part, be derived from trancelike experiences. If this is true, even to a small degree, the major philosophies and religions in the world may owe some of their origins to hypnotic-like states.

Efforts to reproduce, teach, and transfer these conditions probably were the first attempts at hypnotherapy. The early shamans, priests, medicine men, and healers may have been the first hypnotherapists. Modern medicine attributes the initial therapeutic uses of the trance to Anton Mesmer in the late nineteenth century.

The interest in hypnosis has varied in the annals of modern medicine. The pendulum is now probably swinging to a period of extremely high interest, due to the creativity and diversification of its modern practitioners.

DEFINITION

Poets, writers, philosophers, clinicians, and scientists have for centuries alluded to the various levels of awareness that man experiences from day to day. These varying states occur spontaneously and in response to other states. Hypnosis is an altered state of attention which approaches peak concentration capacity. Everyone who has ever experienced a state of trance probably has his own definition for it. For the purposes of this chapter, we would like to define hypnosis as follows: Hypnosis is a response to a signal from another, or to an inner signal, which activates a capacity for a shift of awareness in the subject and permits a more intensive concentration upon a designated goal direction. This shift of attention is constantly sensitive to and responsive to signals from the hypnotist or the subject himself, if properly trained.[1]

Once aware of what hypnosis is, it is time to call our attention to what it is not. The myths surrounding hypnosis may, to a great extent, have retarded its universal acceptance as a useful clinical implement.

MISCONCEPTIONS ABOUT HYPNOSIS

1. Hypnosis is sleep. Sleep and hypnosis are polar opposites. Unfortunately, the word hypnosis is derived from a Greek root, *hypnos,* meaning sleep. There is an illusory similarity between hypnosis and sleep in regard to peripheral awareness. In both, peripheral awareness contracts, but for different reasons. In sleep it contracts because there is a general withdrawal of awareness. In hypnosis it contracts because focal attention is *intensified,* thereby contracting peripheral awareness. In sleep focal attention dissolves, whereas with hypnosis attention increases to peak capacity.

2. Hypnosis transfers something to the subject. In actuality the therapist transfers nothing to the subject, nor does he gain a "magnetic" power over him.

3. Mentally weak people are the only ones capable of being hypnotized. This probably was derived from the second misconception, that the weak mind submits to the strong. In actuality it takes a mentally strong, intact personality to maintain the trance.

4. Hypnosis cannot happen spontaneously. Once a hypnotic trance is experienced it can spontaneously recur, almost as a learned or instinctive response.

5. Hypnosis is dangerous. Hypnosis is not dangerous. We and others have previously mentioned that hypnosis is a state of focal concentration.

The true danger can exist in the strategy of a poor therapist. The trance can be terminated at the subject's will.

6. Hypnosis is a therapeutic regimen. Hypnosis merely creates a therapeutic matrix to facilitate therapy. It is the proposed strategy implemented once trance is achieved that provides the therapy.

7. The hypnotist must be charismatic. The monk Rasputin probably propagated this myth. If the subject will cooperate, the "charisma" is there.

8. Women are more hypnotizable then men. There is no sex or age difference. If the psychophysiological ability exists, the individual, regardless of sex, is hypnotizable.

9. Hypnosis is a psychological phenomenon. Charcot correctly postulated that hypnosis is a profound psychoneurological event that is not learnable.

Examining what hypnosis is not gives us a very definite idea of what it is. The trance capacity exists. It is either genetic, imprinted, or both. It is not subject to debate. The trance exists when focal awareness contracts at the expense of all other peripheral stimuli. People with the trance capacity shift into trance states in the service of pursuing certain goals. The hypnotist, in actuality, merely tests for this trance capacity, and, while measuring it, simultaneously enables the subject to identify this special state of attention as hypnosis. If relevant, the therapist can instruct the subject to knowledgeably shift into the hypnotic state for a given purpose. Technically, the authentic hypnotic state occurs only when knowledgeably induced by the operator and responded to by the subject in a sensitive, disciplined way, and terminated by the operator's signal.

Self-hypnosis differs from formal hypnosis in that there is no actual sensitive reponsivity to an operator during the trance states itself. It differs from spontaneous trance in that it is instigated by conscious design and terminated by the subject himself for a known goal.[2]

PROFILE

The key phrase for effective therapy, mentioned above, stated that the hypnotist simply tests for this trance capacity, and, while measuring it, enables the subject to identify it as hypnosis.

On whom do we elect to use hypnotherapy? In the healing arts and sciences, not oriented to spending long periods of time in multiconsultations, how can we decide when hypnotherapy is a treatment of choice, or even if it is applicable? The answer is some sort of easily administered test that would lend itself to psychometric analysis.

THE HYPNOTIC INDUCTION PROFILE (HIP)

Of the most commonly used scales for hypnotizability, the following three stand out: the Harvard, the Stanford, and the Hypnotic Induction Profile (HIP). The HIP was developed at Columbia University Medical School by Dr. Herbert Spiegel. All three measure the subject's general capacity to enter the trance state. The HIP is the first disciplined clinical approach to testing, enabling the operator to exchange information based upon a standard understood by all and applicable to most cases. The HIP not only tests how readily the subject might enter the hypnotic model but also serves to hint at the appropriate strategy to be utilized in therapy. Again, hypnosis is not therapy; it merely provides a matrix within which a therapeutic regimen is initiated and explored. A link seems to exist between trance capacity and personality or character types. This provocative hypothesis is creating an impact in all of the behavioral sciences.

In both theory and design the HIP is in many ways a departure from the available measures of hypnotizability. Hypnosis should not be considered or defined as a dazed sleeplike state in which the subject readily obeys commands from the hypnotist. The HIP postulates that hypnosis is a complex perceptual alteration involving a receptive, attentive concentrative capacity that is inherent in the patient and can be tapped by the examiner. At one time loss of control was emphasized; today, "executive" control is emphasized.

The HIP was developed to provide a measure useful in the clinical setting where hypnosis is employed to facilitate therapeutic intervention. It evolved out of a need for rapid measurement (5 to 10 minutes) which could easily be integrated into a diagnostic interview. This is of paramount importance in the craniomandibular dental setting.

The present form of the HIP is clinically feasible, rapid, and structured. It is a 5 to 10 minute clinical evaluation of hypnotic capacity using an eyeroll, arm levitation method. The HIP measures one continuous experience that flows from one phase to another.

The first phase involves the measurement of an eyeroll sign (see Fig. 13–2), which is a fixed sign that approximately indicates hypnotic capacity. The eyeroll is the distance between the edge of the lower eyelid and the lower edge of the cornea, measured when the patient looks upward on command as his eyelids close. The induction phase includes instruction for the initial arm levitation and posthypnotic compliance. The formal trance and induction ceremony are terminated and the transition into this testing of posthypnotic responsivity begins. During this next phase the patient's posthypnotic compliance is measured with the posthypnotic arm levitation. This structured situation allows the patient to discover a noninstructed but emergent sensation, a control differential. The control differential is a measurement of the rapidity and style (including measured reinforcement signals) with which the patient raises his arm in response to the posthypnotic signal. The control differential is also a measurement of the patient's sensory experience of relating more control in the "nonhypnotized" arm. The exit phase involves the cut-off, a measurement of the patient's readiness to relinquish the posthypnotic program. The procedure is concluded with the patient's subjective reports of amnesia and the spread of physical sensations from the hand that was touched by the examiner.

The examiner, using a carefully standardized procedure, elects 16 points of information, six of which are used in scoring. Hypnotic capacity is a relatively stable ability or trait for any given individual. As a consequence of this, the HIP score is derived from a matrix of points, a figuration around the same behavior. It appears that this monitoring of one continuous phenomenon can give equivalent, if not more clinically relevant, information than all of the other methods. For this reason we have emphasized the HIP as the method of choice for initiating hypnotherapy in craniomandibular dysfunction.

The instructions for the profile follow. Keep in mind that it is an excellent ready-made induction procedure. We will briefly discuss the scoring of the profile, but, for more comprehensive detailed scoring procedure, we suggest reference to the Manual For Hypnotic Induction Profile by Herbert Spiegel, M.D. (Soni Medica, Inc., New York, N.Y.).[1]

Administering the Profile

If you recall, we mentioned that the HIP uses the trance experience to measure hypnotizability. It will be the only induction procedure that we will describe. It is important that students of hypnosis immediately understand that no one knows all the inductions. They are infinite in number. They range from the clap of the hypnotist's hands, accompanied by the command "pay attention," to the lengthy autogenic phrases introduced by Schultze and Luthe.[1]

What we are saying is that the induction should suit the therapist, his style, his belief systems, and the therapeutic milieu. More will be said about this after the profile has been discussed.

As the profile is discussed a capital letter will appear opposite a direction in the induction. Please refer to the scoring sheet for the scoring area the direction refers to (Fig. 13–1).

The subject should be seated, and you should be seated facing him. Ask the subject to get as comfortable as possible. It helps if the myths previously discussed are first dispelled. The profile now begins.

"Now look toward me. Get as comfortable as you can. As you hold your head in that position, look up toward your eyebrows, now toward the top of your head (A) (Fig. 13–2). As you continue to look upward close your eyelids slowly (B). That's right" (Fig. 13–3). A squint (Fig. 13–4) adds to the score of the roll (C). "Keep your eyes closed and continue to hold your eyes upward. Take a deep breath and hold it. Now exhale, let your eyes relax and your body float. Concentrate on a feeling of floating, floating down right through the chair.* There will be something pleasant and welcome about this feeling of floating. Now, while you concentrate on this floating, I am going to concentrate on your left hand and arm. In a while I am going to stroke the middle finger of your left hand. After I do, you will develop movement sensations in that finger. Then the movements will spread, causing you to feel light and buoyant, and you will let it float upward. Ready?" Perform this stroking act (D4).

"First one finger and then another. As these restless movements develop, your hand becomes light and buoyant, your elbow bends, and your forearm floats into an upright position.

"Just let it go. This is an exercise in your imagination. Imagine your hand feels like a balloon. When you were a seven-year-old child you had

---

*The suggestion of floating down through the chair presents a paradox that suggests something about the trance experience. Floating down through the chair presents a puzzle model that the patient solves by stepping outside his original belief system. The phenomenon of parallel awareness causes the patient to step outside his belief system.

HYPNOTIC INDUCTION PROFILE

Eye-Roll Levitation Method

Patient Name_____ Date_____

Sequence - Initial_____ Previous_____ When_____

Position - Standing_____ Supine_____ Sit_____ Chair-Stool_____

A	Induction - Up-Gaze		0 - 1 - 2 - 3 - 4
B	ROLL		0 - 1 - 2 - 3 - 4
C			- 1 - 2 - 3 (Squint)

Instructions

D	Arm Levitation Right_____ Left_____		0 - 1 - 2 - 3 - 4
E	_Post-Hypnotic Response_ - Tingle	0 -	- 1 - 2
F___	Dissociation	0 -	- 1 - 2

G___	LEVITATION	Immediate	0 - 1 - 2 - 3 - 4	Smile_____
H		Re-enforce (1)	1 - 2 - 3 - 4	Surprise_____
I		Re-enforce (2)	2 - 3 - 4	
J		Re-enforce (3)	3 - 4	
K		Re-enforce (4)	4	
L___	CONTROL DIFFERENTIAL	0 -		- 1 - 2

M___	Cut-off	0 -	- 1 - 2
N	Amnesia to Cut-off	0 -	- 1 - 2
O	No Test_____		
P___	Floating Sensation	0 -	- 1 - 2
Q___	GRADE - continuum	0 - 1 - 2 - 3 - 4 - 5	

_____Increment

_____Average

Minutes_____   Decrement_____   _____Soft

Figure 13-1.

the ability to imagine. Try to recover this feeling. If necessary, help it along. That's right. All the way up.

"Now I am going to position your arm and let it remain in the upright position. (Gently cup the elbow with both hands and position it in comfortable alignment on the chair arm.)

"In fact it will remain in that position even after I give you the signal for your eyes to open. When your eyes are open even when I put your

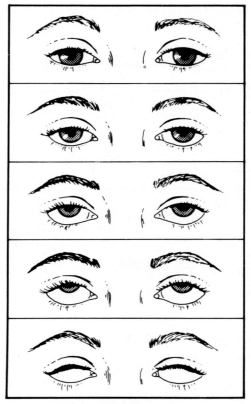

Figure 13–3.

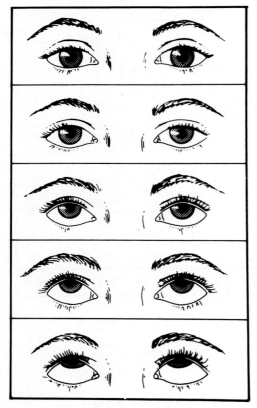

Figure 13–2.

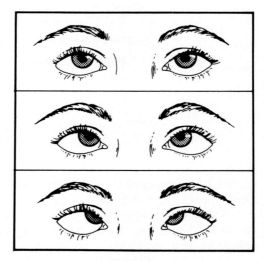

Figure 13–4.

hand down it will float right back up to where it is now. You will find something pleasant and amusing about this sensation. Later when I touch your left elbow your usual sensation and control will return. In the future each time you get the signal for the trance experience, at the count of one, your eyes will roll upward, and by the count of three your eyelids will close and you will be in a relaxed trance state. Each time you will find the experience easier and easier.

"I am now going to ask you to turn your head, open your eyes, and look at your hand. You will find something amusing about it and you will be able to answer all questions concerning it.

"Is it comfortable? Are you aware of any tingling sensation (E)? Does your left hand feel as if it is not as much a part of your body as your right hand (F)? Now note this."

Lower the subject's hand to chair arm. Note any residual levitation (G). Allow the arm to levitate again. If it does not, ask the subject to just put it up, to "fake it."

"While your left arm remains in this upright position, by way of comparison raise your right hand. Now put your right arm down. Are you aware of a difference in sensation in your right arm going up as compared with your left arm? Does one arm feel lighter or heavier than the other (L)? Now note this."

Stroke the subject's elbow (M) (cut-off signal). The arm should float down to the chair; if it does not, firmly press it down. Now the subject is asked why the hypnosis left his hand. If he is not aware of the elbow being touched (N), amnesia to the cut-off may be assumed to be positive. The subject is then asked if the buoyant sensation extended beyond his arm, such as to his shoulder, head, side, or elsewhere (P).

The profile is now completed. In this brief review of the HIP, the student can see the way the hypnotic experience lends itself to psychometric analysis.

"Now you know what it is like to feel hypnotized. You see, it is not sleep, but rather a method of concentration. It is a way of feeling double awareness. You are here, and you are alongside yourself at the same time. A feature about this concentration is that you can shift into this state of buoyant repose; you become more receptive to your own thoughts than you ordinarily are. You are able to mobilize your responses and do something about it in a new way."

PROFILE SCORING

The profile scoring is based upon the hypothesis that the relationship between an inherent potential for experiencing hypnosis and the sustained level of the trance experience will be significant. It involves aligning key items, including upgaze, eyeroll and initial arm levitation dissociation, posthypnotic arm levitation, central differential cut-off, and floating sensation. These measures appear to be indicators of the actual success of maintaining the trance experience once it has been effected through specific instructions. The different profile grades (intacts, decrements, softs, increments, averagings, and special zeros) indicate different kinds of relationship between two factors, the preinduction phase and the trance experience.

The hypnotic profile score describes a response pattern or profile configuration which is established by the patient as his responses to trance are recorded. The purpose of the score is to tap and trace the patient's flow of concentration from a stage of customary awareness or preinduction phase through the trance experience or induction phase. The score is derived from the following three centric components of the HIP: the eyeroll, the control differential, and the posthypnotic arm levitation. Other HIP items are not essential to the profile score. They are part of the induction score and/or fall into the clinical picture outlined by the profile configuration. They form the procedure for entering and exiting the trance state.

Hypnotizability, as reflected by the profile, is not an either-or phenomenon but extends from the nonhypnotizable (grade 0) to the highly hypnotizable (grade 5), including slightly hypnotizable (grade 1), moderately hypnotizable (grade 2), hypnotizable (grade 3), and very hypnotizable (grade 4).

An intact profile greater than intact grade 0 connotes hypnotizability. The intact profile is one in which eyeroll, posthypnotic arm levitation, and control differential all score greater than zero. These scores remain in the zone of attentive concentration. The configuration of straight intacts, increments, averagings, and grades all fall within the zone. The straight intact, increment, averaging, and grade 5 profile all score positive in the eyeroll, posthypnotic arm levitation, and control differential. In a straight intact profile, the eyeroll and posthypnotic arm levitation are within one unit of each other. In an increment profile, the posthypnotic arm levitation is more than one unit greater than the eyeroll score. In an averaging profile, the posthypnotic arm levitation is more than one unit less than the eyeroll score.

All examples of grade 4 are potentially grade 5. A grade 5 is identified by further testing for the following three characteristics: (1) global amnesia; (2) the ability to maintain posthypnotic sensory-motor alternatives; and (3) the ability to experience regression in the present tense. A grade 4–5 subject is a grade 4 who shows some but not all of the grade 5 phenomena. The small frequency of these not-straight variations within the intact zone led them to be grouped with the straight intacts.

A straight zero profile is one in which all of the above three items score zero, thereby forming a profile wholly outside the zone of attentive concentration. Less than 1 per cent of the zero group are special zeros. These people have a zero eyeroll score and either a positive posthypnotic arm levitation score or positive control differential scores, but not both. We hypothesize that these rare cases are caused by specific organic deficits in extraocular muscle innervation. It is considered intact, but it represents nonhypnotizability. The decrement profile begins in the zone of concentration by scoring a positive eyeroll, but it falls out of it with a score of zero for control differential. It is thereby considered a "nonintact" pattern, and it represents a refractory or a dysfunction capacity for trance experience. Decrements are not representative of hypnotizability. They are considerably different structurally and clinically. It is hypothesized that the straight zero nonhypnotizability reflects an absence of the inherent capacity for trance, whereas the decrement profile seems to indicate that the necessary biological substructure is present, but there is a pathological inability to focus through and sustain contact with it for any period of time.

The mechanics of measuring hypnotizability, though seemingly complex, must now take a back seat to the therapeutic matrix hypnosis forms. As a clinician, one must understand that nothing can be done with hypnosis that cannot be accomplished without it. The presence of an intact profile, however, gives therapy a considerable head start (Fig. 13–5).[2]

AN APPROACH TO STRATEGY SELECTION

We mentioned earlier that there was a relationship between trance capacity and personality types, and that we could derive strategic information in regard to therapy from the profile results.

The ancient Romans worshipped in two types of temples. One group of Romans worshipped in the temple of Apollo. These Apollonians were highly analytical and were ruled by their brains. They were the mathematicians and accountants of today. The other Romans worshipped in the temple of Dionysus. The Dionysians were ruled by their emotions and feelings, and their life styles certainly corresponded.

Using the HIP score we can begin to select appropriate strategy in the Apollonian-Dionysian model. The philosopher Pascal may here be paraphrased: "The heart has a mind the brain often does not understand." Assaying in which "temple" our subject "worships" is an invaluable aid in strategy selection.

In general the grades 0–2 are Apollonians and should be considered predominantly mind-oriented. Grades 3–5 are considered Dionysians, and they should be considered dominated by the heart or emotions. A useful way of becoming familiar with the subject's relationship to his environment can be found in Figure 13–6 (Structural Themes and Hypnotizability), a chart Dr. Spiegel uses in his lectures.

The examiner can structure his own questions regarding space awareness, time perception, and so on, to further evaluate his subject. In conjunc-

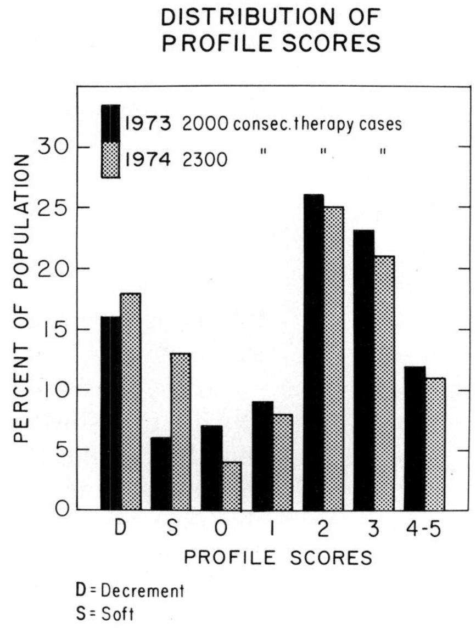

Figure 13–5.

DISTRIBUTION OF
PROFILE SCORES

1973 2000 consec. therapy cases
1974 2300 " " "

PERCENT OF POPULATION

PROFILE SCORES

D = Decrement
S = Soft

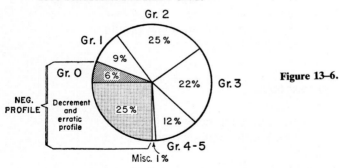

HYPNOTIZABILITY DISTRIBUTION
2000 CONSECUTIVE THERAPY CASES

Figure 13–6.

tion with the profile, the examiner is presented with a comprehensive emotional psychological evaluation of the subject. It is essential to understand and remember that a total Apollonian or a complete Dionysian is rare. Therefore, we have the Odyssean man, the worshiper of the gods.

The therapist has more than one tool he can use during therapy, and that is the patient. Because of the focal awareness that presents itself in trance, the subject will find something to suit him in a strategy in case the therapist should place him in the wrong "temple." Therefore, therapy in the intact profile using the hypnotic model tends to be effective.

A METHOD OF SELF-HYPNOSIS

Hypnosis is an exercise in parallel awareness. In other words, the subject develops the ability to separate from himself and, with executive control, gains some positive movement in his life.

Hypnosis is effective in behavioral modification only if the subject uses a structural ceremony and strategy in his daily routine. We therefore recommend this form of hypnotherapy rather than posthypnotic suggestion, which is subject to extinction. Utilizing only a technique subject to extinction builds failure into the technique. After the subject learns the autohypnotic ceremony, we can then institute therapeutic strategy.

STRATEGY

Once the hypnotic model is selected the therapist presents a strategy that he is comfortable with, one that should fit his style as well as the subject's. Why will it work?

If hypnosis is to occur, a shift in conscious awareness must take place. During this shift there is a physiological enhancement that couples with this shift. In the Dionysian, the shift and the enhancement occur almost immediately; in the Apollonian they occur later in the induction ceremony. At this time the subject becomes acutely aware of the purpose of the session. Hypnosis is goal-oriented, and the goal is now presented. For some reason, the subject becomes "locked" into some aspect of the strategy. It is probably a combination of the goal awareness and the physiological enhancement.

Physiological enhancement may be defined as some physical change occurring during the induction, e.g., arm levitation and lightness.

The enhancement apparently reinforces and reminds the subject of what we are together for. The session is for the patient, and the therapist's ego does not suffer with the success or failure of the patient. Appropriate strategy in the dental environment is the same as the psychological milieu.

TECHNIQUE

After you have completed the Profile, you are now in a position to show the subject how he or she can utilize this capacity to shift into a state of attentive concentration in a disciplined way. The following paragraphs demonstrate how it is done.:

"I am going to count to three. Follow this sequence again. One, look up toward your eyebrows, all the way up; two, close your eyelids, take a deep breath; three, exhale, let your eyes relax and let your body float.

"As you feel yourself floating, *you* permit one hand or the other to feel like a buoyant balloon and allow it to float upward. As it does, your elbow bends and your forearm floats into an upright position. Sometimes you may get a feeling of a magnetic pull on your hand as it goes up. When your hand reaches this upright position it becomes a signal for you to enter a state of meditation and increased receptivity.

"In this state of meditation, you concentrate on the feeling of floating, and at the same time concentrate on this."

Here you insert whatever strategy is relevant for the patient's goal, in a way which is consistent with the trance level the patient is able to experience. It is best to formulate the approach in a self-renewing manner which the subject is able to weave into his everyday style of life. The patient must sense that he can achieve mastery over the problem he is struggling with, by "reprogramming himself," by a self-affirming, uncomplicated, reformulation of the problem, often identified as an "exercise."

"I propose that in the beginning you do these exercises as often as ten different times a day, preferably every one to two hours. At first the exercise takes about a minute, but as you become more expert at it you can do it in much less time.

"You sit or lie down, and to yourself you count to three. At one, you do one thing; at two, you do two things; and at three, you do three things. At one, look up toward your eyebrows; at two, close your eyelids and take a deep breath; and at three, exhale, let your eyes relax, and let your body float.

"As you feel yourself floating, permit one hand or the other to feel like a buoyant balloon and let it float upward as your hand is now. When it reaches this upright position, it becomes your signal to enter a state of meditation.

"In this state of meditation you concentrate on these critical points."

You restate here again, in an abbreviated but even more direct way, what the patient is to review for himself, in as simple a formula as is possible each time he does the exercise.

"Reflect on the implications of these critical points and then bring yourself out of this state of concentration called self-hypnosis by counting backwards in this manner.

"Now, three, get ready. Two, with your eyelids closed, roll up your eyes (and do it now). And one, let your eyelids open slowly. Then, when your eyes are back in focus, slowly make a fist with the hand that is up and, as you open your fist slowly, your usual sensation and control will return. Let your hand float downward. That is the end of the exercise. But you retain a general feeling of floating.

"By doing the exercise ten different times each day, you can float into this state of buoyant repose. Give yourself this island of time—20 seconds, ten times a day, in which you use this extra state of receptivity to reimprint these critical points. Reflect upon it, then return to your usual state of awareness, and get on with what you ordinarily do."

If necessary, demonstrate it yourself. You then repeat the sequence of entering the trance state in order to allow the patient to watch it. Then the patient repeats it again while you supervise with direction.

Camouflage Method

People do not always have the privacy to do the exercise. What follows is a modification of the exercise that can be done in public.

"Now, suppose one or two hours pass and you want to do the exercise. You don't have privacy and you don't want to make a spectacle of yourself. Here's the way you do it. There are two changes. First, you close your eyes and then roll them up so that the eyeroll is private. People seeing the uncamouflaged eyeroll may get frightened. Second, instead of your hand coming up like this (demonstrate arm levitation as it was done in the hypnosis session), let it come up and touch your forehead (demonstrate). To an outsider the exercise looks like you are in deep thought. In 20 seconds you can shift gears, establish this extra receptivity, reimprint the critical points to yourself, and shift back out again.

"You might be sitting at a desk or a table, or you may be in conference, in which case you lean over on your elbow like this (demonstrate). With your hand already on your forehead, you close your eyes, roll them up and shift into a trance state. We'll go over this again, and this time you try it." Repeat the camouflage technique. This time, instead of demonstrating, have the patient try it.

"By doing the basic or camouflage exercise every day for one or two hours, you establish a private signal system so that you're ever alert to a new commitment you are making." (Elaborate on this with reference to the treatment strategy you have used.)

PAIN AND ANXIETY

Pain and anxiety are the primary concerns in treating craniomandibular dysfunction. Some of the strategies that we have found clinically effective for the management of pain and anxiety are presented here. They are by no means all of the effective strategies. We cannot emphasize enough the need for imagination in regard to the formulation of new strategic application.

Dentally, we must be aware of primary gain, secondary gain, and field forces, but in treating craniomandibular dysfunction we have an advantage. Our advantage involves the orthopedic correction of the problem. In other words, there is a physiological enhancement generated by successful treatment. If the patient has the innate feeling of a return to inner equilibrium and balance, the adjunct of hypnosis is even more effective.

Anxiety is a fear of loss of control. Upon the realization that hypnosis is executive control exercised by the patient, the anxiety begins to be allayed. The subject's new-found ability to initiate trance on his own begins to counteract anxiety. The fact that the trance experience becomes easier helps to eliminate the helpless feeling. Trance itself becomes strategic in eliminating anxiety and creating a more positive therapeutic milieu. The therapist should also incorporate some phrase in the session that leads to ego reinforcement. The presence of anxiety actually begins to work for the therapist, since it is the first to abate and reinforces the subject.

HEADACHES

Migraine and Migrainoid-type Headaches

After extensively examining over 200 headache patients whose chief complaint was derived directly from the craniomandibular dysfunction syndrome, a number of things became clear. First, we realized that we were dealing with legalized addiction to analgesics. Secondly, the neurological examination of the suggested headache patients laid the groundwork for migrainoid headaches and a neurological diagnosis of migraine. The nature of the headache history involves suggestion, and the patient in pain is prone to assimilation of the migraine symptoms through suggestion.

True migraine strategy involves the suggestion of a cooling sensation around the head and neck and a warming sensation of the hands. An ice block lowering over the head with electrically warmed mittens is highly effective in the true migraine patient. The strategy counteracts the autonomic sequence of migraine with its carotid artery dilation and peripheral circulation constriction. Concentrated rather than autonomic change is probably the initial factor in this strategy's success.

Tension Headache

According to neurologists, 90 per cent of all head and neck pain is caused by striated muscle tension. This can and should be demonstrated to the patient by asking him to extend his arm and clench his fist as tightly as possible. This ultimately leads to striated muscle pain. Once the patient is aware of this chain of events, he can begin to control or intervene in the sequence. Using the trance experience, profound relaxation can be achieved by the floating suggestion or the suggestion of heaviness. Structuring this strategy offers limitless opportunities to the therapist's imagination.

Comment Regarding the Profile and Craniomandibular Dysfunction

Many headache sufferers unfortunately bear the burden of a diagnosis of psychosomatic disease. Although their headaches are functional in origin, perhaps the term somatopsychic should be applied to their dysfunction. In other words, the target organ or system receives a stimulus overload as a result of the manifestation of tension.

Their pain is real and, as eloquently stated throughout this text, caused by craniomandibular orthopedic imbalance. The stomatognathic system, being imbalanced, becomes the target organ for tension.

The profile not only measures trance capacity but provides information as to the present condition of the patient's emotional health.

Considering 45 HIP profiles, 35 profiles were intact. Not all of these patients were highly hypnotizable, but 77 per cent were able to benefit from their hypnotic capacity. In addition, and statistically more important, the intact profiles indicate a disease causality other than emotional. Seventy-seven per cent of these people were psychologically intact (Fig. 13–6). At this time it is impossible to state that the other 23 per cent were experiencing pain caused by emotional crisis because they did exhibit diagnostic physical signs of CM imbalance.

PAIN

Pain is the most universally reported symptom. It is a very personal experience that is metaphorically described differently by the Apollonians and the Dionysians. If pain becomes the center of one's awareness, it becomes difficult to treat with traditional medical approaches. In hypnosis the shift of awareness helps the patient initiate a change in point of view. Soldiers in combat have been known to sustain and function with injuries that in peace time they could not tolerate. They have in a sense established a parallel awareness. At times the therapist is faced with pain of unknown origin. This emphatically points out that we often cannot control the pain stimulus, but with hypnosis we can control the patient's response to the pain.

If the patient has experienced a limb falling asleep or a dental injection, we can utilize the numbness model. Glove anesthesia (the feeling of a glove of Novocain put on) or numbing cold can be suggested and then applied to the painful area.

Pain can also be controlled by disassociation or a parallel awareness technique. An out-of-body sensation can be suggested to deal with pain, which allows the physical self to experience the pain while the cognitive self is not receptive to it. Asking the patient to view a split screen in his mind's eye is effective here. On one half of the screen he sees himself in pain, on the other half as he would like to be. Fading out the painful side helps restore the patient's self-image and comfort.

Three models have been suggested for pain control. The additional possibilities are endless.

Case History No. 1 (Fig. 13–7)

E. N., female Caucasian, 25 years old, student, residing in Manhattan, referred by an orthopedic physician. Medical history—whiplash injury 3 years previously. Chief complaint—headache (occipital-frontal), earaches, neck pain. Medication—Valium, 5 mg. t.i.d., Fiorinal. Treated for cranial mandibular dysfunction and hypnotically. See profile.

Strategy—Floating in a pool of clear water.

ʀ ℓ c- ʀ ℓ b. ᴠ 2x ʀ ℓ   *col u pm-4 12ʀ 6 74*

HYPNOTIC INDUCTION PROFILE

Eye-Roll Levitation Method

Ⓒase Hist # 1

Patient Name __E.N__   Date _7 | 15 | 76_

Sequence -   Initial __✓__   Previous_____   When_____

Position -   Standing_____   Supine_____   Sit __✓__   Chair-Stool_____

A	Induction - Up-Gaze	0 - 1 - 2 - ③ - 4	
B	ROLL	0 - 1 - ② - 3 - 4	
C			① - 2 - 3 (Squint)

Instructions

D	Arm Levitation Right_____ Left_____	0 - 1 - 2 - ③ - 4	

Post-Hypnotic Response -

E	Tingle 0 -	① - 2
F	Dissociation 0 -	① - 2

G	LEVITATION Immediate	0 - 1 - 2 - 3 - 4	Smile ✓
H	Re-enforce (1)	1 - 2 - 3 - ④	Surprise Amazing
I	Re-enforce (2)	2 - 3 - 4	
J	Re-enforce (3)	3 - 4	
K	Re-enforce (4)	4	
L	CONTROL DIFFERENTIAL 0 -	① - 2	

M	Cut-off 0 -	① - 2
N	Amnesia to Cut-off 0 -	- 1 - 2
O	No Test_____	
P	Floating Sensation 0 -	- 1 - 2
Q	GRADE - continuum	0 - 1 - 2 - ③ - 4 - 5

_____ Increment
_____ Average

Minutes 6.³⁰   Decrement_____   _____ Soft

Figure 13–7.

n l c- n l b· v 2x n l   *col u pm-4 12n 6 74*

HYPNOTIC INDUCTION PROFILE

Eye-Roll Levitation Method

CASE HIST #2

Patient Name G. K   Date 5/15/76

Sequence – Initial ✓   Previous _____   When _____

Position – Standing _____   Supine _____   Sit ✓   Chair-Stool _____

A   Induction – Up-Gaze   0 – 1 – ②– 3 – 4

B   ROLL   0 – 1 – ②– 3 – 4

C   – 1 – 2 – 3 (Squint)

Instructions

D   Arm Levitation Right _____ Left _____   0 – 1 –②– 3 – 4

Post-Hypnotic

E   Response –   Tingle   0 –   – 1 – 2

F___   Dissociation 0 –   – 1 – 2

G___   LEVITATION   Immediate   0 – 1 – 2 – 3 – 4   Smile ✓

H   Re-enforce (1)   1 – 2 – 3 – 4   Surprise ✓

I   Re-enforce (2)   2 –③– 4

J   Re-enforce (3)   3 – 4

K   Re-enforce (4)   4

L___   CONTROL DIFFERENTIAL   0 –   – 1 –②

M___   Cut-off   0 –   – 1 –②

N   Amnesia to Cut-off   0 –   – 1 –②

O   No Test _____

P___   Floating Sensation   0 –   –①– 2

Q___   GRADE – continuum   0 – 1 –②– 3 – 4 – 5

_____ Increment
_____ Average

Minutes ⊆ 10   Decrement _____   _____ Soft

Figure 13–8.

Results—Symptom free.

Comment—Combining craniomandibular dysfunction orthopedic therapy and hypnotherapy diverse muscle spasm was permanently relieved. No medication required.

Case History No. 2 (Fig. 13–8)

G. K., male Caucasian, 43 year old radio announcer residing in Maryland, referred by his attending dentist. Medical history—TMJ pain (left side), headache (left side), earache, tinnitus (left side), severe CL III malocclusion, sleep and dream disturbances, colitis. Medication—Valium, 5 mg. t.i.d., Fiorinal, Tylenol, Cafergot, Sansert. Treated for craniomandibular dysfunction as well as hypnotically. See profile.

Strategy—Split screen.

Results—Pain diminution, sleep-dream problems relieved, colitis controlled.

Comment—Patient experienced a ripple effect.

SUMMARY

The key is in knowing when to use hypnosis and having the confidence to use it. The hypnotic experience neatly fits into the comprehensive intervention in the craniomandibular dysfunction syndrome. We believe that if hypnosis does nothing else it provides a matrix through which the quality of life can be improved. No amount of pharmacological intervention can offer the same thing—independence.

The hypnotic experience is now a scientific tool that belongs in the armamentarium of every health practitioner.

References

1. Spiegel, H.: Manual for Hypnotic Induction Profile. New York, Soni Medica, Inc., 1973.
2. Spiegel, H., Aronson, M., Fleiss, J. L., and Haber, J.: Psychometric Analysis of the Hypnotic Induction Profile. Int. J. Clin. Exp. Hypn., *24*:300, 1976.

14

Biofeedback—The Treatment of Stress-Induced Muscle Activity

ANDREW J. CANNISTRACI, D.D.S., F.A.C.D.
and GEORGE FRITZ, Ed.D.

Since stress is a dynamic state within an organism in response to a demand for adaptation, and since life itself entails constant adaptation, living creatures are continually in a state of more or less stress.

Wolff[1]

Clenching, bruxism, and other forms of stress-induced muscle activity have long been recognized as parafunctional activity of the masticatory muscles. This hyperactivity of masticatory muscles is frequently mentioned in the literature as the destructive component of traumatic occlusion. Although the symptoms are often treated by the dental profession, the direct cause—stress—is seldom mentioned and less often treated.

Chronically rigid styles of attention seem instrumental in the causation of stress-related disorders,[2] including temporomandibular joint (TMJ) dysfunction.[3] Biofeedback-assisted attention training effectively encourages more flexible habits of attention, associated normalization of function, and resulting relaxation.[4] Electromyographic (EMG) biofeedback techniques and adjunctive relaxation exercises also develop more relaxed habits of attention and resulting reduction of stress-induced muscle activity.[5] Since maladaptive temporomandibular response is essentially a stress response,[6] temporomandibular joint dysfunction can largely be overcome with voluntary stress control techniques.

TEMPOROMANDIBULAR DYSFUNCTION AND STRESS

Stress-induced muscle activity in the form of teeth-clenching and bruxism is undoubtedly one of the most important causes of dental disease.[7] Excessive tension of the masticatory muscles is known to aggravate or even cause many common disorders. Prolonged and excessive muscle activity may cause lesions in the hard tissues of the teeth, in their supporting structures, in the temporomandibular joint, and in the tissue supporting a prosthesis. Under such conditions, even the most meticulous dental restoration may deteriorate and fail to give lasting service.

Similarly, painful muscle spasm, tension headache, and general stiffness in the cervical area can frequently be traced to excess muscle activity. When substantial tension persists, the muscles are deprived of needed rest, and surrounding parts of the body are subjected to unhealthy stress.

Stress-induced muscle activity often results in grinding, clenching, or clicking of the teeth in either conscious or sleep states. There is a forceful rubbing together or application of pressure by opposing teeth. Such force is exerted by the contraction of the elevator muscles of the mandible. An exerted force affects the recipient of the force. The recipient can be the teeth, which consequently exhibit excessive wear. The force can affect the supporting alveolar bone, causing periodontal disease. Excessive and prolonged contraction of the masticatory muscles can cause spasm of the muscles surrounding the temporomandibular joint, causing the temporomandibular joint syndrome.

The interaction of psychological stress and occlusal imbalance occurs in the following way:

Ideally, there is a state of harmony and balance between the occlusion of the teeth, the masticatory muscles, and the temporomandibular joints.[8] Such an ideal condition allows the individual to clench and grind teeth evenly. However, when the state of equilibrium between the component parts of the masticatory system is lost or altered, these parts are then in a state of imbalance. In the common case of tooth loss, the teeth adjacent to and opposing the resultant space will drift and rotate, causing abnormal pressures to be exerted on them. The application of such pressure to a tooth initiates a response in the proprioceptors of the periodontal membrane. Through proprioception, the resulting stimulus activates the muscles of mastication to move the mandible so that the teeth occlude in a less traumatic position. In this manner, proprioception can be viewed as a defense mechanism of the teeth.[9]

If the mandible has moved into an abnormal position, certain of its prime mover muscles are placed under stress and tension. Any abnormal and sustained contraction of a muscle leads to overstimulation of the muscle. Muscle fatigue and waste products build up within the muscle, which increases stimulation to the muscle, and a vicious circle ensues. Once the adaptive capacity of the muscle is exceeded, a pathological condition exists. Often, the muscle goes into spasm. Prolonged and sustained hyperactivity of the masticatory muscles past the adaptive capacity of a well-balanced dentition can create the TMJ syndrome. Whatever its form and symptoms, the TMJ dysfunction must be relieved if the patient is to enjoy good dental health and the general comfort which accompanies it.

Traditionally, dentists have employed various methods of overcoming TMJ disorders. The occlusion has been adjusted, or the mandible repositioned with appliances to restore a harmonious relationship between the masticatory components. The muscles have been injected with local anesthetics or sprayed with ethyl chloride. Muscle relaxants and tranquilizers have been prescribed. In many cases, such "administered" techniques are successful, but they more often provide incomplete or temporary relief. Most patients remain unable to cope with tension and emotional stress. These patients continue to clench and grind, maintaining the muscle spasms and perpetuating the TMJ syndrome.

At this juncture, it is necessary for the dentist to consider the psychophysiogical process and the best way to deal with it. A voluntary stress control training program, in our experience, offers the most salutary way to accomplish desired results on a lasting basis.

OVERCOMING STRESS

Recent discoveries about the nature of muscle activity have led to an effective new approach for reducing tension. Methods have been developed in which the patient learns to exercise voluntary control over usually subconscious jaw-muscle activity. Unlike most traditional therapeutic procedures, self-regulation permits the individual to participate constructively in treatment and, with the new personal skill developed, to prevent recurrence of the problem.

Effective self-regulatory training involves the development of more flexible habits of attention, which may be fully transferred by the trainee to everyday life activities. Flexibility of attention is exercised through biofeedback-assisted attention training, which is integrated into moment to moment activity outside the biofeedback situation. Various relaxation procedures offer a somewhat more indirect approach to the development and generalization of self-regulatory skills.

ATTENTION TRAINING

"You must relax!" is often demanded of persons perceived by themselves and others as too tense and consequently suffering a stress-related disorder. They try to relax, but in trying they frustrate themselves. The demand made in the biofeedback training situation—to try to relax—is the same as in everyday life and may be just as self-defeating, regardless of the efforts made by the biofeedback trainer to reduce patient stress. Although some individuals may try to relax and succeed, the same persons can more easily learn to permit relaxation to occur when lower arousal is experienced as a side-benefit of a less controlled style of attention.[10] The additional advantage of an attention training approach has to do with the facility with which the new attentional orientation may be directly transferred to everyday activities and performance.

A series of exercises, called therapeutic awareness, has been devised to guide biofeedback trainees to adopt the attentional disposition or style required in order to increase the occurrence of the physiological concomitants of physical well-being and relaxation.[11] Therapeutic awareness has as its goal an effortless orientation to the biofeedback task, as well as to any wakeful activity. Since concentrated, body-disconnected awareness requires effort and tension, the prerequisite for establishing therapeutic awareness involves opening one's awareness to reconnect with one's whole body all at once.

Ultimately, every perceptible event, whether internal or external, is represented in the nervous system. To establish therapeutic awareness, the subject must allow his awareness to broaden to include *simultaneously* all those perceptible events that are salient in the nervous system.

The experiences reported by attention trainees, as they generalize therapeutic awareness to various life situations, suggest that attention is typified in part by two styles that represent the extreme positions on a continuum of attending. The usual, most habitual, and most generally reinforced attentional mode in our society is concentrated, body-disconnected attention. This refers to the wakeful state in which mental effort is expended to disconnect certain aspects of experience, especially body awareness, in order to concentrate. The reader may observe, for instance, that at this moment the kinesthetic presence of his or her body is largely ignored, while attention is concentrated visually and cognitively in order to grasp the sense of these printed words. An open, whole body–connected style of paying attention and reading these words, however, releases the effort ordinarily necessary for selecting and sorting out experience. The central portion of awareness may be absorbed with reading and understanding these words while *simultaneously* peripheral awareness remains open to the all-at-once presence of the whole body. Therapeutic awareness may be employed similarly in relation to any activity, resulting in physiological normalization and optimization of function.

EMG Biofeedback Training

Let us look at what biofeedback does. As an overall process, biofeedback supplies an individual with information about physiological activities about which he is not normally aware. Biofeedback techniques require instruments which detect bioelectric activity and translate it into information which is easily understood by both the patient and the therapist. Such information can be used by the patient for control skill learning, or by the therapist as an aid in directing the therapy. The body processes which are monitored, singly or in combination, include skin conducting capacity, surface skin temperature, brain waves, and muscle tension.

Physiological studies demonstrate that muscles operate by generating electrical impulses, which are so minute that under ordinary circumstances they cannot be felt. As muscle tension increases, so does EMG activity. To evaluate accurately a muscle's tension level, it is necessary to measure the the muscle's EMG output. We use electromyographic biofeedback, for it can measure muscle tension in the head and neck.

Biofeedback allows the patient to engage in psychomotor re-education and learn to develop internally oriented control systems, as opposed to externally oriented control systems. By attending to the biofeedback signal, be it audio or visual, the patient learns to monitor his own responses. As his response patterns are monitored, the patient begins to relate particular subjective attitudes and emotional states to the corresponding physiological pattern. For example, he discovers that attending in a therapeutic awareness fashion to certain thoughts and feelings regularly accompanies muscle relaxation. This patterned recognition, in turn, promotes the development of voluntary control skills over the physiological response. By altering attentional style, he controls his own physiology, which is a healthy way to regulate excessive stress and its manifestations.

Biofeedback researchers speculate that, through the biofeedback training procedure, individual body organs and systems learn new response patterns. For example, alteration of the activity of sweat glands can be accomplished. Blood vessels in the body's extremities can be made to either expand or contract. The separate motor neurons which control muscle activation levels can be trained to fire or not fire. These changed response patterns occur almost immediately when feedback is supplied and appear to become automatic with repeated practice. Moreover, it is probable that the maintenance of altered bodily response patterns in the face of stressful situations depends on thorough recognition of accompanying attitudinal sets and the capacity to manipulate them at will.

In TMJ dysfunction, the first step toward voluntary tension control involves teaching the patient to recognize EMG variations routinely in the masticatory muscle area. The essential tool in this process is an EMG biofeedback instrument which monitors muscle activity and immediately translates that information to the patient in easily understood audio or visual signals. With this objective indicator of normally subconscious behavior, the patient can begin to learn to modify the styles of attention regularly associated with different tension levels. Thus, he progressively develops his own personalized EMG-monitoring capacity.[5]

RELAXATION THERAPIES

Another aspect of voluntary stress reduction training employs physical and mental exercises which allow the patient to gain willful control over his increasingly familiar EMG patterns and thus to relax the jaw muscles voluntarily at the sensing of an unwanted rise in tension. Here, too, biofeedback plays an essential role by allowing the patient to know instantly the EMG effect of such an exercise. The patient can thereby select that combination which yields the most restful personal results. A trial-and-error approach to finding this combination is necessary because muscle hypertension does not always have the same root causes.

The self-control training programs discussed below may be integrated into biofeedback-assisted attention training. Relaxation therapies have been found most effective when integrated into an open focus strategy of attention.[13] Interestingly, when relaxation exercises are performed simultaneously with an open focus style of attention, the effectiveness of those exercises are ensured.

The most familiar of the relaxation exercises are the following:

1. Progressive relaxation, pioneered by Dr. Edmond Jacobson, involves a structured isometric approach.[12]

2. Autogenic training, derived from work by Drs. Schultz and Luthe, employs adaptive mental imagery.[13]

3. Yogic meditational mantrum and diaphragmatic breathing techniques are adapted from Oriental disciplines.[14]

Despite their different origins and content, all three methods have been shown to have distinctly relaxing, physiological effects upon persons who learn how to use them.

Progressive Relaxation

Progressive relaxation techniques train the subject to achieve deep muscular relaxation throughout the body. The physical exercises deal with skeletal or long muscle groups which the subject can easily manipulate. Progressive relaxation therapy was pioneered by Dr. Edmond Jacobson and his colleagues at the University of Chicago in the 1930s. Dr. Jacobson theorized that, in a state of deep muscular relaxation, it is almost impossible for the subject to experienc an adverse fight-or-flight stress reaction. This technique today offers a proven, systematic path to effective muscle tension control.

When measured with sensitive electromyographic instruments, major muscle groups can be brought to the zero-firing threshold by this method. A successful training program in progressive relaxation can usually be completed in two months—assuming a well-motivated subject, a competent instructor, and regular 30-minute daily practice.

TECHNIQUE. The subject is seated in a comfortable chair. Starting with the arms, the subject is instructed to tense and then relax, in progression, all major muscle areas in the body. He is then instructed in this way by a trainer: "Sit down. . . . Close your eyes, allowing your body to relax as much as possible. Relax for a moment. . . . Now, lift your right arm and hold it out straight in front of you. . . . Clench your right fist just as tightly as you possibly can and hold it until I say to let go. . . . Now, let go, release the tension in your right arm, and allow your arm to drop slowly to your side. . . . Now, lift your right arm again and clench the fist tightly. Hold it, and feel the tension throughout your right hand. . . . Let go and relax the arm by your side. Can you notice a difference in feeling between your right and left arms? If so, you are already experiencing an early effect of progressive relaxation."

To continue the progressive relaxation training, the subject would be instructed to tense and then relax in sequence the voluntary muscles of the head, neck, face, shoulders, chest, stomach, genital area, legs, and feet. The subject exercises this way systematically for about 30 minutes, at the end of which time his entire body should tend to feel warm, calm, and relaxed.

Daily practice of 30 minutes is essential to master this relaxation technique. As the subject approaches self-control over muscle tension, he can apply that skill in daily situations which threaten him with high-anxiety potential. In time this positive adaptation to environment stress becomes second nature to the individual.

Autogenic Training

Autogenic training, another effective method of willfully achieving deep relaxation, was formulated by Dr. Wolfgang Luthe and his associates. This technique involves a self-induced, reprogramming of the subconscious mind to produce psychophysiological tranquility. Autogenic training promotes smooth and skeletal muscle relaxation and teaches the subject to create a sense of personal warmth and heaviness throughout his body.

The subject uses special "autogenic phrases" relating to specific parts of the body while attempting to clearly visualize the parts of the body which are to be influenced. The individual then sets up a "contact" with that particular part of the body. This appears to trigger the chain of psychological events which result in the physiological changes described above. The operative psychophysiological principle which effects these changes affirms that "every change in the physiological state is accompanied by an appropriate change in the mental–emotional state, conscious or unconscious, and, conversely, every change in the mental–emotional state, conscious or unconscious, is accompanied by an appropriate change in the physiological state."[13] This principle, in combination with volition, operates to facilitate psychosomatic self-regulation.

AUTOGENIC TRAINING-TYPE PHRASES. To begin autogenic training, selected exercise phrases are essential. Ideally, the subject visualizes, imagines, and feels that the desired change is happening, and he allows it to happen effortlessly. Ideally, there should be no interference with the body's inherent tendency to cooperate. Ultimately, a very brief recall of a phrase will accomplish the intended physiological change.

The following is a sample instruction from a standard autogenic training program:

The patient is seated in a comfortable chair and instructed to close his eyes. The relaxation trainer then instructs the patient in this way:

"Keeping your eyes closed, listen carefully to my voice. Let my suggestions flow into your mind. . . . Do not force yourself to respond. . . . Just hear what I suggest . . . and allow it to happen. . . . Let your attention drift toward what I say. . . . Let it drift to your body. . . . And feel there what I tell you. . . . No effort . . . just let the feeling form. Relax your body. . . . Now, concentrate effortlessly on these feelings. My right arm feels heavy and warm. . . . I feel heaviness and warmth in my right arm. . . . My left arm is heavy and warm. . . . I can feel the heaviness and warmth in my left arm. . . . Both my arms are heavy and warm. . . . I can feel the heaviness and warmth in my right and left arms. . . . My arms are getting heavier and warmer. . . . I feel peace and calm in both arms. . . . I am at peace. . . . Now, slowly, begin to open your eyes over the next minute . . . slowly . . . very slowly. . . . You can feel peace and quietness from within. . . . The exercise is over."

Similar instruction to calm other parts of the body is given in a 30-minute progression designed for cumulative effect throughout the body. Just as with progressive relaxation technique, the eventual success of autogenic training depends on regular home practice once the patient has mastered the procedure.

Augtogenic training equips the subject to attack tension-related disorders at a primary source—the mind. Furthermore, this training complements progressive relaxation. Since a subject's strong fight-or-flight responses are mental or physical in origin, both realms are involved in maladaptive behavior, and, therefore, an integrated combination of progressive relaxation and autogenic training is useful when teaching a subject to counteract excessive internal tension.

Meditational Techniques

Meditational techniques also promote voluntary stress reduction. The most commonly practiced mantrum-meditational method in the United States is known as Transcendental Meditation.[15] This technique of Yogic derivation was originally taught by the Maharishi Mahesh Yogi, and it has now attracted world-wide attention.

Dr. Herbert Benson notes that four basic elements are necessary to achieve this particular relaxation response: a quiet environment, a mental device, a passive attitude, and a comfortable position.[15]

Dr. Benson reports that the metabolic rate of people engaged in meditation decreases significantly. The heart pumps less frequently and the electrical resistance of the skin increases markedly, demonstrating relaxation. The meditator's body produces smaller amounts of carbon dioxide. Alpha brain waves increase in intensity. (They are a critical parameter of relaxation.) Less lactic acid is produced in the blood, another indication of reduced anxiety.[15]

Lawrence LeShan notes that "technically, meditation seems to bring about a hypometabolic state that is quite opposite to the 'defense-alarm' state described by W. B. Cannon when he analyzed the physiologic state of the 'fight-or-flight' reaction." Mental awareness is increased and is accompanied by a decrease in physiological tension.[16]

Although Transcendental Meditation is one method which incorporates these elements by using a personalized "secret" Sanskrit mantrum, Benson notes that even focusing on a word such as "one" achieves the same results. A basic aspect of meditation, regardless of the method utilized, is focusing on one object, one event. LeShan states: "The signals our body gets as to how it should be responding are simpler and more coherent during meditation than at almost any other time. In meditation we are in the state—or moving toward it—of sending only one set of signals at a time. The effect of this on our physiology is positive, and there is a strong tendency to normalize reactions, to behave physiologically in a more relaxed and healthy manner."[16]

The meditator may stare at an object such as a candle, a star, or a mandala (Oriental symbol of the universe). The meditator may repeat a phrase silently or aloud for about 20 minutes at a time. Also, complete, relaxed, full diaphragmatic breathing, central to all voluntary stress reduction techniques, is practiced. Diaphragmatic breathing involves breathing fully and deeply from the diaphragm instead of the chest, expanding the stomach during inhalation and contracting it during exhalation. Diaphragmatic breathing requires complete body relaxation with each breath cycle.

SELF-REGULATION PROGRAM FORMAT

In our office, a group of dental patients with chronic clenching and grinding of the teeth participate in a ten-session voluntary stress control program. Designed to alleviate maladaptive stress responses through a behavioral conditioning process, the program includes attention training, specific training techniques in EMG biofeedback, progressive relaxation, autogenic training, and meditation.[5]

Most patients exhibit useful muscle control skills after ten 60-minute training sessions. During these sessions, the patient receives systematic instruction and, with the aid of biofeedback, moves through a patterned sequence of EMG recognition and control exercises. The feedback system is used to measure muscular tension in the frontalis region, the area known to correlate with tension headache and bruxism.

Between sessions, the patient practices those techniques which have already proven beneficial. This unassisted phase of training is important, for it progressively lessens the patient's initial dependency upon feedback. Upon successful completion of the program, the patient will have learned to relax his jaw muscles without further external assistance. Thus the instruction and biofeedback will have served their temporary, facilitating purpose.

All patients complete two anxiety or stress scales before and immediately after the training. Results on the Multiple Affect Adjective Checklist test (General Form) usually indicate statistically significant decreases in mal-adaptive stress. Subjective reports by patients indicate that the lowering of stress levels is often associated with less severe day- and night-time grinding of the teeth.[17]

MEASURING BRUXISM

To determine the amount and pattern of bruxism before and after relaxation training, a method is necessary to measure bruxism objectively. This was not possible until the development of the Bruxcore by Dr. Albert Forgione, assistant professor of psychology at Tufts College of Dental Medicine.[18]

The Bruxcore is a plastic-laminated mouthguard composed of four polyvinyl chloride sheets colored white, orange, yellow, and white. Each colored sheet is 0.005 inch thick. They are vacuum-formed to a stone model of the patient's maxillary dentition on a Dentsply vacuum press with 80 pounds vacuum pressure. High-pressure vacuum forming results in a high degree of conformity to the model and a tight, precise fit. When stretched, the final thickness of the laminated mouthguard is 0.015 inch thick.

The topmost white layer is printed in black, edible ink with a halftone dot screen of 14,400 dots per square inch. Each dot is 1/180 inch in diameter. The printed layer is covered with a plastic film 1 ml. thick.

The patient wears the laminated mouthguard for four consecutive nights during sleep. The amount of bruxing is quantified by scoring the number of dots worn away by bruxing and by which colored layer is exposed (Fig. 14–1).

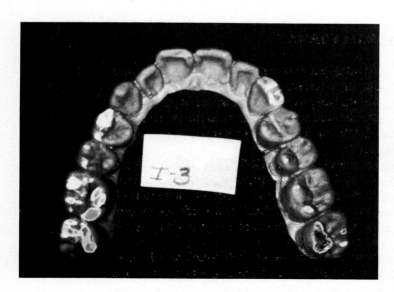

Figure 14–1. Bruxcore. The amount of bruxing is quantified by scoring the number of dots worn away and by which colored layer is exposed.

This procedure is administered once a week for three weeks prior to relaxation training to determine the baseline. After the ten weeks of relaxation training the procedure is repeated again to evaluate the success of the program. It also serves to motivate continued practice by proving to patients that they are indeed grinding their teeth during sleep.

DETERMINING EXAMINATION FOR STRESS CONTROL PROGRAM CANDIDATES

Muscle relaxation programs are *not* appropriate for *all* stressed dental patients. The most critical part of determining appropriate candidates for the stress control program is the dental examination.

The diagnosis of chronic clenching and bruxism is made during the first interview. It is advisable to take the dental and medical history in the business office prior to the oral examination. It is, of course, the dentist's responsibility, both legally and morally, to have a knowledge of the patient's medical history and present medical condition. This process informs the dentist about those patients who have stress-related disorders, among which are tension headaches, gastric problems, high blood pressure, allergies, and many others. The medications patients are presently taking are also indicators of their present physical condition. It is important to know if patients are currently being treated by their physician. The patient should be asked if he has a cardiac condition, is postsurgical, or has bleeding problems, respiratory problems, diabetes, endocrine disorders, neurologic conditions, or hepatitis.

The patient's dental history is also very useful. A knowledge of previous dental experiences supplies a probable indicator of the type of patient the individual is likely to be. Listen carefully to all the patient has to say about his previous dentists and dental experiences.

A most important question involves asking the patient how he reacts to stress. Everyone is subject to stress and tension at times, and the response is widely varied. Some people respond with gastric problems, some get tension headaches, some clench and grind their teeth. It is equally important to explain to the patient at this time that clenching and bruxism are often unconscious actions. Patients must then be made aware of these habits.

This is also the time to educate the patient regarding the serious consequences of stress-induced muscle activity. The patient should be informed that clenching and bruxism generated by stress have a very destructive effect on the oral cavity, causing periodontal problems, wearing of the teeth, bridgework destruction, tooth fracture, difficulty with full dentures, and muscle spasms.

If a patient has very strong, highly calcified teeth, excessive and prolonged muscle activity will cause breakdown of the alveolar bone, muscle spasm of the masticatory muscles, or both. If the alveolar bone is very strong, the breakdown will occur on the teeth, or the muscles will go into spasm. If the teeth and alveolar bone are both very strong, the destructive effects will be found in the temporomandibular joints and the masticatory muscles. When there is prolonged and excessive stress-induced muscle activity past the adaptive capacity, something has to give way.

The patient must be given this information *before* the start of dental procedures, and this information should be woven into the treatment plan.

A comprehensive evaluation of any clenching and bruxing problem will save the dentist a great deal of stress and tension himself in dealing with the patient during any future restorative program.

The patient may then be seated in the dental chair so that radiographs and impressions for study models can be taken.

The next visit includes an examination of the oral cavity. Check for signs of clenching and bruxism, such as flat areas of contacts, wear facets, erosions, cheek biting, and shiny spots on restorations. Then check for muscle spasms. This is one of the most important, and often the most neglected, aspects of the examination procedure. Muscle spasm of any of the masticatory muscles is probably one of the most important symptoms of dental disease. It is an indication of clenching and bruxism.

To examine for muscle spasm, palpate such muscles as the external pterygoid. Move the index finger along the mucobuccal fold above the position of the third maxillary molar. If the muscle is in spasm, the patient will feel unmistakable pain. Then palpate the internal pterygoid. Move the index finger along the median raphe directly behind the mandibular third molar. Finally, palpate the masseter and temporalis muscles, and palpate for neck muscle spasm by checking the posterior cervical, sternocleidomastoid, and hyoid muscles.

Patients with muscle spasm may be considered potentially difficult patients. Make the patient aware of the problems of clenching and bruxism, and explain the fact that the eventual success of the restorative program will be dependent on controlling this habit.

Patients will react to this information in different ways. The majority will understand and agree with the diagnosis once they are made aware of it. The patient is advised that by equilibrating the occlusion and achieving a state of balance and equilibrium between the muscles, the temporomandibular joint, and the occlusion of the teeth, the adaptive capacity of the masticatory apparatus to withstand the stress-induced muscle activity can be increased. The patient can then be advised of the relaxation training program which will aid him in reducing stress.

Many of these patients have obsessive-compulsive personalities. The typical bruxing patient is a controlling, obsessive, rigid, domineering, yet worried person, and shows signs of anxiety and depression. Excessive tension and the bruxing response correlate highly with the idealistic and perfectionist demands that these patients place on themselves.[17]

The characterization of the bruxing patient is typically similar, if not identical, to that of the obsessive-compulsive person who cannot accept anything less than perfection. The usual progression includes perfectionism and rigidity leading to excessive tension, which, in turn, leads to the overt symptoms of bruxing, headache, backache, and other tensional phenomena. Any one, or a combination, of these symptoms continuing over a period of years, or even months, can exhaust the patient's adaptive energy reserve and lead to acute depression and immobilization.

We do find some patients who refuse to admit that they are under stress, or that they clench or grind their teeth. They claim to be perfect, and attribute all their symptoms to inadequate dentistry. These patients are *not* promising candidates for the stress control program. Furthermore, a program of restorative dentistry is likely to fail. Such patients cannot be helped by any complex restorative dentistry, because they refuse to admit that their problem is caused by their own maladaptive response to stress, and thus they will probably continue habits which will eventually destroy the dentist's best efforts.

The best candidate for the stress control program is a person who is motivated and willing to do the necessary homework. Such a patient recognizes the psychological dynamics associated with chronic bruxism and the serious consequences which can result if he does not receive proper treatment. This patient can use a treatment approach which combines traditional dental treatment with self-regulated relaxation or stress control. The stress control program we use emphasizes attention training, progressive relaxation and autogenic training techniques. Electromyographic feedback itself is incorporated to supplement and objectively measure patient progress in stress control for clenching and bruxing.

VOLUNTARY STRESS CONTROL PROGRAM

For appropriate candidates, training is conducted at our office, where patients meet with a certified biofeedback trainer once a week. Throughout the stress control program, an EMG biofeedback instrument is used. This battery-powered unit supplies both audio and visual EMG feedback of muscle activity between 1000 and 3000 microvolts. Variable gain or "shaping" features permit the trainer to adjust feedback signals to assure a manageable challenge to the subject in every session. Frontalis electrode placement is used throughout. Two EMG electrodes, in a headband retainer, are placed approximately 0.5 inch (2.2 cm.) above the right and left eyebrows (at the outer point of densest musculature) and provide the EMG measurement axis, while a third electrode serves as a ground reference (Figs. 14–2, 14–3).

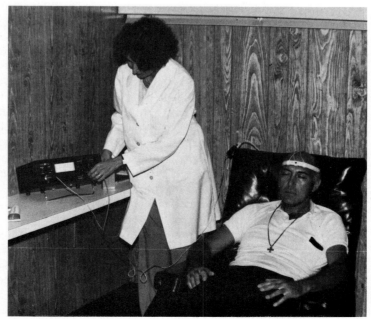

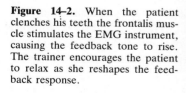

Figure 14–2. When the patient clenches his teeth the frontalis muscle stimulates the EMG instrument, causing the feedback tone to rise. The trainer encourages the patient to relax as she reshapes the feedback response.

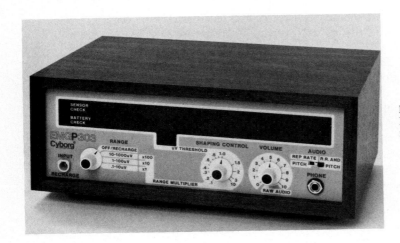

Figure 14-3. P303 EMG Trainer. Electromyographic feedback instrument used in my office.

THE DENTIST AND THE BIOFEEDBACK PRACTITIONER

The dentist, who recognizes the role of stress in the causation of dental disease, will not in most instances treat the stressful habits themselves, except in the most general way. Rather, the dentist usually works in association with a biofeedback practitioner. The role of the dentist, as that of any other medical specialist interfacing with biofeedback treatment, is one of diagnosis, treatment of any organic and structural elements of the disorder, and supervision of other medical aspects of the patient's progress, e.g., medication. Extremely critical variables are the manner in which the diagnosis is presented to the patient, including the clarity of the explanations given regarding the necessity and nature of the treatment and how well they are understood and accepted by the patient, as well as whether a supportive relationship is offered to the patient referred for biofeedback treatment. These are matters of considerable importance for the ultimate outcome of biofeedback therapy.

Consideration of the healing potential of the dentist is not without significance, especially in those instances when the condition of the patient points to deficits in stress management skills and capacity. Here the attention of any medical specialist must shift from a concern for the specifics of the medical disorder to an interest in the person manifesting the same. There is a perceptual shift, in Gestalt terms, from figure to ground. As Pasteur, father of the germ theory of disease, declared on his deathbed, "The pathogen is nothing; the terrain is everything." The oral habits of interest to the dentist, for instance, must include not only the patient's proper cleaning of teeth, but also the effective management of stress-induced muscle activity of the masticatory system.

The biofeedback trainer is an individual well-trained through personal experience as a biofeedback trainee. Many hours of training enable the biofeedback practitioner to understand intimately the subtle processes involved in the mastery of biofeedback skills. Hundreds of additional hours of experience in biofeedback therapy supervised by a licensed professional prepare the biofeedback trainer to communicate effectively the subtleties of voluntary self-regulation to the trainee. The biofeedback practitioner, who has personally mastered the skills of biofeedback and attention training, continually exhibits these skills through the manner in which he or she relates to the trainee. The trainee, therefore, receives nonverbal, as well as explicitly verbal, instruction from the biofeedback trainer.

Psychological Assessment and Program Interview

Stress control patients meet with the biofeedback trainer. Voluntary stress control education and the importance of daily practice are emphasized. The trainer and patient discuss the bruxing problem in depth, and also discuss other psychophysiological symptoms such as headaches, insomnia, and tics; past and present problems with anxiety and depression; personality characteristics such as perfectionism, rigidity, and compulsiveness; and a review of any experience in psychotherapy. Objective baselines of EMG activity are ascertained from the frontalis, temporalis, masseter, sternoclei-domastoid, trapezius, and forearm muscles.

Throughout the program, emphasis is placed on the importance of daily practice of attention, relaxation, and stress control skills. We explain that anxiety and tension result from chronic habits of attention. The patient will develop more flexible and relaxed habits of attention as an adaptive response to daily living, provided that he practices on a daily basis.

The common patient misperception that EMG biofeedback is a magical panacea is quickly refuted. We describe EMG as a new and effective monitor of muscular tension that has proven to be *one* useful aid in our training process. Thus the patient soon realizes that we are not offering a magical or mystical treatment but rather one that demands time and systematic training.

Patients are instructed to keep a daily log to rate the effectiveness of their daily practice sessions. These logs, collected by the trainer at each session, also serve to encourage home practice.

PAIN MANAGEMENT

For persons with chronic temporomandibular pain and dysfunction the pain itself is of as much clinical importance as the dental disorder.[6] These persons become mired in a vicious cycle of muscle tension→pain→increased muscle tension→chronic pain. Already overcontrolled in the manner with which they attend to experience, thus precipitating their tension and related pain, chronic pain patients relate to their pain itself with an even more rigid attentional style. The vicious pain cycle is thus more completely described as follows: overcontrolled attentional habits→tension→pain→chronically rigid attentional habits→chronic pain.

The pain patient knows no alternative for attention to the pain but to alternate between narrow, agitated focus on the pain and effortful focus away from the pain for the purposes of distraction, denial, and disassociation. In either case the pain rules the patient's attention: The person's attention is drawn to focus narrowly and exclusively on the pain or is driven to focus effortfully away from the pain.

Biofeedback-assisted attention training offers to the pain patient an alternative strategy for how to attend to the chronic pain and related symptoms. The person learns that a more broad and evenly distributed scope of attention, an open focus, can be maintained in the face of pain. Rather than allowing the pain to determine the person's attentional style, the person develops attentional flexibility in relation to the pain. Now free to attend in a way that fosters physiological normalization and resulting relaxation of chronically tense muscles, the individual is able to break the vicious cycle of pain. The person is on the way to recovery from both the chronic pain and the associated dental dysfunction.

DIAPHRAGMATIC BREATHING

Training for diaphragmatic breathing can be an important component of any dental practice. There is insufficient appreciation by professional and lay persons alike of the significance of improper breathing habits in the etiology of myofascial tension and related symptoms. Chronic, shallow, thoracic breathing is frequently observed in overcontrolled individuals who habitually brace the muscles of their face, neck, shoulders, and arms. Among the symptoms common to both myofascial pain syndrome and hyperventilation syndrome are dizziness, headaches, chest pain, ringing in the ears, and numbness and tingling of the face.[19] Interestingly, increased reactivity at the myoneural junction of the temporomandibular joint is a diagnostic indicator of hyperventilation syndrome.[3]

Excess involvement of the neck and chest in ordinary breathing can be demonstrated to the patient by asking that one hand be placed on the sternum, the other over the abdomen. Rise and fall of the chest, to the exclusion of the abdomen, suggests the presence of chronic, low-grade hyperventilation. By learning abdominal breathing through relaxing the diaphragm, the patient begins to facilitate relaxation of unnecessary neuromuscular activity in the upper torso and head.

CASE HISTORIES

The first case study involves a patient, Mr. P., who visited my office (A.J.C.) carrying a box containing five sets of full dentures. He was a very well-dressed man in his mid-fifties. Mr. P. was an extremely busy executive with many responsibilities. He complained bitterly about the profession of dentistry. "With all the progress in our modern age of technology and people going to the moon," he stated, "can't dentists make me a set of dentures I can wear?" He was wearing a sixth set of dentures, which were very uncomfortable. He had to pull them out of his mouth constantly to get a few minutes relief. His medical history was difficult to obtain because he saw no relation between his medical condition and his dentures. After obtaining his medical history. I found many symptoms of stress: He had gastric problems; he was on a strict diet; his blood pressure was 190/110; he could not sleep without barbiturates. The oral examination showed severe muscle spasm of the right and left internal and external pterygoids and pain in the back of his neck. The maxillary and mandibular ridges were in excellent condition; there was no evidence of any denture sore spots. Examination of his existing dentures showed very well-constructed appliances with adequate free-way space, good occlusion, and well-developed borders.

I explained to the patient, after a very thorough examination and evaluation of his problem, that I found that he had an excellent set of dentures upon which I could not improve. Owing to the stress he was under in his work, he was clenching his teeth and thereby cutting off the circulation in the underlying tissue, and that was why he was constantly taking them out of his mouth to get relief. His problem was not six bad dentists. I suggested our stress control program which he abruptly refused, stating that he was in complete control of his emotions and business problems and did not need any assistance. This program, he insisted, was for weak people. I refused to make another set of dentures, stating that I could not improve on his existing ones. I also did not want to be the seventh "bad" dentist he went to. He left my office rather despondent.

However, he then began to think about my comments. He became aware that he was indeed clenching his teeth, and he called several weeks later to make an appointment to start his stress control program.

He was repeatedly warned that this program would only be successful if he took it seriously, did his homework, and practiced on a continuing basis. He agreed, and started the program. Once he began stress control training, he cooperated fully and enthusiastically. He more than took it seriously—he exhibited the same obsessive-compulsive traits while learning the various relaxation techniques, that he applied to every other facet of his life. However, as a result of his vigorous attention to the training program, he stopped clenching and became very comfortable with his dentures.

The second case study deals with Mrs. A., who presented with a case of severe clenching and bruxism, accompanied by a history of tension headaches, nervousness, and constant fatigue. Recently divorced, she was caring for three teen-aged children. She was overwhelmed by the responsibility and burden, and she constantly called her former husband for assistance. All her teeth hurt; she had pain in the temporomandibular joint area and occasionally suffered from vertigo. She attempted to control these symptoms with Valium and Dramamine. She was introduced to the stress control program and appeared very receptive. After the second session she began to relax, but, at the same time, she became reluctant about her home practice, started cancelling appointments, and after five sessions dropped out of the program. A review of her case indicates that she apparently did not desire to get well. She probably wanted to keep her reasons for constantly calling her former husband and for being overwhelmed by dependency needs.

A review of these two cases underscores the fact that motivation, daily practice, and a desire to get well are key factors in learning and successfully applying stress control skills.

Where the stress control program is successful, the average bruxing patient is reacting favorably to a non-dental treatment for a problem traditionally thought to be dental. A commitment to the stress control program requires patient recognition and acceptance of maladaptive stress as a major factor in bruxism. Following the training, most patients generally report a dramatic reduction in pain, which is symptomatic of bruxism. This improvement is confirmed by my clinical evaluations so I do consider the stress control training a very helpful tool in the treatment of stress-induced muscle activity.

IDENTIFYING STRESS STIMULI

Since self-destructive oral habits such as clenching and bruxing are usually an unconscious response to stress, reducing their occurrence first requires that the patient be made aware of the habit and the stress situation causing it.[20] John Rugh, of the University of Texas at San Antonio, has designed a portable EMG unit, about the size of a pack of cigarettes, that the patient can wear in his normal environment. The electrodes are attached to the masseter muscle, and the feedback tone is provided via a small transistor radio earphone. The unit sounds a tone when the patient clenches or grinds his teeth.

During the course of relaxation training, the patient is given his instrument and advised to wear it during normal daytime activities for several days to help him identify what stress situation is causing him to clench and the nature and frequency of the habit. To study nocturnal bruxism, the device may be worn during sleep. It will awaken him when he grinds his teeth. Patients are frequently amazed to find how frequently they clench or grind their teeth.

CONCLUSIONS

Biofeedback training for voluntary relaxation of the masticatory system represents a significant advance in both treatment and prevention of many common dental disorders. Extensive clinical experience demonstrates that it promotes a successful cure by bringing the patient's inherent learning capacity to bear on these problems. As a preventive technique, it allows the patient to develop and retain healthy muscle habits. Therefore, this new application of biofeedback technology has a clear place in the practice of modern dentistry.

The methods we have outlined have been refined to the point where they can be offered in dental offices with relative ease. The instruments and training materials required are available at moderate cost and are convenient to use. Biofeedback relaxation procedures can usually be administered by a dental assistant after a short period of instruction. Thus, as the dentist proceeds with his accustomed treatment or prevention program, the patient can develop voluntary muscle control skills to complement the work.

The stress control program we have described combines elements from the disciplines of medicine, dentistry, and psychology. When such interdisciplinary methodology is applied, dentists become more than tooth carpenters: they become doctors of dental medicine.

References

1. Wolff, H.: Stress and Disease, 2nd ed. Springfield, Ill., Charles C Thomas, 1968.
2. Wilson, E.: How stress makes us ill. An invited address to the New Jersey Biofeedback Society, Rutgers University, December 6, 1981.
3. Cannistraci, A. J., and Fritz, G.: Dental applications of biofeedback. In J. Basmajian (ed.): Biofeedback—Principles and Practice for Clinicians, 2nd ed. Baltimore, Md., Williams & Wilkins Co., 1983.

4. Fehmi, L. G., and Fritz, G.: Open focus: The attentional foundation of health and well-being. Somatics, Spring, 1980.
5. Cannistraci, A.: Voluntary stress release and behavior therapy in the treatment of clenching and bruxism. New York, Bio-Monitoring Applications, Tape 5, 1974.
6. Rugh, J., and Solberg, W.: Psychological implications in temporomandibular pain and dysfunction. Oral Sci. Rev., 7:3, 1976.
7. Cannistraci, A.: Procedures for voluntary stress release and behavior therapy in the treatment of clenching and bruxism. New York, Bio-Monitoring Applications, Tape 13, 1975.
8. Shore, N.: Temporomandibular Joint Dysfunction and Occlusal Equilibration, 2nd ed. Philadelphia, J. B. Lippincott, 1976.
9. Cinotti, W., and Grieder, A.: Applied Psychology in Dentistry. St. Louis, C. V. Mosby, 1964.
10. Fritz, G., and Fehmi, L. G.: Open Focus Handbook: Strategies for Attention Training and Transfer to Everyday Activities. Princeton, N. J., Biofeedback Computers, Inc., 1982.
11. Fritz, G.: Therapeutic Awareness: Attention Training Strategies for Biofeedback Therapy. Published by the author, 1983.
12. Jacobson, E.: Anxiety and Tension Control. Philadelphia, J. B. Lippincott, 1964.
13. Schultz, J., and Luthe, W.: Autogenic Therapy, Vol. I. New York, Grune and Stratton, 1969.
14. Proctor, J.: Breathing and meditative techniques. New York, Bio-Monitoring Applications, Tape 12, 1975.
15. Benson, H.: The Relaxation Response. New York, Wm. Morrow & Co., 1975.
16. LeShan, L.: How to Meditate. New York, Bantam Books, 1974.
17. Rappaport, A., et al.: EMG feedback for the treatment of bruxism. (Unpublished.)
18. Forgione, A.: Psychological treatments of nocturnal bruxism. Delivered at the eighty-fourth annual convention of the American Psychological Association, Washington, D.C., September 6, 1976.
19. Compernolle, T., Hoogduin, K., and Joele, L.: Diagnosis and treatment of the hyperventilation syndrome. Psychosomatics, 20:612, 1979.
20. Rugh, J., and Solberg, W.: Electromyographic studies of bruxist behavior. Calif. Dent. Assoc. J., 3:56, 1975.

15

Myofunctional Therapy in the Treatment of the Craniomandibular Syndrome

LAWRENCE A. FUNT, D.D.S., M.S.D.
BRENDAN STACK, D.D.S., M.S.D.
SALLY GELB, B.A., M.F.T.
MAUREEN J. PIVARNICK, C.D.A., M.F.T.

The tongue exhibits a wide variety of special skills, such as taste control, creation of air currents to suck in liquids, and supervision of dental development. It is instrumental in directing the voice into articulated speech and serves as one of the bridges between the internal and external environment for the infant. It guides the food between the teeth during mastication and directs it into the pharynx in deglutition, although not always in the fashion for which it was functionally designed. We manage to abuse it by parching it with smoke, discoloring it with nicotine and antibiotics, freezing it with ice and ice cream, burning it with soup and pizza pies, biting it when frustrated, and sticking it out as a display of aggression.[1]

The term myofunctional therapy was introduced by B. E. Lischer. It was meant to encompass the prevention and treatment of malocclusion through the training and proper use of the head, neck, and tongue muscles, which to a great extent control and constrain the development and movement of the structures of the oral cavity. Orthopedists, as well as physical therapists, have used similar techniques to aid the restoration of muscular function and tonicity. In the field of speech therapy we have heard the term used, and some of these techniques have been applied in treatment. The science and study of speech therapy is a relatively recent evolutionary advance which is superimposed on the more basic mechanisms of respiration, mastication, and swallowing.

The most frequently used term applied to this abnormal behavior pattern is tongue thrust. Other terms used to describe this behavior are deviate swallow, reverse swallow, perverted swallow, deviant deglutition, visceral swallow, infantile swallow, and abnormal swallow. According to Barrett and Hanson[1] the term tongue thrust describes the behavioral problem simply and effectively.

Many authors have noted that teeth are in a state of dynamic balance because the tongue and facial muscles essentially are in equilibrium.[2] Muscle equilibrium can neither anticipate nor correct malocclusion, since malocclusion may also exhibit a state of dynamic balance.

In order to be able to anticipate and correct malocclusion, the total functional phenomenon has to be understood. The teeth and their associated bony structures interact with a network of muscles. A brief review of these muscles is always beneficial.[3] The buccinator muscle attempts to surround the dentition, roughly in the shape of a horseshoe. It is more or less continuous with and anchored into the lips by the fibers of the orbicularis oris muscle, which act as the closing or sphincter muscle of the mouth. It is attached above the alveolar process in the maxilla and below the molars in the mandible, and it is fastened posteriorly on each side of the jaw by the pterygomandibular raphe. The open end of the buccinator envelope posteriorly is closed by the superior pharyngeal constrictor, which anchors on the occipital bone. Three other muscles may be said to affect the mouth; the risorius muscles, which draw the angles of the mouth laterally; the triangularis (depressor anguli oris) muscles, which pull the mouth angles down; and the mentalis muscle, which is attached to the alveolar process just below the lower incisors and to the skin of the chin. The tongue lies within the dentition in the oral cavity and is connected posteriorly to the styloid process through the stylohyoid and digastric muscles. Its anterior support is made up of the geniohyoid, digastric, and mylohyoid muscles.

The jaws close by contraction and open upon relaxation of the masseter, medial pterygoid, and anterior temporal muscles. The masseter attaches above to a special portion of the temporal bone (the zygomatic arch) and at its lower end to the mandibular ramus. The temporal muscles attach to the head and extend downward to the anterior border of the ascending ramus and coronoid process. The medial or internal pterygoid is attached to the medial surface of the angle of the mandible and also to the sphenoid bone (pterygoid fossa) at the base of the skull.

The mouth opens by a combination of gravitational force, contraction of the lateral or external pterygoid muscles, digastric and other hyoid muscles (suprahyoid), and a concomitant controlled relaxation of the temporal, masseter, and (internal) pterygoid muscles. The external pterygoid and temporal muscles also operate to move the mandible from side to side. Closing, essentially a vertical motion of the jaws, is produced by contraction of the temporal, masseter, and internal pterygoid muscles. To move the mandible outward into protrusion, the external pterygoid muscles contract as the opening muscles relax. To move the mandible inward (retrusion) the posterior fibers of the temporal, as well as the hyoid and digastric muscles, contract. The buccinator and constrictor act primarily in a horizontal direction. The tongue, along with its associated muscles, is the main thrusting force opposing the action of the buccinator and orbicularis oris muscles.

When the muscles which close the mouth are relaxed, the tongue sometimes rests on the cingulum of the lower anterior teeth and sometimes on the palate in the roof of the mouth. In normal deglutition the teeth are in contact and the tip of the tongue is positioned just posterior to the anterior teeth on the palate. The middle portion of the tongue presses against the palate. At the same time, the masseters are in a somewhat clenched tension, the buccinator muscles are in normal resting tension, and the orbicularis oris muscles are relaxed. However, during normal breathing (i.e., through the nose), the tongue is in much the same position and the muscles are in normal resting tensions.

When a patient swallows abnormally, the teeth often are out of contact, and the tongue is forced between the teeth. As a result, the masseter muscles contract incompletely and there is a concomitant variable state of tension of the orbicularis oris and buccinator muscles. This lack of coordination is caused by interference created by the tongue being out of position. In abnormal breathing, such as mouth breathing, the tongue is usually depressed and the upper and lower teeth are apart during swallowing. As a result of this pattern, abnormal deglutition ensues. The muscles contract irregularly, resulting in abnormal displacement of the lips and cheeks. Consequently, hundreds of force vectors are created by abnormal swallowing patterns. It then becomes obvious that in the correction or prevention of malocclusion, the coordination of the surrounding muscles is of utmost importance.

HISTORICAL REVIEW

As early as 1839 LeFoulon stated that the many causes of irregularities of teeth were "sounds of speech in which the tongue strikes against the upper anterior teeth pushing them forward."[4] In 1873 Tomes[5] prescribed the concept of balance of labiolingual muscle forces which suggested that the physical forces of the lips and tongue satisfactorily account for the form of the dental arch. It was not until 1906 when Rogers[6] stated that, if children lived in a normal and healthy environment, facial inharmonies and malocclusion would become much less prevalent, and those orofacial organs which were permitted to degenerate would have to be artificially stimulated to restore their normal function. It was Lischer[7] who suggested the name *myofunctional therapy*.

Monson[8] in 1921 called attention to the difficulty occurring in deglutition as a result of a closed bite with a reduction in the mouth space and subsequent lack of tongue room. Nove[9] reported on the reduced mouth space, anthropologically noting that morphological changes of a recessive nature that have taken place in human development result in a tendency toward contraction of the dental arches, which causes a malrelated dentition with a concomitant behavior pattern change in swallowing. He observed further that there is a physiological ideal act of swallowing concurrent with maximal postnasal drainage and an adopted type of swallowing which intends to inhibit postnasal drainage.[10] Regarding the normal act of swallowing, Nove stated: "This effortless synergy of action can take place only when all the structure units connected with mastication, deglutition, and respiration are faultlessly integrated, that is, when the skeletal framework of the 'masticatory face' is fully developed and the maxillae are in correct relationship. When at physiological rest all the musculature concerned (reciprocal antagonists) remains in a state of equilibrium with the mandible, the hyoid bone forming a fulcrum or pivotal centre."[9]

A very comprehensive report describing tongue-thrust swallow as opposed to a normal swallow was published by Truesdell and Truesdell in 1937.[11] They believed that the etiological factor of tongue thrust was related to infected or sore tonsils or to other factors which interfered with the forward movement of the tongue. Their therapy was to instruct the patient to swallow with the teeth in occlusion, "letting nature work out the details." They believed that by telling the patient what the normal swallow is, he or she will learn to do it by direct application under supervision.

Rix[12] in 1946 published the first of a series of articles describing a teeth-apart swallow, which was described as the tongue between the teeth against the tensed muscles of the lips and cheeks. He attributed the etiology of the tongue-thrust swallow to retention of the infantile swallowing pattern, swollen tonsils, or upper respiratory infection. He stated that lisps were always accompanied by abnormal swallowing.

Gwynne-Evans[13] in 1947 experimented with a monoblock for treatment of tongue thrust. He hypothesized that the monoblock would contain the tongue reflexively, thereby correcting the reflex pattern. Seven years later he retracted this hypothesis, noting that the monoblock did not correct atypical swallowing.[14] He thought normal swallowing behavior was somatic and atypical swallowing patterns were visceral, reflecting the visceral origin of the orofacial muscles. He also made a great point of contrasting sucking and suckling. Suckling is the nursing activity of the infant, another inborn reflex, whereas sucking is acquired through a learning process at a later age.

Gratzinger,[15] discussing treatment of periodontal disease, pointed out cases in which "dynamic irritation" was produced by lack of balance between the muscles of the tongue and the muscles of the cheeks and lips. His therapy in these cases included muscle exercises to strengthen the muscles of the cheeks and lips. These exercises consisted of extension and contraction of the orbicularis oris muscle with and without resistance, practiced three times a day, 20 to 50 exercises each time.

Ballard[16] wrote a number of articles relating to the orofacial musculature. He believed that everything affecting orofacial structures occurs reflexively, but his use of the term "reflex" is not as we usually understand it. He felt strongly that all muscle behavior is centrally controlled and impervious to environmental factors. He stated that all muscle forces, normal and abnormal, are inherited, and that reeducation has no useful purpose in orthodontic therapy.

Tulley's[17] research utilizing electromyography and cinefluorography convinced him that certain types of abnormal function are endogenous, but he believed that they were few and might be caused by neuromuscular impairment. He became more optimistic, believing that orthodontic correction of the occlusion would spontaneously correct the adaptive and habitual types, and he suggested that patients with endogenous abnormalities might be helped to reach their growth potential. He worked out a rudimentary classification of eight basic types of abnormal behavior with Gwynne-Evans in 1956.[18]

Straub[19] may be said to have been the individual who started the modern phase of myofunctional therapy. He first presented the theory of bottle feeding as the sole etiological factor of perverted swallowing. He lectured extensively throughout the country, alerting orthodontists to the influence of the tongue on the orofacial musculature. He made many contributions to the literature; some were valid, others misleading, and still others erroneous. Straub[19, 20] grouped abnormal patterns into a classification of types, and he devised a therapy program which was utilized by many clinicians. He stated that treatment should be accompanied by reeducating the 22 muscles that are used in normal swallowing. Retraining was achieved by a series of 16 lessons developed by Straub that "correct not only the habit but also the soft tissues that are involved."

Quantitative estimates were made for maximum lip or cheek pressures by Kydd[21] and for physiological activities by Parfitt[22] and by Winders.[23] Most of these studies dealt with maximum pressure values only. Winders, measuring the forces on subjects with clinically excellent dentitions, found that the tongue exerted more pressure on the dentition than did the buccal tissues. Kydd reported an imbalance in lingual and buccal pressure.

Gould and Picton,[24] using strain gauge pressure transducers, reported considerable variation in lip and cheek pressures in all the series of standard exercises. A later study of theirs[25] showed greater forces acting on the first premolars than on the labial surfaces of maxillary and mandibular incisors or the first molars. All subjects had normal occlusions. Interestingly, more force was recorded on the right premolars than on the left at rest and during the swallowing exercise. In a still later study, Gould and Picton[26] expanded their studies to include groups of ten subjects with Angle's Class II, Division 1, Class II, Division 2, and Class III malocclusions with corresponding skeletal abnormalities. The mean values for Class III and Class II, Division 2 were similar to those for the normal group. However, the Class II, Division 1 group had wider variations of peak pressures. They considered this variation to be related to the subjects attempting to seal the lips in compensation for the skeletal discrepancies and associated incompetence of their lips.

In 1964 Profitt and coworkers,[27] also using strain gauge cantilever transducers, recorded pressures both labial and lingual to the maxillary central incisors and lingual to the maxillary first molars. Consistent patterns of pressure application during swallowing were noted for each person, but there were large differences between individuals. A later study[28] involving five- to eight-year old children showed that each child consistently loaded either the left or the right side of the palate more heavily, being, in effect, right or left "tongued." This was also observed in a study with adults.[29]

Harvold[30] reported on neuromuscular function studies in animals. When a 2-centimeter-long wedge was removed from the center section of the tongue of a rhesus monkey, crowding of the teeth and a deepening of the bite occurred. Another group of animals had a piece of plastic placed in the palatal vault between the right and left molars, but not touching the mandibular teeth during function. The sensation of plastic resulted in an immediate lowering of the mandible. Within a year's time the animals exhibited an anterior open bite and an increased gonial angle, but they showed no evidence of a Class II malocclusion. Another group of animals had a similar piece of plastic placed in the palatal vault between the right and left premolars, but it interfered with the occlusion. The animal had to move the mandible forward 2 to 3 millimeters to masticate easily. Immediate response was a lowering of the mandibles, indentations of the tongues; 8 to

10 months later, with skeletal adaptation, all animals developed a severe overbite, overjet, and Class II malocclusion.

From 1962 to 1973, Subtelny and Subtelny[31] cited cineradiographic studies and demonstrated that protrusion of the tongue through the incisors and incomplete closure of molars are normal. They also stated that tongue thrusting is a maturational problem influenced by age, oropharyngeal level, oral habits, and environmental influences. The Subtelnys said that thumb-sucking is also a causative factor of an open bite because it creates an opening for the tip of the tongue to protrude through during deglutition. They felt tongue thrust was the result rather than the cause of frontal malocclusion.[31] It may be stated that they believed that form determined function. They felt that growth and development could solve occlusal problems, which they called open bite problems. Our experience has shown that it is erroneous to infer that a similar remission will occur in other kinds of occlusal problems in the presence of orofacial muscle imbalance and abnormal swallowing problems. Many cases of occlusal relapse that follow dental intervention have been clearly recognized as related to orofacial muscle imbalance and the abnormal swallowing habit. Our experience has led us to the firm belief that establishing normal function of the orofacial muscles significantly contributes to the successful and permanent correction of occlusal disharmonies.

It was not until the last decade that myofunctional therapy really came into its own. The courses and lectures given by Garliner, Langer, Hanson, and Barrett have helped to educate and train dentists, physicians, speech therapists, and myofunctional therapists. These same individuals have written extensively, and their books are available to all for reference.[1, 32, 33]

We truly owe these individuals a debt of gratitude for the time and effort they have put into teaching us how to deliver a better health service to our patients.

DIAGNOSIS

Without questions there would be no answers and without problems there would be no conclusions. Our problem was that we were presented with various forms of open bite problems in adult dentitions, and these open bite problems had persisted through the following: (1) transitional dentition without treatment; (2) transitional dentition with orthodontic interception; (3) adult dentition without treatment; (4) adult dentition with orthodontic interception; (5) adult dentition with or without orthodontic treatment and with the presence of the craniomandibular dysfunction syndrome (CMDS).

Our initial concern was not with the cause of the open bite, but rather its existence and persistence. In the presence of open bite conditions, how could we even hope to restore these dentitions into functioning units? If we could, what would be the prognosis of stability? For how long? Would other areas become involved? The questions began to mount.

For many years we experienced complete orthodontic closure of open bites only to have them open up in retention! We saw patients with severe anterior open bites (with accompanying anterior tongue thrust) that would almost close with orthodontic treatment but not quite all the way. We also saw patients with moderate to severe anterior open bites (with anterior tongue thrust) that would be completely closed anteriorly; as the anterior bite closure proceeded, however, a posterior open bite emerged. We were aware that approximately 75 per cent of our pain patients had anterior and/or posterior tongue thrust prior to treatment. We also observed the relative stability of our non-open bite non-thrusting CMDS patients and a significant degree of relapse tendency in our CMDS patients with tongue thrust with or without open bite patterns.

Our problems began to become more apparent and also began to fall into various categories.

Diagnostic Criteria

Diagnosis is "the discrimination of diseases by their distinctive marks or symptoms."[34] Did distinctive marks or symptoms exist? If they existed could they be observable differences, distinctive enough to be selective and separable?

Our diagnostic procedures begin as the patient enters our consultation area. We then have the opportunity to view the *entire* patient and to start to collect observable differences.

General Observations

1. **Walking posture.** The position of the head and shoulders (Fig. 15–1) reveals the absence or presence of muscle splinting patterns causing the head to be carried in a tipped position and the shoulders elevated on one side more than the other. A high shoulder position will generally indicate a probable presence of scoliosis. Direct observation or palpation of the spine would be necessary to confirm or deny our initial observation.

2. **Facial movement.** The most apparent visual sign is the "grimace" (Fig. 15–2). Barrett and Garliner both refer to this facial muscle pattern and

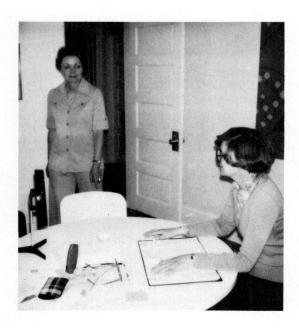

Figure 15–1. Observation of walking posture.

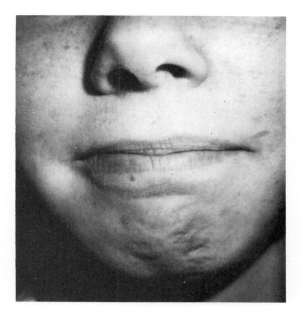

Figure 15–2. Grimace.

it is present in almost all of our muscle imbalance patterns. A tongue thrust can also be present *without* an observable grimace.

3. **EXTERNAL BREATHING PATTERN.** Many times, if the patient is not aware he is being observed, the mandible may then be in a dropped position and the lips apart. If the patient realizes he is being viewed for this problem, he will then try to compensate by tightly holding the lips together in a stressful position (Fig. 15–3).

4. **LIP POSTURE.** A lip roll (eversion) involving either the lower lip (Fig. 15–4) or the upper and lower lips (Fig. 15–5) also begins to suggest deviate swallowing problems. A mentalis crease (Fig. 15–6) can be associated with

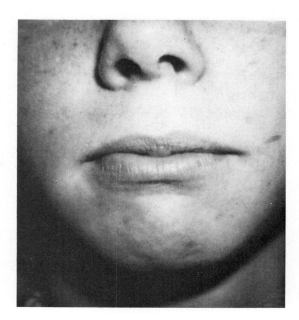

Figure 15–3. Stressed lip position.

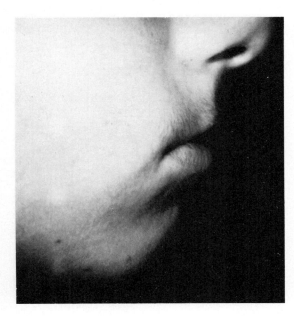

Figure 15–4. Lower lip eversion.

the lower lip eversion. The texture (chapping) of the lip tissue could indicate the presence of mouth breathing.

5. TONGUE POSTURE (EXTERNAL AND INTERNAL). The rest position of the tongue basically involves the following three detrimental positions:

(A) The tongue rests *within* the mandibular arch and the lips are in contact. When swallowing is initiated, the active position of the tongue can then be either: (1) low and within the arch; (2) thrust anteriorly between the teeth; (3) thrust unilaterally between the posterior teeth; (4) thrust bilaterally between the posterior teeth; (5) thrust fully between the maxillary and mandibular dentition.

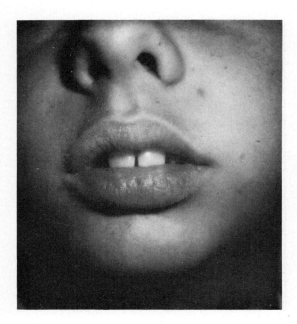

Figure 15–5. Upper and lower lip eversion.

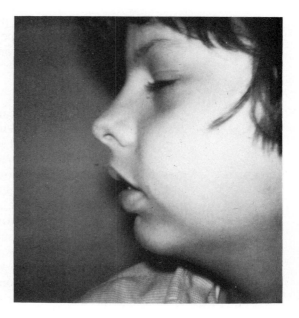

Figure 15–6. Mentalis crease.

(B) The tongue rests *between* the arches, the lips are apart or together. The tongue either fully covers the mandibular incisal and occusal surfaces (Fig. 15–7A) or else it unilaterally covers the incisal and occlusal surfaces, involving segments of the arch extending from the lateral incisor to the most posterior molar, always in direct sequence (i.e., 2–3, 2–4, 2–5, 2–6; 3–4, 3–5, 3–6, 3–7; 4–6, 4–7).

The swallowing pattern in full coverage of the arch can be accomplished with the lips apart or together. Swallowing in unilateral coverage can only be accomplished with full lip closure.

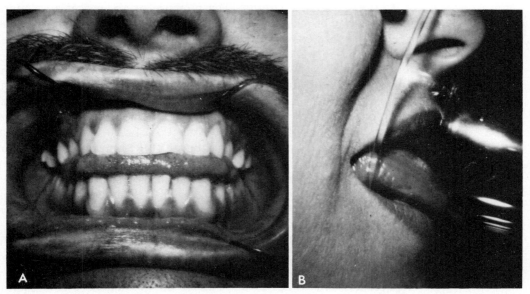

Figure 15–7. *A,* Full coverage of lower anterior and posterior occlusal surfaces. *B,* Tongue position while drinking, observed through a clear glass.

(C) The tongue rests in a position where it is in almost constant contact with the lower lip, and the superior surface of the tongue touches the incisal and/or lingual surfaces of the anterior teeth.

Physical Structures

1. NOSE. A flattened appearance of both alae of the nose should indicate nasal allergies, whereas a flattening of only one side might indicate structural damage or blockage (deviated septum).

2. PALATAL ARCH. The shape of the palatal vault can be normal in the presence of a suspected swallowing pattern. However, if the palate is high and narrow, we may then begin to appreciate the contribution made by the tongue in its rest position and in full deviate swallowing function.

3. PALATAL AND PHARYNGEAL REFLEXES. It has been our experience that the palatal reflex is *not* usually present in tongue thrusters, whereas the pharyngeal reflex is almost always present but in a more diminished dimension. You will also encounter on occasion an anesthetic throat that will not react to any form of stimulation.

4. RUGAE. In the absence of palatal pressure by the tongue, the rugae tend to increase in numbers, developing a deep ridged appearance. Pairs of these rugae extend posteriorly on the hard palate.

Direct Observation

1. DEPRESSING THE LIP. As you place your index finger on the pharyngeal area of the neck and your thumb tip gently on the lower lip, ask the patient to swallow, and as the swallow pattern initiates, quickly but lightly force the lower lip down. You will then note one of the following: (1) the appearance of the tip of the tongue; (2) the tongue will retract and the mandible will elevate to full or partial closure; (3) the inability to depress the lower lip due to extreme lip muscle resistance; or (4) normal function.

2. LATERAL TONGUE THRUST. The presence or absence of a unilateral tongue thrust may or may not be revealed by depression of the lower lip as described above; however, the cheek on the affected side will generally pull in during the initial swallowing pattern.

3. MASSETER-ANTERIOR TEMPORAL REFLEX. The masseters and the anterior portion of the temporalis muscles *do* contract in deviant swallowing patterns, since the jaw has to be postured in order to compensate for the tongue-lip or tongue-lip-cheek seal pattern of the thruster.

4. DRINKING BEHAVIOR. When the patient is asked to drink from a clear glass there are two very typical observations: (1) the tongue tip will rest on the rim and the lower lip will roll (Fig. 15–7B); and (2) just at the moment the cup is lowered, the tongue will remain and then quickly retract.

5. PAYNE'S BLACK LIGHT.[33] A fluorescein dye is placed on the strategic parts of tongue. Patient swallows and by the use of the ultraviolet light we can trace the excursions of the tongue.

6. LIP GAUGE (see Figure 15–18). The force scale is not a scientific instrument but best symptomatic instrument used to measure resistive strength.

7. MYOSCANNER (Fig. 15–8). This is an instrument for measuring physiological strength of muscles. Using the myoscanner, we can measure

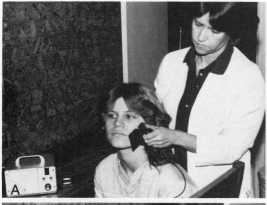
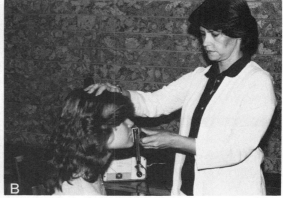
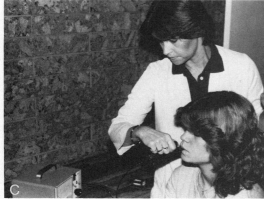

Figure 15–8. Use of a myoscanner.

compressive lip strength, masseters, and tongue muscles. Normal measurements for instrument are as follows:

Masseters (adults)	0.6–0.8 lb
Masseters (children)	0.4–0.6 lb
Tongue (adults)	0.8–1.2 lb
Tongue (children)	0.6–0.8 lb
Compressive Lip Strength (adults)	0.6–0.8 lb
Compressive Lip Strength (children)	0.2–0.4 lb

CLASSIFICATION OF TYPES OF TONGUE THRUST

There are a number of systems used in describing tongue thrust types.[17, 20] *All of these classifications are a description of muscular malfunction, creating oral deformities, and resulting in postural problems!*

The two classifications we find most clinically useful are those of Garliner[33] and Barrett.[1]

Classification of Garliner:
1. Simple anterior swallow.
2. Complete swallow problem.
3. Open bite problem:
   (a) dental.
   (b) skeletal.

4. Bimaxillary protrusion.
5. Class III occlusal problem.
   (a) pseudo class III.
   (b) skeletal class III.
6. Closed bite occlusal problem.
7. Unilateral swallowing problem.
8. Bilateral swallowing problem.

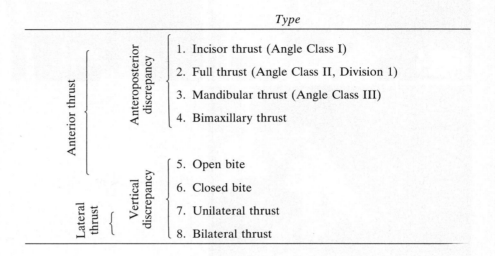

		Type
Anterior thrust	Anteroposterior discrepancy	1. Incisor thrust (Angle Class I)
		2. Full thrust (Angle Class II, Division 1)
		3. Mandibular thrust (Angle Class III)
		4. Bimaxillary thrust
Lateral thrust	Vertical discrepancy	5. Open bite
		6. Closed bite
		7. Unilateral thrust
		8. Bilateral thrust

THE CRANIOMANDIBULAR PAIN SYNDROME

We mentioned earlier that approximately 75 per cent of our dysfunction patients had either anterior or posterior open bites and tongue thrusting habits. A more accurate description of their dental problems would be a *loss of vertical dimension,* usually unilaterally. The diagnosis or even recognition of this type of open bite and concomitant loss of vertical dimension is very apparent. We also found that the vertical loss involved not only *the dentition* but also *adjoining skeletal structures.* We believe this maxillomandibular asymmetry also involves the skeletal developmental pattern of the *whole head, face,* and *mandibular bones.*

The best description and explanation of this aforementioned pattern can be explained by the following quotation of Barrett and Hanson:[1]

Although the minimum level of action potential in the muscle is found during the rest position, we must not consider this state as one of absolute rest. Rather, slight contraction, supplied throughout by the tonus mechanism, maintains the structures in a given alignment. It represents a state of equilibrium between opposing muscles, and between muscles and the force of gravity.

The orofacial rest position is not a constant posture from one individual to the next, nor is it a static condition within the individual. It is a variable relationship influenced by various factors. Muscle tonus, and thus placement, varies with body posture, activity of the moment, age, pathological conditions, etc. It is certainly responsive to function and to the overall development of the musculature.

Posture is the foundation of function: every muscle movement is influenced, to a greater or lesser degree, by the posture from which the movement began and to which it returns. Once deglutition has been retrained, the physiological resting position of the various structures involved form the single greatest determinant of either continued normal function or eventual relapse.

It is our clinical experience that tongue thrusts are a contributing factor to the CMDS, and the persistence of the tongue thrust imprisons the maxillo-mandibular relationship in a state of imbalance and instability.

Myofunctional therapy is therefore very necessary in stabilizing our musculoskeletal relationships and therefore controlling the reflex pain of the craniomandibular syndrome.

TREATMENT

Before treatment commences for orofacial muscle imbalance and an abnormal swallow, all perverse habits must be corrected. The most common of these are thumbsucking, pacifier sucking, lip or finger sucking, tongue sucking, and nail biting. Not to be forgotten is the prolonged keeping of objects in the mouth, e.g., pencils or a pipe. The pressure of the thumb, pacifier, or finger as it hits against the alveolar bone contributes significantly to the anterior protrusion as well as to malpositioning of the tongue during the act of swallowing.[1]

A cross-sectional and longitudinal study was made on 1258 children from the Burlington Growth Center in Burlington, Ontario, evaluating the relationship between oral habits and occlusion. Of the 462 children with a sucking habit, 19.9 per cent were finger suckers, 70.6 per cent were thumb suckers, and 9.5 per cent were blanket suckers. If the sucking habit was stopped before age 6, the effects on occlusion were often transitory. In the serial sample none of the children who stopped a habit after age 6 had a normal occlusion at age 12. Thumbsucking and finger sucking pushed the maxillary teeth and alveolar process forward and produced a greater disparity between the upper and lower teeth. In children who stopped sucking before age 6, the percentage of Class II malocclusions was still higher than that of those in the non-habit group.[2]

Breaking the Oral Habit

There are certain criteria necessary before attempting to correct an oral habit.

1. The patient must be a willing subject, at least 5 to 6 years of age, who can verbalize to the therapist the desire to correct his habit.

2. The parent must be willing to cooperate and to allow extra time with the child, particularly at bedtime.

3. The child must sleep at home for the next two-week period.

Once the above are present, the following materials are needed to begin therapy:

1. A 2″ elastic bandage
2. Three safety pins
3. A ½″ canvas backed adhesive tape
4. A bright magic marker
5. A chart made by the child

The immediate concern of the therapist is to correct night-time sucking habits; therefore, at the initial visit he or she explains that the child is going to be "helped" to conquer the problem with "reminders." The therapist

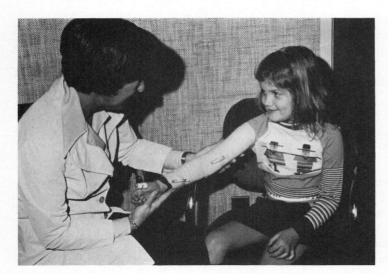

Figure 15–9.

then demonstrates how the parent is to wrap the elastic bandage tightly around the involved arm one-half inch from the shoulder to one-half inch above the wrist (Fig. 15–9). The bandage should be tight enough to make the arm tingle but not so tight as to cut off circulation. Two strips of adhesive tape are then wrapped around the involved finger. One strip is placed above the knuckle and one below. If the child shows no preference between fingers or thumbs, it is best to place a bandage on each arm and to put tape on the involved fingers or thumbs. Then the child is told to put the wrapped finger in the mouth to show that no restraints are being used. A few dots are made on the tape with the magic marker; if they have remained unsmeared in the morning, the child is sure to have had a successful night and should be praised. A star is placed on the chart (Fig. 15–10), and a telephone call should be made to the therapist. There is nothing more exciting to a child than this early morning phone call. If the news is negative, the therapist should be understanding of the difficult task and encourage the child to do

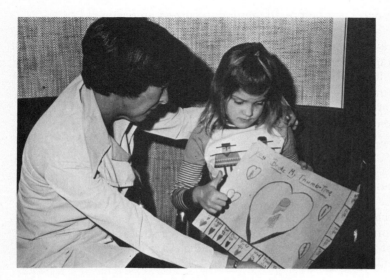

Figure 15–10.

better the following night. The child must complete ten successful nights before he is rewarded. This in itself is too short a period of time to accept as a permanent pattern change, but if the child feels he has conquered the problem he is well on his way to success. It is not unusual for a child to receive two or three stars in a row then suddenly relapse. If this situation occurs, the child must begin the chart again, and, upon completion of the ten successful nights, the chart is brought to the therapist for praise and reward. Gradually the reminders are omitted. The first night after this visit with the therapist the bandage is taken off, and several nights later the tape is removed. (The child must not build up dependency on these aids so that he feels incapable of resisting his thumb or finger without them.) Some children, particularly the older ones, need the reinforcement of speaking to the therapist twice a day during the first week; the therapist should always be receptive and confident in the child's ability to succeed.

Daytime sucking is generally not a difficult habit to break once sucking at night has been conquered. A finger puppet, either purchased or hand-made (with the aid of a tongue depressor and adhesive tape) should be in view at all times (Fig. 15–11). Generally it sits on the TV set or in the child's room, and whenever the child needs to suck a finger he puts on his finger puppet. Parents should try to spend time with the child in the late afternoon and at bedtime, because at these times the child is usually more tired and this leads him to suck his thumb. It is important to note that oral habits do apply to adults as well as children and treatment modality is the same.

Upon the patient's cessation of sucking, an evaluation should be made to determine whether myofunctional therapy needs to be introduced. The case must be evaluated in a "holistic" manner. In some instances, therapy should begin immediately, especially if the incisors have erupted and the tongue is a moving or impeding force and if the orbicularis oris muscles and masseter muscles are weak.

In other cases, it may be desirable to observe the patient periodically to ascertain whether there is spontaneous self-improvement.[4] In situations where lip seal is impossible because of severe labial displacement of upper anteriors, interceptive orthodontic retraction is necessary. When a unilateral

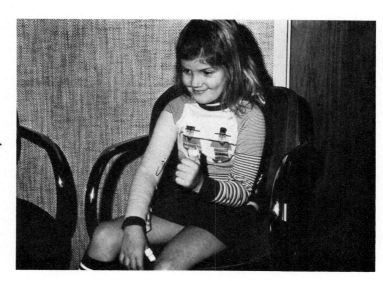

Figure 15–11.

or bilateral cross bite is present, you then either treat the *dental* cross bite or those cases of *skeletal* cross bite orthodontically. (See Chapter 10.)

The full extent of therapy for abnormal deviant swallow lasts one year and consists of the following two phases: (1) the intensive retraining of the tongue and associated muscles, and (2) the follow-up period in which the patient retrains the muscles to make the act of swallowing truly subconscious and automatic.

The first three months consist of 24 semi-weekly sessions in which the patient is given exercises in sequence to retrain and strengthen the tongue. These visits are an important unit unto themselves, a base upon which subsequent therapy is developed and maintained. During this time the patient learns the correct method of swallowing, but it is only after this time period that he can make a habit of what he has learned.

After three months, the patient visits the therapist every week and, as he displays proficiency, the visits become less frequent until the therapist only sees the patient once a month. Occasionally, a patient will relapse if he has not completed or followed up his intensive training program. The therapist must use his or her own judgment to discern how often patients must be seen when they need extra encouragement and reinforcement. During this lengthy nine-month period, the patient must gain experience and total familiarity with his readjusted swallowing position. He should be able to correct himself and to do additional exercises the therapist recommends. But most importantly, by the sixth month or so, the patient should feel that his new swallow is comfortable and right in his mouth, that it is now a subconscious act, a habit. Once the patient achieves automation he has successfully completed treatment.

Exercises for the Tongue

To enhance the function and tonicity of the tongue it is necessary to strengthen the intrinsic and extrinsic muscles.

TONGUE POINTING EXERCISES. Using a hand mirror, patient is instructed to make a "point" with the tongue by pushing it out of the mouth and not allowing the lips to support it. Using the point of the tongue patient is instructed to outline the lips and point the tongue from corner to corner.

Exercises for the Lips

Exercises that reposition lips do not necessarily strengthen them. Angle observed that when lips close in normal alignment the lower lip rests against the labial surface of the upper incisors, and therefore it is the upper teeth that establish the curve of the lower lip, and the lower lip establishes the curve of the upper teeth.

Certain muscles have been overdeveloped and others remain flaccid and underdeveloped. Immediately before practicing lip exercises, the patient should pump hot salt water behind the upper lip, the lower lip, and into each cheek two or three times a day, using 3 or 4 ounces of water (Fig. 15–12). This increases the blood supply and stretches and relaxes the muscles, allowing the lips to gain better tonicity.

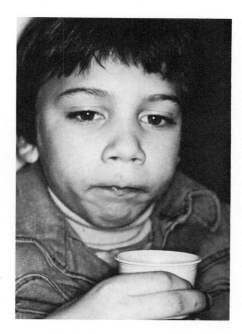

Figure 15–12.

To Extend Upper Lip

STRETCHING THE FIBERS. Place thumbs under the upper lip, directly under the nostrils. Pull down upper lip with force, using the index fingers. Midway through the exercise, wrinkle the nose in order to resist. Continue to stretch upper lip over teeth (Fig. 15–13 A to E).

COTTON ROLLS. For the short upper lip, lower lip, or the overdeveloped mentalis. The cotton roll is wetted and inserted behind the lip to be corrected (Fig. 15–14). These rolls come in different sizes, and many times a small size must be inserted initially. These rolls should be left inside the lip for an hour at a time.

TO STRENGTHEN BOTH LIPS. Two buttons the size of a quarter are tied to either end of a string about a foot long. The button is placed on the labial surface of the incisors, held in place only by the lips themselves. The idea is to pull the button out of the opponent's lips (Fig. 15–15). Adult patients generally prefer doing the exercise by themselves with a single button.

MARSHMALLOW TWIST. Named because it was originally performed with marshmallows. Nowadays special string and discs have been designed. This exercise strengthens both lips; the patient places one end of the string behind his teeth and holds it in place by the tongue (Fig. 15–16). The lips do all the work by stretching over the string and pulling it into the mouth until all the string is in the mouth. The patient begins with one disc at the end of the string, and, as his lips grow stronger, he or she adds a disc at a time, until he is able to pull up all ten. This exercise is done while the patient is bending over at the waist, with hands behind him.

LIP PRESS. This simple exercise can be done by pressing the lips together for several moments and then releasing the pressure (Fig. 15–17). This exercise can be repeated many times during the day to build up pressure in both upper and lower lips. Adults particularly enjoy this exercise and can do it any time during the day.

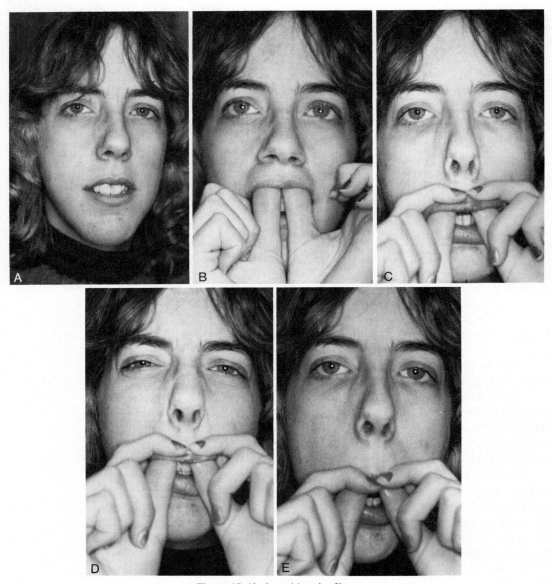

Figure 15–13. Stretching the fibers.

Figure 15–14.

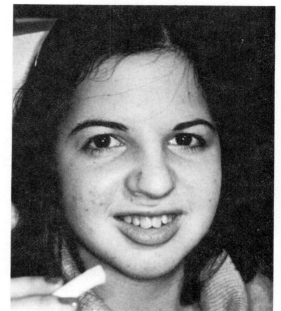

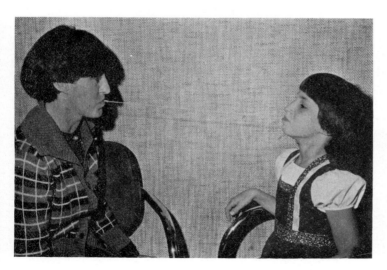

Figure 15–15.

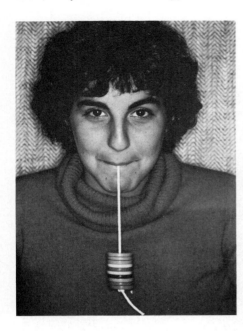

Figure 15–16.

In some instances lips can grow stronger, but the habit of sitting with the lips parted in rest position may still be present. In these cases, additional aids are used. The lip zipper, as this next exercise is commonly called, is a favorite.

LIP ZIPPER. A small disc is placed between the lips against the labial surface of the upper incisors, and an additional disc is added every few days until five discs are being held for at least a half-hour a day. Television watching is an excellent time to practice this exercise (Fig. 15–18).

ORAL SCREEN. This is another habit breaker. A small piece of polyethylene can be cut to fit inside the lips. Teeth and lips must occlude, but now it is impossible for the patient's tongue to thrust out through their mouth. *This should never be used in the presence of nasal blockage.*

Each month the patient is tested with the lip gauge and a chart is kept to show the patient his rate of improvement (Fig. 15–19). During the first

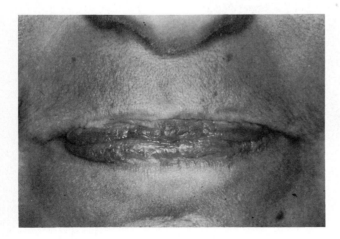

Figure 15–17.

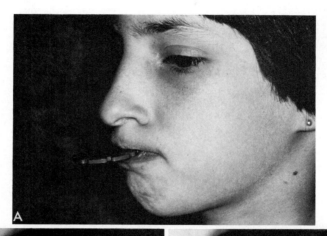

Figure 15–18.

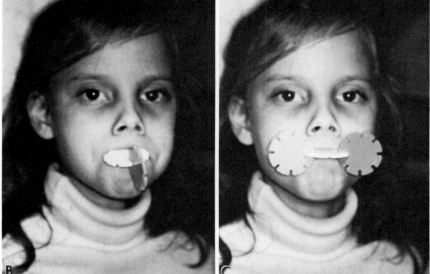

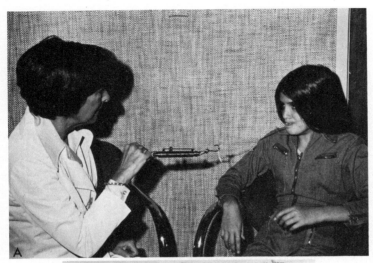

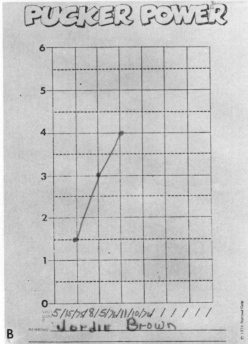

Figure 15–19.

few months this is usually very significant. The chart is exciting for the patient and an immediate way to initiate motivation.

The following exercises are merely guidelines for therapy. It would be impossible to give a specific course of therapy, since each patient presents with different problems.

Repositioning of the Tongue

TONGUE TIP EXERCISES. Tongue push-ups are an initial exercise to strengthen the tip of the tongue and familiarize the patient with the correct placement of the tip of the tongue to an area referred to as "the spot" (Fig. 15–20). This spot is on the anterior palate directly behind the upper incisors on the incisal papilla. The tongue tip is pointed and pressed to the spot, then released, and the exercise is repeated.

SLURP AND SWALLOW. A 5/16-inch elastic is placed on the tip of the tongue. The tongue is lifted and the tip is pressed onto the "spot." The patient is asked to close the back teeth together, then slurp and swallow with the lips remaining open (Fig. 15–21). Next, take the tongue down and check to make sure the elastic is in the same position as before.

ONE ELASTIC SWALLOW. This is exactly like the slurp and swallow exercise, but eliminating the slurp.

TONGUE-HOLD. The tongue is held to the "spot" with an elastic for five minutes. At each session, this time period is extended for an additional five minutes until an hour is reached. This exercise is done with the back teeth gently closed, and the lips closed also.

Certain sounds, such as those made by the letters, T, D, L, and N, raise the tip of the tongue to the incisal papilla. The following words should be repeated with added force to activate the tongue muscle:

TED NUT LET DAD
TEN NOT LEAN DOT
TELL NED LOVE DID

Figure 15–20.

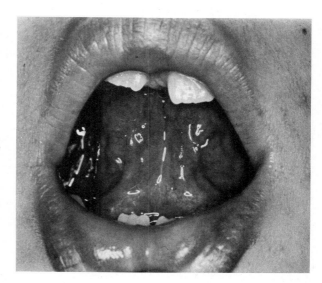

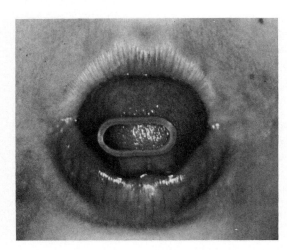

Figure 15–21.

Exercises for the Middle of the Tongue

TWO ELASTIC EXERCISE. One elastic is placed on the tongue tip and one midpoint on the tongue. The tongue tip is raised as before to the "spot" and the middle of the tongue is raised to the palate. The patient swallows with the back teeth closed and the lips open (Fig. 15–22).

HOLD PULL. This exercise is excellent for the tip and middle of the tongue. It stretches the tongue and is a good positioning exercise. The tip and middle of the tongue are placed on the palate and the mandible drops forward, stretching the entire tongue on the palate (Fig. 15–23). If a patient is unable to do this exercise, tongue pops are an easy way to begin. When the hold pull is easily accomplished, the patient is told to do a more complicated exercise. Doing the hold pull exercise, the patient will close the back teeth together, close the lips, swallow, and reverse the procedures. If the tongue remains in the original position, it has already become toned and can work on command.

Sounds that exercise the middle of the tongue are *ch* and *j*. These words should also be repeated forcefully for practice:

CHAP   JACK   PEACH
CHIN   JEEP   TEACH
CHAIR   JAR   REACH

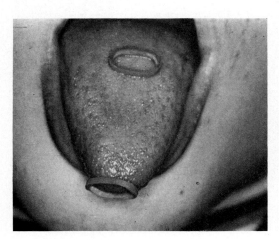

Figure 15–22.

Figure 15–23.

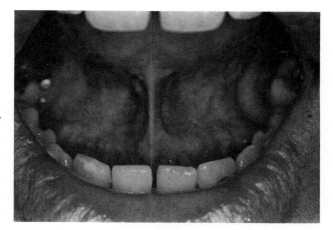

Exercises for the Posterior Part of the Tongue

THREE ELASTIC SWALLOW. The third elastic is placed directly behind the second elastic on the midpoint of the tongue, except in lateral or bilateral swallowing problems (Fig. 15–24). Then the two are placed side by side, midpoint on the tongue in the shape of a triangle. The first elastic is put on the tip of the tongue. The patient swallows with lips open and back teeth together (Fig. 15–24).

K EXERCISE. In a correct swallowing position, the posterior portion of the tongue is placed against the pharyngeal wall. This exercise is designed to activate the movement in the posterior segment of the tongue. Place three fingers vertically between the teeth and forcefully pronounce the letter K, so forcefully that it can be felt posteriorly (Fig. 15–25).

The K and G sounds are for the posterior part of the tongue:

KATE   COOK   GOT   EGG
CAKE   KITE   GET   BEG

In addition to developing the muscles of the lips and tongue, the masseter muscle must also be strengthened. This muscle is often found to

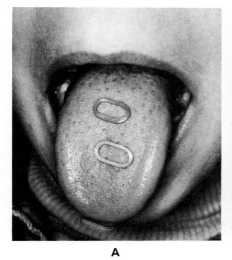
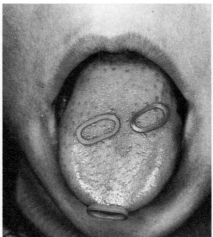

A   B

Figure 15–24.

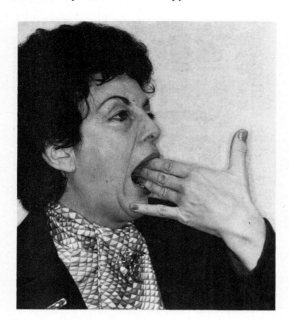

Figure 15–25.

be totally inactive, or very weak owing to disuse. In a correct swallow the posterior teeth occlude and the masseter muscle "pops out" (Fig. 15–26). However, in an abnormal swallow the tongue acts as an impeding force, and the posterior teeth cannot come together. An isometric exercise is done to develop the masseter muscle. The patient should feel the masseter muscle pop out as he bites down on his back teeth, and he should count to ten while holding this position. This exercise is done ten times, at three different periods during the day.

At this phase in therapy, the patient should be evaluated to determine progress. If all exercises can be done with little effort, it is time to introduce food and drink. If there is the slightest difficulty in making a saliva swallow, more time is needed for the intensive part of therapy, and the elastic swallows must be repeated.

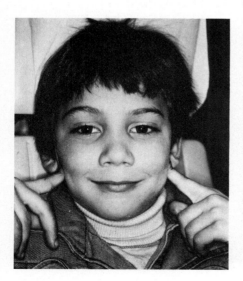

Figure 15–26.

Introduction of Food

The patient is given a cracker and is told to chew but not swallow (Fig. 15–27). Make sure the patient is chewing in the molar area and not in the anterior region of the mouth. The bolus is placed on the middle of the tongue, and the patient is told to proceed with the one elastic swallow, making sure the lips remain open (Fig. 15–28). Following the swallow, the tongue should be checked. It should be clean, with the exception of a few crumbs. The one elastic should remain on the tip, and there should be no facial movement during the swallowing process.

The following week, the patient must divide dinner into two parts. The first party can be eaten with the original swallow, but the second half must be eaten using the one elastic swallow just as the cracker was done in the exercise above. Gradually, all meals are eaten correctly. The most important addition when food is introduced is a "remainder" sign. Young and old patients must make a sign to be kept at the dinner table for every meal eaten at home. This is a must, and when therapy is finished the sign is given to the therapist.

Liquids

People who swallow abnormally generally bring their tongues forward to meet the glass or cup when taking a drink. To change this reflex the patient is told to bite the back teeth together, put the tongue to the spot, siphon the water in between the teeth, and swallow (Fig. 15–29). When this is accomplished, many sips of water are taken and swallowed without any movement of the facial muscles.

SUBCONSCIOUS SWALLOWING. When the patient utilizes the new swallowing pattern for all eating and drinking, it is time to go to the next step—the subconscious phase of therapy. The patient has learned proper posturing and is able to swallow correctly on command. He must now apply what he has learned to all swallowing that occurs day and night, and he must become aware of the rest position of the tongue throughout the day. The success of

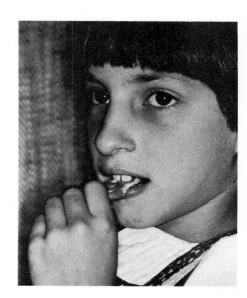

Figure 15–27.

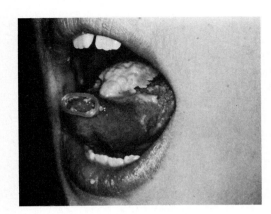

Figure 15–28.

this step depends greatly on the preceding phase of therapy. The ground work is laid with the constant exercises of the tongue. Yet, if these exercises have not been followed, therapy cannot succeed.

Before swallowing can become a subconscious act, it must be a totally conscious one. The patient must therefore keep a time chart as to where the tongue is at six specific times during the day. This serves a dual purpose: (1) to check and see where the tongue is at certain times during the day, and (2) to allow the patient to correct his tongue position if it is not in its proper resting place. Hopefully, it will remain in position until the next time check.

It is important that the patient be especially aware of the tongue during this period, and in order to accomplish this Barrett lists many "reminders" such as viewing:

    (1) a clock or watch—or wearing a watch upside down
    (2) a certain type of car or color
    (3) a reminder sign you have made
    (4) a person with crooked teeth
    (5) one polished fingernail

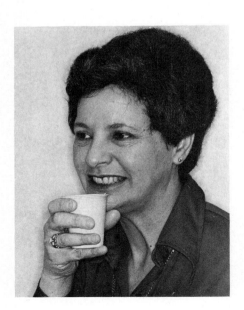

Figure 15–29.

Everytime you hear:
    (1) a bell of any kind—phone, school, door
    (2) a clock ticking
    (3) a horn honk
Everytime you feel:
    (1) a rock in your pocket
    (2) a bracelet on your arm
    (3) a ring on your finger
    (4) a sugarless mint on the tongue
Everytime you:
    (1) go through any doorway
    (2) turn a radio on or off
    (3) turn the TV on or off
    (4) turn a record player on or off
    (5) turn off a light
    (6) practice a musical instrument
    (7) walk up and down the stairs
    (8) smile
    (9) sit down or stand up
One or more of the above can be given to the patient.

Now we come to night swallowing. The following procedure contains elements of autosuggestion, psychosomatic influence, and biofeedback. When the patient is ready to go to sleep he repeats six times "I will swallow right all night long with my lips gently together." Then he proceeds to swallow correctly six times and goes to sleep with the tongue on the "spot." The patient indicates each morning for 14 days where the tongue is located. If the patient forgets this procedure for one night, he must begin all over again until he has 14 successful nights.

Active therapy is herewith concluded. If the patient leaves the office never to return, therapy must fail. Practice and follow-up visits are of utmost importance for success.

The first follow-up visit is 4 months after completing 1 full year of therapy. At this visit there are two main concerns: the rest posture and the subconscious function in swallowing. The therapist begins his or her observation as the patient sits in the waiting room prior to the appointment. The second follow-up is 4 months later, at which time photographs are taken and retesting is done.

Maintenance

In view of the questions, does form determine function or function determine form? A maintenance program is of utmost importance for every patient.
    1. Hold–pull, ten times daily.
    2. Hold tongue to spot for 2 minutes every morning.
    3. Air pumping, ten times daily.

Testing for Correct Swallow

    1. Place a few drops of water on the patient's tongue and ask him to make the seal on the palate. Have him bend over with the mouth open and

then spit out the water with the tongue. If the water is still there he has good control over the tongue muscles.

2. Observe your patient. Tell him to take a small sip of water but not to swallow it. When he has taken the water, study his face for a moment and then quickly depress his lower lip with your thumb. If the water is in the floor of the mouth, there will be a strong resistance in the lip as you attempt to press it down, or you will receive a handful of water. Either way you will know normal swallowing has not yet become a subconscious act. Patients who have the correct habit will instinctively trap the water as it enters the mouth (Fig. 15–30).

3. Have the patient pick up a cup of water and drink. Since he will be swallowing consciously, no doubt he will do it correctly. However, as he lowers the cup, a final clearing swallow should be observed, as this is done subconsciously. If there is the slightest doubt as to the patient's ability to pass these tests, he should be given additional exercises in his needed area and asked to return again the following week. If the patient passes the first recheck period he is dismissed and put on a monthly recall. On subsequent visits the squirt test is used. The patient is given a number and told to count backwards while the therapist periodically squirts water into his mouth. He must not stop counting and must swallow the water at the same time. If the patient gets the numbers confused or the water dribbles down the chin, then you know swallowing correctly is not a subconscious act. The patient must have additional conscious exercises.

Motivation—The Key to Success!

For years the tongue has been a problem to the dental profession. Many techniques have been tried and abandoned by the practitioner as being unsuccessful. Possibly, the problem was a lack of interest and motivation by the dentist. Walter Straub, a prominent orthodontist, sent his patients home with exercise cards, telling them to do the exercises in order to be rid of a deviate or reverse swallow.

All people need to be motivated to undertake a task unfamiliar to them, even though it promises a trimmer figure or, in this case, a more stabilized

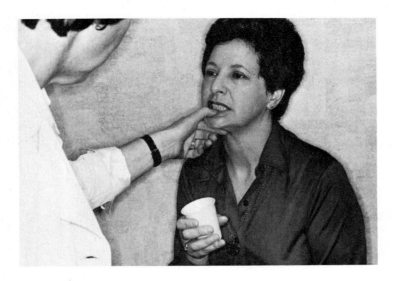

Figure 15–30.

Figure 15–31.

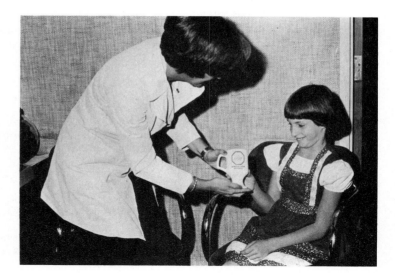

occlusion. It is important for the myofunctional therapist to be interested in his or her patients and to be able to motivate them; he or she must also be well-trained and knowledgeable in his or her field as well as in dentistry and speech (Fig. 15–31). The therapist must realize that he or she cannot motivate everyone, but that motivation is the key to successful therapy. The rapport between a patient and therapist is essential, and if it is not there the therapist is wiser not to accept the case.

Semiweekly visit initiate the program. They are followed by weekly visits, all of which last perhaps 30 minutes; the exercises themselves may take 10 or 15 minutes. The remainder of the time is spent talking with the patient, and it is during this time that the patient becomes encouraged and willing to do his exercises on a daily basis. Children and adults must enjoy a visit to the therapist, and it cannot be stressed enough that it is this relationship upon which success depends.

CONCLUSION

The concern of the dental specialist treating dysfunction of the cranio-mandibular articulation is stabilization of maxillo-mandibular relationships once pain and any associated symptoms have been relieved. Through clinical experience, we have come to the realization that abnormal swallowing patterns do not permit the final orthopedically corrected jaw relationship to be stabilized prior to orthodontic or finishing prosthetic procedures.

It is unfortunate that diagnosis and treatment of myofunctional disorders have been the subject of much controversy. Time will simply demonstrate that, once the air is cleared and additional research done with improved sophisticated instrumentation, the position and practices outlined in this chapter and elsewhere will be substantiated.[1, 32, 33]

This type of therapy can be successfully administered by any therapist who is acquainted with the anatomy and physiology involved, who understands the development of normal speech as well as proper development of the teeth (arch form and eruption patterns) and their surrounding structures, who has knowledge of normal and abnormal behavior, who possesses ability and training in motivational techniques for adults and children, and who is the recipient of advanced training in the newer techniques of myofunctional therapy.

Case History 1

Patient D. O. is a 14-year-old Panamanian girl who was referred by an orthodontist for treatment of an anterior open bite (Fig. 15–32A) thought to be associated with an elongated tongue (Fig. 15–32B). Upon myofunctional examination, a lip locking habit was discovered, which caused a stretching of the tongue muscles. She was also found to have an anterior tongue thrust (Fig. 15–32C) and a lip strength of 2 lb.

The first phase of treatment was to break the lip habit by motivational techniques, followed by myofunctional therapeutic procedures as outlined in this chapter.

Upon completion of treatment the patient was referred to her orthodontist, who completed treatment (Fig. 15–32D). Her final lip strength increased to 5½ lb.

Case History 2

Patient R. R. is an 18-year-old Caucasian college student. Her chief complaint was pain and tenderness in both temporomandibular joints, especially on opening following a visit to her dentist in May, 1976. In February of that

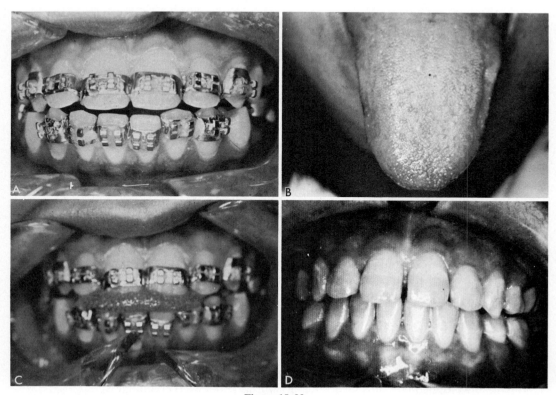

Figure 15–32.

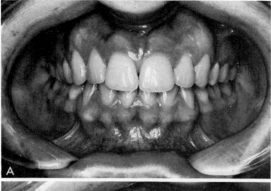

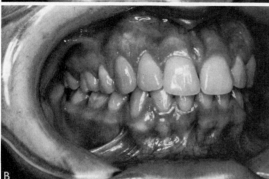

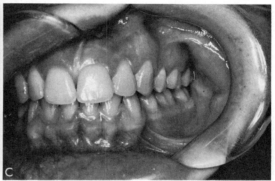

Figure 15–33. *A,* Patient R. R. Frontal view; habitual occlusion. *B,* Right lateral view; habitual occlusion. *C,* Left lateral view; habitual occlusion.

year she had fallen from a horse while riding and landed on her coccyx. She had undergone orthodontic therapy from the ages of 11 through 14 and had four first bicuspids removed (Fig. 15–33; notice lingual version of lower posterior teeth with concomitant loss of vertical dimension). Secondary complaints included popping or whooshing noises on opening and closing on both sides, but more pronounced on the left. She also complained of occasional tinnitus in both ears.

Clinical examination revealed spasm and tenderness on palpation of the anterior, middle, and posterior fibers on the right and left termporalis muscles; the zygomatic, body, and mandibular angle of both masseter muscles; the right and left internal and external pterygoid muscles; the right and left sternocleidomastoid muscles; the right and left trapezius muscles; the right and left posterior cervical muscles; the right and left mylohyoid muscles; the upper middle and lower back muscles on the left; the lower back muscles on the right; and the deltoid muscles on the left side. The left temporomandibular joint was painful, as were both coronoid processes. On palpation of the condylar head through the external auditory meatus, the left was tender.

The mandible deviated to the left on opening. The widest interincisal opening was 42 millimeters.

Radiographic and clinical oral examination revealed a mouth free of caries and an excellent periodontal condition. There was a narrowing of the joint space on both sides in the closed position. The opening position found the condyles in good relation to the eminentia bilaterally. Examination of the face revealed the right eye to be higher than the left. The patient exhibited an anterior thrust swallowing habit, which was more obviously seen in the orthopedically corrected jaw relationship (Fig. 15–34).

After relief of symptoms, myofunctional therapy was instituted, to be followed by additional orthodontic therapy to increase the vertical height of the posterior teeth.

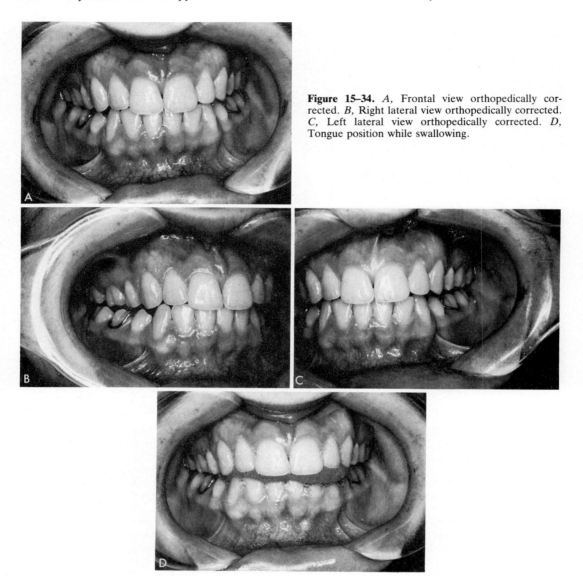

Figure 15–34. *A*, Frontal view orthopedically corrected. *B*, Right lateral view orthopedically corrected. *C*, Left lateral view orthopedically corrected. *D*, Tongue position while swallowing.

Case History 3

Patient M. G. is a 25-year-old accountant, married, Caucasian, female, with no children. Her chief complaint was supraorbital headaches occurring several times a month for the past year and a half. They were at their greatest intensity late at night and when she was tired. She was first seen on December 10, 1976.

She had undergone orthodontic therapy from the ages of 12 until 14 and had four first bicuspids extracted. In addition she exhibited a posterior bilateral tongue thrust habit. Her lip posture was open; the palate was high and narrow; she was a mouth breather and her lip strength was 2 lb at the beginning of therapy (Fig. 15–35). Secondary complaints included double vision and blurring in both eyes. Clinical examination revealed spasm and tenderness on palpation of the anterior, middle, and posterior fibers of the right temporalis; anterior and middle fibers on the left temporalis; the zygomatic, body, and mandibular angle of both masseters; the right and left internal and external pterygoids; the

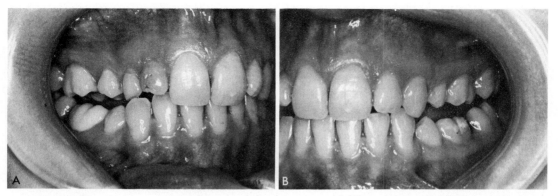

Figure 15–35. *A,* Patient M. G. Right lateral view of patient with bilateral thrust. *B,* Left lateral view.

right and left sternocleidomastoids; the right and left trapezius; the right and left posterior cervicals; the right and left mylohyoids; the upper middle and lower back muscles on the right; the middle and lower back muscles on the left; and the right and left deltoids. The right coronoid process was painful, as were the right and left intercostals and sternum. On palpation of the condylar head through the external auditory meatus, the right was tender.

The mandible deviated to the right on opening and the widest interincisal opening was 40 millimeters.

Examination of the face revealed the right eye to be higher than the left. Since her father had been diagnosed as suffering from multiple sclerosis, she had also been diagnosed as suffering from the same disease by the physicians she had seen with her complaints. No one had been able to resolve her pain symptoms.

After her symptoms were relieved in an approximate two-month period (Fig. 15–36), she was referred for myofunctional therapy. This was to be followed by orthodontic therapy to erupt the depressed posterior teeth.

Case History 4

Patient M. B. is a 14-year-old Caucasian high school student. His chief complaint was bilateral supraorbital headaches occurring at least once a week.

He was a thumbsucker as a youngster and exhibited a full thrust or complete swallowing habit (Fig. 15–37). At the beginning of therapy his lip

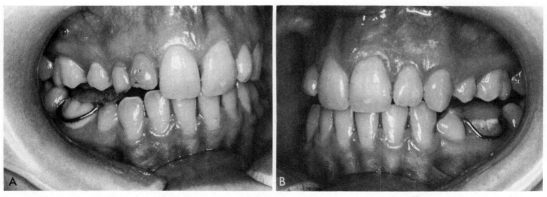

Figure 15–36. *A,* Right lateral view of orthopedically corrected jaw position. *B,* Left lateral view of orthopedically corrected jaw position.

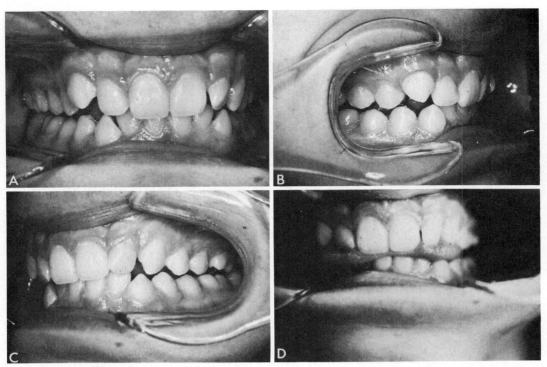

Figure 15–37. Patient M. B. *A*, Frontal view, before. *B*, Right lateral view, before. *C*, Left lateral view, before. *D*, Tongue position while swallowing.

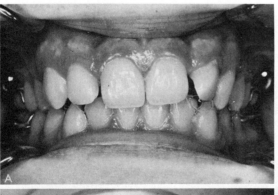

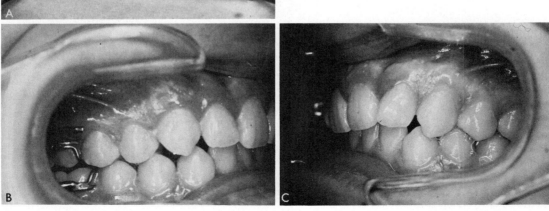

Figure 15–38. *A*, Frontal view of patient M. B. wearing Crozat appliance. *B*, Right lateral view of patient M. B. wearing Crozat appliance. *C*, Left lateral view of same patient wearing Crozat appliance.

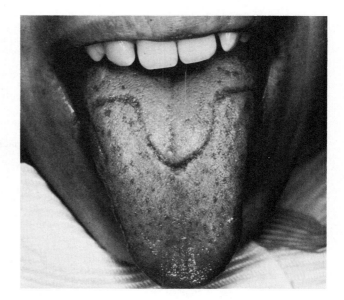

Figure 15–39. Note imprint on tongue of upper Crozat appliance as a result of diligent myofunctional exercising.

strength was 3 lb. Clinical examination revealed spasm and tenderness on palpation of the anterior, middle, and posterior fibers of the left temporalis; the anterior fibers of the right temporalis; the zygomatic, body, and mandibular angle of the left masseter; the right and left external pterygoids; the left internal pterygoid; the left sternocleidomastoid; the right and left trapezius; the right and left posterior cervicals; the left mylohyoids; the right and left deltoids; the left intercostals; the upper, middle, and lower back muscles on the left and the upper back muscles on the right. The right and left temporomandibular joints and the right and left coronoid processes were painful to palpation. The widest interincisal opening was 45.5 millimeters, and there was no deviation of the midline on opening. Examination of the face revealed a high right eye.

After relief of the patient's symptoms by orthopedic correction, orthodontic therapy was initiated using the Crozat technique (Fig. 15–38). Myofunctional therapy was instituted shortly after symptoms were relieved, and orthodontic therapy started (Fig. 15–39). His lip strength was increased to 8½ lb.

EPILOGUE

The material presented in this chapter is a result of an organized and concerted program of myofunctional therapy involving many thousands of hours of treatment in our offices. We have all benefited by the thorough interweaving of the professional disciplines of the doctor and the myofunctional therapist. We especially wish to express our thanks to Thalia R. Funt, myofunctional therapist, for her many supportive contributions.

References

1. Barrett, R. H. and Hanson, M. L.: Oral Myofunctional Disorders. St. Louis, C. V. Mosby Co., 1974.
2. Weinstein, S., Haack, D. C., Morris, L. Y., Snyder, B. B., and Attaway, H. E.: On an equilibrium theory of tooth position. Angle Orthodont., *33*:1–26, 1963.

3. Ravins, H.: Correction of respiratory mechanisms: an integral part of myofunctional therapy. Int. J. Orthod., *14*:1 12–19; 1976.
4. LeFoulon, P. J.: Orthopedic denture. Gaz. Hop., p. 111, 1839.
5. Tomes, C.: The bearing of the development of the jaws on irregularities. Dent. Cosmos, *15*:292–296, 1873.
6. Rogers, A. P.: The Correction of Facial Inharmonies. Read before the Northeastern Dental Association, 1906.
7. Lischer, B. E.: Principles and Methods of Orthodontics. Philadelphia, Lea and Febiger, 1912.
8. Monson, G. S.: Impaired function as a result of closed bite. Natl. Dent. Assoc. J., *8*:823–830, 1921.
9. Nove, A. A.: The physiology and mechanics of swallowing and their clinical significance. Dent. Rec., *68*:28–33, 1948.
10. Nove, A. A., and Schweitzer, J. M.: Oral Rehabilitation. St. Louis, C. V. Mosby Co., 1951, p. 350.
11. Truesdell, B., and Truesdell, F. B.: Deglutition with special reference to normal function and diagnosis, analysis and correction of abnormalities. Angle Ortho., 7:90, 1937.
12. Rix, R. E.: Deglutition and teeth. Dent. Rec., *66*:103, 1946.
13. Gwynne-Evans, E.: The upper respiratory musculature and orthodontics. Br. Soc. Study Orthod-Trans., p. 165, 1947.
14. Gwynne-Evans, E.: The orofacial muscles: their function and behavior in relation to the teeth. Eur. Orthod. Soc. Trans., p. 20, 1954.
15. Gratzinger, M.: Dynamic irritation as a cause of periodontal disease and the means for its elimination. JADA, *37*:294–310, 1948.
16. Ballard, C. F.: The upper respiratory musculture and orthodontics. Dent. Rec., *68*:1, 1948.
17. Tulley, W. J.: Adverse muscle forces—their diagnostic significance. Am. J. Orthod., *42*:801, 1956.
18. Gwynne-Evans, E., and Tulley, W. J.: Clinical types. Dent. Pract., *6*:222, 1956.
19. Straub, W. J.: The etiology of the perverted swallowing habit. Am. J. Orthod., *37*:603, 1951.
20. Straub, W. J.: Malfunction of the tongue: Parts I and II. Am. J. Orthod., *47*:415, 596, 1960, and 1961.
21. Kydd, W. L.: Maximum forces exerted on the dentition by perioral and lingual musculature. JADA, *55*:646–651, 1957.
22. Parfitt, G. J.: The dynamics of tooth in function. J. Periodont., *32*:102–107, 1961.
23. Winders, R. V.: A study of the development of an electronic technique to measure the forces exerted on the dentition by perioral and lingual musculature during swallowing. Am. J. Orthod., *42*:645–657, 1956.
24. Gould, M. S. E., and Picton, D. C. A.: A method of measuring forces acting on the teeth from the lips, cheeks, and tongue. Br. Dent. J., *112*:235–242, 1962.
25. Gould, M. S. E., and Picton, D. C. A.: Forces acting on the teeth from the lips, cheeks and tongue. Br. Dent. J., *112*:235–242, 1962.
26. Gould, M. S. E., and Picton, D. C. A.: A study of pressures exerted by the lips and cheeks on the teeth of subjects with normal occlusion. Arch. Oral Biol., *9*:469–478, 1964.
27. Profitt, W. R., Kydd, W. L., Wilskie, G. H., and Taylor, D. T.: Intraoral pressures in a young adult group. J. Dent. Res., *43*:555–562, 1964.
28. Profitt, W. R., Chastain, B. B., and Norton, L. A.: Linguopalatal pressure in children. Am. J. Orthod., *55*:154–166, 1969.
29. Profitt, W. R., McGlone, R. E., and Christiansen, R. L.: Lingual pressure against anterior and lateral areas of the palate during speech and swallowing. I.A.D.R. Program Abstracts, July, 1965.
30. Harvold, E. P.: The role of function in the etiology and treatment of malocclusion. Am. J. Orthod., *54*:883–898, 1968.
31. Subtelny, J. D., and Subtelny, J. D.: Oral habits—studies in form, function, and therapy. Angle Orthod., *43*:347–383, 1973.
32. Garliner, D.: Myofunctional Therapy in Dental Practice, 2nd ed. Brooklyn, N.Y., Bartel Dental Book Co., 1971.
33. Garliner, D., et al.: Myofunctional Therapy. Philadelphia, W. B. Saunders Company, 1976.
34. Dorland's Illustrated Medical Dictionary, 25th ed. W. B. Saunders Company, Philadelphia, 1974.

16

Applied Kinesiology and the Treatment of TMJ Dysfunction

GEORGE A. EVERSAUL, Ph.D.

The primary objective of this chapter is to acquaint the reader with practical and potential applications of applied kinesiology useful in the treatment of TMJ muscle dysfunctions. In addition, this chapter elaborates on the significance of muscle physiopathology in TMJ disease and its impact upon systemic health. Finally, it is the purpose of this chapter to motivate further research in developing applied kinesiology as a tool in both treatment and preventive TMJ therapy.

DEFINITION

Applied kinesiology is concerned with the dynamics of the smooth and striated musculature, and the impact of those functions on structural entities, healing processes, and disease resistance. In particular, applied kinesiology focuses on the identification and correction of proprioceptive dysfunctions of ligaments and of the muscles' spindle cells and Golgi tendon organs. Finally, applied kinesiology is concerned with the vascular, lymphatic, and other systems supporting proper muscle dynamics as well as the nutritional requirements necessary for those support systems and the muscles themselves.[1]

THERAPEUTIC APPLICATIONS

Briefly summarized, there at at least six major applications of applied kinesiology in TMJ therapy. They are as follows:

1. To improve TMJ musculature function.

2. To further verify the diagnosis of occlusal dysfunction.

3. To facilitate treatment efficiency and effectiveness of mandibular repositioning appliances and of occlusal therapy.

4. To verify the impact and appropriateness for TMJ treatment.

5. To psychologically motivate patient compliance in following the recommended TMJ therapy program.

6. To determine therapeutic needs of TMJ muscle support systems.

The fundamental therapeutic value of applied kinesiology results from the effects that kinesiologic adjustments produce in "strengthening" hypotonic musculature. The impact of such strengthening frequently induces the reduction of spasm in antagonistic musculature, thus achieving a more balanced relationship of the musculature system.

Beyond the reduction of muscle spasms frequently associated with TMJ syndrome, applied kinesiology's improvement of masticatory muscle function will frequently result in other dynamics of benefit in occlusal treatment. For example, these manipulations may stimulate significant changes in vertical dimension and in the patient's bite.

Applied kinesiology is also of diagnostic value in occlusal therapy. As a supplement to traditional methods of muscle palpation, kinesiologic procedures offer the clinician another technique to obtain data regarding the muscular dysfunction which greatly contributes to TMJ disorders.

Improvements in muscular function which result from kinesiologic techniques may facilitate occlusal treatment. In particular, balanced muscular function should enhance the therapeutic effect of mandibular repositioning appliances. With applied kinesiology included in the patient's treatment strategy, such appliances may be needed for shorter periods of time while accomplishing more harmonious occlusion and TMJ balance. In general, such muscular improvements should create an oral environment conducive to quicker and more effective occlusal therapy, whether a repositioning appliance is used or not.

Another diagnostic value of applied kinesiology in TMJ treatment results from the information which kinesiologic muscle testing may provide about the appropriateness of specific occlusal procedures. For example, kinesiologic muscle testing may be used to help evaluate the impact of mandibular repositioning appliances not only upon TMJ musculature but also upon other muscle groups throughout the body. And because of the "relative" degree of dysfunction which muscle testing can discriminate, kinesiologic procedures may be used to help evaluate the progress and direction of specific therapeutic strategies.

Because kinesiologic muscle testing allows the patient to feel significant changes in muscular "energy," applied kinesiology may be very useful to the clinician as a motivational tool. The dramatic and subjective experience of the patient may help some individuals to accept emotionally what they know intellectually about their need for compliance with their doctor's recommended TMJ therapy program.

Finally, applied kinesiology offers therapists a tool to identify and correct problems in the support system of the TMJ musculature. For example, kinesiologic procedures may be used to improve the vascular and lymphatic components affecting TMJ muscular function. In addition, kinesiologic procedures may be used to identify marginal nutritional deficiencies which may be causing the TMJ musculature to function less than optimally.

THEORETICAL CONCEPTS

In brief summary, there are four fundamental concepts which must be understood in order to appreciate the dynamics of applied kinesiology:

1. The concept of physiopathology, which assumes that physiological processes may develop "habits" which may create an environment conducive to organic disease development and/or structural deterioration.

2. The concept of relative dysfunction, which assumes that physiological processes may operate at various degrees of efficiency and may react to stress with varying degrees of response and recovery.

3. The concept of muscle reactivity and reciprocity, which assumes that change in the length and tension of any particular muscle group results in a change of length and tension in some associated musculature.

4. The concept of therapy localization, which assumes that digital contact of any area of the body which has an electromagnetic imbalance will cause all muscle groups of that individual to experience a relative "weakness."

Physiopathology, according to Whatmore and Kohli,[2] "consists of altered physiology for which there is no underlying structural pathology." In TMJ disorders, there are at least three forms of physiopathology which may contribute to the patient's disorder. First, the patient may have developed habituated tension patterns within some of the muscles of mastication. These chronic bracing behaviors of the muscles, medically referred to as "dysponesis,"[2] are easily observed in acute situations such as bruxism. However, dysponetic TMJ musculature may also be present in lesser degrees of severity and frequency. Without electromyographic or kinesiologic techniques, these lesser but significant dysponetic tension patterns and muscle spasm patterns would be difficult to diagnose and quantify.

Second, the patient may have developed physiopathologial processes of the smooth musculature. For example, some individuals demonstrate patterns of habituated vasoconstriction. Such poor circulation is easily identified since the digits and/or lower extremities of these patients have external temperatures which are usually 8° F. cooler than those of normal individuals, given the same environment.[3] However, habituated vasoconstriction may be very localized. For example, the person's hands and feet may be of normal temperatures (indicating normal circulation) while he is suffering from habituated vasoconstriction of the circulatory components providing blood-flow to the TMJ and its striated musculature.

Third, the patient may have developed a physiopathological condition in the proprioceptive functions of various ligaments, spindle cells, and/or Golgi tendon organs. For example, as a result of dysponetic signaling from the reticular formation or as a result of habituated muscle spasm, some antagonistic musculature may develop hypotonic patterns of inappropriate resting length; that is, the proprioceptive components of that hypotonic musculature have learned to "remember" the wrong resting position.

Relative dysfunctions of the TMJ musculature may demonstrate themselves in a variety of ways. For example, some patients seem to have more acute reactions of their smooth musculature, while other patients have more acute responses by their striated muscles, given the same stress stimulant. In addition, these muscular responses vary not only in degree of tension but also seem to occur in specific locations, which vary from individual to individual. For example, some patients may develop extreme vasoconstrictive responses to stress on one side of the jaw while maintaining normal vasoconstrictive responses to the opposing side. For another example, some patients may develop hypertonic patterns of the masticatory muscles which affect mandibular opening, while other patients may develop hypertonic patterns of the masticatory muscles which affect mandibular closing.

These relative dysfunctions of the TMJ musculature seem to be the result of four basic variables. First, there seems to be a genetic propensity by which heredity predetermines the tendency to over-react by specific physiological processes, or at specific "weak link" locations within the body. Second, individuals seem to vary in ability to learn physiological patterns. Some patients quickly learn inappropriate habits, while others learn poor physiological patterns more slowly. Third, experience of the different types and amounts of stimulants which motivate and reinforce the learning behaviors of physiological processes vary from individual to individual. For example, each person experiences different types and amounts of dietary, environmental, and psychological stress. Fourth, the synergistic combination of genetic propensity, learning ability, and reinforcement stimulants also varies in outcome from individual to individual, just as the reactions of chemicals vary by combining different amounts and types of substances.

Muscle reciprocity is important to understand in order to appreciate applied kinesiology because of a fundamental kinesiologic treatment assumption: that every muscle group in spasm has an antagonistic or associated musculature which is hypotonic, and that strengthening the hypotonic muscle will contribute to reduced muscle spasm in the associated musculature.[4]

Historically, treatment of muscles in spasm has addressed itself to the spastic muscle itself. For example, injections would be made into the muscle, systemic muscle relaxants would be given, heat from various physical therapy alternatives would be focused on the spastic muscle, exercise programs would be encouraged which utilized the problem musculature, or biofeedback training would be administered to reduce the muscle tension. In contrast, applied kinesiology focuses on the "weak" musculature and attempts to strengthen these muscles via manipulation and proper nutritional support. The purpose of this strengthening is to reduce the spasm in reciprocal or reactive musculature.

Therapy localization[4] is a technique by which dysfunctioning musculature seems to be quickly identified. Although the physiological mechanisms which account for the dynamics of therapy localization are not understood, the physiological consequences of therapy localization may be replicated with remarkable consistency. In brief, the fundamental observation made by therapy localization is that any strong, normally functioning muscle group will become relatively weak when the individual places his fingers on any dysfunctioning musculature. For example, let us assume that via standardized muscle testing[5] an individual has the ability to resist 300 millimeters of pressure to the quadriceps muscles for a period of 30 seconds. If that same person then placed his fingers on some dysfunctioning muscle group, the masseter for example, and the quadriceps were re-tested while the person maintained digital contact to the masseter, those quadriceps muscles may be able to resist only 200 millimeters of pressure for only 10 seconds.

For reasons which are not fully understood, the weakness of strong muscles induced via therapy localization dynamics is relative from individual to individual; that is, some persons demonstrate an ability to resist less pressure for the same amount of time, while others demonstrate an ability to resist the same pressure for lesser periods, and still others demonstrate combinations of being able to resist lesser amounts of pressure in shorter periods. Because of this relative response, muscle testing, like any other skill, requires practice of precise execution in order to develop clinical competency. In addition, the consequences of this relative response are unknown, but they seem to relate to the severity of dysfunction, although not always.

THE BASIC PROPRIOCEPTIVE ADJUSTMENT

This section describes the basic proprioceptive adjustment which has been found to be of benefit in TMJ treatment. However, it seems important to communicate that the existing state of the art of dental kinesiology is in the embryonic stages. Consequently, the procedures which are about to be described will probably be significantly refined within a very short period of time. Although the techniques and procedures currently recommended seem to be consistently effective, there seems to be no question that the therapeutic methods of applied kinesiology in occlusal therapy will evolve to such degrees of sophistication as to make the following TMJ kinesiologic strategy analogous to a comparison of the Wright brothers' first aircraft with a 747.

OUTLINE OF THE PROCEDURE

1. Identify a strong muscle group.
2. Therapy localize. Have the patient place his fingers on the TMJ hinge. With the jaw *opened*, re-test the originally strong muscle group. If weak, determine whether the problem is on the left or right side, then make the appropriate kinesiologic correction to the side(s) involved.
3. Therapy localize with jaw *closed firmly*. Have the patient place the fingers on the TMJ hinge. With the jaw firmly *closed*, re-test the originally strong muscle group. If weak, determine whether the problem is on the left or right side, then make the appropriate correction on the side(s) involved.
4. After each correction, check the treatment's effectiveness. Have the patient therapy localize the side(s) which were adjusted, and with the jaw in the same testing position, *opened* or *firmly closed*, re-test the originally strong muscle group. If strong, the correction was done properly.

Step 1: Identify a Strong Muscle Group

In Figures 16–1, 16–2, and 16–3 you will see examples of those muscle-testing procedures which have been found to be of most value in the dental environment. Although theoretically you can use any muscle group, the advantages of the muscle groups pictured for the occlusal therapist are six-fold. First, these groups are unusually strong; that is, only rarely will these muscles demonstrate kinesiologic dysfunction. Second, these muscles will not fatigue easily; this is important when multiple testing is necessary. Third, when these muscle groups are made "weak," the strength differential is

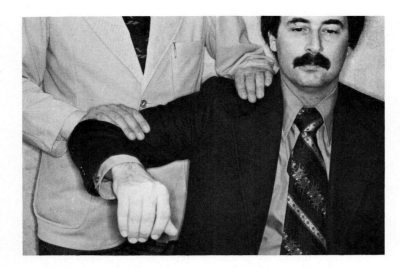

Figure 16–1. Muscle testing: Middle deltoid.

usually gross and readily apparent, which is psychologically impacting on both the therapist and patient. Fourth, testing of the muscle groups shown seems appropriate for the dental setting, causing little discomfort or embarrassment, while being easily done in the standard dental chair. Fifth, it is very difficult for the patient to "recruit" the support of other muscle groups in the muscle-testing process, which could lead the therapist to false positive or false negative conclusions. And sixth, these muscle groups are conveniently measurable using pressure gauge devices.

When testing to identify a strong muscle group, there are three critical dynamics of which the therapist should be aware:

1. To use uniform muscle-testing procedures.
2. To be aware of the relative strength differences between individuals and between different muscle groups of any particular individual.
3. To avoid "accidental" therapy localization.

Muscle testing requires two components to acquire clinical proficiency. First, one must be knowledgeable of standard muscle-testing procedures,

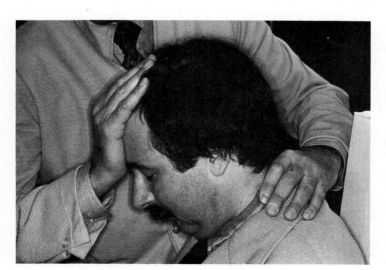

Figure 16–2. Muscle testing: neck flexors.

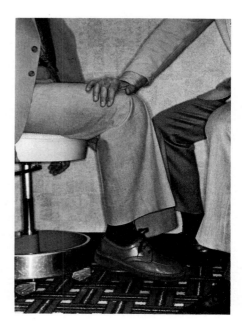

Figure 16–3. Muscle testing: the quadriceps.

such as those advocated by Kendall[5] or by Walther.[6] These texts describe uniform muscle-testing techniques which allow for consistent replication of testing scores for the same musculature of the same individual. Second, muscle testing requires regular practice in order to develop clinical competency, just as it is necessary to develop any skill.

When muscle testing, it is critical to remember that you are testing for the *relative* strength of the particular muscle group of that particular individual. The purpose of muscle testing is not to overpower the patient but to assess the ability of that individual's muscle group to resist pressure for some measured duration of time.

Also when muscle testing, it is critically important for the therapist to be aware that different individuals vary in muscular strength, as do therapists. For example, a 5 feet 1 inch, 95-pound housewife should have significantly less strength in her deltoids than a 6 feet 5 inch, 255-pound football player. In testing data terms, it would be reasonable for the housewife to resist 150 millimeters of pressure for 20 seconds, while the football player may be able to resist 300 millimeters of pressure for better than 30 seconds. (These scores assume that the kinesiologic functioning of both individuals' deltoids is normal.)

As the individuals being tested vary in their relative strength, so do the therapists making the evaluations. For example, one therapist may have sufficient strength to "beat" only the housewife, while another therapist may have the strength to overpower both individuals. Again, however, the purpose is *not* to overpower the patients but to evaluate the relative strength of that particular individual. Simply because the therapist can "beat" the housewife and not the football player does not mean that the therapist may conclude that the housewife has a kinesiologic dysfunction and the football player does not. The 150 millimeter, 20 second score of the housewife may be normal and healthy for that person, while the 300 millimeter, 30 second score for the football player may be significantly weak for that individual.

With kinesiologic corrections, that football player may increase in strength to better than 400 millimeters of pressure resistance for better than 60 seconds. However, it may be important to note that the first therapist would not have been able to "beat" the football player in either case, even when there was kinesiologic dysfunctioning.

In addition, it is necessary to be aware that the relative strength of different muscle groups for any particular individual will also vary. For example, it is normal for the deltoids to be "weaker" than the quadriceps, even when the kinesiologic functioning of both these muscles is normal. In testing data terms, it would be reasonable for an individual to be able to resist 200 millimeters of pressure for 30 seconds to the deltoids while being able to resist 450 millimeters of pressure for better than 60 seconds to the quadriceps.

Finally, when muscle testing, it is important that the therapist avoid accidental therapy localization. Because therapy localization will induce systemic muscle weakness when the hands contact any dysfunctioning body component, the therapist must observe the position of the patient's hands and be sure that these extremities are *not* touching any part of his body. Similarly, be sure that the patient's feet and legs are not crossed in any manner.

Step 2: Therapy Localize with Jaw Opened

After identifying a strong muscle group, have the patient place his three middle fingers on the TMJ hinge, while the little finger and thumb touch one another. As pictured in Figure 16–4, have the patient maintain therapy localization with the jaw opened as far as possible, while the therapist re-tests the originally strong muscle group. Be sure to look directly at the patient's mouth while stressing the muscle being tested, since many patients will instinctively start to close the mouth to clench. This motion of closing the mouth will give you therapy localization information regarding the closing adjustment needs rather than the opening adjustment needs for which you thought you were testing.

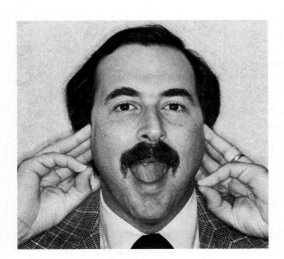

Figure 16–4.

If the originally strong muscle group becomes relatively weak, therapy localize to each individual side. For example, have the patient place the right hand on the TMJ hinge while placing the other hand away from the body. Then re-test the originally strong muscle group. If that muscle group is now relatively weak, you may conclude a kinesiologic dysfunction of the side being therapy localized, in this case the right side. At this point you would make the kinesiologic *opening* correction to the side(s) indicated by therapy localization. (Be sure to test both sides via therapy localization, since it is possible to have a bilateral opening dysfunction, requiring adjustments and treatment for both sides of the mandible.)

For the purpose of clarification, please consider the following hypothetical muscle-testing data regarding the identification of a kinesiologic TMJ opening dysfunction. Let us assume that you originally tested the quadriceps and observed an ability to resist 300 millimeters of pressure for 30 seconds. With therapy localization to the right side of the TMJ hinge, while re-testing the quadriceps, the patient may be able to resist only 200 millimeters of pressure for only 15 seconds. This relative change in muscle strength via therapy localization would kinesiologically indicate a rightsided, TMJ opening problem. Once again, it is important to remember that the relative response of muscle weakness will vary from individual to individual.

In most cases, therapy localization will induce weakness which will be demonstrated by both relative decreases in ability to resist pressure and reduced periods of time. Fortunately, when therapy localization induces such weaknesses, the change in resistance normally drops at least 40 per cent, and/or the time resistance ability decreases by better than 50 per cent. If there is no kinesiologic dysfunction, the originally tested muscle group will re-test with pressure and time endurance within ± 5 per cent of the original score.

Step 3: Therapy Localize with Jaw Firmly Closed

Using any of the strong muscle groups identified in Step 1, have the patient simultaneously therapy localize bilaterally with the jaw firmly closed while re-testing the originally strong muscle. Be sure that the patient has the thumb and little finger of each hand in contact with one another.

If a relative weakness is induced, you would then therapy localize left and right to determine unilateral or bilateral dysfunction, using the same procedure described in Step 2, but with the jaw firmly closed during testing. Again, please be aware of the relative "strength" and "weakness" of any particular individual. Be aware, too, of avoiding accidental therapy localization when trying to establish the side of dysfunction.

At this point, you would make the kinesiologic *closing* correction to the side(s) indicated by therapy localization.

CORRECTION OF KINESIOLOGIC TMJ OPENING PROBLEMS

In the situation where the jaw therapy localizes to the left or to the right in the open position following therapy localization or a lateralization left or right, the mouth is opened and the index finger is directed to the belly of the left external pterygoid (Fig. 16–5). This muscle, which opens

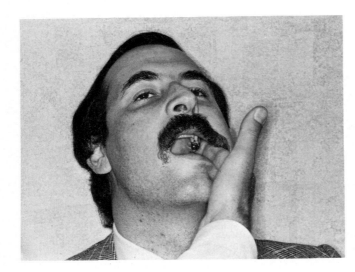

Figure 16–5.

the jaw, and its spindle cell mechanism are quickly and firmly contacted with the index finger and a hard pressure is applied to the spindle cell, first at its posterior position and secondly at its anterior portion. The belly of the external pterygoid is contacted, and a rapid anterior and posterior directional force is then applied to the spindle cell mechanism in the belly of the muscle. Therapy localization is then reapplied with the mouth opened fully. A good response should result under these circumstances. Figure 16–6 shows the position of the index finger contacting the spindle cell mechanism of the right external pterygoid muscle.

CORRECTION OF KINESIOLOGIC TMJ CLOSING PROBLEMS

If therapy localization indicates a left-sided closing dysfunction, you would make the adjustment as depicted in Figures 16–7 and 16–8. At the

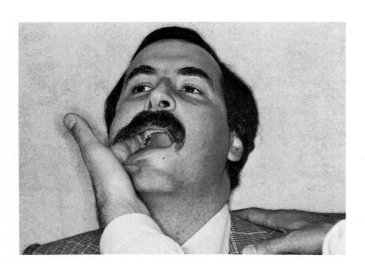

Figure 16–6.

Figure 16–7.

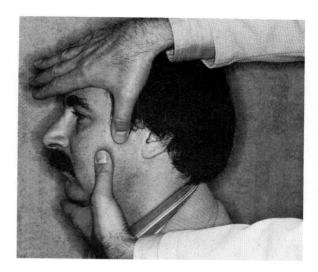

beginning of the adjustment, your left thumb would be placed in the belly of the buccinator, while your right thumb would be at the origin of the masseter. The concluding position of each thumb is shown in Figure 16–8, with the left thumb moving to the origin of the buccinator, the right thumb to the belly of the masseter. Again, the thumbs move parallel to one another and should penetrate into the musculature, not merely massage the skin surface.

Figures 16–9 and 16–10 depict the initial and ending positions of the thumbs in the kinesiologic corrrection of a right-sided closing dysfunction. At the beginning of the adjustment, your right thumb would be placed in the belly of the buccinator, while your left thumb starts at the posterior origin of the masseter. The concluding position, shown in Figure 16–10, has the right thumb ending at the origin of the buccinator, with the left thumb ending in the belly of the masseter.

In Figure 16–11 are shown two common mistakes which result in an improper or less effective kinesiologic correction. Note that the position of

Figure 16–8.

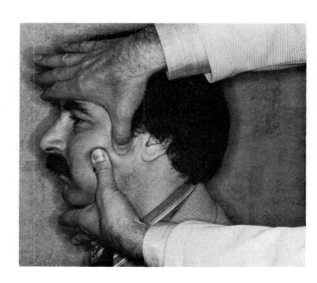

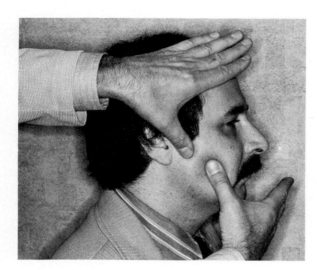

Figure 16–9.

the thumbs is *not* parallel. Also note that the thumbs are positioned flat along the surface of the skin rather than tilted into the musculature to be manipulated.

OCCLUSAL THERAPY APPLICATIONS

The fundamental applications of the basic TMJ proprioceptive adjustment and basic kinesiologic principles in occlusal therapy are described in this section. The applications described probably reflect only the tip of the iceberg in terms of potential applications. Although the techniques and procedures recommended seem consistently effective, there is no question that more sophisticated therapeutic methods will be developed shortly, both improving and replacing existing techniques and procedures.

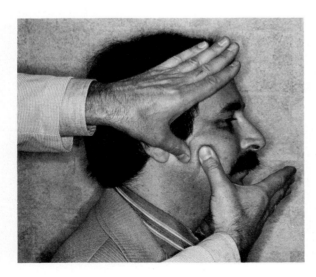

Figure 16–10.

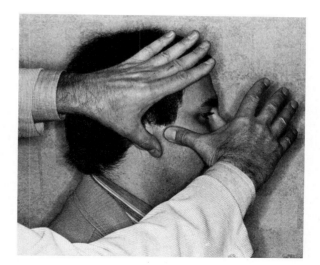

Figure 16–11.

IMPROVING TMJ MUSCULATURE FUNCTIONS

The fundamental application of the basic TMJ proprioceptive adjustment is to improve the functions of TMJ musculature. In particular, applied kinesiology may be used to reduce and prevent muscle spasm. As a result of decreased muscle tension, occlusal therapists will in many cases be able to help their patients improve their jaw opening capabilities and vertical dimension. In addition, decreased muscle tension will help reduce bruxism patterns and TMJ clicking.

In essence, there are two major impacts upon muscle spasm which seem to be affected by kinesiologic corrections. First, the muscle in spasm may be "weakened"; that is, the tension (microvoltage output) of the muscle may be reduced. This tension reduction may be accomplished by applying approximately two pounds of pressure away from the belly of the muscle in the area of the Golgi tendon organs, and/or by applying approximately two pounds of pressure toward the belly of the muscle in the area of the muscle's spindle cells. Second, the hypotonic muscle which is antagonistic to the muscle in spasm may be strengthened. This tension increase may be accomplished by applying approximately two pounds of pressure toward the belly of the muscle in the area of the Golgi tendon organs, and/or by applying approximately two pounds of pressure away from the center of the muscle's belly. (The directions of pressure to strengthen or weaken muscles are diagrammed in Figure 16–12.)

For example, if you wanted to induce a relative weakness to the quadriceps muscles, you could stimulate the spindle cells toward the belly of that muscle, as depicted in Figure 16–13, or you could stimulate the Golgi tendon organ away from the belly, as shown in Figure 16–14. Similarly, you could strengthen that induced weakness by the reverse procedure. Figure 16–15 depicts the strengthening of the muscle by stimulation of the spindle cells away from the center of the belly; Figure 16–16 shows stimulation of the Golgi tendon organs toward the belly. (In doing the correction, be sure to depress your thumbs or fingers firmly into the musculature.)

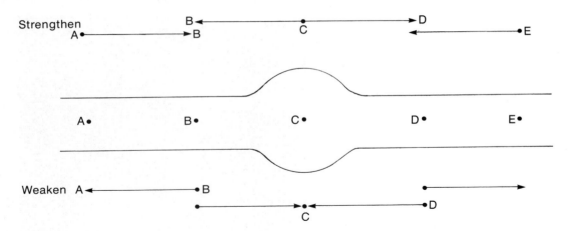

Areas A-B and D-E represent location of Golgi tendon organs.
Area B-D represents location of spindle cells.
Area C is the belly of the muscle.
Area A represents the origin or insertion.
Area E represents the origin or insertion.

Figure 16–12.

As a result of the strengthening and weakening of the various TMJ muscles affected by the basic TMJ proprioceptive adjustment, one of the most consistent jaw function changes observed is that of jaw opening improvement. For example, Drs. Jack Frush and Roy Smudde, of Glendale, California, report an average increase of approximately nine millimeters for over 75 prosthodontic patients. Drs. Frush and Smudde also report that "100 per cent of the edentulous patients we have examined with closed vertical dimension have a kinesiologic TMJ opening problem with severity of different degrees."[8]

In patients who demonstrate inability to open easily, an increase of 20 to 30 per cent is not atypical. For example, if the initial measurement from vermilion border to vermilion border at the center line is 40 millimeters, an increase to over 50 millimeters would not be uncommon.

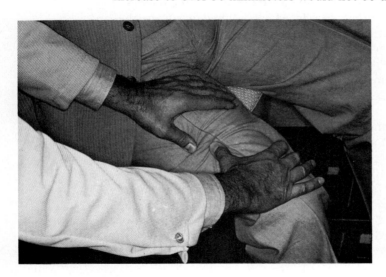

Figure 16–13.

Figure 16–14.

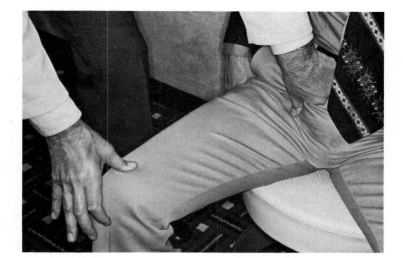

Figure 16–15.

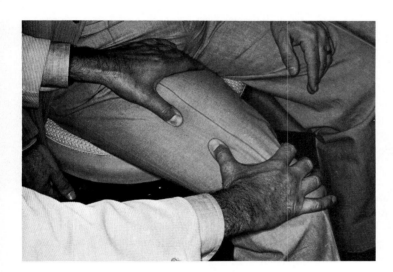

Figure 16–16.

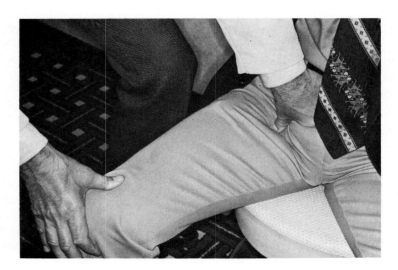

According to Goodheart,[9] "joint clicking on closing would represent a hypertonicity of the buccinator and masseter. This dysfunction could be facilitated by the origin and insertion of the masseter, internal pterygoid, and buccinator being spread apart, stimulating Golgi tendon [organ] activity. This effectively restores lost vertical dimension."

Similarly, the clicking on opening would represent a unilateral or bilateral "weakness" of the temporalis.[9] Pressure into the posterior portion of the temporalis toward the condylar attachment and reciprocating pressure on the condyle would result in increased tonus of the temporalis, thereby reducing the relative protrusive position of the mandible.

Finally, the jaw opening kinesiologic correction seems to consistently result in a reduction of pterygoid tenderness in patients who display sensitivity to palpation of those muscles. This reduction of tenderness seems to be of particular value in helping prosthodontic patients adjust to their appliances.[8] Because of these changes in pterygoid sensitivity, and because of the previously mentioned changes in vertical dimension, it seems reasonable that kinesiologic correction of the TMJ musculature should be made prior to fitting for a prosthodontic appliance.[8]

IMPROVING THE BITE

Another fundamental application of the basic TMJ proprioceptive adjustment is to help improve the bite, and thereby potentially reduce the need for equilibration therapy. Because of the changes in vertical dimension and because of changes in TMJ functions which result from less spasm in specific muscle groups, you may expect changes to occur in tooth-to-tooth relationships.

In some cases, correctly stabilizing the TMJ musculature may help identify a prematurity which may be stimulating the muscle spasm to result. However, in most cases, normalization of the TMJ musculature theoretically should return the bite to its original interarch relationship, thereby "correcting" minor prematurities caused by improper mandibular position and function due to muscle dysfunction.

Since both alternatives may be present in any given individual, it seems necessary first to evaluate muscle function and then determine equilibration needs. This therapeutic strategy logically offers the clinician a more precise technique by which to determine the cause of various prematurities, as well as providing more detailed information which may be used to better plan the execution of equilibration therapy.

VERIFYING THE OCCLUSAL DYSFUNCTION

One fundamental application of kinesiologic testing procedures is to further verify the diagnosis of TMJ dysfunction. As a supplement to the evaluation procedures and techniques discussed throughout this text, kinesiologic testing may help the clinician gain valuable information about the functioning of TMJ musculature which is not available via any other methodology. In addition, the data acquired by applied kinesiology is, in the vast majority of cases, logically consistent in supporting conclusions made through traditional modalities.

TESTING MANDIBULAR REPOSITIONING APPLIANCES

Another fundamental application of kinesiologic testing procedures is to evaluate the effectiveness of mandibular repositioning appliances. In essence, applied kinesiology may be used to test such appliances in two dynamic perspectives. First, if the appliance is appropriate for the individual patient, any kinesiologic TMJ dysfunction should either improve or remain the same when the appliance is used by the patient. If the appliance is not appropriate, kinesiologic testing should demonstrate a relatively greater dysfunction of the TMJ musculature. Second, if the appliance is appropriate for the patient, other muscle groups within the body should improve or remain the same in kinesiologic functioning. If the appliance is not appropriate, other muscle groups within the body will develop relative weaknesses, which logically are not in the best interest of the patient's total health.

For example, let us assume that a patient has a left-sided closing problem which was kinesiologically determined, and that the patient is able to resist only 150 millimeters of pressure for 15 seconds to the quadriceps, while the quadriceps normally test at 300 millimeters for greater than 30 seconds. Assuming that no kinesiologic adjustment was made, and that the patient has now introduced the appliance intraorally, an appropriate appliance would possibly increase the relative strength to 250 millimeters for better than 20 seconds. Although is is possible that some appliances may totally normalize the kinesiologic function of the TMJ musculature, it is more probable that a relative improvement will occur and that kinesiologic treatment will be synergistically beneficial.

It is important to remember that the "weakness" which improved in the quadriceps, as described in the prior paragraph, was assessed via therapy localization to the left side of the TMJ joint. In essence, the improvement in the relative strength of the quadriceps kinesiologically reflects improvement in the function of the TMJ musculature. Had the appliance been inappropriate, you would expect the dysfunction to be relatively greater when therapy localizing the left side of the TMJ and re-testing the quadriceps. For example, the quadriceps would now be able to resist only 100 millimeters of pressure for only 5 seconds.

However, if the quadriceps were originally weak (relatively speaking for that patient), an appropriate appliance may result in strengthening of that or many other muscle groups throughout the body. For example, if the quadriceps tested at 150 millimeters for 15 seconds without any therapy localization, the introduction of the appliance intraorally may have increased the kinesiologic score to the 300 millimeter of pressure for greater than 30 seconds, which would be normal for that individual. In addition to potentially affecting the quadriceps, an appropriate mandibular repositioning appliance may increase the relative strength of any muscle group in the body. For example, such appliances seemingly have generated increases in relative strength of such diverse musculature as the deltoids, psoas, latissimus dorsi, rhomboids, teres minor, and the trapezius. In particular, such appliances frequently seem to affect the function of the abdominal muscles, which in turn may frequently improve vital capacity by 12 to 15 per cent.[1]

When the use of such appliances is made in conjunction with TMJ kinesiologic treatment, more than 50 per cent of previously "weak" muscles will improve in function.[1] For example, if a specific patient demonstrates relative weakness in the deltoids, psoas, abdominals, and trapezius, and if a proper mandibular repositioning appliance were inserted, you would reasonably expect "normalization" of the deltoids and abdominals, while seeing some improvement of the rhomboids and no improvement of the trapezius. However, the improvements may have been normalization in the trapezius with no improvement in the abdominals, or any combination thereof. These reactions of other muscle groups within the body to improvement of TMJ function seem to vary significantly from individual to individual. However, at this time, there has been no clinical evidence to suggest that improving TMJ function will adversely affect any other muscles. Consequently, if a mandibular repositioning appliance induces weakness in a previously strong muscle, it seems reasonable to conclude that the appliance may not be optimal for that individual.

For example, let us assume that a patient without any therapy localization tests at 200 millimeters of pressure to the abdominals for more than 30 seconds. If, with the introduction of the mandibular repositioning appliance intraorally, the abdominals are retested and the appliance is less than optimal, you would possibly expect a decrease in resistance to 100 millimeters of pressure for less than 15 seconds. However, again, the weakness may *not* necessarily demonstrate itself in the abdominals or in any one of the muscle groups previously mentioned. Such weakness may occur within *any* muscle group in the body or within various groups of muscles. For example, such weakness may simultaneously occur in the deltoids, the rhomboids, and the psoas. In addition, such weakness may theoretically demonstrate itself by constriction of smooth musculature, thereby potentially decreasing blood flow to various endocrine glands and affecting their secretion rates.

Motivating Patients Psychologically

Another fundamental application of applied kinesiology is to motivate the patient compliance with the clinician's recommended therapy program. Although an individual may intellectually understand and agree with the need for TMJ treatment, the dramatic subjective experience of applied kinesiology allows many patients to believe emotionally. For example, if you can have the patient concretely experience significant improvements in muscle strength as a result of utilization of a mandibular repositioning appliance, it seems obvious that most individuals would be psychologically reinforced to better utilize that appliance. Similarly, if the patient doubts the need for therapy, you could possibly use applied kinesiology to demonstrate the dysfunction of that person's TMJ. Subsequently, you could make the corrections afforded by a temporary splint or by the basic proprioceptive adjustment, and demonstrate to that patient the impact of maxillomandibular harmony upon general health.

This psychological motivational aspect of applied kinesiology seems particularly important in two major areas of TMJ management. First, during the final stages of treatment after all the major benefits of craniomandibular therapy have been subjectively realized by the patient, and when continued treatment seems to be producing no results from the patient's perspective, applied kinesiology may logically be used to demonstrate the need for continued treatment and compliance by the patient with the doctor's full treatment plan. Second, applied kinesiology seems to have significant potential as a psychological motivator in preventive TMJ dysfunction programs.

Before overt tooth loss, periodontal disease, or other dysfunctions develop as a result of poor or less than optimal occlusion, it seems reasonable that the identification of muscular dysfunctions which could contribute to such disorders and the demonstrative communication of those dysfunctions to the patient would result in more voluntary compliance in preventive occlusal programs.

CRITICISM OF CURRENT PROCEDURES

As previously inferred, dental applied kinesiology is in the embryonic stages of technological development. Consequently, the kinesiologic temporomandibular joint applications and procedures described in this chapter will logically require much sophistication and additional research to cultivate this technology to its optimal utilization of TMJ therapy.

Because of the complexity of the head and neck musculature, it seems obvious that the described basic TMJ kinesiologic adjustments can be significantly refined. In particular, there are several thoughts to consider about improvements which could be made for existing dental applied kinesiology. First, although the manipulative techniques described seem to be consistently effective in improving TMJ function, the degree of improvement could probably be significantly enhanced with better utilization of known applied kinesiology principles. For example, the described adjustments obviously require manipulation of the masseter and buccinator, but they may also affect the temporalis and the pterygoids. It may be therapeutically advantageous to develop adjustments which would specifically affect the individual muscle or muscles that are either hypotonic or hypertonic. It is hoped that further research will establish the effectiveness probabilities of specific spindle cell and/or Golgi tendon organ corrections, given specific TMJ dysfunctions.

Second, future research for a better understanding of the dynamics and interrelationships of the various muscles of mastication will also help develop better kinesiologic applications in TMJ therapy. For example, the described opening adjustment seems to cause a reaction in the functions of the pterygoids. However, the exact degree and extent of this and other reactive dynamics in the kinesiologic functioning of the TMJ musculature have not been adequately investigated.

Third, future research also seems to be needed for better determining the interrelationships of specific muscular dysfunctions to various structural disorders. For example, the role of muscular dysfunctions in the development of prematurities, tooth loss, and periodontal disease logically requires more system investigation. If applied kinesiology and other muscular treatment strategies are used to reduce the need for equilibration therapy, the muscular improvement alternatives seem preferable to the permanent loss of enamel.

Fourth, much additional research is needed to better establish the interrelationships between masticatory functions and systemic health. It is hoped that the pioneering investigations of Goodheart,[9] May,[10] and Fonder[11] will be of value in developing a concept of optimal individual occlusion. For example, an individual may have an occlusal relationship and TMJ muscular functions within the range of adaptability which would allow that person to enjoy good dental health. However, minor imperfections of the occlusal function may cause other muscular or structural dysfunctions throughout the individual's body. In addition, further research would be valuable in establishing how physiological processes and nutrition relate to less than optimal occlusal harmony and TMJ muscular functioning. For example, the chronic ingestion of refined carbohydrates should logically lower muscular stress thresholds, thus allowing habituated tension problems to develop more frequently.

Fifth, definitive understanding of the physiological dynamics by which therapy localization works, and which would account for the changes in tonicity affected by kinesiologic adjustments, would also help develop more sophisticated applications of applied kinesiology in occlusal therapy. In particular, understanding the dynamics of therapy localization, which are thought to be electromagnetic,[1] may lead to the development of electronic sensing equipment which could be used to diagnosis TMJ muscular dysfunctions very accurately. More importantly, such measuring capabilities could be used to evaluate both the need for preventive therapy as well as the progress of TMJ treatment.

PHYSIOLOGICAL RATIONALE AND CONJECTURES

Goodheart[9] has speculated that spindle cell and Golgi tendon organ manipulations result in a change in proprioceptive dynamics of the muscle being manipulated. However, it seems important to note that such ideas have been neither experimentally verified nor denied.

In brief summary, it is argued that each muscle has a resting length which is proprioceptively "remembered." This resting length is determined by the amount of contraction in the spindle cells and by the amount of relaxation of the Golgi tendon organs. It is speculated that within the belly of the muscle, and within the areas of the origin and insertion, are proprioceptive units which determine the number of spindle cells and/or Golgi tendon organs which will be firing, thus determining the resting length of that muscle.

For a multitude of reasons, including minimum diet and stress exposure, it is further argued that some muscles learn to be fatigued; that is, they learn a hypotonic resting length. This hypotonicity in turn contributes to the antagonist muscle acquiring a hypertonic resting length, which functionally means that the muscle is in spasm.

The theorized purpose of the kinesiologic adjustment is to strengthen the hypotonic muscle, thus inducing a weakening in the antagonistic, spastic muscle. This is theoretically accomplished by affecting extreme function of either the muscle's spindle cells or Golgi tendons, or both. For example, let us assume that the normal resting length of a muscle requires a balance between the tension levels of the spindle cells and the Golgi tendon. Let us further assign an arbitrary value of 10 units of force being exerted by the spindle cells, balanced by 10 units of force being exerted by the Golgi tendon, a total of 20 units.

In the case of a hypotonic muscle, it is speculated that the proprioceptive dynamics could represent a value of 18 units being exerted by the Golgi tendon, while the spindle cells would exert only minimal tension, such as 2 units. However, the combined tension between the spindle cells and the Golgi tendon still totals the 20 units originally observed.

It is theorized that the kinesiologic adjustment functions in the same manner as the psychological procedure called overcorrection. This suggests that in order to normalize a desired behavior it is necessary to overcorrect for that particular position. For example, if a child knocks over a chair next to a table, he would be required to straighten up all the chairs surrounding the table rather than just correct the position of that one chair. In analogy, in order to attain a balance of 10–10 between the spindle cells and the Golgi tendon, it will be necessary to overcorrect each of those dynamics. This means that the spindle cells, hypotonically with a setting of 2, would be manipulated to a stretching position of 18, which, when the pressure was released, would theoretically return to the normal position of 10. Similarly, the Golgi tendon organs, hypotonically with a setting of 18, would be stimulated to a position of 2, which, when the pressure was released, would theoretically return to the desired normal of 10 units of force.

To summarize briefly, various stimulants cause a specific muscle to fatigue, whereby it learns a posture of hypotonicity which subsequently causes its antagonist muscle to go into a degree of spasm. The fundamental purpose of the kinesiologic adjustment is to affect the proprioceptive units within that muscle's structure to allow the muscle to assume its natural resting position length.

How Long Does It Last?

The most frequent question raised by clinicians after seeing the improvements in TMJ functioning resulting from the appropriate applied kinesiology adjustments is "How long does that improvement last?"

The answer to this question varies from patient to patient, for a variety of different reasons. Obviously, patients with more severe occlusal problems may require more intensive kinesiologic therapy, with only short-term results during the initial periods of treatment. As with any treatment regimen, some patients will respond significantly more favorably than others. However, beyond individual differences, the permanency of the TMJ kinesiologic adjustment basically depends upon the major and minor systems which support muscle function.[1]

In particular, there are three muscle support systems which need to operate at certain levels of efficiency in order to provide an environment conducive to permanent, proper TMJ muscular functioning. The first major support system is the nutrition available to the musculature. The second major support system is the neurolymphatic, which concerns itself with the removal of waste materials generated by muscle function. The third is the neurovascular, which concerns itself with the blood flow available to the musculature.

If any of these three major support systems is operating below a certain level of efficiency, which logically varies from patient to patient, the kinesiologic correction will probably not last for a significant period of time. For example, if a patient consumes a large amount of refined sugars and refined carbohydrates while consuming minimal amounts of foods with calcium, magnesium, vitamin C, and vitamin E, the poor nutrition of that patient may significantly decrease the operating dynamics of the TMJ musculature. This less than optimal functioning thereby may create an environment in which those muscles learn and maintain inappropriate hypotonic and hypertonic relationships.

In summary, to insure proper muscle function and the permanent retention of kinesiologic corrections, evaluation and appropriate actions are necessary to maintain proper functioning of the muscle support systems. In particular, it is critical to ensure that your patient significantly reduces the intake of refined carbohydrates and refined sugars. In addition, it is also necessary to motivate your patient to eat a diet which provides the necessary minerals, vitamins, amino acids, and so forth, which are needed for proper functioning of both the TMJ muscles and their various support systems.

PHYSIOPATHOLOGY AND OCCLUSAL DISEASE

The concept of physiopathology has been implied throughout this text. Because this concept may provide significant value in understanding the development of jaw imbalance and in understanding the need for appropriate muscle therapy in occlusal treatment, this section will briefly attempt to describe the causes and types of physiopathological processes which may affect TMJ syndromes.

Definition

Physiopathology is concerned with the effect of physiological functions, or more specifically dysfunctions, in the development of pathological disease. To grossly oversimplify, the basic notion of physiopathology is that chronic poor function provides an environment which is conducive to the development of structural deterioration or organic disease. For example, chronically tense TMJ muscles may cause the mandible to be held in a position and to function in a position of malocclusion, subsequently resulting in tooth wear and/or loss.

Physiopathology should not be confused with pathophysiology, whereby abnormal body structure acquired congenitally, by trauma, or by disease, causes a physiological process to operate below maximal efficiency. For example, a gross prematurity may stimulate chronic spasm in TMJ musculature on one side of the mandible, which could interfere with the individual's ability to open his mouth.*

TYPES OF DENTAL PHYSIOPATHOLOGY

Although there are many forms of physiopathology, two are of special significance for occlusal therapy—neuromuscular and vascular.

Neuromuscular physiopathology may demonstrate itself basically in three manners within the TMJ muscular complex. First, an individual may overreact to a stress stimulant in terms of neuromuscular tension. For example, a stressor such as the sound from a high-speed drill may cause most individuals to respond with 25 microvolts of tension in the masseter muscles, while an individual with an abnormal condition may respond with more than 100 microvolts of masseter tension.

---

*For a brilliant description differentiating pathophysiology and physiopathology, see Whatmore and Kohi.[2] This concludes that "pathophysiology consists of physiologic alterations that are the result of structural abnormalities . . . whereas . . . physiopathology, by contrast, consists of altered physiology for which there is no underlying structural pathology."

Second, an individual may develop patterns of habituated tension. For example, the normal resting tension of the masseter muscles may be 5 microvolts, while an individual may have an abnormal resting tension level of 25 microvolts.

Third, an individual may develop patterns of habituated hypotonicity. For example, because of atrophy or other causes, including exhaustion due to stress, any muscle may become relatively "weak" in comparison with its normal ability to function. In other words, any chronically hypotonic muscle would be able to accomplish less effort before reaching a point of fatigue. Quantitatively, this "weakness" could be measured with a hypotonic muscle that is able to resist only 150 millimeters of pressure for less than 5 seconds, while the same muscle group under normal functioning capabilities would be able to resist over 300 millimeters of pressure for more than 30 seconds.

It may be useful to conceptualize that chronic hypotonicity and chronic tension patterns are a form of proprioceptive physiopathology, since the common characteristics of these two muscular habits is that the resting length and position of the involved musculature are inappropriate. Although it may be commonly thought that proprioceptive dynamics of musculature are "fixed and permanent," the concept of physiopathology argues that proprioceptive functions are changeable. For example, the proprioceptive characteristics of the periodontal ligament may change with tooth loss.

Vascular physiopathology also may demonstrate itself basically in three manners within the TMJ muscular and structural complex. First, an individual may over-react to a stress stimulant in terms of smooth muscle contraction in the form of vasoconstriction. Quantitatively, this decrease in bloodflow can be expressed by measuring the surface temperature above the vasoconstricted area, with colder surface temperatures reflecting greater vasoconstriction. For example, a normal person may demonstrate a decrease in bloodflow as measured by a carotid surface temperature of 94° F., down from 95° normal where the drop in temperature was stimulated by a stressor. An abnormal individual may demonstrate a drop to 89° F. to the same stressor at the same carotid surface measurement point. Second, an individual may develop patterns of chronic vasoconstriction. For example, instead of maintaining the 95° F. carotid temperature, an abnormal individual may maintain a carotid surface temperature of only 90° F. Third, because of stress responses, as described by Selye,[12] an individual may develop patterns of chronic inflammation.

CAUSES OF PHYSIOPATHOLOGY

To understand the development of physiopathology, it may be helpful to understand a few basic concepts of psychophysiology. In summary, there are seven behavioral and psychological characteristics of physiological processes necessary to appreciate in order to acquire a fundamental knowledge of the dynamics of physiopathology in occlusion. They are as follows:
1. Muscle function is largely autonomic.
2. Autonomic responses may be psychologically conditioned.
3. Stress causes physiological responses.
4. Responses to stress may become habituated.
5. Abnormal stress responses may be reconditioned (re-educated).
6. Autonomic processes may be brought under cognitive control.
7. What is "normal" may not be healthy.

It seems obvious that the vast majority of muscle functions are autonomic, with very little cognitive effort normally made in the performance of muscle movement. Whether muscle activity is unconscious or deliberate, the neural control of that activity is mostly involuntary. Information regarding the muscle's length, speed of contraction, range and angle of motion, and its antagonist muscle(s) functions must be sorted, analyzed, and then converted into an outflow of signals from brain centers in order to have the precise regulation of mobility and stability of body parts necessary for human movement. The autonomic regulation of muscle function is basically accomplished by information provided by proprioceptors within the muscles' spindle cells and Golgi tendon organs, with signal outputs for muscle function and movement being generated from the premotor and motor cortex and sent into the reticular activating system, the hypothalamus, and the limbic system.[2]

Since Pavlov's classical experiments in conditioning dogs to salivate at the sound of a bell, it has been psychologically accepted that autonomic responses in general may be similarly conditioned. This technology and concept are important in understanding physiopathology, since muscle functions are largely autonomic and consequently may be conditioned to maintain inappropriate tension patterns. The fundamental aspect about conditioning which relates to the development of physiopathology is that a neutral event (the ringing of a bell) may be associated with a natural stimulus (the food placed in front of the animal). By analogy, the environment (neutral) may become associated with the sound of the high-speed drill (anxiety stimulus), so that an individual may learn to demonstrate bracing (muscle tension) behavior whenever he is in that particular environment.

It also seems obvious that stressors produce physiological responses. In particular, a stressor may cause responses in an individual's neuromuscular system as well as in the vascular system. In addition, stress in general, as described by Selye,[12] affects the adrenal, the thymus, and the gastrointestinal tract.

There has been an abundance of literature in recent years which clearly substantiates the theory that abnormal stress responses may be reconditioned via a psychological process called desensitization. In addition, there has been much literature describing how habituated tension patterns and other inappropriate physiological habits may be conditioned and/or brought under cognitive control via biofeedback training.[13] Finally, diet, applied kinesiology, and occlusal therapy seem to be useful tools in creating an environment which is conducive to re-educating abnormal stress responses and in changing habituated tension patterns.[1]

Because of the large amounts of stress to which most members of an industrialized society are subjected, and because of poor diet, it seems highly probable that the vast majority of individuals have some neuromuscular or vascular physiopathological process. In particular, it seems likely that most people may develop physiopathology of the TMJ musculature because these muscles are among those most consistently responding to stress stimulants. In conclusion, it seems probable that it is currently "normal" or "average" to have a physiopathological condition of the TMJ complex, although it is obviously not healthy to have these physiological habits.

Since physiological responses to stressors are a significant component in the development of neuromuscular and vascular TMJ physiopathological states, it may be useful to understand the basic forms of stress stimulants.

In simplified summary, the following four major groups of stressors may motivate or reinforce the learning of physiopathological muscular patterns:

1. Diet
2. Environment
3. Psychological (emotional) factors
4. Trauma and disease

Various foods may stimulate tension responses of the smooth and/or striated muscles. For example, most people demonstrate such tension responses to the ingestion and digestion of refined sugars and refined carbohydrates. Other common food sensitivities which may produce such tension responses are corn, wheat, dairy products (especially processed milk), red meats, coffee, cola products, and refined white flour products.

In addition, if an individual's diet provides insufficient amino acids, minerals, and/or vitamins necessary for that particular person, such nutritional deficiencies may lower stress tolerance thresholds, which could have two major effects in the development of physiopathological conditions. First, the frequency of any specific physiological response to stress could increase. For example, some stressors may not cause response by the TMJ neuromuscular complex when the diet is nutritionally adequate; however, with an insufficient diet, these muscles may respond to that particular stimulant. Second, the intensity of the response may be more acute if the person's nutritional intake is inappropriate.

Environmental stressors may also stimulate tension responses, contributing to the development of physiopathological conditions. These stressors include both natural stressors, such as weather, and man-generated stressors, such as noise, air conditioning, pollutants, and so on. Weather may motivate vasoconstrictive responses in particular. In cold climates, for example, people tend to acquire habituated vasoconstrictive patterns much more frequently than do people in warmer climates. In addition, loud noises or sounds of specific frequencies seem to cause some people to respond with neuromuscular tension. For example, the sound of high-speed drills may motivate some individuals to develop significant tension responses.

Psychological stressors also contribute to the development of physiopathological states. When an individual "worries," he probably engages in what Whatmore and Kohli[2] term "re-representing error" or "flow error" behavior, which leads to dysponetic signaling producing muscular tension. In others words, repetitive thinking about dreaded events, unpleasant situations which currently exist, the responsibility of who or what is to be blamed for a current plight, or about prior decisions or actions, will hyperactivate limbic and other neurological circuits, which will excite skeletal-muscle bracing.

Trauma and disease may also motivate the development of physiopathological conditions. For example, a patient who undergoes a cervical fusion of C5–7 may develop neck muscular tension patterns in order to help hold the vertebra in place while healing progresses. Note that this phase of neuromuscular tension is not physiopathology, but pathophysiology—that is, a structural problem causing a change in physiological function. However, if that tension pattern maintains itself after the healing process is complete, a physiopathological condition exists. Similarly, following trauma or disease, an individual may develop vasconstrictive patterns locally to the injury or disease process, or systemically, and he may subsequently maintain this circulation behavior after the structural or pathological involvement abates.

In TMJ treatment, the understanding that physiopathological states may exist after structural alterations have been made may be a very valuable concept. In essence, you cannot assume that equilibrating a prematurity that motivated detrimental tension patterns of the TMJ musculature will automatically return those muscles to normal function. Although many patients may have their TMJ muscular function normalized, some may maintain tension patterns and will subsequently need muscle correction therapy, such as exercise, biofeedback, and/or applied kinesiology. For example, if masseter physiopathology develops as a result of a prematurity, following equilibration the patient may still suffer excessive tooth wear of the molars as a result of the remaining habituated masseter tension, although that wear will be even.

In conclusion, physiopathology is *not* a muscular problem; the smooth or striated muscular dysfunction is simply a symptom. Physiopathology is basically a neurological problem in which various brain centers have learned or been conditioned to generate inappropriate signals. These inappropriate signals, operating from the premotor and motor cortex, hypothalamus, reticular formation, and/or the limbic system, are called dysponesis.[2] It would be the purpose of applied kinesiology, proper diet, exercise, biofeedback, and other tools of TMJ therapy to correct this neurological disturbance.

RELATIONSHIP BETWEEN JAW POSITION AND INCREASED STRENGTH AND ENDURANCE

Many dentists treating patients with craniomandibular disorders as well as athletes have reported increased strength and performance in their subjects as a result of changing their maxillo-mandibular relationships.[15–17] This concept has caused much controversy between various scientific and clinical investigators.[18, 19]

The criticism directed at the group in favoring positive changes relates to the following aspects: (1) lack of adequate controls in the research design (such as double-bind experimental designs); (2) a lack of proper statistical analysis and (3) lack of knowledge of strength testing.

On the other hand, the research that indicates that the maxillary or mandibular orthopedic repositioning appliance (MORA) is ineffective for strength increases has been critized because (1) the research did not allow adequate time for the MORA to work; (2) the MORA will only work on subjects with TMJ problems or occlusal problems, and (3) it is not known whether or not the appliance has placed the mandible in its optimal physiologic relationship.[20, 21]

One of the first articles to appear was by Smith,[16] who did a sample study of professional football team players with an emphasis on the temporomandibular joint and associated musculature. The effect of proper jaw and masticatory muscle balance was then related to arm muscle strength. It was ascertained that there was a correlation between the jaw posture and the ability of the arm to give strong contraction. This was measured with the teeth together first, and then with a wax bite position, which was fabricated by bringing the player's lower jaw from physiological rest position toward the closest speaking space with midlines evenly aligned. The measurements were made using a Cybex II Dynamometer as well as the kinesiologic deltoid press method.[8, 9]

Similar observations had been made in the 1950s and 1960s by Dr. John Stenger,[22] who reported improvements in the performance of a number of Notre Dame football players fitted with custom-made mouthguards that were designed both to protect the anterior teeth and to match or exceed the thickness of the player's interocclusal "free-way" space. Similar results have been reported by Dr. William Osmanski, a former professional football player who had fitted mouthguards to a specified thickness for a group of athletes.[23]

In 1980, Dr. Richard Kaufman fabricated and positioned several splints for the United States Olympic luge and bobsled teams. He found that headaches previously suffered by luge athletes during their runs were alleviated to varying degrees in some of the athletes by use of these splints. Some of the athletes also indicated an increase in strength when pushing off at the start. He has since continued to research in the area of sports medicine at C. W. Post College.

A controlled double-blind field study[24] was conducted to observe the effects of the mandibular orthopedic repositioning appliance (MORA) on football players on the 1982 C. W. Post College football team. Forty players were randomly divided into two groups, one wearing the MORA [21] and the other wearing the Conventional Mouthpiece (CM).[19] They were tested to discover the effects of the MORA on performance, number, type, and severity of injuries and on three measures of physical fitness, which included strength, jumping ability, and balance and agility.

Overall results were positive and in favor of the MORA. Significant findings favored use of the MORA in that there was lesser severity of injuries, decreased numbers of knee injuries, and greater strength and satisfaction. No significant findings favored the CM. The findings show the importance of the MORA to football players. The authors suggest that the study be replicated with planned periodic readjustments to the mouthpiece.

Several recent research projects[9, 25] have reported that repositioning appliances have merely a placebo effect on strength and performance of the normal population. On reading the design and testing procedures of these studies, it becomes obvious that further research is necessary before the final verdict will be made. In these studies, none of the subjects included were TMJ patients at the time of testing, but several experimental subjects had symptoms of TMJ. Clinical findings and changes in total body strength of the experimental group indicated that the mandibular orthopedic repositioning appliance might help increase strength for TMJ dysfunction patients. It was also stated that strength is a very difficult physiological parameter to measure accurately. Strength can be easily affected by such factors as temperature of the room, tester's voice, color of the room, time of day, presence of other people, emotional state of subject, blood sugar level, and fear of the testing situation. Future research in this area should take these factors into account.[25] It should be noted that another experiment[26] involving TMJ patients using the Cybex II–Data Acquisition System could not measure muscular strength changes with vertical dimension of occlusion variations, which Eversaul,[8] Stenger[22] Goodheart,[19] and Smith[16] suggest. However, subjective clinical measurements of the isometric break test have provided data on changes in muscular strength of patients whose occlusions and jaw relationships are considered to be normal at the TMJ Clinic at the Medical College of Georgia. It is suggested that further research into the neuromuscular system responsible for developing maximum strength and instrumentation capable of measuring isometric break strength are necessary to clarify this kinesiologic concept.

Two recent studies conducted at well-known teaching institutions showed a positive correlation between changes in jaw relationship and increases in strength and muscle efficiency. One study showed a highly significant increase in muscle efficiency (power) of a group of athletes recorded by vertical jump and grip tests. In one study, there was no significant increase in strength recorded by maximum hip sled and bench press tests.[27] The other study tested 23 athletes, comparing mandibular position with appendage muscle strength. Three different mandibular positions were tested, as were all four appendages. Results indicated that mandibular position affects appendage muscle strength and may be important to total well-being. However, considerable variability of optimum muscle strength by muscle groups and mandibular positions was observed.[28]

Another recent double-blind study[29] performed at the University of Illinois involved 20 randomly undergraduate students. Two appliances were constructed: a mandibular orthopedic repositioning appliance, which repositioned the mandible in three dimensions as described in this book, and a placebo splint, which did not alter the individual's normal bite. Data were collected using a Cybex II dynamometer with the subjects seated in a stabilized chair. Information was obtained for three bite conditions: a normal bite, a normal bite with the placebo splint inserted, and a normal bite with the MORA splint inserted. Statistically significant results were recorded between the MORA and normal bite condition for shoulder extension, peak torque; shoulder extension, average torque; and external rotation, average torque. No statistical differences were observed between the placebo and the normal bite condition.

References

1. Eversaul, G. A.: Biofeedback and Kinesiology: Dental Applications. Las Vegas, privately published, 1977.
2. Whatmore, G., and Kohi, D.: The Physiopathology and Treatment of Functional Disorders. New York, Grune & Stratton, 1974.
3. Eversaul, G. A.: Practical and Potential Applications of Feedback Thermometer Training and Nutrition in Crisis and Preventive Medicine. In New Dynamics of Preventive Medicine, Houston, IAPM Press, 1975.
4. Goodheart, G. J.: Applied Kinesiology. Annual Laboratory Manuals. Detroit, Michigan, privately published, 1971–1976.
5. Kendall, JH. O.: Muscles, Testing and Functions, 2nd ed. Baltimore, Williams and Wilkins, 1971.
6. Walther, D.: Applied Kinesiology. Pueblo, Colorado, D.C. Systems, 1976.
7. Goodheart, G. J.: Applied Kinesiology. 1976 Workshop Procedure Manual, 12th ed., 1976.
8. Eversaul, G. A.: Biofeedback and kinesiology: Technologies for preventive dentistry. J. Am. Soc. Prevent. Dent., 6:19, 1976.
9. Goodheart, G. J.: Kinesiology and dentistry. J. Am. Soc. Prevent. Dent., 6:16, 1976.
10. May, W. B.: Exclusive Interview, Dr. W. B. Mays, DDS. The Healthview Newsletter, Vol. 1, Nos., 7 and 8, Manasquan, New Jersey, 1976.
11. Fonder, A. C.: The Profound Effect of the 1973 Nobel Prize in Dentistry. Basal Facts, May, 1976.
12. Selye, H.: The Stress of Life. New York, McGraw-Hill, 1956.
13. Barber, T. X. et al., eds.: Biofeedback and Self-Control: Annual Readers. Chicago, Aldine Publishing Company, 1975.
14. Goodheart, G.: Applied kinesiology in dysfunction of the temporomandibular joint. Dent. Clin. North Am., 27:527, 1983.
15. Eversaul, G.: Applied Kinesiology. Las Vegas, Nev., Box 19476, privately published.
16. Smith, S.: Muscular strength correlated to jaw posture and the temporomandibular joint. N.Y. State Dent. J. 44::278–285, 1978.

17. Schwartz, R., and Novich, M.: The athlete's mouthpiece. Am. J. Sports Med., *8*:357, 1980.
18. Jakush, J.: Divergent views: Can dental therapy enhance athletic performance? JADA, *104*:292, 1982.
19. Moore, M.: Corrective mouthguards: Performance aids or expensive placebos? Physician Sports Med., *9*:127, 1981.
20. Burkett, L. W., and Bernstein, A.: Strength testing after jaw repositioning with a mandibular orthopedic appliance. Physician Sports Med., *10*:101, 1982.
21. Greenberg, M. S., Cohen, S. G., Springer, P., Kotwick, J. E., and Vegso, J. J.: Mandibular position and upper body strength: A controlled clinical trial. JADA, *103*:576, 1981.
22. Stenger, J.: Physiologic dentistry with Notre Dame Athletes. Basal Facts, *2*(1), Spring 1977.
23. Kaufman, R. S.: Case reports of TMJ repositioning to improve scoliosis and the performance by athletes. N.Y. State Dent. J. *46*:206, 1980.
24. Kaufman, A., and Kaufman, R. S.: An experimental study on the effects of the MORA on football players. Unpublished article.
25. Burkett, K. N., and Bernstein, A.: The effect of mandibular position on strength, reaction time and movement time on a randomly selected population. N.Y. State Dent. J., *49*:281, 1983.
26. Hart, D. L., Lundquist, D. O., and Davis, H. C.: The effect of vertical dimension on muscular strength. J. Orthopaed. Sports Physical Ther., *3*:57, 1981.
27. Bates, R. F., and Atkinson, W. B.: The effects of maxillary MORA's on strength and muscle efficiency tests. J. Craniomandib. Pract., *1*:37, 1983.
28. Williams, M. O., Charcomas, S. J., and Bader, P.: The effect of mandibular position on appendage muscle strength. J. Prosthet. Dent., *49*:560, 1983.
29. Verban, E. M., Jr., Groppel, J. L., Pfautsch, M. S., and Ransmeyer, G. C.: A biochemical analysis of the effects of a mandibular orthopedic repositioning appliance on shoulder strength. J. Craniomandib. Pract. (in press).

Supplementary Reading

Smith, Stephen D.: *Atlas of Temporomandibular Orthopedics: Interrelationships of Jaw/Joint Function and Dysfunction to Whole Body Medicine.* Philadelphia College of Osteopathic Medicine Press, Philadelphia, Pa., 1981.

17

The Osteopathic Management of Temporomandibular Joint Dysfunction

EDNA M. LAY, D.O., F.A.A.O.

Three basic tenets of osteopathic medicine are that the human body functions as a total biologic unit in both health and disease, that the body possesses self-regulatory mechanisms, and that structure and function are reciprocally interrelated. All these tenets apply in the osteopathic management of temporomandibular (TM) joint dysfunction.

The temporomandibular joint syndrome may include pain in and around the TM joint, pain in the ear, above and behind the ear, along the side of the head and neck, ear involvement as diminished hearing, stuffiness, tinnitus, vertigo, burning or discomfort in the throat, tongue, along the side of the nose, disturbances in vision, jaw locking, muscle imbalance, trismus, bruxism, accelerated wear, hypermobility, hypersensitivity of the oral mucosa, dryness of the mouth, and herpes of the oral mucosa, external ear canal, and face.

The usual approaches to this problem, including use of occlusal splints, build-up of deficient teeth, adjusting the occlusion, muscle training, anesthetizing muscle trigger points, and so forth, may give partial or temporary relief of symptoms. But they are not complete, because they do not address the underlying cause of this enigmatic problem. In this chapter another aspect of temporomandibular joint dysfunction will be described and explained.

ANATOMICAL CONSIDERATIONS

In analyzing the source of pain in the structures related to the temporomandibular joint, a review of the anatomic and physiologic relations of the trigeminal nerves is in order. Each of the trigeminal nerves possesses three peripheral divisions—the phthalmic, the maxillary, and the mandibular. By way of these three divisions, the peripheral branches of the axons of the somatic afferent cells are distributed as nerves of common sensation to the face, the front of the scalp, the eyeball and conjunctiva, the nose and nasal cavity, parts of the interior of the mouth (including the palate, the teeth, and the anterior portion of the tongue), and the external ear. All motor fibers join the mandibular division and are distributed through it, chiefly to the masticatory muscles.

The trigeminal nerves arise from the sides of the brain stem. Each has a large sensory and much smaller motor root. The sensory nucleus (general somatic afferent) extends throughout the whole length of the brain stem as far as the upper end of the midbrain; below, it reaches down into the second cervical segment of the spinal cord. The motor nucleus lies in the floor of the upper part of the fourth ventricle. It represents the upper end of the column of cells from which the branchial musculature is innervated, for its fibers supply the musculature derived from the first branchial arch. Since this musculature is mainly concerned with the movements of the mandible, the motor root of the fifth nerve is sometimes called the masticator nerve. Boyd and associates[1] stated that

the trigeminal nerve terminates in three nuclei, the main sensory nucleus, the descending or spinal nucleus and the mesencephalic nucleus. . . . The main sensory nucleus and the spinal nucleus have important functional differences. In the main sensory nucleus terminate the relatively coarse sensory fibers of the trigeminal nerve which convey tactile impulses. . . . The spinal nucleus receives mostly fibers of fine calibre which convey impulses related to pain and temperature sensation. . . . The mesencephalic nucleus is concerned with the reception of impulses from stretch receptors in the masticatory muscles and pressure receptors related to the teeth and hard palate. It appears that these impulses, in constituting the afferent side of masticatory reflex arcs, play a part in the coordination and control of chewing movements.

The motor and sensory roots of each trigeminal nerve have their superficial origin from the corresponding side of the pons. . . . From here the two roots pass forward and laterally, beneath the anterior part of the tentorium, and enter a recess of the dura mater in the middle fossa of the skull by passing over the upper edge of the petrous part of the temporal bone and under the superior petrosal sinus. The dural recess (cave of Meckel) contains the trigeminal, or semilunar, ganglion into which the sensory root passes.

The semilunar ganglion occupies a cavity in the dura mater covering the trigeminal impression near the apex of the petrous part of the temporal bone. It is lateral to the internal carotid artery and the posterior part of the cavernous sinus. The ganglion receives, on its medial side, filaments from the carotid plexus of the sympathetic nerves. It gives off minute branches to the tentorium cerebelli and to the dura mater in the middle fossa of the cranium. From its anterior border, three large nerves proceed—the ophthalmic, maxillary, and mandibular.

Associated with the three divisions of the trigeminal nerve are four small ganglia. The ciliary ganglion is connected with the ophthalmic nerve, the sphenopalatine ganglion with the maxillary nerve, and the otic and submaxillary ganglia with the mandibular nerve.

The ophthalmic nerve, a sensory nerve, supplies branches to the cornea, ciliary body, and iris; to the lacrimal gland and conjunctiva; to part of the mucous membrane of the nasal cavity; and to the skin of the eyelids, eyebrows, forehead, and nose. It arises from the semilunar ganglion, passes forward along the lateral wall of the cavernous sinus, and, just before entering the orbit through the superior orbital fissure, it divides into the lacrimal, frontal, and nasociliary nerves. The ophthalmic nerve is joined by filaments from the cavernous plexus of the sympathetic nerves and communicates with the oculomotor, trochlear, and abducent nerves, giving off a recurrent filament which passes between the layers of the tentorium cerebelli and supplies that structure.

The maxillary nerve, the second division of the trigeminal nerve, also is a sensory nerve. It passes forward from the semilunar ganglion and leaves the skull through the foramen rotundum. It then crosses the pterygopalatine fossa, inclines laterally on the back of the maxilla and enters the orbit through the interior orbital fissure. It traverses the infraorbital groove and canal in the floor of the orbit and appears in the face at the infraorbital foramen. A meningeal branch within the cranium supplies the dura mater of the middle cranial fossa. In the pterygopalatine fossa some of its branches pass through the sphenopalatine ganglion. Branches of the maxillary nerve supply the mucous membrane of the roof of the pharynx, posterior ethmoidal and sphenoidal sinuses, and the roof, septum, and conchae of the nose, soft and hard palate, maxillary sinuses, upper teeth and gums, the skin on the side of the nose, cheek, and upper lip, the skin and conjunctiva of the lower eyelid, and the periosteum of the orbit.[2]

The mandibular nerve is the largest division of the fifth nerve and is made up of two roots: a large sensory root proceeding from the inferior angle of the semilunar ganglion, and a small motor root that passes beneath the ganglion and unites with the sensory root just after its exit through the foramen ovale. A small branch is given off just outside the cranium (nervus spinosus), reenters the cranium through the foramen spinosum, and supplies the dura mater and the mastoid air cells. The mandibular nerve supples all the muscles of mastication, the tensor tympani, tensor veli palatini, and mylohyoidus muscles, the anterior belly of the digastric muscle, the temporalis muscle, and the temporomandibular joint. The mucous membrane of the cheek, lower lip, mouth and anterior two thirds of the tongue, the lower teeth and jaw, the skin and fascia of the cheek, the upper half of the ear, the external auditory meatus and tympanic membrane, the skin of the temple and scalp, the skin over the jaw, chin, and lower lip, and the parotid, sublingual, and mandibular glands are supplied by the mandibular nerve.[3]

With this extensive nerve supply to most of the dura mater in the cranium, the sensory supply to the entire anterior portion of the head and face, and all of the muscles of mastication as well as the TM joint capsule, it is necessary to seek any and all stresses on these nerves in our endeavor to relieve TMJ pain and muscle dysfunction. Therefore a study of the dura mater and the temporal bone logically follows.

Dura Mater

The dura mater is the outermost envelope of the central nervous system, a tough membrane of two layers in the cranium. The external layer serves as the internal periosteum for the cranial bones and is continuous through the sutures with the periosteum on the external surface of the skull. The internal layer has four reduplications or folds: the falx cerebri, the tentorium cerebelli, the falx cerebelli, and the diaphragma sellae. There are spaces between the folded layers that contain several important structures, listed as follows by Magoun:[4]

1. Meckel's cave for the semilunar ganglion;
2. the endolymphatic sac;
3. the venous sinuses, into which most of the blood from the brain drains;
4. the meningeal vessels;
5. the nerve supply to the dura from the trigeminal and vagus nerves.

The falx cerebri is a sickle-shaped partition which descends between the cerebral hemispheres. Its anterior end is attached to the crista galli of the ethmoid; its upper border is attached to the cranial vault along the median line from the crista galli to the internal occipital protuberance. The anterior two thirds of its lower border is free, and the posterior third of this border is attached to the tentorium cerebelli along the straight sinus.

The tentorium cerebelli is a large crescentic partition (shaped like a double sickle) which forms a membranous, tentlike roof for the posterior cranial fossa, and this separates the cerebral hemispheres and the cerebellum. Its highest point is in front at the median line where it is attached to the falx cerebri. It slopes downward and backward to its posterior border, which is attached to the internal occipital protuberance and along the transverse ridges, across the mastoid angles of the parietal bones, and all along the petrous ridges of the temporal bones. The anterior termination of these borders on either side is called the petrosphenoid ligament and attaches firmly to the posterior clinoid process of the sphenoid bone. This portion of the dura mater is placed under marked strain in dental traumatic lesions between the petrous portion of the temporal bone and the sphenoid bone. The roots of the trigeminal nerve ascend from the side of the pons, pass beneath this dural band and over the petrous ridge, and enter the semilunar ganglion on the anterior surface of the petrous portion of the temporal bone.

The anterior, or free, border of the tentorium is concave, and within it lies the midbrain. The free edges run forward, cross over the converging petrosphenoid ligaments, and insert firmly into the anterior clinoid processes of the sphenoid bone.

Around the foramen magnum and on the floor of the cranial cavity the dura mater is firmly adherent to the bone. This is particularly marked in the projecting parts of the cranial floor, such as the petrous ridges and clinoid processes. The firm dural adherence in these regions is strengthened by sheaths of the fibrous dura mater that accompany the nerves as they leave the cranium through the various foramina. Outside the cranium the prolongations of the membrane blend with the fibrous sheaths of the nerves. Thus articular strains between the sphenoid, occiput, and temporal bones may put a pull or drag or tension on the second or third division of the trigeminal nerve by way of the nerve sheath, as an overly tight sleeve does on an arm.

The internal layer of cranial dura mater is attached firmly to the cranium at the foramen magnum, is then continuous into the spinal canal as the tough covering of the spinal cord (spinal dura), and extends to the second sacral segment, where it is attached firmly to the bone on the anterior surface of the sacral canal. The spinal dura is attached firmly to the second and third cervical vertebrae and attached loosely within the spinal canal to allow for spinal motion. In the sacral canal the filum terminale, which pierces the dura and drags off a sheath from it, extends downward to blend with the periosteum on the back of the coccyx. The inferior end of the tube is thus securely anchored and held in place.[5]

Thus it is evident that a distubance in position or physiological motion of the sacrum (pelvis) can directly affect the base of the skull and the tension of the cranial dura and its reduplications. Similarly, a structural strain involving the first, second, and third cervical vertebrae and the occiput places the spinal dura under tension that may extend into the entire base of the cranium. Conversely, a dental traumatic strain between the sphenoid and temporal bones may affect the occiput and the upper cervical vertebrae.

TEMPORAL BONE

The anatomy of the temporal bone is complex and will be described only briefly here, highlighting certain aspects which are pertinent to the symptoms and treatment of TMJ dysfunction. The temporal bone consists of four parts, the squamous, petromastoid and tympanic parts, and the styloid process.

The temporal squama is thin and scalelike, its superior surface having a very wide internal bevel for articulation with the inferior border of the parietal bone, which it overlaps. The anterior inferior border is thin above and thick below. Its upper part is bevelled internally, the lower part externally for articulation with the great wing of the sphenoid.[6] The zygomatic process projects forward and articulates with the zygoma. The mandibular fossa, which is smooth, oval, and deeply concave, articulates with the articular disc of the temporomandibular joint and head of the mandible.

The petromastoid may be considered in two parts. The mastoid part forms the posterior part of the temporal bone, houses the mastoid air cells, and articulates with the posterior-inferior angle of the parietal and the occiput. The sternocleidomastoid, splenius capitus, and longissimus capitus muscles attach to the mastoid process. The petrous portion projects medially and forward between the occiput and sphenoid in the base of the skull and articulates with both bones. The articulation between the temporal and occiput is a mechanically complex articulation. The petrous portion articulates with the lateral border of the basiocciput. Posterior to the petrobasilar articulation is the jugular fossa, which, with the jugular notch of the occiput, makes up the jugular foramen. Posterior to the jugular foramen, the jugular surface of the temporal bone articulates with the jugular process of the occiput with an intervening cartilaginous plate. Posterior to that pivotal area, the mastoid portion of the temporal articulates with the inferolateral border of the squama of the occiput (occipitomastoid suture).

Nine of the 12 pairs of the cranial nerves are in close relation to the temporal bone. The oculomotor nerve emerges from the brain, runs forward, and lies in the triangular interval between the free and attached borders of the tentorium cerebelli. Piercing the inner layer of dura mater on the lateral side of the posterior clinoid process, the nerve traverses the roof and further forward descends into the lateral wall of the cavernous sinus, where it lies above the trochlear nerve. The trochlear nerve pierces the dura mater immediately below the free border of the tentorium cerebelli, a little behind the posterior clinoid process. It then passes forward in the lateral wall of the cavernous sinus, below the oculomotor and above the ophthalmic division of the trigeminal nerve. In this part of its course it is closely adherent to the tentorial branch of the ophthalmic nerve, which lies below it.

The course of the trigeminal nerve has been reviewed. Its close relationship to the petrous apex and the dural bands and envelopes are extremely significant in TMJ dysfunction. The abducent nerve pierces the dura lateral to the dorsum sellae of the sphenoid and then bends sharply forward as it crosses the superior border of the petrous temporal close to its apex. In this situation it is inferior to the petrosphenoidal ligament—a fibrous band which connects the lateral margin of the dorsum sellae to the upper border of the petrous temporal near its medial end. The facial nerve enters the internal acoustic meatus, makes a circuitous route through the interior of the petrous portion, and emerges from the bone at the stylomastoid foramen having numerous communications with other nerves. The vestibulocochlear (acoustic) nerve enters the petrous at the internal acoustic meatus, along with the facial, to supply the vestibular apparatus (organ of equilibrium) and the cochlea (organ of hearing). The membranous labyrinth of the inner ear continues into the blind-ended saccus endolymphaticus, which expands under the dura mater on the posterior surface of the petrous temporal bone.[6]

The glossopharyngeal, vagus, and accessory nerves are closely related to the temporal and occiput as they exit from the skull through the jugular foramina along with the jugular veins. Eighty-five to 90 per cent of the venous blood from the brain leaves the cranial cavity through these two foramina. The arterial supply to the brain is likewise related to the temporal bones. The internal carotid artery enters the carotid canal on the inferior surface of the petrous temporal, curves forward and medially, emerges from the canal between the petrous apex and the carotid sulcus in the sphenoid, and enters the cranial cavity, taking with it the sympathetic plexus of nerves. The middle meningeal artery crosses the articulation between the great wing of the sphenoid and the squama of the temporal as well as the parietosquamous suture.

The styloid process projects downward and forward from the under surface of the bone. Three muscles attach to this process, the stylohyoid, styloglossus, and the stylopharyngeus. The stylomandibular ligament passes from the apex of the styloid process to the posterior border of the angle of the ramus. The sphenomandibular ligament attaches to the spine of the sphenoid and descends to attach to the lingula of the mandibular foramen. The capsular ligament and the lateral ligament support the temporomandibular articulation and its articular disc. Thus the mandible is hanging from the inferior surface of both temporal bones and the sphenoid by ligamentous support. The anatomy of the muscles of mastication will not be described here, as that subject has been covered elsewhere in this book.

In order to understand the causes of TMJ dysfunction, it is necessary to understand that the temporal bones from which the mandible is suspended are not in a static or fixed position. The assumption that the sutures of the cranium are immovable is incorrect. They are immovable in cadavers and anatomical specimens. They are *movable* in the *living* human body.

THE DYNAMIC CRANIUM

The cranium is a *dynamic mechanism* in the living human. This dynamic function was discovered by William Garner Sutherland, D.O., D.Sc. (Hon.). By the year 2000 the scientific world may realize that this was one of the foremost discoveries of the twentieth century in the field of human physiology.

Dr. Sutherland made this discovery through the simple modes of keen observation and astute palpation. His study persisted throughout his professional life, from 1900, when he graduated from the American School of Osteopathy in Kirksville, Missouri, until his death in 1954. His studies led him through the complex *design* of the articular surfaces of each of the bones of the cranium and face. His attention was first drawn to the bevel (internal) of the squama of the temporal bone as it overlaps the great wing of the sphenoid and inferior border of the parietal (external bevel). Upon further study of the temporal bone, he noted the "tongue-and-groove" design of the lateral border of the basilar portion of the occiput as it fits into the groove on the medial side of the anterior one third of the petrous portion of the temporal. The jugular process of the occiput articulates with the jugular notch of the temporal, with a cartilaginous plate intervening between the bones and allowing for a pivotal motion. This intricate architecture of the osseous cranium led Sutherland to question: Why this design for motion? What is moving the osseous structure?—a motion he detected by palpation. The anatomy books stated that the joints (sutures) of the skull were immovable. Medical and dental educators had assumed and taught that the osseous cranium is a solid, immovable structure housing and protecting the brain and cranial nerves. They believed the upper jaw was a rigid and fixed osseous structure projecting from the anterior portion of the skull, and, except for the mandible, that all the bones of the head and face were in a *fixed* or *static* position.

Disregarding the rigid thinking of his contemporaries and the erroneous conclusion of the entire scientific world, Sutherland continued his observation and study of the *living* human body. Gradually he came to understand the inherent activity of the central nervous system and its protective elements; the cerebrospinal fluid, the meninges, and the osseous structures, which function as a movable, bony armor to which the meninges attach. He named this dynamic functioning unit the *primary respiratory mechanism*.

Ordinarily we think of respiration as the physiological activity of the lungs and heart in the thorax and the diaphragm moving rhythmically up and down with alternating changes of shape during inhalation and exhalation. In addition to this gross movement of air and exchange of gases, there is *tissue* respiration. This takes place at the cellular level with the constant exchange of metabolites and catabolites through a fluid medium and across cell membranes.

The brain especially demands efficient *tissue* respiration. Its need for oxygen is the greatest of any organ in the body. This tissue in the floor of the fourth ventricle must be functioning efficiently for the body to remain alive because the physiological centers that regulate vital processes of the body are located in the floor of the fourth ventricle. Among these is the respiratory center.[7] The brain is in control of all the functioning processes, including heart action and pulmonary respiration. Thus the rhythmic activity of the brain and its protective elements was named the primary respiratory mechanism.

The term mechanism, from "mechanical" or "machine," implies a functioning unit made up of a number of integrated parts working synergistically. The primary respiratory mechanism includes the following structures and motions:

1. The inherent motility of the brain and spinal cord;
2. the fluctuation of the cerebrospinal fluid;
3. the mobility of the intracranial and intraspinal membranes;
4. the articular mobility of the cranial bones;
5. the involuntary mobility of the sacrum between the ilia.

THE INHERENT MOTILITY OF THE BRAIN AND SPINAL CORD

Every organ in the body exhibits the phenomenon of pulsation or rhythmic action, and the brain is no exception. Lassek[8] describes it as being "vibrantly alive. . .incessantly active. . .dynamic. . .highly mobile, able to move forward, backwards, sidewards, circumduct and to rotate." He further stated: "The normal, human brain is a wondrous, enormously complex, master organ which can be only made by nature. . . . There are probably about twenty billion neurons in the central nervous system of man and it runs on a mere 25 watts of electrical power."

The normal motion of the brain and spinal cord is a slow, wormlike movement. It will be recalled that during the embryonic growth of the neural tube two anterior evaginations, which curl up like a ram's horns in their development, become the cerebral cortex.[4] The normal activity of the brain, which Sutherland observed, is a slow, rhythmic coiling and uncoiling of the hemispheres in the pattern of the ram's horn, whereas the spinal cord moves longitudinally within the spinal dura. This slow rhythmic movement of the CNS may be a function of the glial cells, although this is not yet known.

THE FLUCTUATION OF THE CEREBROSPINAL FLUID

The cerebrospinal fluid is formed in the choroid plexuses within the ventricles. It circulates through the ventricles, over and around the surface of the brain and spinal cord in the subarachnoid spaces and cisternae. Thus the CSF, within and without the central nervous system, is bathing, protecting, and nourishing it.

Fluctuation is defined as "the wavelike motion of fluid in a natural or artificial cavity of the body observed by palpation or percussion." Sutherland observed this subtle rhythmic activity by palpation, and he determined by observation that its normal rate is 10 to 14 cycles per minute. This phenomenon is called the *cranial rhythmic impulse* (CRI). The combined motility of the central nervous system and the fluctuation of CSF manifests as a hydrodynamic activity as well as a bioelectrical interchange. Simply stated, they function as a pump as well as a dynamo.

THE MOBILITY OF THE INTRACRANIAL AND INTRASPINAL MEMBRANES

Surrounding, supporting, and protecting the central nervous system are the meninges. The outermost layer is the dura mater, which is composed of tough fibrous tissue. The intracranial dura mater consists of two layers which blend or fuse together in some areas and which are separated in certain areas by the intradural venous sinuses. The outer layer of dura lines the intracranial cavity, forming a periosteal covering for the inner aspect of the bones. Through the various cranial foramina, and through the fibrous tissue joining the skull bones along the sutural lines, it becomes continuous with the periosteum on the outer surface of the skull. It provides an investment for the cranial nerves as they issue from the intracranial cavity, which is continued into the epineurium of these nerves in their peripheral course. The falx cerebri and tentorium cerebelli have been described, as has the attachment of the spinal dura to two cervical vertebra and to the sacrum. The cranial and spinal dural membranes move in a particular functional pattern in response to the inherent motility of the living brain and cord and fluctuation of cerebrospinal fluid (Fig. 17–1).

THE ARTICULAR MOBILITY OF THE CRANIAL BONES

The erroneous belief that the skull is a rigid osseous structure and that the sutures are immovable arose from the observation and study by anato-

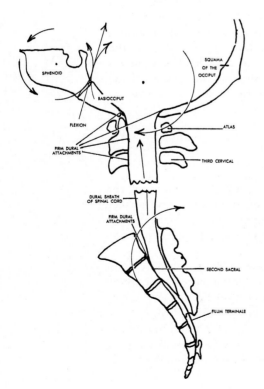

Figure 17–1. Diagram of the cranial and spinal dura mater or reciprocal tension membranes. (From Magoun, H. I.: Osteopathy in the Cranial Field, 2nd ed. Kirksville, Mo., Journal Printing Co., 1966. Reprinted by permission.)

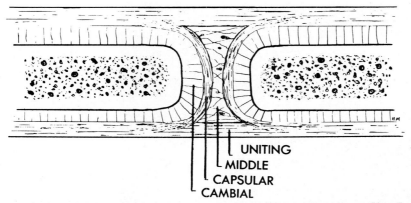

Figure 17–2. Histology of cranial sutures. The two uniting and five intervening layers between the edges of adjacent bones, found only in the skull, suggest a strong bond of union, but one which will permit definite but limited movement. (From Magoun, H. I.: Osteopathy in the Cranial Field, 2nd ed. Kirksville, Mo., Journal Printing Co., 1966. Adapted from Pritchard, Scott, and Girgis by H. I. Magoun.)

mists of dried specimens from cadavers and skeletons stripped of periosteum. Try to erase that false mental conception from your mind and visualize live osseous tissue. The bones of the vault have an inner layer and an outer layer of compact bone with an intervening cancellous layer, which are permeated with fluid (blood) and hematopoietic red bone marrow, and they are encased in an envelope of tough fibrous tissue (periosteum and dura mater). Thus *live* bone is designed to have a slight resiliency.

Pritchard, Scott, and Girgis have described five intervening layers of tissue between the edges of adjacent bones (sutures) of the vault (Fig. 17–2). This design permits a definite, although small, amount of movement of the sutures.[4]

Retzlaff and associates[9] reported on cranial bone mobility using the squirrel monkey. "It is of particular interest," they wrote, "to note that in the 10 adult monkeys from which the bone tissue was removed there was no evidence of suture ossification." They went on to explain:

The general pattern of the suture was similar to that reported by Pritchard et al. In each sample studied the sutures displayed five distinct layers of cells and fibers between the articulating edges of bone. The outer-most layer is a zone of connective tissue which bridges the suture and is designated the sutural ligament. The next layer consists of osteogenic cells. These two layers appear to be continuous with that of the periosteum of the skull bones. This modified periosteal layer, the sutural ligament, is found on both the outer and inner surfaces of the suture. The space between the ligaments is loosely filled with fibrous connective tissue.

The reticular connective tissue portion is seen in the space with extensions into the sutural ligaments. This may provide an inner and outer binding structure which serves to hold the sutures, but still permits some movement of the skull bones.

In addition to the connective tissue seen in the central space blood vessels and nerve fibers are evident. The function of these nerve fibers is not known, but it is possible that they may be involved in the physiological effects of cranial treatment.

The question whether suture obliteration, by ossification, ever occurs in man cannot be answered by this study. We do know that the sutures between the parietal bone and the adjacent bones in the adult squirrel monkey show no evidence of closure in the specimens we have studied.[9]

Space does not permit a detailed description of the direction of motion of each of the bones of the vault and face. Briefly, the osseous structure is moved rhythmically 10 to 14 times per minute by the pull of the dural

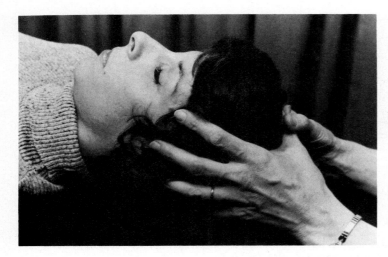

Figure 17–3. Observing the Cranial Rhythmic Impulse with light palpation.

membranes, the fluctuating cerebrospinal fluid, and the inherent motility of the central nervous system. This activity is observable by light palpation (Fig. 17–3).

The key articulation of the cranium is the sphenobasilar symphysis, which has a cartilaginous union up to the age of 25 years and thereafter has the resiliency of cancellous bone. This articulation is slightly convex on its superior surface. Flexion of this joint is a slight increase in this convexity, and extension is a slight decrease in the convexity. Flexion and extension are the normal motions of all the midline bones of the cranium (occiput, sphenoid, ethmoid, and vomer). The paired bones (temporal, parietals, maxillae, etc.) move in external rotation and internal rotation synchronously with the midline bones (Fig. 17–4).

THE INVOLUNTARY MOBILITY OF THE SACRUM BETWEEN THE ILIA

The spinal dura extends from the foramen magnum through the vertebral canal into the sacral canal, attaching to the second sacral segment. A careful

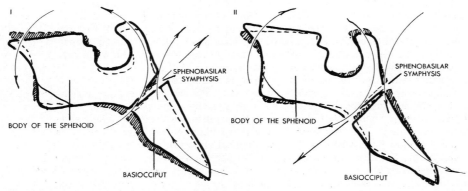

Figure 17–4. Diagrammatic mechanics of the sphenobasilar symphysis. I. Flexion. Viewed from the side, flexion of both sphenoid and occiput (increase of the dorsal convexity) results in elevation of the sphenobasilar symphysis towards the vertex. The deviation from the neutral position is shown in the shaded areas. II. Extension of both sphenoid and occiput is just the reverse. (From Magoun, H. I.: Osteopathy in the Cranial Field. 2nd ed. Kirksville, Mo., Journal Printing Co., 1966. Reprinted by permission.)

study of the design of the articular surfaces reveals that the sacrum may move on one or several postural axes in relation to the ilia. In addition to these voluntary or postural movements, the sacrum also responds to the inherent motility of the central nervous system, the fluctuation of the cerebrospinal fluid, and the pull of the intracranial and intraspinal membranes, with an involuntary movement which is palpable in the living body (Fig. 17–5). This is a slight rocking motion around a transverse axis, called the respiratory axis. Normally the involuntary motion of the sacrum is synchronous with the involuntary motion of the occiput, each bone being influenced by the rhythmic pull of the spinal and cranial dura mater.

Thus we can visualize this physiological unit of function, which Sutherland named the primary respiratory mechanism, with all five components moving slightly but steadily in the living body from before birth until death. Becker[10] summarized its influence on the total body economy thus:

Health requires that the PRM have the capacity to be an involuntary, rhythmic, automatic, shifting suspension mechanism for the intricate, integrated, dynamic interrelationships of its five elements. It is intimately related to the rest of the body through its fascial connections from the base of the skull through the cervical, thoracic, abdominal, pelvic, and appendicular areas of the body physiology. Since all of the involuntary and voluntary systems of the body, including the musculoskeletal system, are found in fascial envelopes, they, too, are subjected to the 10-to-14-cycle-per-minute rhythm of the craniosacral mechanism in addition to their own rhythms of involuntary and voluntary activity. The involuntary mobility of the craniosacral mechanism moves all the tissues of the body minutely into rhythmic flexion of the midline structures with external rotation of the bilateral structures and, in the opposite cycle, extension of the midline structures with internal rotation of the bilateral structures 10 to 14 times per minute throughout life.

All credit and honor for making this discovery of a very complex, physiological unit of function belongs to William G. Sutherland, D.O. He not only discovered the intricacy of its function, but he developed and taught methods of diagnosis for recognizing dysfunction of the *mechanism* and osteopathic manipulative techniques of treatment for restoring normal function.

Dysfunction of the primary respiratory mechanism is present in every case of temporomandibular joint pain and dysfunction.

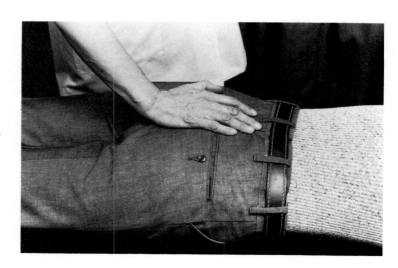

Figure 17–5. Palpation of the involuntary motion of the sacrum.

ETIOLOGICAL CONSIDERATIONS

The position and mobility of the temporal bones must be fairly normal and balanced for proper function of the temporomandibular joints. The physiological motion of the temporal is external rotation and internal rotation (referring to the petrous ridge). The axis for this motion runs from the petrous apex to the jugular surface. In external rotation the temporomandibular fossa, being below the axis, moves slightly posteromedially. With internal rotation it moves anterolaterally.[11]

Obviously the mandible must reflect the position of the fossae. Should both temporal bones be in an exaggerated position of internal rotation, a degree of mandibular protrusion would be present. With both fossae in a posteromedial position from external rotation of both temporal bones, a degree of retrusion would be present. However, the common finding is a combination of one temporal in anterolateral and the other in posteromedial position. This position is of the greatest significance in TMJ problems (Fig. 17–6).

Stone, Dunn, and Rabinov[12] noted that in TMJ pain–dysfunction syndrome the most common clinical sign in 80 per cent is deviation of the mandible laterally during opening, usually toward the involved side and the side on which the click occurred. In addition there is deviation of the symphysis menti to that side. Why? What better explanation than a shift in the fossae?

In addition to external and internal rotation, the temporal bones may be deviated in other planes. One may be inferior to the other, one may be posterior to the other, or combinations of these malpositions may occur. They may occur as a result of force applied directly to the temporal or to bones which articulate with the temporal. They occur when the sphenobasilar symphysis is forced by trauma into abnormal strain patterns and the temporals are moved unphysiologically to accommodate to the distortion or asymmetry of the base of the skull. This brings us to a consideration of the development of the cranium in the perinatal period.

Developmental problems of the osseous cranium of infants may arise in utero or during the birth process. At birth the occiput is in four parts, the sphenoid in three parts, the temporal in three parts, the maxilla in two, the mandible in two, the ethmoid in three, and the frontal in two. The growth

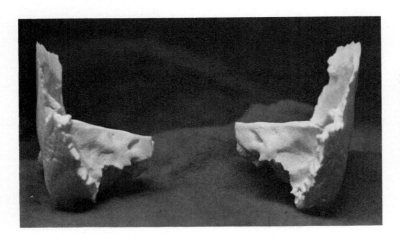

Figure 17–6. Model of temporal bones viewed from back of head, showing the right temporal bone in external rotation (with the mastoid process caudad, the petrous apex high, and the squama temporalis deviated laterally) and the left temporal bone in internal rotation.

of bone responds to stresses applied. These preosseous elements may suffer distortion of shape or disturbance in growth potential, with serious consequences to the bones they become.[13] If the sphenobasilar symphysis maintains an exaggerated convexity (flexion pattern), the maxillae will be maintained in a position of external rotation, the hard palate is low, and the upper teeth will tend to flare a bit. If the sphenobasilar symphysis maintains an exaggerated position of extension, the maxillae will be in internal rotation, the roof of the mouth is narrow, and the hard palate is high. With growth, the upper teeth become crowded. The narrowed alveolar arch may be so extreme that there is not room for the tongue, and mouth breathing results. As growth progresses and the maxillae fail to widen, the premaxillae, carrying the four incisors, grow anteriorly to assume the position known as buck teeth. If one maxilla is maintained in external rotation and the other in internal rotation, other problems or malocclusions result. The mandible, being in two parts with a fibrous union at the symphysis, may have strain or distortion between the parts. Strain between the developing osseous, cartilaginous, and membranous elements of the neonatal cranium are common. Frymann,[14] in a study of 1,250 newborns, found that severe visible trauma was inflicted on the head—either before or during labor—in 10 per cent of the infants. Membranous articular strains, which could be detected by the physician proficient in the diagnostic techniques of osteopathy in the cranial field, were present in another 78 per cent. Thus nearly nine of ten infants in the study had been affected.

There are eleven patterns of strain which may be imposed on the sphenobasilar symphysis. They may occur as a single strain pattern or as combinations of patterns. The position and motion of the occiput influence the temporals and parietals; the position and motion of the sphenoid influence the frontal and all the bones of the face. The bones of the vault and face, being formed in membrane, accommodate to the pattern in the base which is formed in cartilage. A strain pattern may be imposed in utero, during the process of birth, when compressive forces may be severe, or in early infancy from falls and bumps (referred to as birth patterns).[15] Or they may be induced by trauma at any time during the life of the individual (traumatic patterns).

The term trauma is used in this chapter to denote any force applied to any part of the body. It may be physical or psychological. It may vary in magnitude from microtrauma to macrotrauma. Examples of microtrauma to the primary respiratory mechanism are sleeping in a prone position with the face turned to one side habitually, thumb sucking, wearing a tight swim cap for prolonged periods, carrying a brief case in one hand habitually, and similar habits. From infancy throughout childhood and into adult life the body is subjected to many types of trauma. Examples include accidental bumps and falls, contact sports, auto accidents, blows to the face, jaw, or any part of the head, or falls in a sitting position in which the force is transmitted through the spine into the base of the skull.

Some types of trauma which cause strain of the bones and temporomandibular joints may be iatrogenic in nature. The apparatus used by a physician, chiropractor, physical therapist, or a self-treatment for traction to the cervical spine has a head halter with a strap under the chin and another under the occiput. An upward pull is applied to both straps, forcing the mandible into the mandibular fossae and impacting the temporal bones, usually into extreme internal rotation. The occipital strap forces the occiput upward and forward, jamming the occipitomastoid and lambdoid sutures and forcing the temporals into internal rotation. This combination of compressive forces locks the primary respiratory mechanism so that its normal motion is almost obliterated. If there is an imbalance in the position of the temporal bones present before the traction is applied, the strain pattern is exaggerated and so are the patient's symptoms.

Another type of iatrogenic trauma which may induce or aggravate TMJ pain and dysfunction is forceful or ineptly applied manipulative techniques to the cervical spine and suboccipital region. A thrusting force on the occiput with the head and neck in extreme rotation can drive the occiput into the temporal, creating an occipitomastoid strain locking the temporal bone on that side. Or the operator can inadvertently apply force to the mastoid portion of the temporal. The use of the laryngoscope or bronchoscope with the patient's mouth wide open and the head and neck in a backward-bending position for a period of time may induce strain.

A prolonged period in the dental chair with the mouth held open while the dentist pries, drills, scrapes, or hammers may be traumatic. The forces used to extract molar teeth may cause a particular strain referred to as the dental traumatic lesion. Magoun[4] describes this strain as follows:

There is usually marked internal rotation of the temporals. Both bones are held in internal rotation and displaced slightly medially by the V-shaped headrest compressing the mastoid area on either side. This strain is further exaggerated by the thrust of the condyles into the glenoid fossae with the mouth held open and the jaw pulled upon by the muscles of mastication, as well as the force exerted upon the jaw on the side of a lower extraction.

The inward side leverage used to pull a lower tends, however, to disengage the mandible from the glenoid (mandibular) fossa on the opposite side. Since this is opposed by the sphenomandibular ligament running from the angular spine of the sphenoid inferolaterally to the lingula on the jaw, there is sufficient ligamentous traction on the angular spine to twist the sphenoid on its anteroposterior axis as in torsion. We then have, on the side opposite from the extraction, the basisphenoid elevated (petrosal process of the dorsum sellae) while the petrous apex is lowered because of the excessive internal rotation of the temporal. A severe petrobasilar separation results, producing tension on the root, the ganglion or the branches of the fifth cranial nerve, as well as disturbance in the metabolic function of the cerebrospinal fluid to these important structures because of the induced stasis [Fig. 17–7].

The picture is somewhat different but the result can be the same in the extraction of an upper. Here the leverage is downward both medially and laterally but usually ends in a lateral pull. Thus the tuberosity of the maxilla, taking the palatine and the pterygoid with it, is lesioned inferiorly and laterally. As a result of this the sphenoid greater wing is elevated on the side of the upper extraction, instead of the opposite side as with a lower. Since both temporals are in marked internal rotation, the petrobasilar separation occurs on the side of the extraction and also the facial neuralgia [Fig. 17–8].

The diagnosis is rather obvious. Both temporals are slightly medial and in marked internal rotation. The pterygoid process is elevated laterally on the side opposite to a lower extraction but on the same side as an upper extraction and may even crowd the coronoid process of the mandible. The maxilla is inferior on the side opposite the lower extraction but on the same side as the upper extraction, sometimes as much as one eighth of an inch. The mandible is malaligned in any case and tends to protrude slightly because of the internally rotated temporals. The results can be quite widespread. In addition to being separated from the basisphenoid, the petrous apices are jammed medially and posteriorly against the basilar process of the occiput, augmenting the restriction imposed upon the tentorium and the junction with the falx cerebri and so retarding cerebrospinal fluid fluctuation and primary respiratory

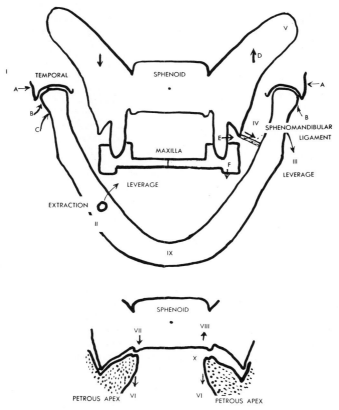

Figure 17–7. Sphenopetrous lesion produced by extraction of a lower tooth. Diagrammatic representation of the sphenoid, temporal, maxilla and mandible.

  I. Temporal rotated internally and compressed medially by
    A. The headrest on the dental chair.
    B. The thrust on the condyles by the muscles opposing opening the jaw.
    C. Increased internal rotation from the extraction on the same side.
 II. Extraction, with inward side leverage.
III. Inward side leverage on the one side tends to disengage the opposite condyle.
 IV. This disengagement is opposed by the sphenomandibular ligament from the angular spine of the sphenoid to the lingula of the jaw.
  V. This traction rotates the sphenoid with the
    D. Greater wing upwards on the side opposite the extraction.
    E. The pterygoid process laterally on this side, sometimes sufficiently to crowd the coronoid process of the mandible.
    F. The maxilla rotated externally and so low on this side.
 VI. The petrous apices inferior with marked internal rotation of the temporals.
VII. The basisphenoid inferior on the side of the extraction.
VIII. The basisphenoid superior on the site opposite the extraction.
 IX. The mandible malaligned with the temporals and maxillae.
  X. A severe sphenopetrous lesion (separation) on the side opposite the extraction. (From Magoun, H. I.: Osteopathy in the Cranial Field. 2nd ed. Kirksville, Mo., Journal Printing Co., 1966. Reprinted by permission.)

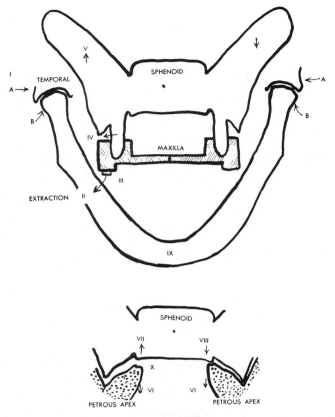

Figure 17–8. Sphenopetrous lesion produced by extraction of an upper tooth. Diagrammatic representation of the sphenoid, temporal, maxilla and mandible.

    I. Temporal rotated internally and compressed medially by
        A. The headrest on the dental chair.
        B. The thrust on the condyles by the muscles opposing opening the jaw.
    II. Extraction with downward and lateral fixation.
  III. Maxilla lesioned inferolaterally on the side of the extraction.
  IV. Pterygoid process carried with the maxilla towards the side of the extraction, sometimes sufficiently to crowd the coronoid process of the mandible.
    V. Sphenoid rotated on its anteroposterior axis by the maxilla through the palatine to carry the greater wing up on the side of the extraction.
  VI. The petrous apices inferior with the marked internal rotation of the temporals.
 VII. The basisphenoid superior on the side of the extraction.
VIII. The basisphenoid inferior on the side opposite the extraction.
  IX. The mandible malaligned with the temporals and maxillae.
    X. A severe sphenopetrous lesion (separation) on the same side as the extraction. (From Magoun, H. I.: Osteopathy in the Cranial Field, 2nd ed. Kirksville, Mo., Journal Printing Co., 1966. Reprinted by permission.)

mechanism function in general. Twisting of the medial two thirds of both Eustachian tubes invites ear complications such as tinnitus or deafness. The sphenoid fixation tends to disturb the venous drainage through the ophthalmic veins or restrict orbital movement, giving rise to eye complications. Maxillary malalignment crowds the ethmoid, turbinates, vomer and palatine bones, inviting nose and throat complications.

That the apex of the petrous portion may be elevated on one side or depressed on the other is supported by Gardner,[16] who reported on cases of trigeminal neuralgia. In a roentgenographic study of the petrous ridges of 130 patients with trigeminal nerve pain and 200 adults (controls) who did not have trigeminal neuralgia, he stated:

For ease of comparison in the data that follow, measurements and percentages in the controls are indicated in parentheses. In the patients the apex of the right petrous bone was higher than that of the left in 46 per cent (controls 47.5 per cent). . . The left was higher than the right in 34 per cent (controls, 29 per cent). . . . They were of equal height, *i.e.*, less than 1 mm. difference, in 20 per cent (controls, 23.5 per cent). These figures show that the apex of the right petrous bone is likely to project farther into the cranial cavity than that of the left regardless of the presence of trigeminal neuralgia. This finding may be related to the fact that more persons are right-handed and therefore inclined to use the right hand for lifting. In carrying a suitcase, for instance, the contraction of the neck and shoulder muscles, particularly the trapezius, exerts a downward pull on the skull so that in effect the suitcase is partially suspended from the skull. . . . In the trigeminal neuralgia series the pain was on the side of the higher petrous apex in 60 per cent and on the side of the lower in 20 per cent. In other words, trigeminal neuralgia occurred 3 times more often on the side of the higher petrous apex than on the side of the lower [Fig. 17–9].

In osteopathic terminology, the temporal with the high petrous apex is in external rotation, the side with the low apex is in internal rotation. This asymmetry is common in the populace and may occur when the sphenobasilar

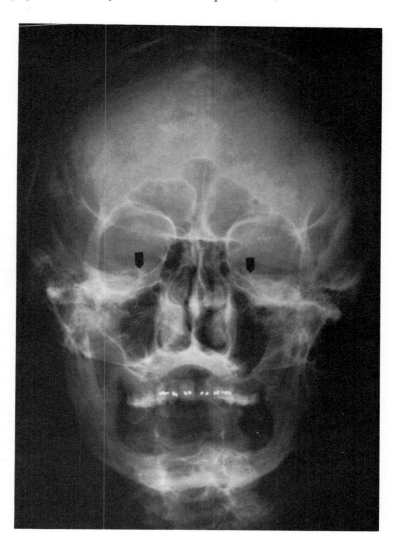

Figure 17–9. Posteroanterior roentgenogram of the skull, showing the apex of the petrous portion of the right temporal bone superior to the left.

symphysis assumes a strain pattern of side-bending rotation or torsion. The question which naturally arises is: Why did some of the patients in Gardner's study have trigeminal nerve pain and others have no pain? Based on this author's clinical experience, the answer lies in whether or not the temporal bones had some degree of physiological motion present or whether one or both temporals were immovable. The presence or absence of motion can be determined only by gentle palpation by a skilled physician trained in the intricate mechanism of the primary respiratory mechanism.

If one temporal bone is restricted in its motion, there is a deleterious effect on all of the primary respiratory mechanism. Let us assume the right temporal has been forced by trauma into extreme external rotation and maintained in that position. Any combination of these signs and symptoms tends to develop. The petrous apex is elevated, the mandibular fossa is posteromedial, the midline of the chin deviates to the right as the mouth is opened wide. The tentorium cerebelli is unable to move physiologically on that side, the petrosphenoid ligament becomes taut, the rhythmic fluctuation of the cerebrospinal fluid is disturbed or static. There may be dysfunction of the third, fourth, or sixth cranial nerves as eye strain, venous congestion, and the like. One or more of the divisions of the trigeminal may be involved with pain in the head and face and spasm or trismus of the masticatory muscles. The venous drainage through the dural venous sinuses related to the falx and right side of the tentorium is disturbed, and drainage through the right jugular vein may be slowed, resulting in congestive headache. Vestibular function may be disturbed, manifesting as dizziness or vertigo; hearing may be disturbed and expressed as stuffiness of the ear (auditory tube malfunction), deficient hearing, tinnitus, or pain in the ear. Malfunction of the ninth, tenth, or eleventh nerve may bring symptoms of discomfort in the throat and tongue, larynx, gastrointestinal tract, cardiorespiratory system, or muscle tension in the sternocleidomastoid or trapezius. It is quite evident that this is an amplified description of TMJ dysfunction.

The spine, pelvis, and extremities also affect the head and temporomandibular joints. The direct dural attachment of the sacrum to the cervical spine and occiput has been described. The action of muscles, ligaments, and fasciae throughout the body from the head to the feet coordinates it as a functioning unit. Time and space in this chapter do not allow for a detailed description of the pelvis and spine and their relation to the base of the skull and TM joints. Suffice it to say that all the supportive structures below the head influence it. The position and motion of the sacrum directly affects the function of the primary respiratory mechanism. The pull of muscles and ligaments which attach the base of the skull to the spine affects the position of the occiput and temporals. Thus faulty mechanics of the pelvis (including a short lower extremity), spine, rib cage, and cervical spine may affect TM joint function. Realizing that the cranium has slight mobility and thereby can compensate to some degree to the forces from below, it is clear that a scoliosis or the habitual use of one arm (carrying a brief case) has a direct influence on the position and motion of the temporal bones and the function of the TM joint.

PHYSICAL EXAMINATION AND AIDS

A general osteopathic structural examination is paramount and should include the following:

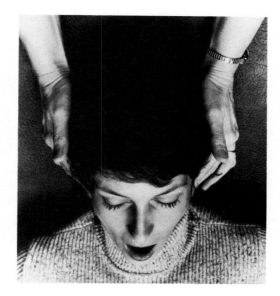

Figure 17–10.

1. Palpatory evaluation of the primary respiratory mechanism as to position and involuntary motion of its components. This is done with *light* palpation of the various osseous components of the cranium and the sacrum, noting position, symmetry, and involuntary motion present. The reciprocal motion or abnormal tension of the dural membranes is assessed. The rate, amplitude, and direction of the fluctuant motion of the CSF is observed—all with light palpation. *Heavy palpatory pressure is definitely contraindicated.*

2. Observation and palpation of the excursion of the mandible. With the patient's mouth closed, his temporomandibular joints are palpated gently for symmetry, tenderness, and tension of the masseter muscles bilaterally. With the operator seated at the head of the table, lightly palpating over the TM joints, the patient is directed to open his mouth slowly (Figs. 17–10, 17–11). The excursion of the mandible, deviation of the midline of the chin, and smoothness of the glide are noted. Travell[17] stated that the full excursion

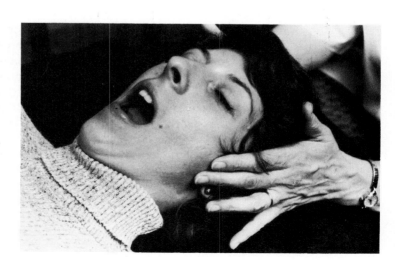

Figure 17–11.

of the mandible can be gauged by the ability of the patient to insert the knuckles of three fingers between the upper and lower incisors. Some patients with TMJ dysfunction will tolerate almost no motion of the mandible. *No force should be applied* in an attempt to elicit motion. If there is marked pain and/or muscle spasm of one or both sides, do not pursue motion testing of the mandible. In that case, the osteopathic physician should begin treatment of the cranium, releasing the membranous (dural) strain within the cranium which is maintaining stress or pressure on the mandible branch of the trigeminal nerve. Completion of the structural examination can be done at a subsequent visit.

3. Observation and palpation of the musculoskeletal system from the feet, through the lower extremities, pelvis, spine, thoracic cage, shoulder girdle into the neck and base of the skull seeking structural deviations, tissue changes, and motion changes.

A general physical examination is needed for an overall evaluation of the patient's state of health. An examination of the eyes, ears, nose, mouth, throat, and cervical lymph glands is necessary for locating any foci of infection, irritation, or abnormality. Blood chemistry should be checked. X-ray films of the skull are helpful in viewing the nasal sinuses and the relative positions of the petrous ridges. Roentgenograms do not reveal cranial articular strains but may reveal bony asymmetry or erosion, osteoporosis, arthritic degeneration, malignant change in bone, or Paget's disease.

A dental examination is indicated seeking foci of infection, malfitting prostheses, malocclusion, and so on. That examination is discussed by other authors.

An evaluation of the patient by a dentist and an osteopathic physician working coordinately before a treatment program is started is essential for thorough evaluation of the TMJ problem. For the dentist to pursue extensive studies in equilibration, building up or grinding off of teeth, designing splints and prostheses, while ignoring the structure from which the mandible is suspended is inadequate diagnosis which results in incomplete and unsuccessful treatment, with much physical and monetary suffering by the patient. For the osteopathic physician to treat and release the strains of the cranium and musculoskeletal system while ignoring the patient's dental health and occlusal relationship also results in incomplete diagnosis and inadequate care of the TMJ problem.

Baker[18] reported on a case in which a good result was accomplished by the cooperative effort of a dentist and an osteopathic physician. His research work demonstrated that "serially measured models of maxillary teeth over six months of combined osteopathic treatment and occlusal equilibration in a patient with traumatic malocclusion showed lateral overall dimensional changes between permanent maxillary second molars of as much as 0.0276 inch, which is nearly nine times the possible error in measurement. In this patient the head bones moved along their sutures." It is interesting to note that this patient had no recent trauma. He had been a paratrooper and had sustained multiple fractures of his left foot in a parachute jump several years before he came under treatment for severe headache, which preceded seizures, nausea, vomiting, and TMJ dysfunction. The osteopathic physician found that the parachute jump, which had caused fractures of the foot, had compressed his entire left side into various strains (including the cranium), and malocclusion was present to the left at the midline of the mandible.

DIAGNOSIS

The patient's history and symptoms suggest the initial diagnosis of TMJ dysfunction. The osteopathic structural findings combined with the dental findings as just described establish the diagnosis. X-ray findings give information concerning osseous degeneration or disease, which is essential in differential diagnosis in some cases.

Observation and palpation of the excursion of the mandible has been described. Observation and palpation of the temporal bones and occiput is done by placing both hands cupped under the occiput with the thumbs lying along the mastoid portions of the temporal bones just behind the ears (Figs. 17–12 and 17–13). The physician determines whether the occiput is level or if one side is nearer the shoulder (more caudad) than the other. The tips of the mastoid processes are compared as to position (superior–inferior, medial–lateral, and anterior–posterior). The general contour of the lateral sides of the head are noted.

Testing motion of the primary respiratory mechanism requires a knowledge of the physiological motion of each of the cranial bones, a matter too intricate to be included in this chapter.

TREATMENT

The aims of osteopathatic management of TMJ dysfunction are as follows:

1. To release the membranous (dural) articular strains of the cranium, cervical spine, and sacrum in order for the patient's primary respiratory mechanism to function at optimum efficiency and his level of health to improve. With this release the temporal bones (and other cranial osseous elements) automatically resume their physiological motion and assume a balanced position for the pattern in that individual's cranium and craniosacral mechanism. The stresses on the cranial nerves are automatically released and the irritability of the masticatory muscles is automatically lessened. As

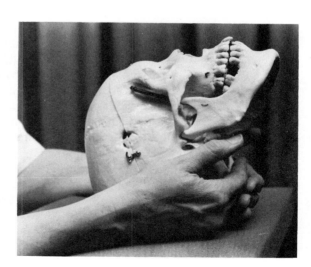

Figure 17–12.

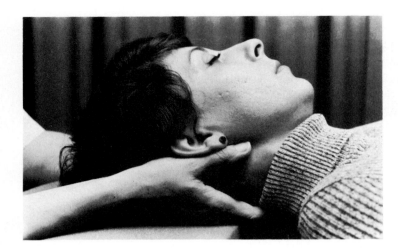

Figure 17–13.

the involuntary motion of the temporal bones normalizes, the function of all the related structures tends to normalize.

2. To release the ligamentous strains and fascial imbalances of the TM joints.

3. To treat the somatic dysfunction throughout the musculoskeletal system, which may contribute to the ligamentous and/or muscular strains affecting the cranial base. This may include a lift under the heel of an anatomical short leg.

4. To advise the patient to have a dental evaluation and treatment as needed.

5. Educate the patient concerning faulty posture, habits which are creating the strains in the craniofacial structure and general spinal structure. These may include faulty habits of chewing and swallowing, sleeping in a prone posture, cradling a telephone between the ear and shoulder, carrying a brief case or suitcase on the same side, and similar habits.

Learning osteopathic techniques for treatment of the craniosacral mechanism requires persistent study and prolonged practice. To diagnose and treat the primary respiratory mechanism requires that the physician have a thorough knowledge of the anatomy and physiological motion of each of the osseous elements and its relationship to the involuntary motion of the total mechanism. In addition to the anatomical knowledge, he must (with proper direction) gain the manual skill, sensitivity and dexterity to palpate the minute rhythmic motion of the living cranium, diagnose membranous strains, and release them. It is essential to use *light* palpation in diagnosis and treatment. Any forceful manipulative techniques to the cranium, the upper cervical spine, or the temporomandibular joint are definitely contraindicated. Forceful osteopathic manipulation or chiropractic "adjustment" of the occipito–atlanto–axial complex may traumatize the spinal and cranial dura mater, forcing the occiput into the temporal(s), thereby causing further dysfunction between the occiput and the temporal at the occipitomastoid suture, a very crucial area to normal cerebral function.

The intention of treatment is not to force the bones of the cranium and face into a particular pattern of symmetry, but to release the stresses in the intracranial membranes which tend to maintain the articular strains between the various bones. In order to release the strain within the cranium, one must have a thorough knowledge of the primary respiratory mechanism and how to employ the intrinsic forces within the mechanism for release. Keeping in mind that the mechanism functions as a unit, a strain may originate at the sacral end of the mechanism, along the spinal structure at any level, or within the cranium.

With the foregoing explanation of the underlying causes of TMJ dysfunction, it is evident that *prevention* is of prime concern in the overall consideration of this common dysfunction.

As physicians, our first opportunity for prevention is to examine and treat the neonate within the first few days after birth for release of the membranous and cartilagenous strains which establish the osseous birth pattern of the individual. This examination and, if indicated, treatment should be a part of the neonatal care before the infant and mother are dismissed from the hospital, not only for the dental aspects but also for the total health care of the infant and the development of its brain and nervous system.

It is imperative that all professionals who care for patients develop an awareness that the human body, particularly the cranium, is a dynamic mechanism, vulnerable to trauma of any kind. With that awareness, they will automatically induce the least possible trauma when necessary and seek professional help for release of the recognized strains early in the course of the dysfunction. As with many human ailments, prevention is of the essence.

CONCLUSION

This chapter is intended to broaden the knowledge of the scientific community concerning temporomandibular joint dysfunction. The assumption that the temporal bones are static is erroneous. They are part of a dynamic functioning unit, the primary respiratory mechanism. The chief etiological factor in TMJ dysfunction is trauma, both micro- and macrotrauma. Treatment (multidisciplinary) through the cooperative effort of an osteopathic physician trained in treatment of the craniosacral mechanism and a dentist provides the patient with a much better result.

References

1. Boyd, J. D., et al.: Textbook of Human Anatomy. Hamilton (ed.): London, Macmillan Co., 1957, p. 745.
2. Gray, H.: Anatomy of the Human Body, 29th ed. C. M. Gross, (ed.): Philadelphia, Lea and Febiger, 1973, pp. 915–919.
3. Romanes, G. J.: Cunningham's Textbook of Anatomy, 11th ed. London, Oxford University Press, 1972, pp. 722–724.
4. Magoun, H. I.: Osteopathy in the Cranial Field, 2nd ed. Kirksville, Mo., Journal Printing Co., 1966, p. 19.
5. Lay, E. M.: The osteopathic management of trigeminal neuralgia. J. Am. Osteopath. Assoc., *74*:373, 1975.
6. Warwick, R., and Williams, P. L. (eds.): Gray's Anatomy, 35th British edition. Philadelphia, W. B. Saunders Co., 1973, p. 293.
7. Wales, A. L.: The work of William Garner Sutherland, D.O., D.S. (Hon.). J. Am. Osteopath. Assoc., *71*:788, 1972.
8. Lassek, A. M.: The Human Brain. Springfield, Illinois, Charles C Thomas, 1957, p. 27.

9. Retzlaff, E. W., et al.: The structures of cranial bone sutures. J. Am. Osteopath. Assoc., 75:607, 1976.
10. Becker, R. E.: Craniosacral trauma in the adult. Osteopathic Annals. 4:43, 1976.
11. Magoun, H. I.: Dental equilibration and osteopathy. J. Am. Osteopath. Assoc., 74:981, 1975.
12. Stone, S., Dunn, J. J., and Rabinov, K. R.: The general practitioner and the temporomandibular pain-dysfunction syndrome. J. Massachusetts Dent. Soc., 20:262, 1971.
13. Magoun, H. I.: Osteopathic approach to dental enigmas. J. Am. Osteopath. Assoc., 62:110, 1962.
14. Frymann, V. M.: Relation of disturbances of craniosacral mechanisms to symptomatology of the newborn: study of 1250 infants. J. Am. Osteopath. Assoc., 65:1059, 1966.
15. Frymann, V. M.: The trauma of birth. Osteopathic Annals, 4:22, 1976.
16. Gardner, W. J.: Trigeminal neuralgia. Clin. Neurosur., 15:1, 1968.
17. Travell, J.: Lecture on head pain. Convocation of American Academy of Osteopathy. Colorado Springs, May 25, 1973.
18. Baker, E. G.: Alteration in width of maxillary arch and its relation to sutural movement of cranial bones. J. Am. Osteopath. Assoc., 70:559, 1971.

18

Arthrokinematics of the Temporomandibular Joint

MARIANO ROCABADO, P.T.

In order to understand how a joint that maintains such a close environment can become unstable, lose its normal mechanics, and start functioning against the rules of synovial joints (movable, frictionless, and pain-free joints), we must understand the normal physiology of joints and of periarticular connective tissue, mainly, ligaments and capsules.

The temporomandibular joint (TMJ) is a synovial joint and has three elements that are related to each other for normal function: the condyle of the mandible, a disc, and the eminentia articularis ossis temporalis. These three elements relate so that the areas that are built to support pressure are facing for normal function. The condyle has a major area of trabecular bone in the anterior joint surface; the disc, which is a biconcave structure, is highly innervated and highly irrigated in the anterior and mainly the posterior edges. The middle portion where the biconcave surfaces meet is avascular and noninnervated. One surface of the disc (inferior) relates to the anterior portion of the condyle. The opponent surface (superior) faces the middle third of the eminentia articularis ossis temporalis, which has the major area of trabecular bone at that point. These three surfaces—the anterior portion of the condyle, the biconcave joint surfaces of the disc, and the middle third of the eminentia articularis facing each other in maximal intercuspation of the teeth during the position of the mandible at rest—are kept together by periarticular connective tissue and muscle in a physiological state of functional rest. This relationship is called, according to physiology of joints, a loose-packed position (Fig. 18–1).

Normal periarticular connective tissue is ligament, tendon, capsule, and fascia, and as its name implies, its function is to connect tissues together. Particularly on the TMJ, the purpose is to maintain the joints together and to limit the range of motions of the joint.

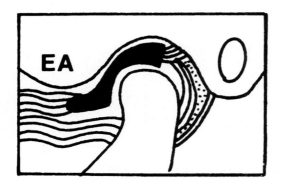

Figure 18–1. Loose pack. EA = eminentia articularis ossis temporalis.

PHYSIOLOGY OF PERIARTICULAR CONNECTIVE TISSUE

Connective tissue is one of the four basic tissues of the body, and collagen is the major structural component of these tissues that make up 80 per cent of the total dry weight of the periarticular connective tissue. There are four types of collagen, each varying slightly in the arrangements of its alpha chains and having different distributions in the body.

COLLAGEN

Type I collagen is found in ordinary connective tissue and bone. Connective tissue can be divided in two different types: (1) Dense, which consists of ligaments, tendons, aponeuroses, capsules, and the deep connective tissue layer of the skin; and (2) loose, ordinary connective tissue, which consists of areolar tissue filling between body parts, surrounding fascia, blood vessels, nerves, and muscles. Type II collagen is found in the hyaline cartilage; type III, in the fetal corium and arteries; and type IV, in the basement membrane. This discussion will focus mainly on type I collagen fibers of ordinary connective tissue which are intimately related to the biomechanics of the TMJ.

Type I Collagen

Dense, ordinary connective tissue is commonly classified into two main types: (1) the irregularly arranged and (2) the regularly arranged fibers.

The irregularly arranged type has collagen fibers running either in different directions in the same plane or in every direction. This is quite functional for capsules, aponeuroses, and sheaths that need to withstand stretching in all directions, including along the direction of the fibers. A common example of this is the oblique fibers frequently seen traversing a joint capsule. Such multidirectional fibers are responsible also for the stretchability of the corium of the skin.

The regularly arranged type I collagen fibers all run more or less in the same plane and same direction in a linear fashion. This arrangement gives great tensile strength to ligaments and tendons. These structures can withstand tremendous pulling without stretching. The cells in the dense regular connective tissue are mainly fibrocytes located between the parallel bundles of collagenic fibers. Collagen forms the fibrous portion of connective tissue. The nonfibrous portion, often referred to as ground substance or matrix, is composed of acid mucopolysaccharides, or glycosaminoglycans, and water. It is important to be familiar with glycosaminoglycans and their functions to understand the changes that occur with some types of immobilizations or even with rest of the joints. The main glycosaminoglycan of connective tissue is hyaluronic acid. Generally, the glycosaminoglycan is bound to a protein and is collectively referred to as proteoglycan. In connective tissue, proteoglycans combine with water to form a proteoglycan aggregate.

Water makes up the 60 to 70 per cent of the total connective tissue's wet content. The glycosaminoglycans, with their large surface, have an enormous binding capacity and are responsible for this large water content of connective tissue. Together the proteoglycans and water form a gel that acts as a lubricant between the collagen fibers. Hyaluronic acid with water is believed to play the most active role in lubrication. The gel also maintains a space between the fibers known as the critical fiber distance, which allows free sliding of the fibers with adequate lubrication.

In summary, dense ordinary connective tissue of the regular type consists of collagen and fibrocytes imbedded in a gel of glycosaminoglycans and water.

The proteoglycans with protein dispersed between the collagen fibers give tissue its rigidity and maintain the critical fiber distance. Free gliding of individual collagen fibers is essential for mobility of normal connective tissue. All connective tissue displays viscoelastic properties to that found when we test the joint with passive stretch techniques to see the condition of the joint, this viscoelastic property will give a typical gummy-end feel in the joint.

On microscopic examination, the ligament is crimped and almost looks like a wave, which gives the ligament the possibility of expanding by 20 to 30 per cent more of its actual length. This imparts a quasi-elasticity to the ligament. This means that there can be elongation of the ligament without actual stretching of the collagen fibers. This is a very important concept to understand when we are dealing with TMJ dysfunctions, in which 70 or 80 per cent of the actual length of the ligaments is in the elastic condition, allowing functional range of motion to the joint, where stress and strain are proportional and can be taken by connective periarticular tissue. As the stress is increased, the strain is also increased, and if it goes beyond the range of elasticity of the ligament toward the plastic or early failure region of connective tissue, the material will elongate at its own speed independent of the rate of the load that is applied. If at any time during the range of elasticity the stress is removed, the tissue would return down the line to its original length without permanent elongation. Beyond the range of elasticity, connective tissue has time-dependent creep properties; the material will elongate at its own speed, independent of the rate at which the load is applied, whether slowly or rapidly. If stress continues, failure will start to appear as the result of another important property of the viscoelastic material. When a certain point is reached elongation continues with less stress. The tissue undergoes a reduction in its cross section before it actually reaches ultimate failure. Failure, as the name implies, is when the tissue breaks or tears. It is important to remember that each collagen fiber has its own stress-strain curve and will respond differently. This explains the

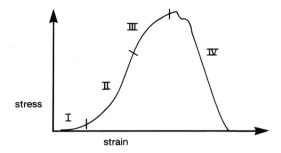

Figure 18–2. Stress-strain curve of connective tissue. I, toe region; II, elastic/linear region; III, plastic/early failure region; IV, failure region.

extended range of failure in which some fibers may stretch considerably before finally failing. This is the point at which the TMJ becomes very loose and unstable with a typical bulging disc; there is reciprocal clicking, a locking, or different sounds in the joints associated with excessive protrusive movements of the mandible and large anterior translatory glides of the condyle.

This concept of viscoelasticity is schematically shown with a stress-strain curve that also illustrates the importance of keeping in mind the 70 or 80 per cent elastic condition of the connective tissue, especially when treating hypermobile joints with lost synovial joint properties (Fig. 18–2). In order to maintain this healthy elastic joint in a normal relationship, we must understand some other characteristics of synovial joints.

PHYSIOLOGY OF SYNOVIAL JOINTS

We know that the joint is kept together in a relationship in which the condyle, disc, and the temporal bone (eminentia articularis ossis temporalis) are facing each other. It is kept together by periarticular connective tissue in range of elasticity in which the structures that can give joint pain are mainly the intercapsular structures, located posteriorly to the condyle. These structures are the posterior edge of the disc, the disc attachments to the capsule, the capsule itself, and the retrodiscal fat pad. Anterior to the joint are the muscular attachments and the superior and inferior bellies of the lateral pterygoid muscles. With these concepts in mind concerning the way the joint is kept together and the characteristics of the posterior and anterior structures of the joint, we will consider the physiology of synovial joints.

In any synovial joint we have what is called a close-packed position. This is a position in which the joint is maximally congruent and cannot accomplish any further movement, and the ligaments surrounding the joints are tightened. Most of the fractures and maximal derangements of the joints

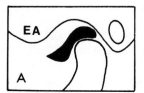 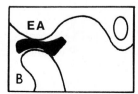 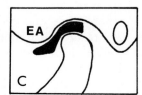

Figure 18–3. A, Posterior close pack. B, Anterior close pack. C, Loose pack. EA = eminentia articularis ossis temporalis.

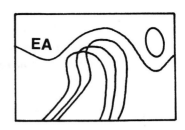

Figure 18–4. Loose-packed positions—any position away from the posterior and anterior close-packed positions. EA = eminentia articularis ossis temporalis.

occur in this position. The TMJ has two close-packed positions (Fig. 18–3). One is in the most retruded position of the condyle, where the condyle cannot go any farther back and where the ligaments are maximally tightened (Fig. 18–3A). The second close-packed position is in the most anterior position of the condyle on the eminentia articularis with maximal opening of the mouth in which no further opening can be accomplished (Fig. 18–3B).

If there are two close-packed positions, one in the most posterior position of the joint and one in the most anterior position of the condyle in relation to the apex of the eminentia articularis, this means that the condyle must be placed in a position in the joint that will be a loose-packed position (see Figs. 18–1 and 18–3C). This loose-packed position is any position away from the posterior and anterior close-packed positions (Fig. 18–4) in which the periarticular connective tissues will maintain their normal elastic condition in that 70 or 80 per cent range of their normal viscoelastic property.

As a summary, we can say that the condyle of the TMJ, according to physiology of joints, cannot be placed in the posterior close-packed position because the intercapsular structures that can give joint pain are located posteriorly to the condyle. The condyle has to be placed in a loose-packed position in the fossa or slightly anteriorly, facing the middle third of the eminentia articularis and the biconcave surface of the disc (see Fig. 18–1). At this point the connective tissue will maintain normal viscoelastic properties and any changes of condylar position will be acknowledged by the receptor system that will react because of stimulation of the mechanoreceptors I, II, and III, or the nociceptive receptor system.

The TMJ has its own nervous system located around the periarticular connective tissue of the joint. This concept of neurology of joints and of the receptor system of the TMJ is fundamental when changes of condylar position are applied. These changes are sensed by the receptors of the joint and will be transmitted to the cranium by the capsules and ligaments of the joints.

RECEPTOR SYSTEM OF THE TMJ

NEUROLOGY OF JOINTS

Traumatic, degenerative, and inflammatory lesions and mechanical derangements of the TMJ make a significant contribution to the production of craniofacial pain. Therefore knowledge of the innervation of the TMJ appears relevant to an understanding of the cause, differential diagnosis, and treatment of some of the varieties of craniofacial pain that are encountered so frequently in the TMJ in clinical practice. Articular tissues are not the only ones that may contribute to pain in the head and face. Other tissues in the craniofacial area and its adnexa, especially the capsules (periarticular connective tissue in general), muscles, and aponeuroses, may be involved in the production of this common complaint, in addition to its association with irritative lesions involving the cervical spine and its functional relationship to the craniomandibular system.

Pain in the TMJ, like pain anywhere else in the body, is an emotional disorder that is provoked by activation of a specific afferent system, the nociceptive system. Pain is not a primary sensation in the same way as are vision, hearing, touch, and kinesthesia. Instead, pain is an abnormal affective state, experienced in the limbic sectors of the cerebral cortex, that is evoked by activation of the nociceptive afferent system that projects through the thalamus and the reticular system of the brain stem to the cerebral cortex as a result of mechanical or chemical abnormalities involving the various tissues of the body that irritate the nociceptive receptor system located therein. However, the intensity of such peripheral irritation of the nociceptive receptor system as it affects the flow of afferent cortex may be modulated up or down by a variety of facilitating and inhibiting influences operating at the various synapses along the central nociceptive afferent pathways, including those derived from the mechanoreceptors located peripherally in joint capsules. These general considerations are applicable to pain arising from any other tissue in the body as well.

ARTICULAR RECEPTORS

It is well established that all the synovial joints of the body are provided with a quadruple array of corpuscular (mechanoreceptors) and noncorpuscular (nociceptor) receptor endings with individually characteristic properties of behavior and differing distributions in the articular tissues.[6, 7]

Type I Receptor System

The type I receptor system consists of clusters of small, thinly encapsulated globular corpuscles located in the peripheral layers of the fibrous joint capsule, each such cluster being innervated by a small myelinated afferent fiber that enters the related articular nerves. These corpuscles behave as low-threshold, slowly adapting mechanoreceptors whose frequency of discharge is a continuous function of the tension prevailing in the part of the joint capsule in which they lie. In addition, they have an inhibitory effect on the transsynaptic centripetal form of nociceptive activity from the type IV articular receptor system. Their activity also exerts powerful tonic reflexogenic influences on the motor neuronal pool of the muscles of mastication, as well as on the cervical and limb musculature; they contribute significantly to postural and kinesthetic sensation.

The mechanoreceptor population is denser in the posterior region of the joint capsule than elsewhere. Consequently, the mechanoreceptor contribution to the reflex regulation of postural tone in the mandibular musculature must be greater from this region. The duration of the evoked discharges increases with increases in the load applied to move the joint. Variations in applied load produce differences in the rate of change in capsular tension. The duration of mechanoreceptor discharge is independent of the direction of the mandibular-movement sequence.

It appears that the major articular contribution to the reflex regulation of motor-unit activity in the mandibular musculature is provided by the type I mechanoreceptors. These contribute to reflex regulation of postural muscle tone, to coordination of muscle activity (reinforced by the type II mechanoreceptors) guiding mandibular movement, and to perceptual awareness of mandibular position.

Type II Receptor System

The type II receptor system is represented by larger, thickly encapsulated conical corpuscles that are embedded in the deeper parasynovial layers of the posterior fibrous joint capsule and that are innervated from thicker myelinated afferent fibers in the articular nerves.

The type II corpuscles operate as low-threshold, rapidly adapting mechanoreceptors that fire brief bursts of impulses only at the onset of changes in tension in the joint capsule, or in response to vibratory stimulation, the effect of which is to generate phasic reflex changes in the activity of the musculature and transient inhibitory effects on the centripetal flow of nociceptive afferent activity from the tissues of the mandible.

The posterior capsule mechanoreceptors exhibit a relatively uniform threshold over the entire population of these receptors in all regions of the joint capsule so that at the onset of any mandibular movement, all type II mechanoreceptors in the stressed region of the joint capsule are stimulated more or less simultaneously. Their behavior in this respect suggests that they function as acceleration-deceleration receptors,[2-7] providing a transient reflex contribution to the regulation of motor unit activity in the prime movers of the joint. The activity of the type II mechanoreceptors has usually adapted before the incremental type I mechanoreceptors' discharge becomes apparent.

The disc in its central portion has no nerve endings of any description and hence cannot be the source of pain in the TMJ.

Type III Receptor System

Neurohistological studies[1] established that type III mechanoreceptors are sparsely distributed in the superficial layers of the lateral capsule ligament of the TMJ. The type III receptors may, by inference, be regarded as high threshold. Since the lateral articular nerve is the only nerve to the TMJ containing type III mechanoreceptor afferent fibers, it follows that only during high capsular tension will type III receptors evoke discharges. The evoked discharges from the lateral articular nerve are higher than those evoked by the anterior articular nerve. This may be due to the fact that the population density of the type I mechanoreceptor is greater in the lateral capsule than in the anterior capsule so that when the lateral capsule is stretched, a greater number of receptors are stimulated; the higher discharge frequency may be due to greater contributions from the type III mechanoreceptors at higher levels of tension. This process will appear when the tension is able to induce distraction (to separate joint surfaces) in the joint that will induce muscle relaxation and pure lateral glides of the condyle of the joint without distraction (refer to the section on hypomobile joints later in this chapter).

Type IV Nociceptive Receptor System

The type IV nociceptive receptor system is a plexiform array of unmyelinated nerve fibers distributed three-dimensionally throughout the fibrous joint capsule. No nerve endings of this or any other kind are present in the articular cartilage, synovial tissues, or central portion of the disc. This type IV receptor system is activated when its constituent nerve fibers are depolarized by the generation of high mechanical stresses in the joint capsule containing it—for example, whiplash injuries, dislocations, trauma, exposure to chemical agents, or accumulations of K^+ ions, lactic acid, and kinins in high concentrations in the fluid of the interstitial tissue in the joint capsule in circumstances of acute or chronic inflammatory involvement of joints.

Excessive translatory glides of the TMJ with or without a click or subluxation are considered high mechanical stresses in the joint capsule that will induce trauma, a possible inflammatory response, and pain from type IV depolarized nerve fibers contained in the joint capsule.

DYNAMICS OF THE TMJ

In normal dynamics of the TMJ, there are two definite arthrokinematic movements. This is because the TMJ is a disc joint and therefore must have two independent movements. The rotation movement occurs at the beginning and during the midrange of the movement that takes place between the condyle and the inferior joint surface of the disc. The second movement is an anterior translatory glide that occurs when the collateral ligaments of the joints—which are relating, specifically, the lateral and medial aspect of the disc to the lateral and medial aspects of the neck of the condyle—tighten. At this point, rotation between condyle and disc ends, and the condyle and disc move together with the superior surface of the disc on the eminentia articularis to complete a functional range of motion, with a short anterior and caudal translatory glide.

If an average osteokinematic mandibular movement of maximal opening is approximately 50 mm (measured from the ridge of the upper and lower incisors), this means that the descending movement of the mandible took the periarticular connective tissue (capsules and ligaments) to 100 per cent of their length, which is not a functional position. The periarticular connective tissue should not exceed 70 or 80 per cent of its total length in a functional joint. Therefore the functional range of opening of the TMJ is approximately 40 mm. If rotation is 50 per cent of the total range of opening (50 mm), 25 mm of opening is rotation. To complete the 40 mm of functional opening, 15 mm more of anterior translatory glide is needed. This is a very important factor to keep in mind when treating TMJ. One must emphasize a large amount of rotation taking place between condyle and disc and a short anterior translatory glide in order not to overload the eminentia articularis. Rotation is the most important movement taking place at the TMJ; it implies rest in the joint and avoids disc-condyle derangements.

In normal arthrokinematics (intimate relationship between joint surfaces) of the TMJ, because of the convex-concave relationship between the condyle and inferior joint surface of the disc, when the condyle joint surface glides anteriorly the disc will have a relative posterior glide on the condyle until the collateral ligaments tighten. At this point rotation ends, and to

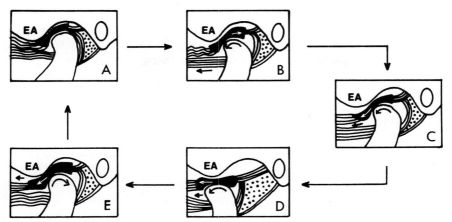

Figure 18–5. TMJ arthrokinematic steps. *A,* Rest position. *B,* Rotation: mid-opening. *C,* Functional opening. *D,* Translation: full opening. *E,* Closure. EA = eminentia articularis ossis temporalis.

complete the functional range of motion, an anterior translatory glide starts to take place in the superior joint surface of the disc and the eminentia articularis (Fig. 18–5).

ARTHROKINEMATIC STEPS OF THE TMJ

REST POSITION. The rest position is the first step. In this, the joint is in a loose-packed position, the connective tissue is at rest, and the upper and lower lateral pterygoid muscles are at rest.

ROTATION. In the second step, rotation, there is a mid-opening, the condyle joint surface glides forward, the inferior joint surface of the disc has relative posterior glide, the upper lateral pterygoid relaxes, the lower lateral pterygoid contracts, and the posterior connective tissue is in a functional state of rest.

FUNCTIONAL OPENING. In functional opening, the disc and condyle experience short anterior translatory glide, the upper and lower heads of the lateral pterygoid contract to guide the disc and condyle shortly forward, and the posterior connective tissue is in functional tightening.

TRANSLATION. In translation, there is a full opening, the disc and condyle glide anteriorly and, caudally guided by the joint surface of the eminentia articularis, the upper and lower heads of the lateral pterygoid contract in order to guide the disc and condyle fully forward, and the posterior connective tissue tightens.

CLOSURE. In closure, the surface of the condyle joint glides posteriorly, the disc glides relative to the anterior surface, and the upper head of the lateral pterygoid contracts, in order to monitor the return of the condyle and the disc together back to the normal loose-packed position. The lower head of the lateral pterygoid relaxes, and the posterior connective tissue returns to a functional rest position.

When the joint loses the normal physiological position, the capsules and the ligaments become loose because of the lack of viscoelastic properties of the periarticular connective tissue. The joint becomes hypermobile, characterized by excessive protrusive movements of the mandible. The patient shows large anterior translatory glide at the beginning of the opening, where rotation should be taking place. This condition can easily be observed in a lateral view in which the patient performs mandibular dynamics. Also, from an anterior view, it can be seen that the patient is constantly talking in a protruded fashion, not allowing for dynamics of rotation during midrange of motion.

This condition of excessive protrusive movements is aggravated by a muscle imbalance that will cause bilateral or unilateral deviations of the mandible during opening and closing movements.

This unstable condition of the TMJ may lead to a bulging disc that reacts inconsistently according to different demands of mandibular functions, such as mastication and speech. The patient will complain of having difficulties in finding a comfortable position for the mandible, which will induce abnormal mandibular movements for accommodation. This predisposes to further loosening of ligamentous structures.

INTRACAPSULAR DYSFUNCTIONS OF THE TMJ

One of the most common intracapsular dysfunctions of the TMJ is the internal derangement or displacement of the articular disc. Internal derangement of the disc and condyle is characterized by anterior displacement of the disc and a posterosuperior displacement of the condyle. If the relative position of the condyle to the fossa changes in a closed position, the position of the disc must change also because of the convex-concave relationship. The posterior attachments are highly vascularized and innervated and can be overstretched if the joint is subjected to trauma or condylar changes and if the force is such that the condyle is forced posterosuperiorly. The posterior attachments (connective tissue) will elongate, and as a consequence of this, the articular disc will be displaced anterior to the condyle. If this condition continues, the attachments will become elongated and will tend to go into the early failure or failure condition of the ligaments (refer to the earlier section on the physiology of the periarticular connective tissue), which will get thinner and weaker, and the disc will migrate even farther anteriorly. The disc is loose, out of its normal relationship with the condyle and the temporal bone, and it will click during the different movements of the mandible that include normal or functional openings of the mouth. The most common conditions of internal derangements of the TMJ are mainly these three: (1) the reciprocal clicking, (2) the locking condition, and (3) the degenerative processes such as osteoarthritic conditions. The many causes of disc displacement can be placed into two major categories: acute and chronic trauma.

Acute trauma includes a sudden traumatic episode that displaces the condyle posteriorly and stretches the posterior attachments of the disc, affecting its normal elasticity and producing a loosened effect. Typical conditions of an acute trauma are a whiplash injury, which is a soft-tissue injury; traumatic extractions of teeth; trauma during intubation of anesthesia; or any long-term anterior close-packed position of the condyle.

Chronic trauma includes repetitive microtraumas extended over long periods of time. Here there are forces that cause the mandible to move into the posterior close-packed position. This could be caused by loss of posterior teeth, incisal interferences, or occlusal contacts that produce a posteriorly directed jaw position, generally with loss of vertical dimension.

In both of these categories one must maintain the concept of functional range of the TMJ, which is between 70 or 80 per cent of the maximal range of motion, in order to restore the viscoelastic property of the connective tissue and the stable relationship of the joints. For example, for maximal opening of 50 mm, the functional opening will be 70 or 80 per cent of 50 mm, 35 or 40 mm.

RECIPROCAL CLICKING OF THE TMJ

The first sign of dysfunction occurring in the TMJ is a click. This click is evidence that the TMJ is going against the rules of synovial joints, which are frictionless joints. The most common type of joint clicks are described as reciprocal clicks. During the phase of opening, a click occurs when the condyle moves beneath the disc and the posterior attachments, snaps under the posterior band of the disc, and falls into its normal relationship on the concave surface. The closing click occurs at the end of the closing movement as the condyle slides posteriorly to the posterior band of the disc and the disc becomes displaced anteriorly.

When a pure clicking sound disappears and a grinding sound appears in the joint, this indicates a possible degenerative arthritis, and further studies should be made.

Reciprocal clicking is classified as early, intermediate, or late, depending on the degree of opening at which the click will occur. In reciprocal clicking, the closing click will not occur unless it is preceded by the opening click. A joint that has a clicking sound is not a locked joint because a locked joint does not click.

If the click occurs at the beginning of mandibular movements, the degree of anterior displacement is small, but if the click occurs close to the maximal opening position, this indicates that the disc has been displaced further anteriorly. When the degree of displacement becomes such that the disc lodges anteriorly to the condyle, the patient experiences locking. This may become intermittent, with the patient experiencing clicking and locking, and is common in patients who have a bulging disc with very loose ligaments. This is characterized by a large thrust and anterior translatory glide at the beginning of the opening or during speech. Also, the patient will show an excessive amount of opening beyond the point of average opening. Under these conditions, the patient may experience two different types of situations. One is a permanent close-locked condition in which the disc is lodged anteriorly to the condyle and will not allow normal opening. Only rotation in the joint can be performed and anterior translatory glide is lost. The second condition is a dislocation or a luxation of the joint in which the condyle and the disc seat in front of the eminentia articularis, and the patient is unable to close his mouth.

In close-locked conditions, one must differentiate between two types. The first is in relation to a permanent anterior displacement of the disc and does not allow the condyle to roll forward into the concave surface of the disc and continue a further anterior translatory glide. This close-locked condition has a "hard-end feel" in the joint. This hard-end feel is typically noted when one tries to induce a passive stretch to the joint, further movement cannot be accomplished, and there is a hard stop at maximal restricted opening.

The second is a close-locked condition with restriction of opening in which only rotation is taking place in the joint but there is passive stretch. The joint increases the amount of range of motion and has a gummy-end feel that indicates that the relationship of condyle, disc, and temporal bone is possibly normal but that the capsule and the ligaments are short, not allowing the normal anterior translatory glide. The periarticular connective tissue is responsible for the shortening and the limitation of opening.

Both close-locked conditions, whether occurring by anterior displacement of the disc or by shortening of the periarticular connective tissue, are considered capsular patterns because approach to treatment involves work on distraction of the joint surfaces (separate joint surfaces). To accomplish distraction, one must realign the collagen fibers of the capsule and ligaments, which will allow restoration of the normal relationship of the disc to the condyle or will restore the viscoelastic property of the collagen fibers for full range of motion.

In both situations one must "get the joint moving." In one case the retraction of the periarticular connective tissue takes the condyle to a posterior position in the close-packed position (see Fig. 18–3A), which is pathological and may induce degenerative processes. Also, when the disc is displaced, the bony elements of the joints are not protected by the cushioning effect of the disc and degenerative processes may start to appear. The end result of this condition if untreated or improperly treated is a degenerative arthritis, and the probability that the posterior attachments of the disc will become permanently elongated with no possibility of realigning the fibers because of the loss of the creep properties of the connective tissue.

In the close-locked position the patient typically opens to around 25 mm or less, the joint does not click, the condyle is only allowed to rotate in the joint, and no anterior translatory glide is taking place. Secondary muscle spasm may be present in a close-locked condition, but this should not be mistaken for a muscular trismus. This can be confirmed by the passive stretch technique and also by specialized radiographic studies.

In summary, we have two very specific pathological conditions of the TMJ. One is in relation to a hypermobile joint with excessive translatory glide that induces sounds in the joints like reciprocal clickings, subluxation, or dislocations. The second is locking in the joint that is characteristic of a hypomobile joint, that is, a joint that has limitation of opening mainly restricted to rotation in the joint with an average of opening of 25 mm. The locking of the joint, or a close-locked position, can be of two major types. One is the shortening of the periarticular connective tissue as a defensive mechanism. The joint will respond to trauma through the mechanoreceptors producing a shortening and a retraction of the fibers of the capsular ligaments. With passive stretch one sees a considerable increase in range of motion with a gummy-end feel. The second situation is a close-locked position caused by an anterior displacement of the disc. This is characterized by a posterosuperior displacement of the condyle with a limitation of opening and with a hard-end feel. When the passive stretch is practiced, there will be little or no increase in range of motion. Approaches to treatment in these two situations of hypermobile and hypomobile joints are quite different.

TREATMENT OF HYPERMOBILE JOINTS

Hypermobile joints are treated mainly by avoiding the excessive anterior translatory glides of the condyle, controlling rotation, stabilizing the joint, and restabilizing normal head, neck, and shoulder-girdle posture.

ROCABADO'S 6 × 6 PROGRAM

If the diagnosis establishes an interrelated biomechanical dysfunction of the craniocervical and craniomandibular systems, then both an active treatment plan and a home self-mobilization program should be developed. The home program, or the "6 × 6 program," is based on the sequence of exercises the patient must perform. This 6 × 6 exercise program will typically follow along with an active treatment program that the therapist provides in the office during the beginning stages of treatment. The important elements of emphasis in the home program are the postural relationship of (1) the cranium to the upper cervical spine; (2) the cervical spine (anterior, posterior, and lateral aspects) to the shoulder girdle; and (3) the mandible to the maxilla. These important relationships make up the key elements that determine the orthostatic equilibrium of the entire upper body, and it is not possible to successfully treat one area without the other.

The objectives of the home self-mobilization program are that the patient should:

—learn a new postural position,
—fight the "soft-tissue memory" of the old position,
—restore original muscle length,
—restore normal joint mobility,
—restore normal body balance, and
—initiate this exercise program whenever symptoms of dysfunction return (in other words, fight back!)

TABLE 18–1. Summary of 6 × 6 Program for Prevention of Dysfunction and Stabilizing the Joint

THE SIX BASIC TEMPOROMANDIBULAR DYSFUNCTION PREVENTIVE PROCEDURES	THE SIX BASIC TEMPOROMANDIBULAR STABILIZING PROCEDURES
1. Prevent isometric parafunctional muscle activities.	1. Induce functional isometric muscle activity. Rhythmic Stabilization. Contract-Relax.
2. Prevent excessive translatory movements of TMJ.	2. Induce rotation = rest. Angular (hinge) movement.
3. Prevent condylar movements into anterior and posterior close-packed positions.	3. Keep the joint in a loose-packed position (mandibular rest position).
4. Prevent or avoid excessive wide opening of the mouth.	4. Do not force range of motion over a functional opening. 70–80% of actual connective tissue length (35 mm. approx.).
5. Prevent or avoid posterior rotation of the cranium (extension or backward bending).	5. Induce only 15° of cranial anterior rotation (flexion or forward bending).
6. Prevent forward head and neck posture.	6. Induce axial extension of head and neck: − 15° cranial flexion. —Extension of inferior cervical spine, maximum 6 cm. from tangent line of the apex of thoracic kyphosis.

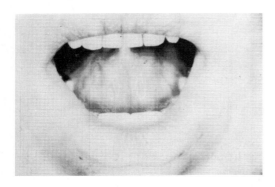

Figure 18–6. Rest position of the tongue.

To accomplish these objectives without an active treatment program is quite difficult. Most patients will not exercise if the exercises increase pain; therefore, the therapist must initially help the patient achieve some relief of the symptoms. One of the therapist's objectives is to teach the patient how to avoid activities that are injurious to the synovial joints involved. Once the symptoms have decreased, then the patient will have incentive to keep the dysfunction from returning. The 6 × 6 program is not meant to be a time-consuming regimen. These exercises should be able to be performed in any position and should not last more than a minute or so. The program is termed "6 × 6" because (1) there should be no more than six instructions, (2) they should be repeated six times each, and (3) they should be performed six times a day.

Although the patients should be constantly trying to correct their posture with these exercises, they should not overdo them and increase the pain—just enough to keep them out of dysfunction during the day is recommended. Within these limitations, the patient should be able to easily devote a minute, six times a day. It is helpful to use visual reminders of the exercise program placed in various areas of the patient's home or work. Visual cues will help patients remember to perform the exercises.

Although each exercise program should be individually designed to the patient's complaints, there are six fundamental components commonly used for head-neck-mandibular dysfunction patients.

REST POSITION OF THE TONGUE. In order to reestablish a correct position of the tongue during rest, it is necessary to teach the patient the correct position of the tongue against the palate (Fig. 18–6). Advise the patient to place the tongue against the anterior palate then to make a "clucking" sound. This positions the tip of the tongue in a position similar to that which occurs during swallowing and also results in the correct mandibular rest position. After finding this position, teach the patient to maintain the anterior third of the tongue against the palate with a slight pressure. This is basic to accomplishing a normal swallow and a rest posture with the least amount of muscle activity. Furthermore, instruct the patient to breathe through the nose and to use the diaphragm muscles for respiration. The patient should not be using the accessory respiratory muscles (that is, pectoral, scalene, sternocleidomastoid, and intercostal muscles) for breathing. When overactive, accessory muscles will act to maintain a forward head-and-shoulder posture.

CONTROL TMJ ROTATION. The TMJ rotation exercise is used to reduce any tendency for an early translation of the TMJ and to reposition the condyle correctly in the fossa. Instruct the patient to place and hold the anterior third of the tongue flat aginst the palate during a hinge-opening movement of the mandible. Maintaining this tongue position limits the range of opening to rotation only and reduces the tendency for a protrusive movement. This exercise stops the joint sounds and serves to protect the joint components against wear and tear. Patients can monitor the joint rotation by placing the finger over the TMJ region. After the patient is able to perform this exercise adequately, additionally instruct him to chew in this nontranslatory manner or with a short translatory glide, just enough to maintain health of the superior joint of the TMJ (Fig. 18–7).

RHYTHMIC STABILIZATION TECHNIQUE. This technique is adapted from the Proprioceptive Neuromuscular Facilitation technique[8] used for many years in other parts of the musculoskeletal system. Primarily it consists of a method to increase muscular control or dexterity by proprioceptive sensory activation. The rhythmic stabilization technique is a series of isometric contractions of the jaw opening, closing, retraction, protrusion, and lateral excursion against light resistance in order to break down the parafunctional muscle activity of the craniomandibular musculature. The patient must contract a group of muscles and immediately after contract the antagonistic muscle in order to induce muscle relaxation through the principle of reciprocal innervation and functional isometric muscle contraction of short duration. Begin with the patient's mandible in rest position and then instruct the patient that there should be no movement of the mandible from this position. Show the patient how to apply opening, closing, and even lateral forces to the chin of the mandible while making sure he or she resists these movements to maintain a constant jaw position (Fig. 18–8). Do not use excessive force or mandibular movement will result. This exercise will help

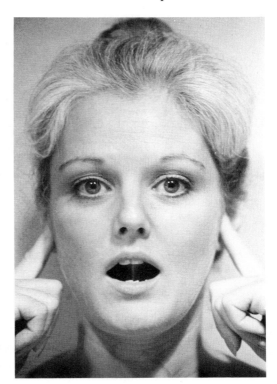

Figure 18–7. TMJ rotation exercise.

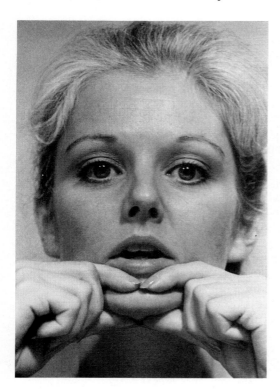

Figure 18–8. Rhythmic stabilization technique.

the patient increase proprioceptive control over the mandible and reeducate the neuromuscular system to avoid unconscious abnormal postural positionings.

CERVICAL JOINT LIBERATION. The main objectives of this technique are to induce a distraction of the upper cervical vertebrae, relieve any mechanical compressions, and elongate the posterior cervical muscles. These mechanical compressions primarily occur between the occiput-atlas, atlas-axis, and axis-C3 joints. Distraction of the craniovertebral joints can be produced by instructing the patient to hold both hands behind the neck to stabilize the C2 to C7 region and then bend the head, stabilizing the cervical spine and inducing *not more than 15° of cranial flexion* six times (Fig. 18–9). This forward pressure stabilizes the cervical spine while flexing of the head relieves any neurovascular compression in the upper cervical region. Specifically, this flexion distracts the occiput from the atlas to counteract the extension produced by a forward head posture. This movement is not a flexion of the neck but a flexion of the head on the cervical spine (15°).

AXIAL EXTENSION OF THE CERVICAL SPINE. The objective of this technique is to improve the functional and mechanical relationship of the head to the cervical spine. This is accomplished by inducing a distraction of the cervical vertebrae by a combined movement of flexion of the occiput (15° of cranial flexion) on the upper cervical spine and extension of the lower cervical spine relative to the thoracic region (6 cm of lordosis) (Fig. 18–10). This movement will position the head into an ideal orthostatic position. With an abnormal forward head posture, the sternocleidomastoid muscle maintains an almost vertical relationship. When axial extension is accomplished this reduces the tension of the suprahyoid and infrahyoid muscles and enhances the ability of the craniomandibular muscles to relax. The sternocleidomastoid

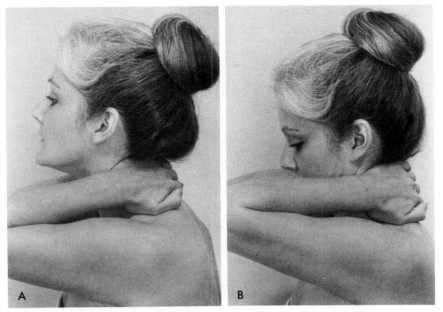

Figure 18–9. Cervical joint liberation (15° of cranial flexion). *A,* Step 1. *B,* Step 2.

muscle takes a more normal posterior angulation and thus reduces unnecessary cervical muscle activity required to maintain this position anteriorly, laterally, and posteriorly.

SHOULDER GIRDLE RETRACTION. The objective of this exercise is the restoration of the shoulder girdle to an ideal postural position to establish stability of the entire head-neck-shoulder complex. To do this, the patient must be shown how to move the shoulder girdle back and then down relative

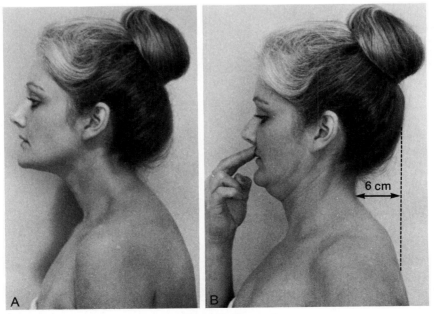

Figure 18–10.

to the rib cage. This accomplishes the correction of the abnormal scapular abduction, reduces tension in the acromioclavicular joint, and relieves compression in the sternoclavicular joint. However, the patient must be aware that more activity is required in the larger upper back muscles, such as the rhomboids and the inferior trapezius, to keep the shoulder girdle in the correct position to prevent head, neck, and shoulder girdle forward relapse (Fig. 18–11).

MAINTENANCE

If no irreversible degenerative joint changes have occurred, a return to a more normal craniocervical posture and improved mandibular function

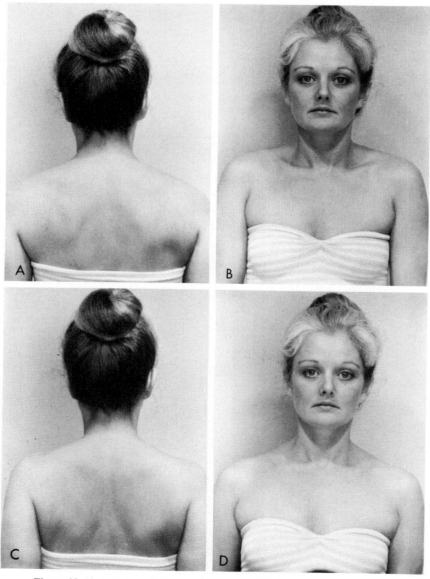

Figure 18–11. Shoulder girdle retraction. *A* and *B*, Step 1. *C* and *D*, Step 2.

will result. The release of any compression in the upper cervical vertebrae will also decrease the referred pain symptoms. Have the patients follow the 6 × 6 exercise program to maintain a dysfunction-free state. Relapse will usually result in restoration of the symptoms, so periodic recall and evaluation is helpful as a preventative measure for these patients.

TREATMENT OF HYPOMOBILE JOINTS

The goal of this treatment technique is to restore functional range of motion of the joint. To accomplish this, a technique called joint liberation is used that relies on the effect of restoring the normal physiological condition of the joint by realigning the collagen fibers and restoring the normal relationship of disc and condyle. Joint-liberation techniques are passive movements applied to the joint in all planes in order to realign the collagen fibers of the capsule that are shortened in a multidirectional fashion. The first approach will be to accomplish the following.

DISTRACTION. Separate the joint surfaces of the TMJ to allow the disc to start repositioning on the condyle and to start realigning the fibers of the connective tissue caudally (Fig. 18–12).

DISTRACTION WITH ANTERIOR GLIDE. One must accomplish a distraction with anterior glide to start restoring the anterior translatory glide that has been lost because of the capsular retraction or by the anterior displaced disc (Fig. 18–13).

DISTRACTION, ANTERIOR GLIDE, LATERAL STRETCH. To maintain this more normal relationship, one must distract, anteriorly glide, and laterally stretch the joint to the opposite side in order to realign the fibers in all three planes of space (Fig. 18–14). (This is especially true if the disc is displaced anteriorly and medially by the action of the superior lateral pterygoid muscle.)

LATERAL GLIDE WITHOUT DISTRACTION. A lateral glide without distraction must be accomplished to restore lateral joint play (Fig. 18–15).

SELF-DISTRACTION. Finally, we must instruct the patient to maintain self-distracting techniques or self-mobilizing techniques in the joint with opening, protrusion, and lateral excursions of the mandible as a home exercise program (refer to the Rocabado 6 × 6 treatment approach discussed earlier) (Figs. 18–6 to 18–11).

In summary, in a hypermobile joint, the main objective is to stabilize the joint and avoid excessive anterior translatory glide by controlling rotation in the joint. In a hypomobile joint, the main objective is to restore the lost

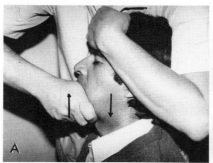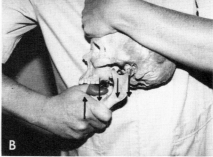

Figure 18–12. *A* and *B*, Distraction.

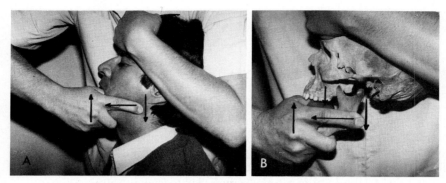

Figure 18–13. *A* and *B*, Distraction with anterior glide.

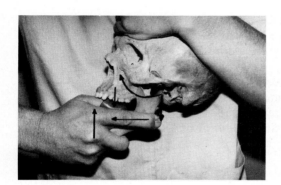

Figure 18–14. Maintenance of position of distraction with anterior glide.

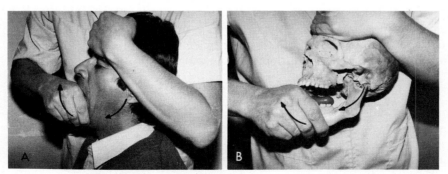

Figure 18–15. *A* and *B*, Lateral glide without distraction.

anterior translatory glide by mobilizing the joint in distraction, by translatory glides with distraction, and by inducing protrusive movements of the mandible to maintain collagen-fiber alignment in the three planes of space.

References

Periarticular Connective Tissue

Akeson, W., et al.: Immobility effects of synovial joints, the pathomechanics of joint contracture. Biorheology, *17*:95, 1980.

Akeson, W.: Collagen crosslinking alterations in joint contractures: Changes in the reducible crosslinks in periarticular connective tissue collagen after nine weeks of immobilization. Connect. Tissue Res., *5*:15, 1977.

Akeson, W., et al.: Value of 17-β-oestradiol in prevention of contracture formation. Ann. Rheum. Dis., *35*:429, 1976.

Amiel, E., et al.: Effects of nine weeks' immobilization of the types of collagen synthesized in periarticular connective tissue from rabbit knees. Trans. Orth. Res. Society, vol. 5, 1980.

Betsch, D., and Baer, E.: Structure and mechanical properties of rat tail tendon. Biorheology, *17*:83, 1980.

Clark, D., et al.: The influence of triamcinolone acetonide on joint stiffness in the rat. J. Bone Joint Surg., *53A*:1409, 1971.

Enneking, W., et al.: The intra-articular effects of immobilization on the human knee. J. Bone Joint Surg., *54A*:973, 1972.

Evans, E., et al.: Experimental immobilization and remobilization of rat knee joints. J. Bone Joint Surg., *42A*:737, 1960.

Ham, A., and Cormack, D.: Histology. Philadelphia, J. B. Lippincott, 1979.

Meyer, K.: Problems of the structure and chemistry of the ground substance of connective tissue. Presented at the International Connective Tissue Symposium, Lyon, France, 1965.

Noyes, F.: Functional properties of knee ligaments and alterations induced by immobilization; a correlative biomechanical and histological study in primates. Clin. Orthop., *123*:210, 1977.

Noyes, F., et al.: Effects of intra-articular corticosteroids on ligament properties: A biomechanical and histological study in rhesus knees. Clin. Orthop., *123*:197, 1977.

Neuberger, A., et al.: The metabolism of collagen from liver, bones, skin, and tendon in the normal rat. Biochem. J., *53*:47, 1953.

Owen, H.: Effects of immobilization on normal periarticular connective tissue. Atlanta, Ga., Institute for Graduate Health Sciences, 1981.

Peacock, E.: Comparison of collagenous tissue surrounding normal and immobilized joints. Surg. Forum, *14*:440, 1963.

Schiller, S., et al.: The metabolism of mucopolysaccharides in animals. Further studies on skin utilizing C^{14} glucose, C^{14} acetate, and S^{35} sodium sulfate. J. Biochem., *218*:139, 1956.

Schiller, S., et al.: The metabolism of mucopolysaccharides in animal studies in skin utilizing labeled acetate. J. Biochem., *212*:531, 1955.

Warwick, R., and Williams, P. L. (eds.): Gray's Anatomy. 35th ed., Philadelphia, W. B. Saunders Co., 1973.

Temporomandibular Joint

Blaschke, D. D.: Arthrography of the T.M.J. *In* Temporomandibular Joint Problems. Chicago, Quintessence Publ. Co., 1980.

D'Ambrosia, R. D.: Musculo Skeletal Disorders. Philadelphia, J. B. Lippincott Co., 1977.

Farrar, W. B., and McCarty, W. L.: The T.M.J. dilemma. J. Alabama Dental Assoc., vol. 63, 1979.

Farrar, W. B.: Diagnosis and treatment of anterior dislocation of the articular disc. N.Y. J. Dent., *41*:348, 1971.

Farrar, W. B.: Characteristic of the condylar path in internal derangements of the T.M.J. J. Prosthet. Dent., *39*:319, 1978.

Gelb, H.: Clinical Management of Head, Neck and TMJ Pain and Dysfunction. Philadelphia, W. B. Saunders Co., 1977.

Mahan, P. E.: The Temporomandibular Joint. Philadelphia, J. B. Lippincott, 1979.

Mahan, P. E.: The Temporomandibular Joint in Function and Pathofunction. Chapter II, Temporomandibular joint problems. Chicago, Quintessence Pub. Co., 1980.

McCarthy, W.: Diagnosis and Treatment of Internal Disengagements of the Articular Disc and Mandibular Condyle. Chapter III, Temporomandibular joint problems. Chicago, Quintessence Pub. Co., 1980.

Rocabado, M., and Cabeza y Cuello: Tratamiento Articular. EDIT. Intermedica, Buenos Aires, Argentina, 1979.

Rocabado, M.: Biomechanical effect of periarticular connective tissue. Head, Neck, and T.M.J. Manual. Tacoma, Wash., Rocabado Institute, 1981.

Rocabado, M.: Temporomandibular joint disc pathology. Head, Neck, and T.M.J. Manual. Tacoma, Wash., Rocabado Institute, 1981.

Rodriguez, E., and Rocabado, M.: Algias Craneofaciales de Origen Cervical y por Disfuncion del Sistema Estomatognatico. Facultad de Odontologia, Universidad de Chile, 1980.

Solberg, W. K., and Clark, G. T.: Temporomandibular Joint Problems. Chicago, Quintessence Pub. Co., 1980.

Standler, A.: Kinesiology of the Human Body. Springfield, Ill., Charles C Thomas, 1977.

Warwick, R., and Williams, P. L. (eds.): Gray's Anatomy, 35th ed., Philadelphia, W. B. Saunders Co., 1973.

Zarb, G. A.: Temporomandibular Joint Function and Dysfunction. St. Louis, C. V. Mosby Co., 1979.

Neurology of Joints

Franks, A. S.: Study of the innervation of the temporomandibular joint and lateral pterygoid muscles in animals. J. Dent. Res., *43*:947, 1964 (Proc).

Gardner, E. D.: Physiology of moveable joints. Physiol. Rev., *40*:127, 1950.

Greenfield, B. E., and Wyke, B. D.: The innervation of the cat's temporomandibular joint. J. Anat. (Lond.), *98*:300, 1964.

Greenfield, B. E., and Wyke, B. D.: Reflex innervation of the temporomandibular joint. Nature, *211*:940, 1966.

Kawamura, Y., and Majima, T.: Temporomandibular joint's sensory mechanisms controlling activities of jaw muscles. J. Dent. Res., *43*:150, 1964.

Kawamura, Y., Majima. T., and Kato, I.: Physiologic role of deep mechanoreceptor(s) in temporomandibular joint capsule. J. Osaka. Univ. Dent. Sch., *7*:63, 1967.

Klineberg, I. J., Greenfield, B. E., and Wyke, B. D.: Stimulus-response characteristics of temporomandibular articular mechanoreceptors. Int. Assoc. Dent. Res., 48th General Meeting. Abstract 626, 1970a.

Klineberg, I. J., Greenfield, B. E., and Wyke, B. D.: Evoked discharges from articular mechanoreceptors in the cat's temporomandibular joint. Int. Assoc. for Dent. Res., 18th Meeting, Brit. Div. Abstract 130, 1970b.

Klineberg, I. J., Greenfield, B. E., and Wyke, B. D.: Afferent discharges from temporomandibular articular mechanoreceptors. An experimental study in the cat. Arch. Oral Biol., *15*:935, 1970c.

Klineberg, I. J., Greenfield, B. E., and Wyke, B. D.: Contributions to the reflex control of mastication from mechanoreceptors in the temporo-mandibular joint capsule. Dent. Practit., *21*:73, 1970d.

Larsson, L. E., and Thilander, B.: Mandibular positioning. The effect of pressure on the joint capsule. Acta Neurol. Scand., *40*:131, 1964.

Ringel, R. L., Sakman, J. H., and Brooks, A. R.: Oral perception II. Mandibular kenaesthesia. J. Speech Hearing Res., *10*:637, 1967.

Thilander, B.: Innervation of the temporomandibular joint capsule in man. Trans. Roy. Sch. Dent. Unmed. (Series 2), *7*:1, 1961.

Wyke, B. D.: Neurophysiological aspects of joint function, with particular reference to the temporo-mandibular joint. J. Bone Joint Surg., *43B*:396, 1961.

Wyke, B. D.: The neurology of joint. Ann. Roy. Coll. Surg. Engl., *41*:25, 1961.

19

Arthrography of the Temporomandibular Joint

RICHARD W. KATZBERG, M.D.
STEVEN G. MESSING, D.M.D.
CLYDE A. HELMS, M.D.

Temporomandibular joint pain and dysfunction present difficult diagnostic and therapeutic problems. Only within the last half decade has an appreciation developed for the significance of internal derangements and abnormalities of an important structure called the meniscus.[4, 6, 9, 10, 16, 17] Indeed, many of the clinical signs and symptoms are directly attributable to displacements and detachments of this structure.

The current era of understanding is largely attributable to improved techniques in the radiographic imaging of the temporomandibular joint. The technique used is known as arthrography and it allows an objective assessment of internal derangements of the temporomandibular joint. At a growing number of institutions across the United States, TMJ arthrography is gaining hold as a routine procedure in the evaluation of patients with TMJ pain and dysfunction.[1, 2, 4, 6, 7, 9, 11, 14, 16, 17] The ability to depict a specific abnormality responsible for the symptoms of an organic disease allows a more rational approach to patient management. It is the purpose of this chapter to outline the capabilities and potential of TMJ arthrography for clinical diagnosis and case management, as well as further exploration of the pathophysiology of joint disease.[3, 5, 15]

ANATOMY

The mandibular condyles act as a unit in their articulations with the glenoid fossae and articular eminences of the temporal bones (Fig. 19–1 A). Each condyle of the mandible is elliptical, with its long axis oriented mediolaterally and at right angles to the plane of the mandibular ramus. The

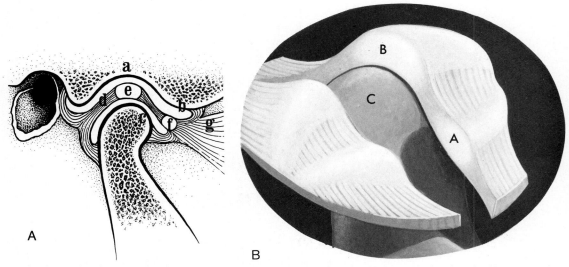

Figure 19–1. *A,* Sagittal diagram of the osseous and soft tissue anatomy of the temporomandibular joint. *a,* Roof of the glenoid fossa; *b,* apex of the articular eminence; *c,* condyle; *d,* bilaminar zone of the meniscus; *e,* posterior band of the meniscus; *f,* anterior band of the meniscus; *g,* superior head of the lateral pterygoid muscle. *B,* Temporomandibular joint meniscus with longitudinal slice for cross-sectional detail shows normal relationship of condyle to meniscus. Note the thickened anterior *(A)* and posterior *(B)* ridges. The superior surface of condylar head *(C)* is visualized beneath the meniscus.

upper articulating surface to each TMJ is composed of the glenoid fossa and the eminence of the temporal bone. The inferior surface of the articular eminence is saddle-shaped along its posterior slope (anterior aspect of the glenoid fossa). It has a convex curvature in the sagittal plane and a slightly concave curvature in the coronal plane. Farther anteriorly, the eminence forms the infratemporal surface of the temporal bone.

A funnel-shaped capsule encases and is loosely attached to the TMJ, and it is tapered at its lower end, where it attaches to the condylar neck. A strong lateral ligament reinforces the joint capsule.

Unlike other joint articulations (which are covered by hyaline cartilage), the articulating surfaces of the TMJ are covered by a fibrous connective tissue, which may contain a variable amount of cartilage cells (fibrocartilage). The rich vascular supply to the joint arises predominantly from the superficial temporal artery. Additional perfusion reaches the anterior portion of the joint by the masseteric branch of the maxillary artery. Innervation is primarily via the auriculotemporal branch of the third division of the trigeminal nerve with additional nerve fibers from the masseteric nerve and posterior deep temporal nerves.

MENISCUS

The meniscus is a fibrocartilaginous structure with specialized shape and function. It has a central zone which is considerably thinner than the peripheral ridges. These ridges are formed by the thicker posterior and anterior edges (Fig. 19–1 B), with the posterior edge generally thicker than the anterior edge. The upper surface of the meniscus adapts to the contour of the eminence of the temporal bone, and the lower surface of the meniscus adapts to the contour of the mandibular condyle. The lower surface is a concave ovoid with its long axis running mediolaterally. The central thin zone of the meniscus is the articulating surface between the convexity of the condyle and the convexity of the eminence. The meniscus forms a complete partition dividing the joint space into two distinct synovial compartments.

The meniscus has important supporting and functional attachments. The specialized posterior attachment (bilaminar zone or retromeniscal pad) consists of fibrovascular connective tissue with laminar elastic and collagenous tissue components. The superior lamina is composed of abundant elastic fibers attached to the postglenoid tubercle and squamotympanic fissure. The inferior lamina contains an elastic collagenous tissue and is attached to the posterior aspect of the condylar neck. An interlaminar zone occupies the space between the superior and inferior laminae, and this is well innervated and quite vascular. Both medially and laterally, the meniscus attaches to the condylar neck. The meniscus blends with the joint capsule anteriorly and is attached to the superior head of the lateral pterygoid muscle anteromedially.

FUNCTION

The temporomandibular joint is a combined hinge-gliding articulation of the mandibular condyle with the glenoid fossa and eminence of the temporal bone. The muscles of mastication (masseter, medial pterygoid, lateral pterygoid, and temporalis) and the suprahyoid muscles (digastric, geniohyoid, and stylohyoid) act bilaterally and simultaneously to produce two distinct types of movement. The first, while opening, is pure rotation around a horizontal axis through the condylar heads. The second is a gliding motion with the condyle and meniscus functioning as a unit and translating anteriorly beneath the articular eminence of the temporal bone. During the anterior gliding action of the condyles, the thin zone of the meniscus remains the articulating surface between the convexity of the condyle in the inferior joint compartment and the convexity of the articular eminence in the superior joint compartment. As forward translational rotation proceeds, the anterosuperior, then the superior, and finally the posterosuperior aspects of the condylar head articulate with the central thin zone of the meniscus.

The normal TMJ functions bilaterally and synchronously. The mandibular midline remains in the sagittal plane during opening and closing of the mouth in the normal condition.

INDICATIONS AND OBJECTIVES

The overall objective of the arthrogram is to assess the position of the meniscus and extent of meniscal movement and integrity. Primary indications for arthrography include pain associated with symptoms of dysfunction (i.e., clicking or locking), vague or persistent complaints not responding to symptomatic therapy, and evaluation of patients undergoing splint therapy. Less common indications include the delineation of loose bodies within the inferior or superior joint spaces, postoperative evaluation, acute injury, and diagnostic aspiration of joint fluid. Patients presenting with symptoms suggesting internal derangements of the TMJ are selected for arthrographic evaluation if conservative methods of therapy have been unsuccessful. The most common symptoms in these patients include TMJ pain and/or muscle tenderness, headaches, joint clicking, and limitation of jaw movements.

CONTRAINDICATIONS

Arthrography should be performed with caution in patients who have a history of prior, severe reactions to iodinated contrast media. Arthrograms have been performed on several such patients without untoward reaction. Serious or life-threatening reactions are exceedingly rare.

Excessive apprehension can lead to a vagal reaction during arthrography, and every attempt should be made to allay patient fears.

Bleeding disorders and anticoagulant therapy are relative contraindications to arthrography, and anticoagulants should be discontinued prior to the procedure.

Arthrography should not be performed in the presence of local skin infections owing to the risk of introducing infection. Joint infection per se is not a contraindication because aspiration may actually be useful for diagnostic purposes and joint fluid analysis.

PLAIN FILMS OF THE TEMPOROMANDIBULAR JOINT

In preparation for arthrography of the temporomandibular joint, linear or multidirectional tomograms are obtained of both TMJs with the head in the lateral position and the mandible in closed and maximally opened positions. The tomographic radiographs are inspected for evidence of degenerative arthritis, for assessment of joint space size and for the presence of intra-articular calcifications (Fig. 19–2 A, B, C). The plain radiographs are

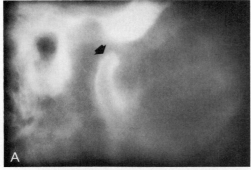
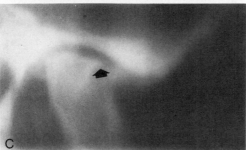
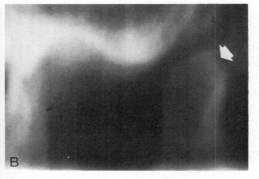

Figure 19–2. *A,* Plain tomogram through the temporomandibular joint with the jaw in the mid-opening phase shows early erosions of the condylar surface posteriorly (arrow). Note that the condyle is very thin, probably representing evidence for regressive remodeling. *B,* Tomogram through the joint space and condyle with the jaw in the maximal opening position. Note the deep erosion in the anterior surface of the condyle (arrow). *C,* Tomogram through the temporomandibular joint shows anterior osteophyte formation (arrow), condylar flattening, and joint space narrowing.

rarely, if ever, diagnostic of meniscal derangements but are useful for disease staging in combination with the arthrographic findings.

ARTHROGRAPHIC TECHNIQUE

PREPARATION OF THE PATIENT

The procedure is explained carefully to the patient before beginning. The objective of the arthrogram is explained briefly as a radiographic study employing the injection of material to assess the soft tissue components of the joint, and to evaluate the position, dynamics, and integrity of the joint.

The patient is placed on a fluoroscopic table in the laterally recumbent position, the head tilted on the table top (Fig. 19–3 A). This allows the joint to project over the skull above the facial bones. The side of the face to be examined is thus uppermost and accessible for skin preparation and draping. Instructing the patient to open and close the mouth several times while under fluoroscopic observation allows rapid identification of the condylar head on the affected side.

NEEDLE PLACEMENT AND FLUOROSCOPY

Under fluoroscopic guidance, the posterior aspect (posterior upper quadrant) of the mandibular condyle is identified. Local anesthetic (lidocaine, 1 per cent) is infiltrated into this region. A ¾ inch or 1¼ inch scalp vein needle and its attached tubing is filled with contrast material (Fig. 19–3 B); care is taken to eliminate air bubbles. Perpendicular to the skin and roentgen beam, the 23-gauge needle is introduced to the predetermined region of the condyle with the jaw in the closed position (Fig. 19–3 C). After advancement of the needle, fluoroscopic observation assures proper positioning (Fig. 19–3 D). When the condyle is encountered, the patient is instructed to open the jaw slightly, and the needle is guided off the posterior slope of the bony margin. The needle will easily advance into the space behind the condyle, without resistance. On fluoroscopic observation the needle will appear to be contiguous with the posterior condylar margin.

Three milliliters of diatrizoate meglumine (282 mg. of iodine content plus 0.03 ml. of 1:1000 epinephrine) are loaded in a 5 ml. syringe. A 0.2 to 0.3 ml. test injection of contrast material will be observed to flow freely anterior to the condyle when the needle is properly placed in the lower joint compartment. A total of approximately 0.5 ml. of contrast material completes the injection. If there is simultaneous filling of the upper joint compartment, with instillation of contrast into the lower joint compartment, another 0.5 ml. of contrast material is usually needed for optimal visualization. Fluoroscopic observation is used to determine the optimal quantity of contrast material to introduce.

The needle is immediately withdrawn and fluoroscopic evaluation and arthrographic recording completed. If multidirectional tomograms are needed for a more complete evaluation, the patient is moved immediately to the multidirectional tomographic unit for arthrotomography.

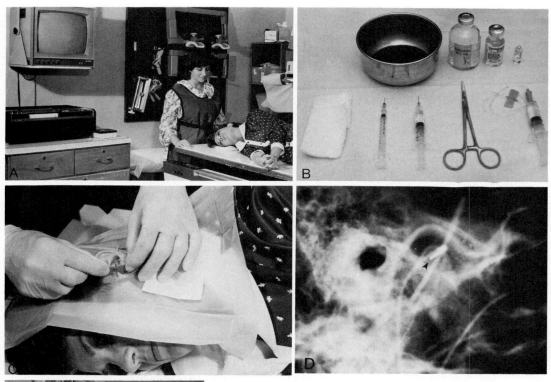

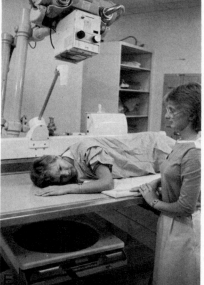

Figure 19–3. Arthrographic technique. *A*, Laterally recumbent position of the patient on the fluoroscopic table top allows the joint space to project over the skull and above the facial bones for optimal fluoroscopic visualization. *B*, The sterile tray. From left to right in the foreground: 1 ml. syringe for epinephrine, 3 ml. syringe for 1 per cent lidocaine, metal hemostat, and 5 ml. syringe with 3 ml. of contrast material and attached 23-gauge scalp vein needle. *C*, The 23-gauge scalp vein needle is introduced into the lower joint space. *D*, Spot radiograph under fluoroscopic guidance confirms proper needle placement with the bevel of the needle at the posterior superior condylar margin (arrowhead). *E*, The patient now lies prone on a tomographic table with the head oriented in a lateral position and with the injected side down. We utilize a multidirectional tomographic unit with a hypocycloidal motion to obtain images of the TMJ in the closed and opened positions.

ARTHROTOMOGRAPHY

The patient lies prone on the roentgenographic table with the head oriented in a lateral position or in such a way that the flat surface of the ramus of the mandible is parallel to the table top (Fig. 19–3 E). Experience has shown no difference in diagnostic accuracy between these positions. A multidirectional tomographic unit is utilized with a hypocycloidal motion to obtain images of the TMJ in the closed and opened positions. The images are approximately 3 mm. in thickness. Three tomograms at 3 mm. intervals are obtained in each position of the jaw. The objective of the tomogram is to survey the joint space from medial to lateral compartments. Rare earth film-screen combinations are utilized throughout the entire roentgenographic protocol to minimize radiation exposure of the patient. These film-screen combinations permit a 75 per cent reduction in radiation exposure compared with conventional film-screen combinations.

In arthrograms of patients with clicking of the TMJ, images are obtained in the closed and maximally opened positions as well as just before the click occurs. The roentgenographic protocol is tailored to the clinical presentation and fluoroscopic-arthrographic impression. As shown in the flow chart, TMJ dynamics in patients with painful clicking of the TMJ are evaluated thoroughly with videotape recording of the session to allow review at a later time (Fig. 19–4). Spot radiographs are obtained during fluoroscopy as a permanent record and the video tape record is available for review during subsequent, more detailed evaluation. In those patients with a reducible click, splint therapy is guided arthrographically using the fluoroscopic image to position the condyle beneath the anteriorly displaced meniscus. This establishes a good starting point for the design of a therapeutic splint that can be shown to have recaptured the meniscus.

In those patients with meniscus displacement without reduction or with meniscus displacement associated with perforation, we obtain arthrotomograms for a more detailed assessment of the anatomical derangement. If an arthrogram appears normal or is indeterminent by fluoroscopy, arthrotomograms are necessary for definitive evaluation.

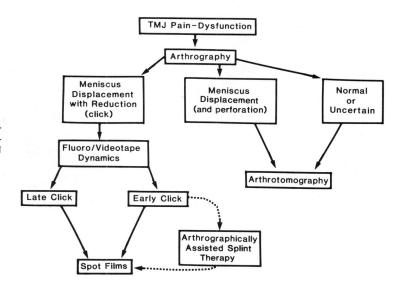

Figure 19–4. Flow chart of arthrographic protocol in patients presenting with symptoms of TMJ pain-dysfunction.

NORMAL APPEARANCE

The position and integrity of the meniscus is interpreted indirectly by its relationship with the joint spaces. A normal meniscus allows no communication of contrast medium between the upper and lower joint spaces.

LOWER JOINT SPACE

The lower joint space is contiguous with the articular surface of the mandibular condyle. In the closed jaw position the posterior aspect of the joint space has a curvilinear, thin configuration along the posterior and superior aspects of the mandibular condyle (Fig. 19–5 A, B). The lower joint space is widest anteriorly, forming a small, smooth teardrop configuration directed obliquely downward. The superior margin of the teardrop delineates the inferior margin of the anterior ridge of the meniscus. Contrast material flows posteriorly, and the joint space opens behind the condyle. Only a thin curvilinear rim of contrast material now remains along the

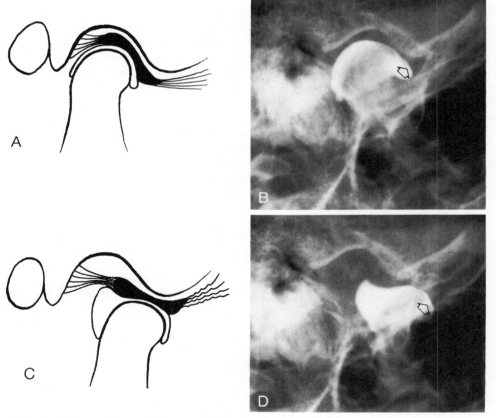

Figure 19–5. *A, B,* Normal. Lower joint space in closed mouth position. Anterior recess of lower joint space in small teardrop configuration (arrow) delineates margin of anterior ridge of meniscus. Central thin zone of meniscus articulates between anterior convex surface of condyle and inferior convex slope of eminence. *C, D,* Normal. Lower joint space in opened mouth position. Joint space widens posteriorly. Only a thin curvilinear rim of contrast material is now noted along the anterosuperior aspect of the condylar head (arrow). Thin zone of the meniscus articulates with the convex surface of the condyle and convex surface of the eminence.

anterosuperior margin of the condyle (Fig. 19–5 C, D). The joint space behind the condyle is smoothly convex inferiorly, and the superior margin is slightly concave.

UPPER JOINT SPACE

The upper joint space is contiguous with the glenoid fossa and articular eminence of the temporal bone. In the closed jaw position, the posterior aspect of this space conforms closely to the margin of the glenoid fossa. The inferior margin of the upper joint space in the region of the middle to posterior aspect of the glenoid fossa delineates the posterior ridge of the meniscus. The anterior aspect of the upper joint space has a teardrop shape, horizontally directed beneath the eminence. This delineates the anterior ridge and the thin central zone of the meniscus.

ABNORMAL FINDINGS

MENISCUS DISPLACEMENT WITH REDUCTION (CLICKING)

Clicking of the TMJ is usually the result of a frictional bind between the posterior edge of the meniscus and condylar head as these structures cross each other in an irregular fashion, momentarily moving in opposite directions. This represents a form of mechanical dysfunction (meniscocondylar incoordination), during which the meniscus is anteriorly positioned relative to the oncoming condylar head during jaw opening. A wide spectrum of meniscocondylar incoordination is often observed. Many patients have asymptomatic, early clicking and do not present for treatment. Arthrograms are performed in those patients, with clicking associated with pain, muscle tenderness and headaches. By arthrographic methods, one may determine the position of the condylar head, during opening at the point of clicking (Fig. 19–6 A, B) and just after clicking occurs (Fig. 19–6 C, D). In general, the later the clicking occurs in the opening phase, the greater the severity of internal derangement.[1, 6, 10] Thus, early clicks are more amenable to splint therapy. Late opening clicks are less easily managed by conservative means, and surgical intervention is often considered. This is because the degree of permanent tissue damage is more severe with late opening clicks and the required splint is often too bulky for satisfactory patient compliance. Meniscus displacement with reduction (clicking) is often a precursor to complete anterior displacement of the meniscus that will not reduce.

Meniscus displacement with reduction (clicking) is only rarely associated with a perforation or tear. The displacement and folding of the anteriorly displaced meniscus is easily diagnosed by lower joint space arthrography, usually not requiring arthrotomography or upper compartment opacification.

The plain radiographic changes in patients with meniscus displacement and reduction may be manifested as superficial erosions or depressions on the posterior surface of the mandibular condyle.[12] Posterior condylar defects may also be associated with recurrent dislocation of the jaw.

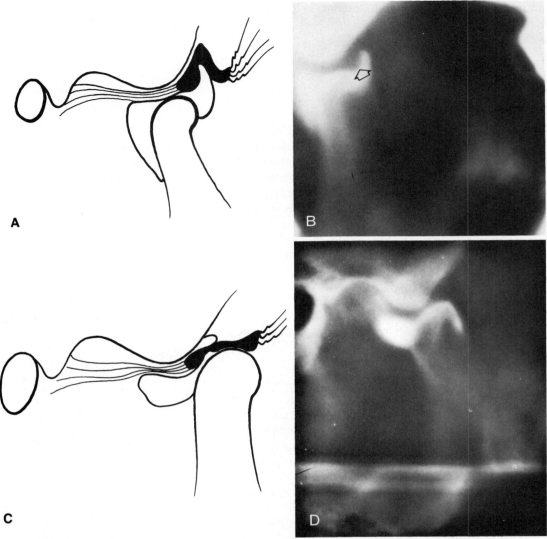

Figure 19–6. *A, B,* Meniscus displacement with reduction (click). Arthrotomogram in a 21-year-old patient experiencing pain and a late opening click, obtained just before the patient experiences the click on opening the mouth. The meniscus remains forward of the condyle. Note that the meniscus is folded upward. The posterior edge of the meniscus (arrow) is anterior to the anterosuperior condylar surface. *C, D,* Diagram and arthrotomogram with further jaw opening and, following the audible click, now demonstrating reduction of the displaced meniscus. The click and dysfunction are produced by the sudden force of the posterior edge of the meniscus moving in an opposite direction to condylar motion.

MENISCUS DISPLACEMENT WITHOUT REDUCTION (CLOSED LOCK)

This is the most significant mechanical dysfunction, which is caused by displacement of the meniscus and is often preceded by painful clicking of the temporomandibular joint. This condition is manifested as an acute, unilateral limitation of opening with deviation of the jaw to the affected side upon opening. This condition is associated with pain, tenderness, and headaches. The patient will frequently relate that prior episodes of clicking are no longer present and that limitation of jaw opening is now a prominent concern.

When a displaced meniscus forms a physical barrier to anterior translation of the condyle, the result is a "closed lock." Incompetency of the posterior attachment (bilaminar zone) of the meniscus is the pathophysiologic mechanism and this may be associated with damage to the elastic tissue and fibrosis.[4, 10, 16, 17] The pressure of the condyle upon the richly innervated posterior meniscal attachment may well be a major cause of pain in this condition.

The arthrographic findings for this type of derangement are highly diagnostic. In the closed jaw position the entire meniscus is anterior to the condylar head (Fig. 19–7 A, B). The anterior recess of the lower joint space is much larger, with a more horizontal orientation than in the normal condition. A concave upper margin is most often apparent and delineates the inferior portion of the posterior ridge of the meniscus. The concave joint space configuration may be quite large when there is thickening of the posterior ridge of the meniscus. With attempted jaw opening the impression of the meniscus upon the anterior recess becomes more prominent and there is greater distortion (angulation) of the most anterior and superior portions

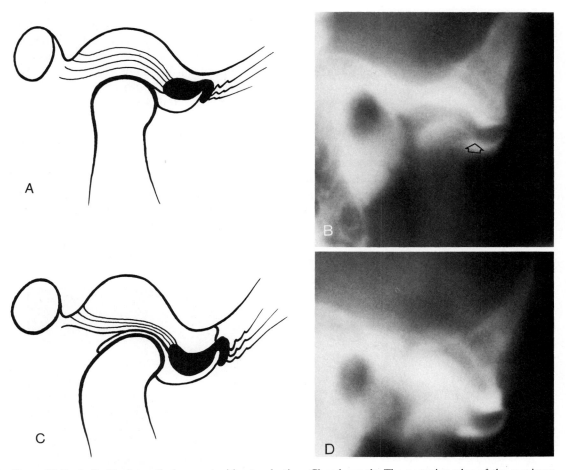

Figure 19–7. *A, B,* Meniscus displacement without reduction. Closed mouth. The posterior edge of the meniscus (arrow) anterior to condyle causes concave impression on the anterior recess. Contrast material is also noted in the upper joint compartment, indicating a perforation. *C, D,* Maximal opening. Decreased condylar translation with accentuation of concave impression on anterior recess created by the displaced meniscus.

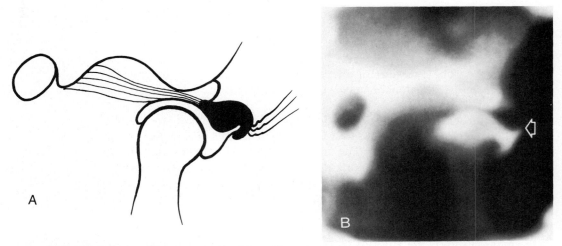

Figure 19–8. *A, B*, Meniscus displacement without reduction. Maximal opening. The meniscus is displaced anteriorly and is folded at the central thin zone in an upward direction. Note the sharp "beak" or angulation in the anterior recess (arrow).

of the anterior recess (Fig. 19–7 C, D). This represents a progressive folding due to pressure of the meniscus against the anterior surface of the condyle.

The "beak" or angulation in the lower joint space is formed by upward folding of the meniscus as it bends at its central thin zone (Fig. 19–8 A, B). The meniscus may actually be completely folded with only a dimple of contrast material between the apposed anterior and posterior meniscal ridges (Fig. 19–9 A, B).

A very large, smooth impression upon the anterior recess of the lower joint compartment represents a markedly thickened and deformed meniscus, which may not be amenable to surgical repair (Fig. 19–10).

Some patients are able to manipulate their jaws into a position such that a click can be converted into an anterior meniscus displacement without reduction (Fig. 19–11 A, B). However, condylar translation does not decrease in these patients and slight self-manipulation of the jaw by the patient will reduce what had appeared to be a displacement without reduction (Fig. 19–11 C).

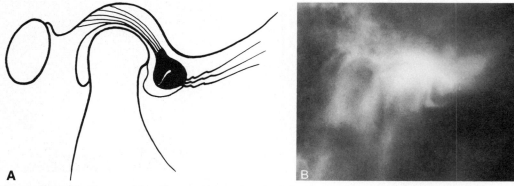

Figure 19–9. *A, B*, Trauma. This 23-year-old man sustained fractures of the mandible and pelvis following an automobile accident. The condyle is noted to be ankylosed with no translation during maximal opening. The arthrotomogram shows anterior meniscus displacement with the meniscus completely folded upon itself.

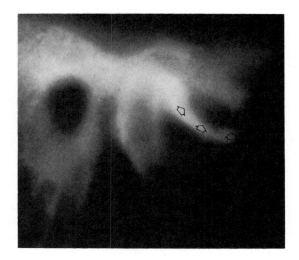

Figure 19–10. Thickened and deformed meniscus. Arthrotomogram demonstrates very prominent contrast-opacified anterior recess of the lower joint compartment. The large concave impression upon the anterior recess is diagnostic of a markedly thickened and deformed meniscus (arrows).

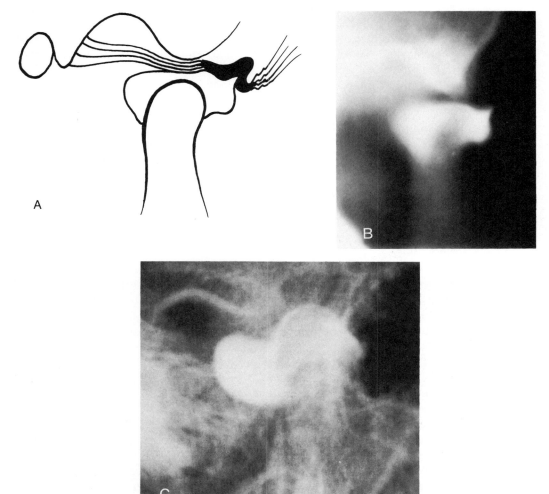

Figure 19–11. *A, B,* Arthrotomogram with the lower joint space opacified, demonstrating anterior meniscus displacement without reduction. Note the upward "beak" configuration of the anterior recess of the lower joint compartment and the diagrammatic representation of the displaced meniscus. *C,* Spot radiograph obtained during arthrography in the same patient now demonstrating reduction of the displaced meniscus. This 23-year-old man is able to manipulate the jaw into a position that can create complete anterior meniscus displacement without reduction as depicted here.

There are multiple configurations of the lower joint space in patients presenting with meniscus displacement without reduction, yet all conform to generally similar patterns. These patterns are clearly indicative of forward positions of the meniscus with various types and degrees of folding. These are usually so clearly distinguishable from the normal that there is little confusion in interpretation.

MENISCUS DISPLACEMENT WITH PERFORATION

The vast majority of patients with perforations of the meniscus also have anterior meniscus displacement without reduction.[10] Indeed, most of these patients have suffered for years from symptoms suggestive of internal derangements. A very high percentage of these patients will show osseous abnormalities of degenerative arthritis on plain tomographic evaluation. A recent prospective survey identified signs of degenerative arthritis in approximately two thirds of these patients.[12] Flattening of the condyle with osteophytosis and flattening of the articular eminence appear to be classic radiographic changes.

Another interesting aspect is that condylar translation may be normal, but these patients do report a history of chronic limitation of opening, which slowly resolved over a long period of time.

Arthrographic detection of a perforation is demonstrated by simultaneous opacification of the upper joint space when contrast material is introduced into the lower joint compartment. Anterior meniscus displacement without reduction will usually also be demonstrated (Fig. 19–12 A, B). This requires arthrotomography for complete evaluation, as the upper joint compartment may obscure the lower joint compartment in conventional radiographs (Fig. 19–12 C). If a complete column of contrast material is noted posteriorly, a diagnosis of complete meniscus detachment is likely (Fig. 19–13 A, B).

Arthrography cannot demonstrate the actual site of the perforation, but in those patients with surgical confirmation, most perforations and detachments have been noted to occur in the bilaminar zone region. This is the posterior attachment of the meniscus to the temporal bone.[7, 10] Other perforations have been noted to occur in the lateral thin region of the meniscus itself.

There is approximately a 15 per cent incidence of false positive perforations by arthrography. This might be due to straddling of the needle bevel between the upper and lower joint spaces with simultaneous opacification or improper needle positioning. It is fortunate, however, that virtually all of the perforations are associated with anterior meniscus displacement without reduction. Therefore, we present the primary diagnosis as a displaced meniscus and a secondary diagnosis of possible perforation.

A recent two-year prospective investigation that compared the preliminary plain tomograms with the arthrographic diagnosis found an overall incidence of arthritis in 22 per cent of patients presenting with signs and symptoms of internal derangements.[12] The average age of these patients was 29 years, with an 8:1 female predominance. Those patients with the most severe internal derangements diagnosed by arthrography had the greatest incidence and severity of degenerative joint disease. Erosions of the condylar surface were an early finding (Fig. 19–2 A). Abnormalities of greater severity

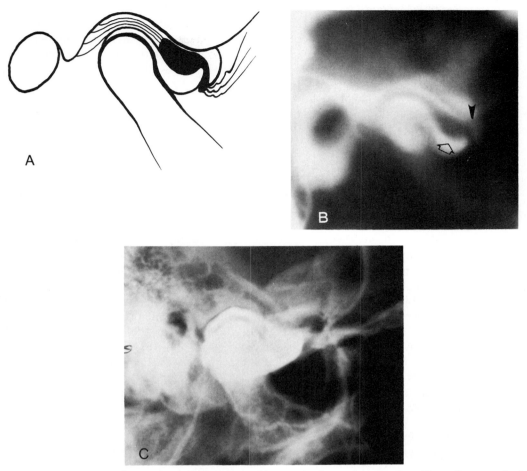

Figure 19–12. *A, B,* Anterior meniscus displacement without reduction and perforation. The arthrogram depicts filling of both lower (arrow) and upper (arrowhead) joint compartments associated with anterior meniscus displacement without reduction. *C,* Spot radiograph of the same patient is difficult to interpret without the arthrotomogram demonstrated in *B.*

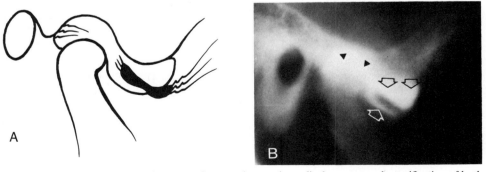

Figure 19–13. *A, B,* Arthrotomogram demonstrating anterior meniscus displacement and opacification of both upper (arrows) and lower (arrow) joint compartments. A complete column of contrast material (arrowheads) is noted posteriorly, suggesting detachment of the meniscus.

were manifest as deep erosions in the anterolateral pole of the condyle with or without sclerosis (Fig. 19–2 B). Those patients with meniscus displacement of long duration by history, and with a greater frequency of perforations, were associated with condylar flattening, osteophyte formation, and joint space narrowing (Fig. 19–2 C). Erosions and flattening of the apex of the eminence occurred with the most severe grades of internal derangements as depicted by arthrography.

ARTHROGRAPHICALLY ASSISTED SPLINT THERAPY

Splint therapy is a mode of treatment currently used for those patients known to have symptomatic meniscus displacement with reduction (clicking) that occurs during the early to mid-opening phase of mandibular movement. The intraoral splint is utilized to advance the mandibular condyle anteriorly and inferiorly to a position that is normal in relationship to the anteriorly displaced meniscus. Clinically, splint therapy has required a subjective deduction of the relative position of the condyle to meniscus using the position of the mandible when the click occurs as a guide. The arthrogram objectively documents the position of the anteriorly displaced meniscus (Fig. 19–14 A) and is then used to guide mandibular positioning so that the condyle lies underneath the thin zone of the meniscus (Fig. 19–14 B, C). This method allows objective establishment of the optimum meniscus-to-condyle relationship at the very outset of splint therapy. A temporary splint may be fashioned during the arthrography session and a more permanent splint can then be constructed, using the temporary appliance as a model. The clinical value of this new approach is enormous and yet to be fully explored.

ARTHROGRAPHY FOR MISCELLANEOUS CONDITIONS

MANDIBULAR TRAUMA

The relationship between TMJ disease and direct trauma to the mandible severe enough to cause fractures of the mandible or condylar process has not been systematically evaluated. Experience with patients who have previously sustained mandibular fractures suggests a very high incidence of internal derangements. Ankylosis of the temporomandibular joint has been noted in patients evaluated by arthrography (Fig. 19–15). The ankylosis is a result of both intra- and periarticular fibrous adhesions and related to meniscus displacement without reduction (Fig. 19–16 A, B). A greater awareness of the possibility of internal derangements with mandibular fractures is anticipated.

INFLAMMATORY ARTHRITIS

The diagnosis of inflammatory arthritis is usually established on clinical grounds. Rheumatoid arthritic patients generally have multiple involved joints, an elevated erythrocyte sedimentation rate, and elevated levels of rheumatoid factor. Other forms of inflammatory arthritis occur in association

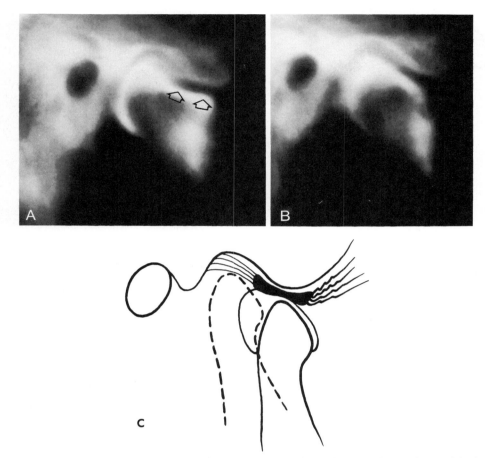

Figure 19–14. *A*, Arthrotomogram depicts anterior positioning of the meniscus relative to the condyle (arrows). This patient was experiencing painful clicking with jaw opening and had the arthrographic diagnosis of anterior displacement with reduction. *B*, *C*, Arthrotomogram demonstrating optimal relationship between condyle and meniscus following splint therapy. Diagram depicts the change in relationships of the condyle prior to splint therapy (dashed outline) and condyle in recaptured relationship relative to meniscus (solid condyle outline).

Figure 19–15. Trauma. This patient sustained severe trauma to the mandible with mandibular fracture. Arthrotomogram demonstrates markedly irregular upper joint compartment (arrows). This patient had severe limitation of mandibular opening. The lower joint compartment could not be opacified. Subsequent surgical observation demonstrated complete ankylosis of the joint compartment with obliteration of the lower joint space. Fibrous adhesions were present.

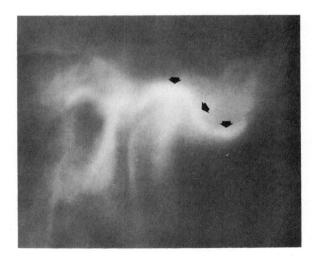

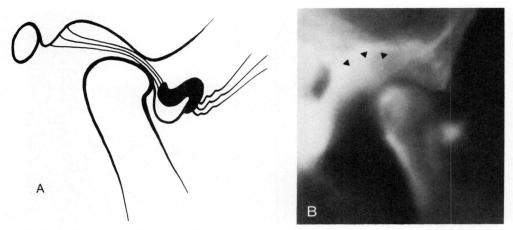

Figure 19–16. *A, B,* Trauma. The patient is in the closed mouth position. Note that the mandibular condyle is seated inferiorly and anterior to the glenoid fossa (arrowheads). Only a rotational component of the condyle was noted at fluoroscopy with jaw opening and closing. Contrast material introduced into the lower joint compartment demonstrated anterior meniscus displacement without reduction.

with skin lesions (psoriasis) or other stigmata, such as inflammatory bowel disease. The temporomandibular joint is rarely the presenting complaint but may be coincidentally involved. Occasionally patients will present with TMJ symptoms and equivocal plain radiographic findings that require differentiation from actual internal derangements. The arthrogram can clearly distinguish the synovial changes of an inflammatory arthritis from an internal derangement secondary to meniscus dysfunction (Fig. 19–17). The physician must be alert to the possibility that patients with inflammatory arthritis may also have a coincidental internal derangement.

Capsular Damage

Acute injuries to the temporomandibular joint may lead not only to anterior meniscus displacement and perforations or tears of the meniscus, but also to capsular damage. Indeed, capsular damage is often associated with severe grades of meniscus displacement.[11] Capsular damage may occur in association with internal derangements or may be the sole abnormality (Fig. 19–18).

COMPLICATIONS

Serious complications following TMJ arthrography are extremely rare. The temporomandibular joint is quite resistant to infection, and there have been no reported instances of TMJ infection secondary to arthrography.

Allergic reactions to intra-articular contrast media are exceedingly rare, and we are unaware of any such occurrence in TMJ arthrography.

The most frequent complication of TMJ arthrography is contrast medium extravasation into the capsule and soft tissues around the joint with mild to moderate patient discomfort. Meglumine salts are recommended rather than sodium salts to reduce discomfort.

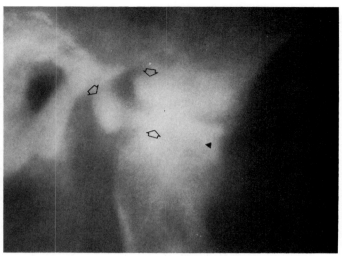

Figure 19–17. Psoriatic arthritis. This 56-year-old man experienced an acute limitation of mandibular opening, more severe on the left than on the right. Internal derangement related to meniscus dysfunction was suspected. Arthrotomogram shows severe derangement of the upper and lower joint compartments secondary to an inflammatory arthritis (arrows). The meniscus was in a normal relationship to the condyle. The anterior band of the meniscus is faintly identified (arrowhead).

Intravasation of contrast material occurs infrequently, but this theoretically increases the risk of an idiosyncratic reaction. Epinephrine, in a dose of 0.03 ml. (1:1000) per 3 ml. of contrast material, is recommended because there is a risk of an acute hypertensive episode with intravasation of higher doses. A case of parotitis has been reported following arthrography with larger needles and cannulas. A cannula tip can be lost in the region of the joint with this technique.[17]

Transient facial nerve palsy may result from vigorous infiltration of lidocaine. A nerve block is usually not attempted during the arthrographic procedure, and therefore some patients will experience a moderate degree of pain with needle placement upon the periosteum of the condyle and with joint distension following the injection of contrast material. The discomfort is quite transient in the majority of cases. If persistent joint pain occurs following the procedure we recommend an oral anti-inflammatory agent (aspirin; acetaminophen) and cold compress applications to the affected area.

Some patients show a great deal of anxiety before the arthrographic procedure, and these patients will occasionally experience a vagal reaction

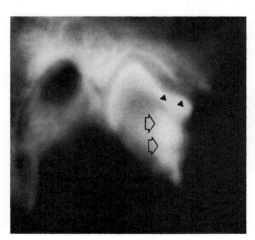

Figure 19–18. Capsular damage. Arthrotomogram demonstrates anterior meniscus displacement (arrowheads). There is suggestion of lateral capsular damage noted as extravasation of contrast material along the anterior surface of the condylar neck (arrows). The extravasation is remote from the injection site.

(fainting episode). If such a response should occur and is serious enough to lead to hypotension and bradycardia, intravenous atropine may be administered. In our experience with TMJ arthrograms, it has not been necessary to administer this medication.

COMPUTED TOMOGRAPHY (CT) OF THE TEMPOROMANDIBULAR JOINT

Initial experiences with computed tomographic evaluation of the temporomandibular joint have been very encouraging[8, 11, 13] (Fig. 19–19 A, B). The technique involves either axial tomograms through the base of the skull with sagittal reconstruction in the area of the temporomandibular joint or direct sagittal CT of the TMJ. Both methods appear to have a potential of visualizing the meniscus itself and do not require a percutaneous injection of contrast material.

Another benefit of the CT technique is that it allows a thorough assessment of the osseous structures along with an adequate evaluation of the soft tissue components. Bilateral CT scans can be obtained with ease and without patient discomfort.

A disadvantage of the CT scan, however, is that it can produce only static images and thus cannot record the soft tissue dynamics. Although displacements of the meniscus are distinguishable, perforations cannot be detected.

CT scanning of the TMJ shows great promise in the evaluation of the temporomandibular joint for internal derangements. Large clinical studies are now under way at several major medical centers, and these studies will establish more definitive diagnostic guidelines. CT scanning of the temporomandibular joint may someday gain acceptance as a noninvasive alternative to TMJ arthrography.

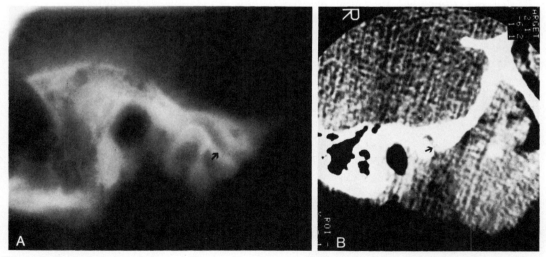

Figure 19–19. *A,* Arthrotomogram in a 33-year-old patient with the jaw in the closed position showing the meniscus (arrow) to be displaced anterior to the condyle. *B,* Direct sagittal computed tomographic scan of the same patient performed on a different date and without the injection of contrast material into the joint compartment shows the anteriorly displaced meniscus (arrow) with good correlation to the arthrotomographic findings. This scan was performed with the jaw in the closed position and with a window width optimal for soft tissue.

SUMMARY

Temporomandibular joint arthrography is gaining wider acceptance as a diagnostic tool which complements clinical evaluation and aids treatment of TMJ pain and dysfunction. In a growing number of medical centers it is performed as a routine procedure. TMJ arthrography is highly accurate in depicting internal derangements of the temporomandibular joint and in the differential diagnosis of patients with TMJ pain. TMJ arthrography is an outpatient procedure that can be performed with local anesthesia and is devoid of serious complications. TMJ arthrography will continue to gain in popularity as its full value in both diagnosis and treatment become more widely recognized.

References

1. Bronstein, S. L., Tomasetti, B. J., and Ryan, D. E.: Internal derangements of the temporomandibular joint: Correlation of arthrography with surgical findings. J. Oral Surg., *39*:572, 1981.
2. Blaschke, D. D., Solberg, W. K., and Sanders, B.: Arthrography of the temporomandibular joint: Review of current status. JADA, *100*:388, 1980.
3. Choukas, N. C., and Sicher, H.: The structure of the temporomandibular joint. Oral Surg., *13*:1203, 1960.
4. Dolwick, M. F., Katzberg, R. W., Helms, C. A., and Bales, D. J.: Arthrotomographic evaluation of the temporomandibular joint. J. Oral Surg., *37*:793, 1979.
5. El Mahdy, A. S.: Intra-articular tissue in the temporomandibular joint. J. Prosthet. Dent., *26*:396, 1971.
6. Farrar, W. B., and McCarty, W. L.: Inferior joint space arthrography and characteristics of condylar paths in internal derangements of the TMJ. J. Prosthet. Dent., *41*:548, 1979.
7. Helms, C. A., Katzberg, R. W., Dolwick, M. F., and Bales, D. J.: Arthrotomographic diagnosis of perforations of the temporomandibular joint. Br. J. Radiol., *53*:283, 1980.
8. Helms, C. A., Morrish, R. B., Kircos, L. T., Katzberg, R. W., and Dolwick, M. F.: Computed tomography of the meniscus of the temporomandibular joint: Preliminary observations. Radiology, *145*:719, 1982.
9. Katzberg, R. W., Dolwick, M. F., Bales, D. J., and Helms, C. A.: Arthrotomography of the temporomandibular joint: New technique and preliminary observations. Am. J. Roentgenol., *132*:949, 1979.
10. Katzberg, R. W., Dolwick, M. F., Helms, C. A., Hopens, T., Bales, D. J., and Coggs, G. C.: Arthrotomography of the temporomandibular joint. Am. J. Roentgenol., *134*:995, 1980.
11. Katzberg, R. W., Dolwick, M. F., Keith, D. A., Helms, C. A., and Guralnick, W. C.: New observations with routine and CT-assisted arthrography in suspected internal derangements of the temporomandibular joint. Oral Surg. Oral Med. Oral Pathol., *51*:569, 1981.
12. Katzberg, R. W., Keith, D. A., Guralnick, W. C., Manzione, J. V., and Ten Eick, W. R.: Internal derangements of the temporomandibular joint and arthritis. Radiology, *146*:107, 1983.
13. Manzione, J. V., Seltzer, S. E., Katzberg, R. W., Hammerschlag, S. B., and Chiango, B. F.: Direct sagittal computed tomography of the temporomandibular joint. Am. J. Neuroradiol., *3*:677, 1982.
14. Murphy, W. A.: Arthrography of the temporomandibular joint. Radiol. Clin. North Am., *19*:365, 1981.
15. Sicher, H., and DuBrul, E. L. (eds.): Temporomandibular articulation: *In* Oral Anatomy. St. Louis, C. V. Mosby Co., 1975, p. 160.
16. Wilkes, C.: Structural and functional alteration of the temporomandibular joint. Northwest. Dent., *57*:287, 1978.
17. Wilkes, C.: Arthrography of the temporomandibular joint in patients with the TMJ pain dysfunction syndrome. Minn. Med., *61*:645, 1978.

20

The Significance of Computed Tomography (CT Scanning) of the Temporomandibular Joint

ERIC PAUL SHABER, D.D.S.
CLYDE A. HELMS, M.D.

Historically, disorders of the temporomandibular joint (TMJ) and its adnexal structures have perplexed the medical, surgical, and dental specialties. This is in part due to the unique morphokinetics of the condyle-disc-eminentia assembly and its unique relationship with myofascial, psychophysiologic, and systemic factors that exert significant influence on the stomatognathic apparatus.[1]

As members of an increasing number of professional (and paraprofessional) disciplines become interested in facial pain syndromes (both acute and chronic), an enormous emphasis has been placed on the region of the TMJ.

Soon after the clinical applicability of TMJ arthrography was demonstrated, it became consummately clear that "a new breed of cat" had emerged: positional disorders (internal derangements) of the meniscus of the TMJ.[2-11] It is our intention in this chapter to briefly describe the "state of the science" diagnostic tool for evaluating the component elements of the condyle-disc-eminentia assembly of the temporomandibular joint—computed tomography (CT scanning).

MECHANICS OF COMPUTED TOMOGRAPHY

A conventional radiograph is obtained by recording the differences in attenuation of an x-ray beam through an object onto an x-ray film. This process has been only modestly improved on since its inception by Conrad

Roentgen in 1895 to the current state of the art; such improvements include magnification films, fine detail films, and dozens of other types of techniques, each of which enhance a particular area of interest.

Several problems exist with conventional radiography when applied to the temporomandibular joint (TMJ). First, subtle changes in soft tissue density cannot be appreciated. Therefore, the meniscus of the TMJ cannot be visualized on plain films. In order to visualize the meniscus it must be coated with a high-density contrast agent—hence, arthrography must be performed. Second, plain films record only the total attenuation of an object and tell nothing of the object's homogeneity. Thus, an object of high density peripherally and low density centrally may appear identical to another object of moderate density throughout.

Computed tomography (CT) suffers from neither of these shortcomings and has the advantage of being able to reconstruct an image in any desirable projection once the data have been acquired by the computer (Fig. 20–1).

In first generation EMI scanners (EMI was the first company to produce and market scanners, in 1973), a thinly collimated x-ray beam is passed through the object to be studied and its attenuation is recorded by a detector (usually made of sodium iodide; however, more advanced scanners now use other detector substances, such as xenon). The detector sends an electrical transmission to the computer based on the amount of attenuation, which the computer sends along with the exact position of the detector. The x-ray beam and detector then move through the object making recordings of the attenuation at multiple points, which are stored by the computer. After a complete "pass" or "translation," the x-ray tube and the detector are shifted or rotated 1 degree, and the process is repeated (Fig. 20–2). After 180 degrees of recordings are obtained, the data accumulation is complete and the patient can be removed. Note that the multiple intersecting x-ray beams through the object form small honeycomb-like sections. The more x-ray passes used, the smaller these units become, which essentially determines the resolution size of the scan. Current scanners can resolve objects 0.6 to 0.25 mm in size.

A problem with the early scanners was that it took quite a long time to obtain all the data, and patient motion would severely degrade the image.

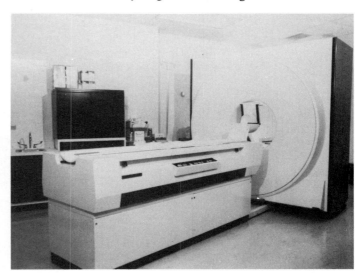

Figure 20–1.

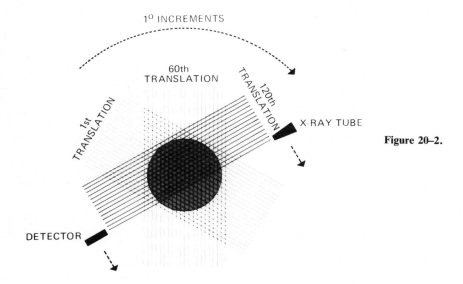

Figure 20–2.

More recent scanners use larger detector arrays and fan-beams (Fig. 20–3) to eliminate the time-consuming "translation" process and can perform scans in less than 10 sec.

The attenuation data are recorded digitally by the computer and an acceptable reproduction is made by assigning shades of gray (and even color in some scanners) to each attenuation value. This gives a picture not unlike a conventional x-ray, except that now cross-sectional anatomy, subtle differences in tissue density, and inhomogeneity of an object can be appreciated.

CT OF THE TMJ

Computed tomography has shown itself to be extremely useful in evaluating complex joints, such as the hip and shoulder. These joints are often difficult to examine with conventional films because of their complex anatomic configuration. The same is true of the TMJ.

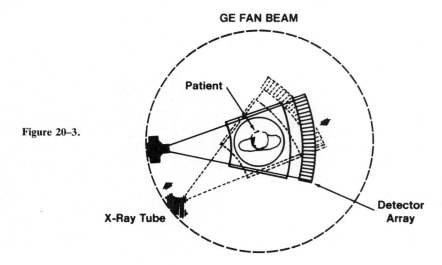

Figure 20–3.

In evaluating tumors of the jaw, especially their soft tissue extent, and when evaluating trauma, CT has been shown to be superior to plain films and tomography.

CT can be used to evaluate degenerative disease of the TMJ (Fig. 20–4). In the case illustrated, tomograms (Fig. 20–5A,B) failed to reveal the extent of degenerative disease present. The CT examination showed severe joint space narrowing, subchondral sclerosis, and osteophytosis. At surgery this was confirmed.

Early attempts to visualize the meniscus of the TMJ were unsuccessful. The size of the meniscus is not a limiting factor (since modern scanners can resolve structures as small as 0.25 mm); therefore, it was determined that the difference in density from the surrounding tissue was so subtle as to not allow separation of the meniscus from the lateral pterygoid muscle. Histologic sections of menisci showed that the meniscus is definitely denser than the surrounding soft tissues and less dense than the bone, and thus it should be seen on CT.

Most CT scanners can give actual density readings or attenuation values of any desired tissue on a scan. Therefore, the anatomic region of the meniscus can be sampled and compared to the adjacent soft tissues. When this was done, it was shown that the meniscus is indeed increased in density over the surrounding soft tissues. This can be shown on many scanners by use of the procedure identified as "blink mode," which causes all the tissue on a scan that is of any particular density to be highlighted by blinking on and off. The density can be changed at random so that either low tissue density (fat) or high tissue density (bone) can be blinked. This is helpful when trying to distinguish between two nearly identical but separate densities, which have differences too subtle to be distinguished easily by the human eye. Hence, the meniscus of the TMJ can be blinked separately from the lateral pterygoid muscle and its attachments.

METHOD OF SCANNING

Patients with suspected internal derangements of the TMJ who would otherwise have had a TMJ arthrogram are studied in an axial position with the mouth open. This exacerbates the displacement of the meniscus and makes it more prominent, thus making it more likely to be seen. If the patient is experiencing clicking or popping, it is imperative that the patient be studied with the mouth open *prior* to the click. Once the joint pops or clicks, presumably the meniscus reduces and returns to its normal position atop the condyle, and the CT scan would therefore be normal. To demonstrate a displaced meniscus in a person whose joint clicks, therefore, the scan must be performed *before* meniscus reduction.

A bite splint or several gauze sponges are placed in the patient's mouth to allow the patient to relax and to eliminate motion. A frequent error in positioning occurs when the mouth is opened to a point just before the click and then, when putting in the bite splint or gauze, the patient opens further and the click occurs. To avoid having the patient open the mouth beyond the click point, it is best to place the bite splint or gauze in the patient's mouth while feeling the TMJ for a click. If a palpable click occurs, merely start again. The patient's forehead is then taped to the table to reduce motion.

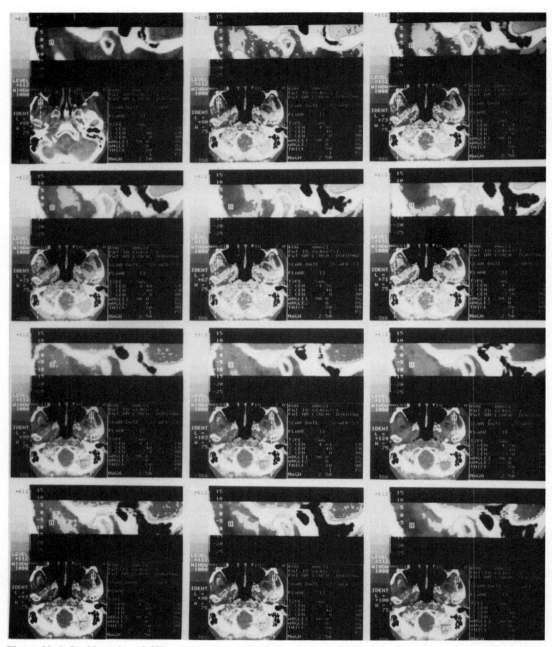

Figure 20–4. In this series of CT scans the upper six views are the right TMJ and the lower six views are the left TMJ. The TMJ has been scanned from medial to lateral aspects, with a concentration on the medial surface, since herniated discs usually occur anteromedially. This case demonstrates bilaterally displaced TMJ discs. Also note that the medial to lateral scans on the left (bottom three films) show gross osteophytic formation: Compare these scans with the tomographs shown in Figure 20–5 (same patient).

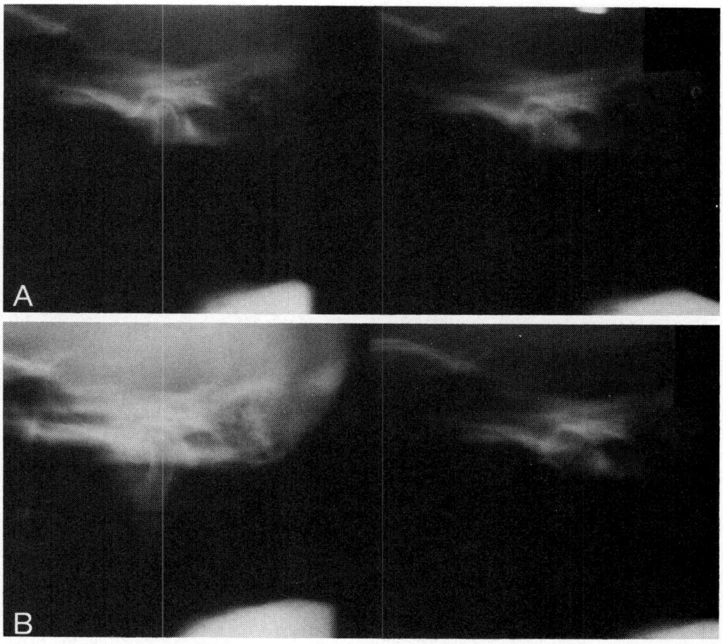

Figure 20–5. *A,* Medial and central tomograms of patient in Figure 20–4. Note obvious osteoarthritic changes and condylar position. *B,* Lateral view of the left TMJ. Although a hint of osteophyte formation can be seen, it is not nearly as clearly visualized as on the CT scan (see Fig. 20–4, lower three views).

A lateral scout view is obtained to mark the area to be studied. Cursor lines are placed throughout the area from just below to just above the TMJ, which correspond to the scan slices which will be made. The external auditory canal is a helpful landmark for localizing the TMJ on the scout film.

Scan slice thickness is 1.5 mm, with scans done every 1.5 mm. Other protocols, such as 5 mm thickness done overlapped at every 3 mm, can be performed, but the former protocol has been found to be preferable by the authors on empirical grounds. About 14 to 16 scans are obtained. The radiation dose for CT scans of the head has been documented multiple times in the literature and is felt to be within the diagnostic range. It certainly provides less radiation than an arthrogram with several minutes of fluoroscopy and tomograms.

Once the scan is completed (it takes about 20 min of the scanner's time per examination), the data must be reformatted from an axial plane to a parasagittal plane. The computer will allow easy and rapid reformations through each condyle, and the menisci are shown by use of the blink mode, as mentioned earlier.

In the normal, nondisplaced meniscus, no increase in the tissue density anterior to the condyle should be present (Fig. 20–6). Care should be taken to show that the soft tissue anterior to the condyle is truly isodense to the surrounding soft tissues.

In the anteriorly displaced meniscus, the blink mode should demonstrate an increased tissue density anterior to the condyle, which corresponds to the displaced posterior bond of the meniscus.

Arthrograms were performed on 12 or so patients who had CT scans several weeks later, and these were compared for accuracy. In all instances the correlation was accurate.[12]

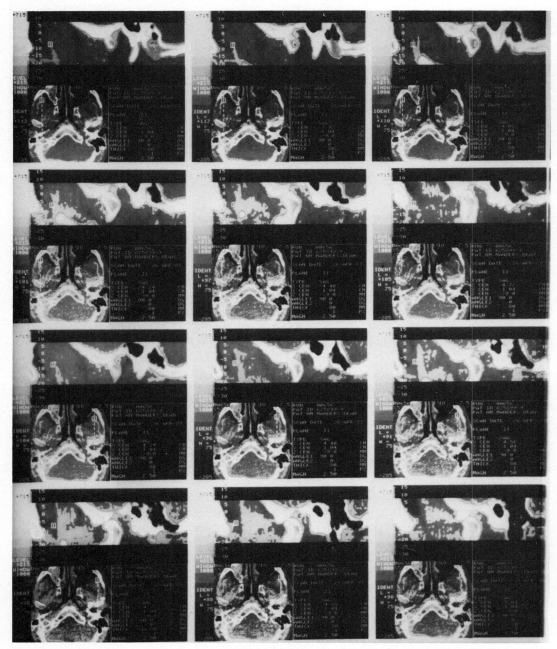

Figure 20–6. Normal CT scan of the bilateral TMJ. Note that compared with the scan in Figure 20–4, there is no increase in tissue density on the parasagittal reformation.

ADVANTAGES AND DISADVANTAGES OF THE CT SCAN

The main advantage of the CT scan over the arthrogram is that the CT scan is noninvasive and thus there is no associated morbidity. Another advantage is the ability to examine both joints simultaneously. Almost half of the CT scans performed by us have shown bilateral abnormalities, which, with clinical follow-up, have proved to correlate well in most cases. The lower amounts of radiation used with the CT scan is another advantage. Evaluation of the osseous structures is also far superior with the CT scan as compared to the arthrogram.

A disadvantage of CT is the cost. Currently a CT scan is almost twice as expensive as an arthrogram unless a bilateral arthrogram is performed. Also, CT scanning capabilities are not as readily available as arthrograms would be at most institutions. Finally, perhaps the most serious limitation to the CT scan is that it fails to evaluate the dynamics of the meniscus, as does an arthrogram. Also, it will not diagnose a perforation of the meniscus. Fortunately, most oral and maxillofacial surgeons merely want to know the position of the meniscus.

A potential pitfall in performing CT of the TMJ was mentioned earlier: a patient who is studied *after* a click or pop, which indicates that a meniscus has reduced, will appear normal.

Another problem area is the blink mode. A displaced meniscus can appear normal when only very high density tissue is blinked when in reality the meniscus is displaced and can be shown by blinking lower tissue densities. It must be emphasized that the meniscus is only subtly increased in density over the surrounding tissue, and because of this the surrounding tissue should be blinked first; then slowly adjust the blink mode to blink higher densities until the meniscus is observed.[12]

CLINICAL IMPRESSIONS

When a patient presents to our office with pain or dysfunction, certain questions must be asked. Is the dysfunction etiologically related to muscular incoordination or to internal derangement(s) of the meniscus within the TMJ? More appropriately, are the dysfunction excursions of the jaw of an extracapsular origin or an intracapsular origin, or both? Do the pain referral patterns with which patients present more closely resemble masticatory muscular pain patterns or joint pathology? Very often these are difficult questions that may never be answered with even the best of clinical examinations. By utilizing CT scanning, we can rule out the most serious possible dysfunctional etiologic factor—the anteromedially displaced TMJ meniscus. Once we know diagnostically that the disorder is extracapsular, intracapsular, or both, we may then formulate a suitable treatment regime.

TREATMENT OF FACIAL PAIN AND TMJ DYSFUNCTION

A brief overview of the most frequent forms of TMJ pain and dysfunction is shown in Figures 20–7 through 20–10. This diagrammatic sequence is presented with the intention of availing the practitioner of a procedural context in which to render treatment.

Acknowledgment: The authors would like to gratefully acknowledge Victoria Seltner for her research assistance and manuscript preparation.

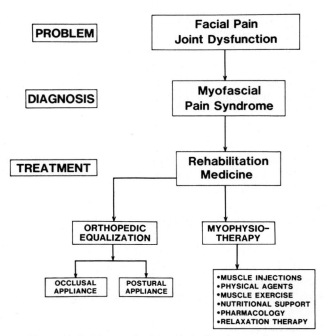

Figure 20–7. The myofascial pain dysfunction syndrome.

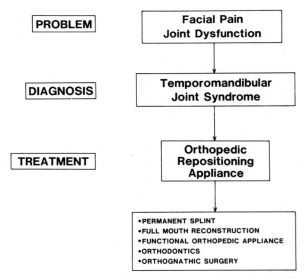

Figure 20–8. The temporomandibular joint syndrome (orthopedic position disease).

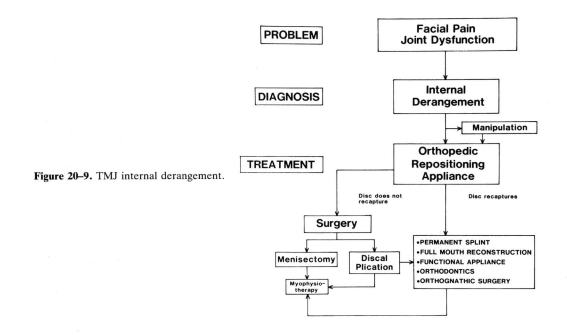

Figure 20–9. TMJ internal derangement.

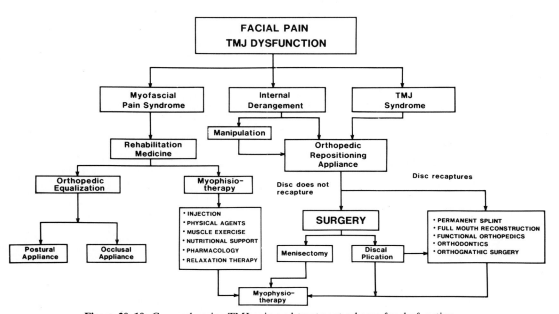

Figure 20–10. Comprehensive TMJ pain and treatment scheme for dysfunction.

References

1. Shaber, E. P.: Temporomandibular joint disorders. The California Institute of Continuing Education, Vol. 4, Article 3.
2. Katzberg, R. W., Dolwick, M. F., Helms, C. A., Hopens, T., Bales, D. J., and Cobbs, G. C.: Arthrotomography of the TMJ. A.J.R., *134*:995–1003, 1980.
3. Blaschke, D. D., Solberg, W. K., and Sanders, B.: Arthrography of the temporomandibular joint: Review of current status. J. Am. Dent. Assoc., *100*:388, 1980. Presented at the meeting of the International Association of Dental Research, New Orleans, March 1979.
4. Katzberg, R. W., Dolwick, M. F., Bales, D. J., and Helms, C. A.: Arthrotomography of the TMJ: New technique and preliminary observations. A.J.R., *132*:949–955, 1979.
5. Murphy, W. A.: Arthrography of the temporomandibular joint. Radiol. Clin. North Am., *19*:365–378, 1981.
6. Farrar, W. B., and McCarty, W. L., Jr.: Inferior joint space arthrography and characteristics of condylar paths in internal derangements of the TMJ. J. Prosthet. Dent., *41*:548–555, 1979.
7. Katzberg, R. W., Dolwick, M. F., Helms, C. A., and Bales, D. J.: Arthrotomography of the temporomandibular joint. *In* Dalinka, M. K. (ed.): Arthrography. New York, Springer, 1980.
8. Toller, P. A.: Opaque arthrography of the temporomandibular joint. Int. J. Oral Surg., *3*:17–28, 1974.
9. Lynch, T. P., and Chase, D. C.: Arthrography in the evaluation of the TMJ. Radiology, *126*:667–672, 1978.
10. Norgaard, F.: Temporomandibular arthrography (thesis). Copenhagen: Elinar Munksgaard, 1947.
11. Dolwick, M. F., Katzberg, R. W., Helms, C. A., and Bales, D. J.: Arthrotomographic evaluation of the temporomandibular joint. J. Oral Surg., *37*:793–799, 1979.
12. Helms, C. A., Katzberg, R. W., and Dolwick, M. F.: Internal derangements of the temporomandibular joint. University of California, San Francisco, Radiology Postgraduate Education.

21

Traditional and Modern Acupuncture Modalities in the Diagnosis and Treatment of the Temporomandibular Joint Syndrome

PETER V. MADILL, M.D.

This chapter is written to introduce the reader to the possibilities that traditional and modern acupuncture modalities offer in the evaluation and treatment of the temporomandibular joint syndrome. The chapter will provide an introductory account of the opportunities for treatment made available by traditional acupuncture and auricular therapy (ear acupuncture). It will also contain a summary survey of the potential for diagnosis, etiological analysis, and treatment of the temporomandibular joint syndrome afforded by German electroacupuncture, also known as electroacupuncture according to Voll (EAV). Relative to this last named body of knowledge, it must be pointed out that the possibilities it offers still await extensive investigation in the American medical and dental context. However, it is hoped that this discussion, along with the increasing interest among members of the dental profession, will stimulate skilled and open-minded researchers, in funded institutions, to undertake serious investigation and testing of these possibilities.

Any practitioner attempting to offer comprehensive treatment for the temporomandibular joint syndrome soon becomes embroiled in a number of intriguing clinical paradoxes, as well as encountering an already bewildering array of different therapeutic options. Among the many questions that occur to such practitioners, the following are common:

1. If altered (non-physiological) vertical dimension, maxillomandibular

relations, or malocclusion is the predominant cause of TMJ problems, why doesn't each TMJ patient who can be clearly demonstrated to have this condition complain of the accepted and described symptoms?

2. If stress-induced maladapted neuromuscular habit patterns instigate the TMJ syndrome in one individual, what causes such stress-induced habits to arise or locate in different neuromuscular structures in other individuals?

3. In two individuals complaining of typical TMJ symptoms to roughly equal degrees, why does one respond to splint therapy while the other does not?

4. Why do some patients respond initially to occlusal and neuromuscular relaxation therapies, then continually relapse?

5. What methods might be used to determine which patients are more likely to respond to splint equilibration therapies and which are not?

6. What other factors of potential significance in individual cases of the TMJ syndrome are not commonly considered?

These questions and others are often not easily answered using the traditional approaches to diagnosis and therapy and thus have led thoughtful practitioners outside the traditional fold for answers. Acupuncture and more specifically German electroacupuncture (perhaps better called acupuncture point diagnosis) has, among other newer disciplines, been the focus of attention because it may offer novel ways of providing answers to these questions. This chapter will not attempt to present electroacupuncture as a system of diagnosis and therapy that is consistent, proved, and sufficient unto itself. Rather, it will attempt to demonstrate why there is genuine interest in its potentialities, why there is substantive potential, how it can and should be integrated with other traditional and nontraditional approaches to diagnosis and therapy, and how future research efforts might explore, validate, refine, or even refute the claims made by its advocates. It is important for the reader to realize that while electroacupuncture (or, better, acupuncture point diagnosis) clearly has its roots in traditional acupuncture, it is not a species of traditional acupuncture. Nor is it a variant of electroacupuncture as commonly conceived, in which needles are inserted into various acupuncture points and are connected to electronic pulsing devices. A brief review of the history and principles of acupuncture will give better insight to contemporary use of the modality in the treatment of TMJ dysfunction.

TRADITIONAL CHINESE ACUPUNCTURE

Any health practitioner intending to acquire skill in one of the schools of acupuncture practice should begin study by becoming acquainted with the general philosophy and rudiments of practice of traditional acupuncture. Chinese medicine, of which traditional acupuncture is but one—albeit the best known—division, is the original holistic medicine in terms of its emphasis on prevention, its acknowledgment of an ecologic perspective, and its insistence on the integral interaction of mind and body in the determination of health. Like all traditional cultures, Chinese medicine postulates that the body is essentially electromagnetic in character and is animated and integrated by "Qi" or "Chi," which can be loosely translated as life force or bioenergy. This "Qi" is held to flow through the body in rhythmic and orderly fashion through channels or energy conduits that have become most commonly known as "meridians" in Western cultures. Each of these meridians follows a specific course over the surface of the body, which can be characterized in terms of specific anatomical landmarks. Twelve major meridians are described, which are held to relate to individual internal organ systems (see Fig. 21–1). Also, a number of other, minor vessels are described, such as the "extra" and "muscle" vessels. Along the course of the meridians lie the acupuncture points where the "Qi" is held to be most available to the external environment and, therefore, most readily influenced by the acupuncturist's needles, massage, burning of moxa (an aromatic herb, known in this country as mugwort), or electronic impulses (new in this century). The acupuncture points are serially numbered as they occur along the meridians and prefixed by the abbreviation of the name of the meridian. Thus we have Lu (Lung) 1, Lu 2, Lu 3, and so forth, as well as St (stomach) 36, St 37, St 38, and so forth.

Just as body function is conceptualized in energetic terms, so also are disease processes. Thus, the Chinese physician making use of acupuncture is mainly concerned with grasping excesses and deficiencies of this energy and blockages or obstructions to its orderly flow. His or her fundamental emphasis in treatment is not to focus on the disease process as an entitity in and of itself, but to rebalance the body's energy, his understanding being that when this is achieved, the body will naturally rid itself of the disease process and health will be restored. A number of laws are described in Chinese medicine. These define the flow of this "Qi" or bioenergy through the body, describe the relationships and patterns of interactions of the body's internal organs and meridian systems, and summarize the many ways in which external environmental influences can impact on normal body function. The most important task confronting the prospective student of acupuncture is to learn the location and course of the most commonly used acupuncture points found along these meridians, especially those on the extremities.[1, 2]

Despite the continued reticence on the part of the American medical establishment to acknowledge the clinical usefulness of traditional and modern acupuncture modalities, there are now a sufficient number of well-designed and controlled studies that confirm the usefulness of traditional acupuncture[1, 3–5] and auricular acupuncture[1, 5, 6] in both acute and chronic pain syndromes. The use made of traditional acupuncture and auriculotherapy, in the context of a broader treatment program for the temporomandibular joint syndrome, will be predominantly to treat the pain associated with this syndrome, both acute and chronic. The treatment program should, of course, always include emphasis on muscle rehabilitation involving muscle stretching therapies. Such an approach helps ensure participation in the treatment program that demands responsibility on the patient's part.

Other uses for which traditional acupuncture and auriculotherapy hold promise in the dental context are in the treatment of other pain syndromes associated with the oral cavity and dental pathology, and also as an alternative or supplemental pathway of providing satisfactory analgesia for the performance of various dental surgical procedures. This latter possibility holds considerable promise for the future, as analgesia in the oral cavity can be induced with a high degree of reliability using manual or electrical acupuncture needle stimulation of indicated points. Acupuncture also holds promise for postoperative pain relief in both hospital and outpatient settings, as well as hope for improved postoperative morbidity.[1, 2, 7]

Traditional acupuncture and auriculotherapy as treatment modalities for acute and chronic pain can be placed alongside or offered as alternatives to ethyl chloride spray, galvanic stimulation, application of hot or cold packs, massage, osteopathic, chiropractic, or kinesiological adjustment, trigger point injection, transcutaneous electrical nerve stimulation (TENS), and other bioconductive therapies. Some practitioners skilled in the application of a number of these modalities indicate a preference for trigger point injection therapy using procaine or other short-acting local anesthetic for the relief of acute pain and spasm, and the use of traditional and auricular acupuncture for more chronic types of pain; other practitioners prefer acupuncture in both situations. A number of clinicians feel that acupuncture treatment offers more profound and long-lasting pain relief than TENS.[4, 8, 9] However, there are as yet no convincing, well-documented, carefully designed, and properly controlled studies that substantiate this clinical impression. It is to be hoped that such studies will soon be forthcoming, so that clinicians can make prudent choices concerning the best pain control modalities in which to acquire competence.

Just as debate persists over the efficacy of acupuncture in the treatment of acute and chronic pain, so also is there continued and lively controversy over the physiological mechanisms that underlie acupuncture-induced pain relief. It is beyond the scope of this chapter to embark on a detailed discussion of this issue. Recent research has focused on the intriguing and important role of endorphins and enkephalins in the mediation of the acupuncture effect. Despite the central role of this mechanism it is probably also true that there are other important mechanisms involved. The interested reader is referred to other sources for further information.[1, 4, 6, 10,11]

Besides acquiring a working knowledge of the theory and philosophy that underlies Chinese medicine and learning the course of the meridians and location of at least the commonly used acupuncture points, the student of acupuncture must also learn how to use the needle and to select proper points for therapy. Treatment of specific conditions using traditional acupuncture involves in most circumstances the selection of points from three broad groupings, used either in combination with each other or independently of the others.[1, 2] The three categories of points are as follows:

1. Local points found in the vicinity of the pain or other pathologic condition to be treated. A number of investigators have noticed similarities between local acupuncture point therapy and certain features of trigger point injection.[7]

2. Distal points on the meridians that course through the area of pain or pathologic feature to be treated.

3. Points chosen because of their proven usefulness in the treatment of particular syndromes. These points are generally located distal to the area of pain or pathologic lesion being treated. Examples are Large Intestine (L.I.) (Fig. 21–1) for the treatment of toothache, and Bladder (Bl) 54 for the treatment of low back pain.

Local points that have been found useful in the treatment of pain and spasm in the TMJ area include Stomach 6 and 7, Gallbladder 41, Triplewarmer 22, and Small Intestine 19, as well as trigger (Oh Yes!) points located in the area by careful palpation (Fig. 21–2). Distal points that might prove useful in the treatment of TMJ syndrome could include Stomach 42, Gallbladder 41, Triplewarmer 3, and Small Intestine 3 or 4. Points known to be of special use in the treatment of pain and spasm in the TMJ include L.I. 4, which is also known to be useful in the treatment of toothache and in the induction of dental analgesia, and Stomach 44, also well known for

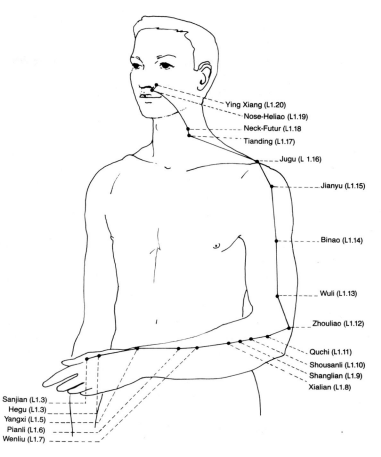

Figure 21–1. The left large intestine meridian.

Ying Xiang (L1.20)
Nose-Heliao (L1.19)
Neck-Futur (L1.18
Tianding (L1.17)
Jugu (L 1.16)
Jianyu (L1.15)
Binao (L1.14)
Wuli (L1.13)
Zhouliao (L1.12)
Quchi (L1.11)
Shousanli (L1.10)
Shanglian (L1.9)
Xialian (L1.8)
Sanjian (L1.3)
Hegu (L1.3)
Yangxi (L1.5)
Pianli (L1.6)
Wenliu (L1.7)

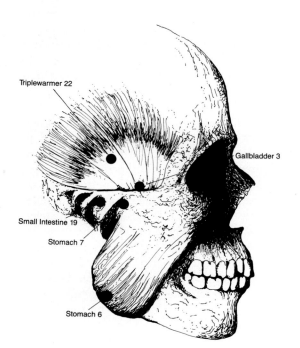

Figure 21–2. Local points of use in traditional acupuncture treatment of TMJ syndrome.

Triplewarmer 22
Gallbladder 3
Small Intestine 19
Stomach 7
Stomach 6

its usefulness in the treatment of pain in the temporal region and spasm of the muscles around the TMJ. Treatment using local and distal acupuncture points is usually performed two or three times a week to begin with, and once clear progress is being made, then generally once a week until a cure is effected, or until a plateau of pain relief has been reached. The number of needles used depends on the experience, biases, and skill of the acupuncturist, but usually varies from as few as three or four to as many as 10 to 15. When electrical stimulation is applied, along with needle insertion, usually fewer needles are required, and electrical stimulation is usually applied in the area from which the symptoms arise.[12] A typical acupuncture treatment will last anywhere from 20 to 30 minutes.

Many clinicians skilled in acupuncture combine the points of traditional acupuncture with one or a number of points chosen from the ear on the same side of the body as the pain or pathology is found. Other practitioners prefer to confine themselves to treatment with only auricular points or the body points of traditional acupuncture. Although different clinicians have their preferences, it must be admitted that there is no sound body of evidence indicating the relative efficacy of body points alone, auricular points alone, or the combination of body and auricular points. Considerable usefulness in the relief of pain and spasm associated with the TMJ syndrome can be gained by the practitioner by learning to use electronic point location and treatment equipment manufactured specifically for auricular therapy or found in combination with other modalities in more comprehensive pain treatment devices. This generally is a much easier task than learning how to treat auricular points with needles.

AURICULOTHERAPY OR EAR ACUPUNCTURE

As with traditional body acupuncture, the practitioner studying auricular therapy must first learn the location of significant and useful points on the ear and then the protocols in common use for the selection of appropriate points for the treatment of specific syndromes.[1, 2, 13, 14] Unlike the traditional acupuncture points on the body, the points on the ear can vary slightly in location from one individual to the next. Thus, it is generally advised that the practitioner learn to identify points through acquiring skill in the use of an electronic point locator.

Like the points commonly used in German electroacupuncture (acupuncture point diagnosis), the points on the ear generally correspond to different anatomical structures in the body[6] (Fig. 21–3). The display or distribution of these points is very interesting and is described as being like, or following the pattern of, an imaginary inverted fetus superimposed on the outer surface of the ear, with the head lying in the area of the lobule, the vertebral column extending up the antihelix, the viscera in the concha, the skin represented on the helix, and the extremities lying in the areas on the ear between the helix and antihelix (Fig. 21–4). Besides points that represent specific anatomical structures, there are also a lesser number of points identified and commonly used in the ear, which are known by some auricular therapists as master points.[13, 14] Examples of these include Shenmen, in the apex of the triangular fossa, and point zero on the root of the helix. Most practitioners skilled in the use of auricular therapy use a combination of master points and points that relate to the anatomical area of pain or pathology.

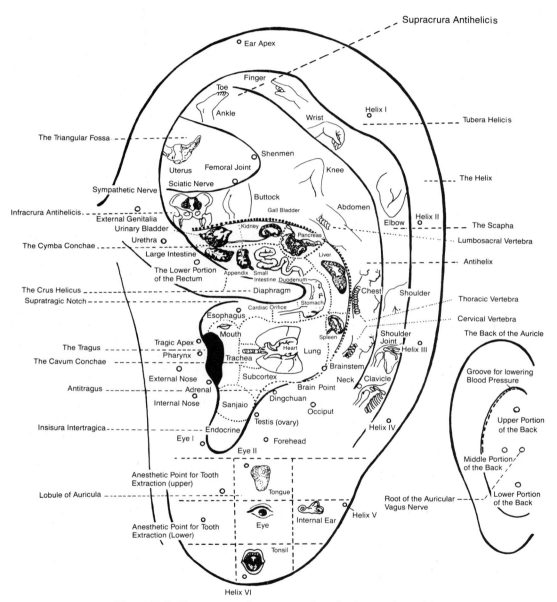

Figure 21–3. The somatotopic representation of points on the auricle.

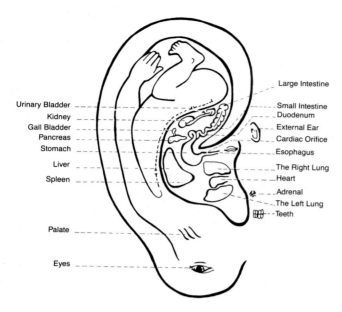

Urinary Bladder
Kidney
Gall Bladder
Pancreas
Stomach
Liver
Spleen

Palate

Eyes

Large Intestine
Small Intestine
Duodenum
External Ear
Cardiac Orifice
Esophagus
The Right Lung
Heart
Adrenal
The Left Lung
Teeth

Figure 21–4. The somatotopic representation of points on the external ear summarized as the inverted fetus.

Points on the ear differ from body points in one important respect: when the anatomical structure that they are thought to relate to is functioning within normal limits, they cannot be differentiated electrically from surrounding areas of the skin on the ear. However, when there is pain or a pathologic condition in specific areas of the body, then the corresponding auricular points become increasingly tender, discolored, and electrically active. In this case specialized electronic probes can be safely and painlessly passed over the surface of the ear to detect the presence of any active points that indicate the area of pain or pathology. A recent study completed at University of California, Los Angeles, confirms the considerable accuracy available in the identification of a variety of pain-related problems, and confirms the somatotopic mapping of different anatomical structures on the surface of the ear.[6]

Although there are occasional references to the use of auricular points in the early literature of traditional acupuncture, the potential usefulness of ear acupuncture was first brought to the attention of the medical community by an observant French neurologist named Paul Nogier.[13, 14] Since this time, both the French and the Chinese have brought increasing sophistication to this intriguing area of acupuncture endeavor.[1, 2, 6, 13, 14] Relative to treatment of the TMJ syndrome, points known to be useful in the treatment of pain and spasm in this area include the points for the upper and lower jaw, the points for subcortex, temple, and cheek, and the points for the upper and lower teeth, used commonly along with the indicated master points. Some of these points are also very useful in promoting dental analgesia.

ACUPUNCTURE POINT DIAGNOSIS (GERMAN ELECTROACUPUNCTURE OR ELECTROACUPUNCTURE ACCORDING TO VOLL, EAV)

Acupuncture point diagnosis had its birth in the early 1950s, when Dr. Reinhold Voll and his colleagues were attempting to discover more specific and reliable ways through which they could determine which meridians were dysfunctional and therefore required treatment. Besides gleaning hints from a comprehensive history, the Chinese had traditionally resorted to pulse diagnosis to make this determination. This is an art that is more intuitive and subjective than objective, difficult to communicate, and therefore a practice with little general appeal to the intellectual demands of the majority of Western health practitioners. At this time it had already been established that acupuncture points had different electrical properties than neighboring areas of the skin, and that these could be characterized in terms of altered resistance or conductivity. It was suspected that if the electrical resistance or conductivity of the acupuncture points could be reliably and reproducibly measured in a clinically practicable fashion, these investigators would be able to offer to the acupuncture community a more valid and appealing method for determining the functional (energetic) status of each of the meridians of the body, an essential prerequisite to successful therapy. It was as a consequence of the pursuit of this goal that Dr. Voll and his co-workers made the discoveries that form the foundation of this new body of knowledge and research called EAV, German electroacupuncture, or, perhaps better, acupuncture point diagnosis. The discoveries of Dr. Voll and his co-workers can be approached through a description of five areas of investigation.

1. The first area of discoveries involves the relationship of individual acupuncture points to organ systems and physiological processes. Since the earliest records of Chinese medicine, practitioners within this discipline have postulated that linear aggregates of acupuncture points, which we call meridians, relate to individual organ systems. Dr. Voll and his co-workers reasoned that if it proved possible to measure the electrical properties of acupuncture points, the information thus generated might prove useful in making inferences as to the functional status of the related organ or tissue system. This in fact proved to be the case. Through exhaustive corroborative studies, they established the relationships of the distal acupuncture points of each of the meridians to specific anatomical components of the organ systems (Fig. 21–5A and B shows the anatomical relationships of the distal points of the large intestine meridian). Not only did they discover the anatomical relationships of those points found on the traditionally described meridians, but they also established a division of labor among the different points so that categories of points could be established with different functions found from meridian to meridian in typical positions (Fig. 21–6). Another important discovery pertains to the vacant sites on the digits where meridians where not commonly found. This discovery is of new linear aggregates of points, called vessels, in contradistinction to meridians; points for these have been established only on the extremities, and they relate to the tissue systems and major physiological functions that are not reflected in the traditional meridians. Figures 21–7 and 21–8 illustrate the meridians and vessels by means of their control measurement points. Among the points described are points for the dental structures, the temporomandibular joint, and the muscles supplying the TMJ. The chapter will conclude with an introductory discussion of the use of these points in relation to the temporomandibular joint syndrome.[15-25]

2. The second area of discovery involves the development of a specific methodology for reliable and clinically practicable point measurement, methods of electronic point treatment, and the provision of accessory treatment modalities, the latter of which share features in common with transcutaneous nerve stimulation (TENS), galvanic stimulation, and other

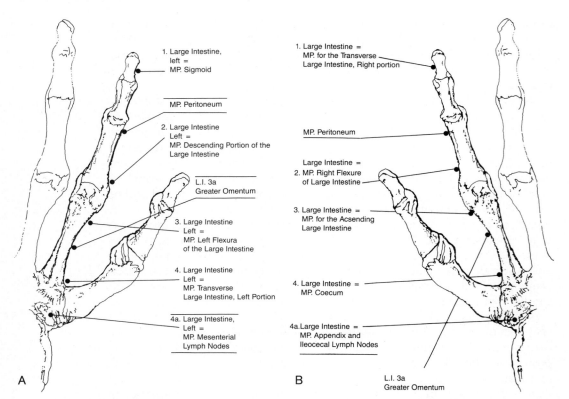

1. Large Intestine,
   left =
   MP. Sigmoid

MP. Peritoneum

2. Large Intestine
   Left =
   MP. Descending Portion of the
   Large Intestine

L.I. 3a
Greater Omentum

3. Large Intestine
   Left =
   MP. Left Flexura
   of the Large Intestine

4. Large Intestine
   Left =
   MP. Transverse
   Large Intestine, Left Portion

4a. Large Intestine,
    Left =
    MP. Mesenterial
    Lymph Nodes

1. Large Intestine =
   MP. for the Transverse
   Large Intestine, Right portion

MP. Peritoneum

Large Intestine =
2. MP. Right Flexure
   of Large Intestine

3. Large Intestine =
   MP. for the Ascending
   Large Intestine

4. Large Intestine =
   MP. Coecum

4a. Large Intestine =
    MP. Appendix and
    Ileocecal Lymph Nodes

L.I. 3a
Greater Omentum

A

B

Figure 21–5. The points along the large intestine meridian. *A*, Left hand. *B*, Right hand.

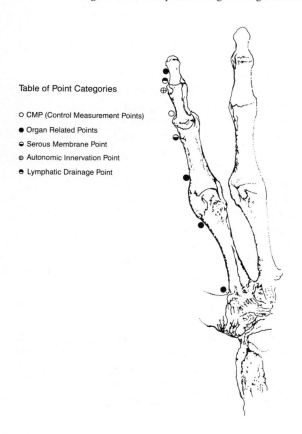

Table of Point Categories

○ CMP (Control Measurement Points)

● Organ Related Points

◒ Serous Membrane Point

⊕ Autonomic Innervation Point

◓ Lymphatic Drainage Point

Figure 21–6. Schema of typical point locations.

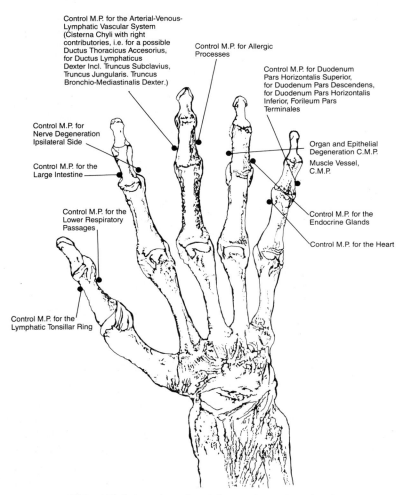

Control M.P. for the Arterial-Venous-
Lymphatic Vascular System
(Cisterna Chyli with right
contributories, i.e. for a possible
Ductus Thoracicus Accesorius,
for Ductus Lymphaticus
Dexter Incl. Truncus Subclavius,
Truncus Jungularis. Truncus
Bronchio-Mediastinalis Dexter.)

Control M.P. for Allergic
Processes

Control M.P. for Duodenum
Pars Horizontalis Superior,
for Duodenum Pars Descendens,
for Duodenum Pars Horizontalis
Inferior, Forileum Pars
Terminales

Control M.P. for
Nerve Degeneration
Ipsilateral Side

Control M.P. for the
Large Intestine

Organ and Epithelial
Degeneration C.M.P.

Muscle Vessel,
C.M.P.

Control M.P. for the
Lower Respiratory
Passages

Control M.P. for the
Endocrine Glands

Control M.P. for the Heart

Control M.P. for the
Lymphatic Tonsillar Ring

Figure 21–7. Location of meridians and vessels on hand.

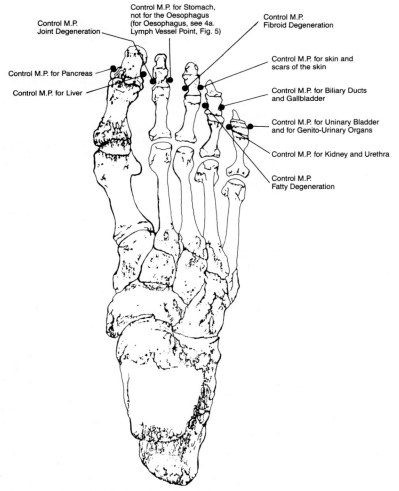

Figure 21–8. Location of meridians and vessels on foot.

bioconductive therapies. Besides the development of a specific method for point measurement, a further achievement in this area of discovery was the elucidation of the clinical significance of the different readings that might be obtained. It is beyond the scope of this chapter to discuss in detail the biophysics of point measurement or the implications for differential diagnosis of the different point measurements that can be obtained. For a full discussion of this topic the reader is referred to the report by Madill and Tiller.[26] For the purposes of this discussion the principle of point measurement can be stated as follows: When a healthy or normally functioning organ system is challenged, via its associated measurement point, with a constant stimulus (in acupuncture point diagnosis the constant stimulus is a tiny amount of DC current generated by the point measurement device), it will be able to offer a constant response to the challenging stimulus, whereas a dysfunctional organ system, when challenged in the same fashion, will not be able to mount a constant response to the same challenging stimulus. In the former case, the needle on the diagnostic dial (a sensitive voltmeter), will rise promptly and remain stable at 50 or just above 50 on the diagnostic dial. However, in the latter case, the inability of the organ system to mount a constant response to the challenging stimulus is reflected on the diagnostic dial by a changing pattern of resistance. In this instance, the needle will rise, usually to a point somewhere between 50 and 100, a position known as the maximal labile position, then fall off to reach a stable lower position, a point known as the minimal stable position. This phenomenon of decreasing conductivity or increasing resistance of the acupuncture point to the constant challenging electrical stimulus is the prime index of dysfunction in acupuncture point diagnosis, and is called the indicator drop. The diagnostic meter on the acupuncture point measurement device is graduated from 0 to 100. Values obtained during point measurement that approach 0 are believed to signify increasing degrees of degeneration, whereas values progressively approaching 100 represent increasing degrees of inflammation.

The point treatment facilities made available by acupuncture point measurement devices provide current of two different waveforms with adjustable intensity and frequency. The different currents are used for raising or lowering the values obtained in the course of point measurement to the norm of 50 on the diagnostic dial. In my experience these currents have limited usefulness in therapy in comparison with other therapies available, but they play an important role in differential diagnosis using acupuncture point measurements, especially in testing of hypotheses relating to fields of disturbance. For further discussion of point treatment and the accessory treatment modalities, the interested reader is referred to other sources.[15, 16, 19, 24, 26]

3. The third area of discovery in acupuncture point diagnosis can be described as medicine selection, medicine testing, and medicine administration. It is at the same time possibly the most interesting and certainly the most controversial area of innovation. Having established the anatomical relationships of the individual acupuncture points, and having developed a reliable and practicable method of measuring points, Dr. Voll and his co-workers realized that they had a useful method of following the course and thus of assessing the usefulness of any therapy directed to pathophysiology that could be detected through careful point measurement. They frequently observed that although patients might report symptomatic improvement, the administration of many of the commonly prescribed allopathic pharmacological drugs made little difference to the point measurements reflecting the underlying pathologic condition. In order to see whether there existed any category of medicines that do influence the underlying pathologic lesion by provoking a regenerative response, instigating a more potent degree of immune resilience, mobilizing organ reserve, inducing a return to immune homeostasis, and strengthening the body's eliminative mechanisms, they tested a number of different types of medicinal preparations. Through repeated observations they determined that items drawn from the homeopathic pharmacopeia seemed to perform this function most reliably and effectively, their use entailing no serious or long-lasting side effects. During the subsequent years of investigation, considerable experience has established the indications for the use of these preparations in the electroacupuncture context. Voll and co-workers also discovered that medicines could be tested prior to their administration by having the patient hand-hold the preparation and remeasuring the point indicating the dysfunction to be treated. A move of the needle on the diagnostic dial toward 50 on remeasuring the point with the patient hand-holding the intended medicinal preparation is accepted as another piece of corroborative evidence supporting

the likely usefulness of the preparation in question. This whole area remains a very fertile area for experimentation. It is hoped that as the possibilities of acupuncture point diagnosis receives a wider hearing the therapeutic principle that underlies the use of the serially diluted preparations of the homeopathic pharamacopeia will receive wider appreciation.[25-28]

4. The fourth area of discoveries relates to the diagnosis and treatment of maladaptive reponses to a wide variety of commonly encountered environmental chemicals and foods, as well as the diagnosis and treatment of the more traditionally defined allergic responses, such as hay fever, asthma, and atopic dermatitis. This includes the study of adverse responses to dental materials, which will be discussed further later in this chapter. Not only does acupuncture point diagnosis open a new pathway for the diagnosis and treatment of allergies and environmentally related disorders, but it also offers health practitioners the opportunity to study the role of such reactions in instigating or exacerbating a wide variety of chronic disorders, such as migraine headaches, nocturnal enuresis, inflammatory arthritis, and connective disorders, among many others.[21, 26, 29, 30]

5. The fifth and final area of discoveries relates to what are known as field disturbance phenomena. The careful consideration of these phenomena along with observations as to the possible systemic effects of certain dental materials has helped to rekindle a renewed appreciation of the very important interaction of medical and dental factors. A field of disturbance is believed to exist when it is determined, through careful point measurement, that an inflammatory or infective focus that is not necessarily symptomatic or easily observed is found to be inciting or exacerbating dysfunction or a pathologic condition in an organ system or other anatomical structure elsewhere in the body. These fields of disturbance are believed to be of considerable significance in a high proportion of chronic pain syndromes and various arthritic conditions, as well as other disorders. The most common sites of distal foci that give rise to these fields of disturbance include the paired tonsils of the oropharyngeal cavity (Waldeyer's ring), the teeth, gums, and periodontal tissues, the middle ear, eustachian tube and mastoid tissue, and the nose and paranasal sinuses. It must be remembered that other anatomical structures can also be the site of distal foci giving rise to fields of disturbance. The concept of fields of disturbance is another fertile field for experimentation and application in both medicine and dentistry.

The fact that the oral cavity, including the dental structures, was on occasion found to be the site of a distal focus inciting a field of disturbance elsewhere in the body led Dr. Voll and his co-workers to vigorously seek out the potential applications of the tools of acupuncture point measurement to diagnosis and treatment in the dental sphere. Their efforts resulted in the development of two other evaluative procedures of potential usefulness to contemporary dentistry. The first is the use of a sensitive ammeter and voltmeter to locate the source and measure the magnitude of "vagrant" oral galvanic currents generated by metallic restoration materials either singly or in juxtaposition in the mouth.[31, 32] It is believed by a number of investigators in West Germany that intraoral galvanic currents may prove to be of etiological significance in a number of different chronic pain and other syndromes (e.g., vasomotor problems), especially in the head and neck. Among the negative effects these currents may prove to have is the electrogalvanic release of potentially toxic heavy metal ions, such as mercury from silver amalgam fillings, or nickel from nonprecious metal alloys, which permits their local or even distal migration. Although considerable controversy surrounds these issues, especially the continued widespread use of silver amalgam as a universal restoration material, I believe the issue of electrogalvanism in the oral cavity is deserving of further research.

The second evaluative procedure made possible by acupuncture point measurement devices is a vitality test that can be used to expose latent areas of lowered or absent vitality in the pulps of teeth, periapical areas, or old extraction sites. Such nonvital sites can on occasion prove to be significant distal foci inciting fields of disturbance. This procedure may also prove to be of use in helping the dentist to decide on the most prudent course of therapy in attempting to deal with such foci.[22, 31–37]

ACUPUNCTURE POINT MEASUREMENT AND THE DIAGNOSIS AND TREATMENT OF THE TMJ SYNDROME

Of what use might the possibilities just described be in establishing diagnosis, causation, and treatment of the TMJ syndrome? Space precludes a detailed discussion of this question, but nevertheless an attempt will be made to summarize briefly the potential usefulness of acupuncture point measurement relative to the TMJ syndrome. It must be clear that the remarks that follow do not present proven facts, but instead suggest experimental possibilities.

The differential diagnosis of head and neck pain syndromes presents a difficult challenge to both physicians and dentists alike. An almost exclusive reliance must in most cases be placed on careful history-taking, a task that time considerations very often compromise. Notwithstanding the patient's complaints, the clinician is often left with a dearth of signs detectable by careful physical examination. This, coupled with a general lack of appreciation of the temporomandibular joint syndrome, especially on the part of physicians, adds to the difficulties met with in this area and often delays significantly institution of care appropriate to the condition.

It is believed that careful acupuncture point measurement, along with an appropriate history and physical examination, offers the medical and dental community the possibility for improvements in diagnosis relative to the area of head and neck pain syndromes and the evaluation and etiological understanding of the TMJ syndrome in particular. I have evaluated many patients with head and neck pain syndromes, including the TMJ syndrome, and have found that each of these syndromes presents a unique pattern of acupuncture point measurement values of potential usefulness in differential diagnosis.

Acupuncture point measurement offers not only possibilities for the diagnosis of the TMJ syndrome but also potential for improvements in understanding its causation and a nonbiased feedback system to monitor the course, and thus to judge the usefulness, of any of the many therapies offered for the treatment of this syndrome. Following a careful history and physical examination, the clinician making use of acupuncture point diagnosis begins his evaluation of the patient with suspected TMJ syndrome by performing what is called in this school of acupuncture practice a "meridian search," on those meridians that course through the area of dysfunction—in this case the area of the TMJ. The purpose of this procedure is to test for the presence of any dysfunction in the organ system relating to the meridian being studied. The meridian search is always performed because one of the fundamental beliefs of both traditional acupuncture and German electroacupuncture is that although a certain degree of dysfunction may exist within a particular organ system, the patient may experience this dysfunction as symptoms at any point along the course of the related meridian in a manner that may not be easily related to the organ system in which dysfunction originates. The phenomenon of referred pain shares some common elements with this basic postulate of traditional acupuncture theory.

Having performed a careful meridian search, the practitioner then proceeds to measure specific acupuncture points known to be of special use in the evaluation and determination of causation of suspected TMJ syndrome. These points include Lymph (Ly) 2 for the dental structures, Muscle Vessel (MV) 3 (Fig. 21–9) for the skeletal muscles of the upper neck and head, Joint Vessel (JV) 3 (Fig. 21–10) for the joints of upper neck and head, connective tissue vessel (CTV) 3 for connective tissue of the upper neck and head, Triplewarmer (TW) 1a for the sympathetic innervation of the head and neck, and Nerve Vessel (NV) 3a for the parasympathetic innervation of the head and neck. Careful comparative measurement of these points and others enables the practitioner to make certain assumptions regarding etiology as well as differential diagnosis. If on one side (one hand) the practitioner obtains readings from point measurement of the points Ly 2 and MV 3 in a patient complaining of unilateral facial pain, this represents further evidence of a possible case of TMJ Syndrome. If the point Ly 2 has the highest maximal labile reading or the greatest indicator drop, or both, the practitioner might conclude that occlusal factors are of prime etiological significance in a particular case, and thus begin management of this case with the provision of a splint. If, on the other hand, the highest maximal labile reading or the greatest indicator drop is obtained on the point MV 3, the practitioner might suspect that stress factors manifesting as increased tonus, even spasm, in the muscles of the TMJ are of prime etiological significance. He might then begin to approach this patient with therapies that focus on muscle relaxation and reeducation. Measurement of the points Ly 2 and MV3 also offer the clinician another potentially useful tool to evaluate the adequacy of splint adjustment. A high reading obtained in a patient complaining of unilateral facial pain from the point JV 3, for the joints of the upper neck and head, would alert the practitioner to consider the possibility of inflammatory or arthritic changes in the temporomandibular joint itself, and to focus on the protocols unique to acupuncture point diagnosis for the evaluation of arthritis in a particular joint. High readings from the points Tw 1a or NV 3a will alert the practitioner to consider vasomotor factors or the possible role of chemical sensitivities as significant etiological factors in the patient presenting with symptoms suggestive of TMJ syndrome. It must be remembered that a reading from the point Ly 2 indicating dysfunction does not necessarily imply TMJ involvement, but merely that there is some disturbance in the ipsilateral dental structures, and that further efforts will have to be made to discern the precise implications of this reading. A detailed presentation of the applications of acupuncture point diagnosis will be published in the future.

It has already been indicated that the system of acupuncture point diagnosis is not tied to any particular therapeutic modality. Rather, it is presented as an evaluative tool that, it is hoped, will in the future help clinicians to make wiser and more expedient choices concerning what

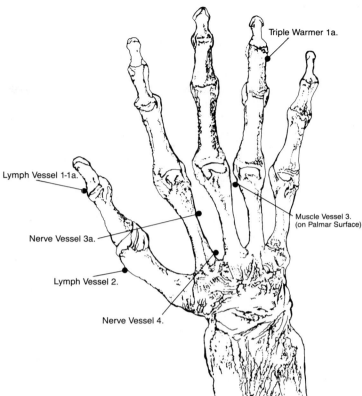

Figure 21–9. Points on the hand for TMJ evaluation.

Triple Warmer 1a.

Lymph Vessel 1-1a.

Nerve Vessel 3a.

Lymph Vessel 2.

Nerve Vessel 4.

Muscle Vessel 3. (on Palmar Surface)

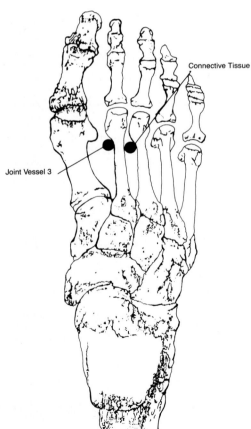

Connective Tissue

Joint Vessel 3

Figure 21–10. Points on the foot for TMJ evaluation.

particular therapies are best suited to the individual case. Therapy with nosodes and accompanying remedies, as evolved by Dr. Voll and his co-workers drawing from the tradition of classic homeopathy and adding their own unique insights and innovations, is thought to be most useful relative to the treatment of chronic inflammatory, allergic, and autoimmune phenomena. Thus, with respect to the TMJ syndrome, therapy with these agents will probably prove to be of most use in those cases in which there is an inflammatory process in the muscles associated with the TMJ or tendencies to arthritis in the joint itself. Compared with other therapies that are available, including the possibilities offered by traditional and auricular acupuncture, the treatment of peripheral points and the accessory treatment modalities made available by the acupuncture point measurement device of German electroacupuncture await further broad-based testing.

References

1. O'Connor, J., and Bensky, D.: Acupuncture in Medical Practice. Reston, Virginia, Reston Publishing Co., 1980.
2. Beijing College of Traditional Chinese Medicine, et al: Essentials of Chinese Acupuncture. Beijing, China, Foreign Languages Press, 1981.
3. Chou, S. N.: Acupuncture. Mayo Clinic Pract., *55*:775, 1980.
4. Ulett, G. A.: Acupuncture treatments for pain relief. JAMA, *245*:768, 1981.
5. Editorial: How does acupuncture work? Br. Jed. J., *283*:746, 1981.
6. Oleson, T. D. Kroenig, R. J., and Bresler, D. T.: Diagnostic accuracy of examining electrical activity at ear acupuncture points for assessing areas of the body with musculoskeletal pain. Pain Abstracts, *1*:185, 1978.
7. Vanderschot, D. O.: Trigger points v. acupuncture points. Am. J. Acupuncture, *4*:233, 1976.
8. Fox, J. E., and Melzak, R. Transcutaneous electrical stimulation and acupuncture: Comparison of treatment for low-back pain. Pain, *2*:141, 1976.
9. Brandweis, A., and Corcos, J.: Cutaneous and transcutaneous electroacupuncture. Am. J. Acupuncture, *4*:161, 1976.
10. Editorial. Endogenous opiates and their actions. Lancet, *2*:305, 1982.
11. Sjolund, B., Terenius, L., and Eriksson, M.: Increased cerebrospinal fluid levels of endorphins after electroacupuncture. Acta Physiol. Scand., *100*:382, 1977.
12. Wensel, L. O.: Acupuncture in Medical Practice. Reston, Virginia, Reston Publishing Co, 1980.
13. Nogier, P. F. M.: Treatise of Auriculo-Therapy. Mainsonneuve, France, 1972.
14. Wexu, M.: The Ear, Gateway to Balancing the Body. A Modern Guide to Ear Acupuncture. New York, ASI Publishers, Inc. 1975.
15. Voll, R.: Twenty years of electroacupuncture diagnosis in Germany. A progress report. Am. J. Acupuncture, *3*:7, 1975.
16. Voll, R.: Twenty years of electroacupuncture therapy using low-frequency current pulses. Am. J. Acupuncture, *3*:291, 1975.
17. Voll, R.: Energetic reactions between organ pairs and paranasal sinuses, odontons and tonsils in electroacupuncture according to Voll. Am. J. Acupuncture, *5*:101, 1977.
18. Voll, R.: Topographic Positions of the Measurement Points in Electroacupuncture. Vol. I. D-3110 Uelzen, West Germany, ML-Verlag, 1976.
19. Voll, R.: Topographic Positions of the Measurement Points in Electroacupuncture. Textual Vol. I. 1977. D-3110 Uelzen, ML-Verlag GmbH, West Germany, 1977.
20. Voll, R.: Topographic Positions of the Measurement Points in Electroacupuncture. Illustrated Vol. II. D-3110 Uelzen, ML-Verlag GmbH; West Germany, 1977.
21. Voll, R.: Topographic Positions of the Measurement Points in Electroacupuncture. Textual and Illustrated Vol. III. D-3110 Uelzen, ML-Verlag GmbH, West Germany, 1978.
22. Voll, R.: Interrelations of Odontons and Tonsils to Organs, Fields of Disturbance, and Tissue Systems. D-3110 Uelzen, ML-Verlag, West Germany, 1978.
23. Voll, R.: First Supplement to the Four Volumes on the Topographic Positions of the Measurement Points in Electroacupuncture (E.A.V.). 3110 Uelzen, ML-Verlag GmbH, West Germany, 1978.
24. Werner, F., Voll, R.: Electroacupuncture Primer. ML-Verlag GmbH, 3110 Uelzen, West Germany, 1979.

25. Madill, P.: Electroacupuncture: A true and legitimate preventative medicine. Am. J. Acupuncture, 7:279, 1979.
26. Madill, P., and Tiller, W.: The five areas of discoveries of German electroacupuncture or electroacupuncture according to Voll (E.A.V.). Am. J. Acupuncture (in press).
27. Voll, R.: The phenomenon of medicine testing in electroacupuncture according to Voll (E.A.V.). Am. J. Acupuncture, 8:22, 1980.
28. Boericke, W.: Pocket Manual of Homeopathic Materia Medica. New Delhi, India, B. Jain Publishers, 1976.
29. Randolph, G.: An Alternative Approach to Allergies. New York, Lippincott and Crowell, 1980.
30. Dickey, D.: Clinical Ecology. Springfield, Ill., Charles C Thomas, 1976.
31. Madill, P.: First, doctor to the whole body. E.A.V. and the cause of holistic dentistry. Am. J. Acupuncture, 8:299, 1980.
32. Rane, H.: Vagrant Buccal Currents from Dental Filling Materials: The Use of the Potentiometer in the Electroacupuncture Dental and Medical Practice (Privately published).
33. Bauer, J., and Fist, H.: The toxicity of mercury in dental amalgam. J. Califor. Dent. Assoc., June, 1982, p. 47.
34. Nilner, K.: Electrochemical Action in the Oral Cavity. Swedish Dental Journal. Supplement 9, 1981.
35. Thomsen, J: The frequent involvement of "vital teeth" in focus disturbances. Am. J. Acupuncture, 8:44, 1980.
36. Thomsen, J.: Energetic remote effects of odontons on organs measured by electroacupuncture (E.A.V.). Am. J. Acupuncture, 9:63, 1980.
37. Voll, R.: Electroacupuncture (E.A.V.) diagnosis and treatment results in odontogenous focus events. Am. J. Acupuncture, 9:293, 1980.

22

Functional Jaw Orthopedics: Mastering More Than Technique

JOHN W. WITZIG, D.D.S.
IRA M. YERKES, D.M.D., M.S.

OBJECTIVES OF ORTHODONTICS

In modern orthodontics, the total patient must be considered, not just the teeth. Therefore, the face, the teeth, and a functional occlusion, without TMJ problems afterward, must be considered in the diagnosis and treatment plan for each patient.

In a sense, the goals of modern orthodontics can be distilled to four principles:
1. Pleasing *face*.
2. Attractive *full smile*.
3. *No TMJ problems*.
4. *No relapse* later.

RECENT DEVELOPMENTS IN ORTHODONTICS—THE NEW TREATMENT MODALITIES

Unfortunately, more is required than mastering the technical aspects of fixed appliances in order to successfully practice orthodontics today. To achieve these objectives, the practitioner must also possess a firm background in both functional jaw orthopedics (FJO) and temporomandibular joint (TMJ) treatment. This chapter will deal with several important issues that are frequently overlooked. These include the importance of tracing and treating cause as well as effect and the necessity of supplementing many traditional therapies with new techniques.

It is in the best interest of the patient for the doctor to examine these issues thoroughly. Even if you now think that you are doing everything possible for your patients, read on.

THE ONE HUNDREDTH MONKEY PHENOMENON

There is an interesting phenomenon recorded by Lyall Watson in his book *Lifetide*,[1] reprinted by Avrom King in *Nexus*. King says, "In it may lie our only hope for the future of our species."[2]

The Japanese monkey, *Macaca fusata,* has been observed in the wild for a period of over 30 years. In 1952, on the island of Koshima, scientists were providing monkeys with sweet potatoes that were dropped in the sand, a new food previously unknown to the monkeys. The monkeys liked the taste of the raw sweet potatoes, but they found the grit unpleasant.

An 18-month-old female named Imo found she could solve the problem by washing the potatoes in a nearby stream. In monkey terms, this is a cultural revolution almost comparable to the invention of the wheel. It involves abstraction, the identification of concept and deliberate manipulation of the environment. She taught this trick to her mother. Her playmates also learned this new way and they taught their mothers, too.

This cultural innovation was gradually picked up by various monkeys before the eyes of the scientists. Between 1952 and 1958, all the young monkeys learned to wash the sandy sweet potatoes to make them more palatable. Only the adults who imitated their children learned this social improvement. Other adults kept eating dirty sweet potatoes.

Then something startling took place. In the autumn of 1958, a certain number of Koshima monkeys were washing sweet potatoes—the exact number is not known. Let us suppose that when the sun rose one morning there were 99 monkeys on Koshima Island who had learned to wash their sweet potatoes. Let's further suppose that later that morning, The Hundredth Monkey learned to wash potatoes.

Then it happened: By that evening almost everyone in the tribe was washing sweet potatoes before eating them. The added energy of this hundreth monkey somehow created an idealogical breakthrough.

But notice. The most surprising thing observed by these scientists was that the habit of washing sweet potatoes then spontaneously jumped over the sea. Colonies of monkeys at Takasakiyama began washing their sweet potatoes.

Thus, when a certain critical number achieves an awareness, this new awareness may be communicated from mind to mind. Although the exact number may vary, The Hundreth Monkey Phenomenon means that when only a limited number of people know of a new way, it may remain the conscious property of these people. But there is a point at which if only one more person tunes in to a new awareness, a field is strengthened so that this awareness reaches almost everyone.[1]

FUNCTIONAL JAW ORTHOPEDICS AND
TEMPOROMANDIBULAR JOINT THERAPY TODAY

This chapter will set out to describe why orthodontics has not yet reached the end point in the One Hundredth Monkey Phenomenon. Although the number of FJO and TMJ proponents is growing daily, these new treatment methods have yet to gain general acceptance. You, the reader, might prove to be that one more person that makes all the difference.

Some background on the history of the newer appliances and their application may be helpful here in illustrating why these newer forms of treatment have yet to gain total acceptance. One of the best brief summaries explaining this is given by Graber and Neumann.[3]

Before and after World War II, when the development of modern removable appliances was just beginning, the number of trained orthodontists in Europe was negligible. Active plates and activators, introduced mainly in the Germanic-speaking parts of the continent, were very simple devices. Since for socio-economic reasons there had been no way to treat an appreciable portion of the child population, the new possibilities aroused great enthusiasm and the results achieved were grossly overestimated and judged prematurely.

In Great Britain, the sudden expansion of the responsibilities of the Dental Health Service, which included orthodontic treatment, necessitated that it be done by the rank and file of the profession. Quite understandably, the results of these activities on both sides of the English Channel did not appeal to American orthodontists. The opinion became firmly entrenched that removable appliances are vastly inferior and not worth studying at all. Second rate service with removable appliances in the hands of orthodontically unqualified dentists in the United States and Canada strongly supported this prejudgment.[3]

This attitude was responsible for retarding the growth of the use of the newer appliances in the United States for many years.

THE FIRST STEP—DEBUNKING THE MYTH OF THE PROTRUDED MAXILLA

Although documented studies have shown the effectiveness of functional appliances in patient treatment, many practitioners are hesitant to use them for another reason not yet mentioned—the long-held belief that mandibles cannot "grow." Some growth does take place at the head of the condyle with the use of functional appliances. This growth is limited by age and mandibular position, however. The most logical explanation for the "growth" where the mandible is concerned it is not growth at all, but merely the reposturing of the mandible for a long enough duration to allow muscle and joint changes to take place. This basic tenet of FJO and TMJ therapies is integral to the practitioner's success, and gains even greater importance when debunking the myth of the protruded maxilla.

A recent article by Luzi seriously questions the concept that there are fixed "ideal" SNA and SNB angles of 82° and 80°, respectively.[4] In traditional orthodontics, an SNA greater than 82° indicated a clear-cut protruded maxilla. Now, however, findings indicate that it is almost never the maxilla that is protruded (in fact, it is often retruded), but the mandible is retruded.

In Luzi's study, SNA and NSar angles were clearly found to vary in an inverse ratio (Fig. 22–1). The combined variation (CV) value is virtually constant at 205°, regardless of the SNA angle. Because of this unique relationship, the conclusion may be drawn that it is the maxilla that is in harmony with its environment, as opposed to the mandible.[4]

This concurs with results of another study by Jarvinen,[5] and with the findings of Enlow, who wrote in his textbook that in most cases of Class II malocclusion, "it is not the maxilla itself that 'protrudes,' rather it is the mandible that is actually retrusive."[6]

Luzi, in his article, gives an example of how this new knowledge of the CV value may be applied in analyzing patient problems:

We are dealing with a Class II malocclusion and find an SNA angle of 85 degrees with an SNB angle of 80 degrees (ANB = +5 degrees). If we limit our research to these data, we could jump to the conclusion that the large SNA angle is responsible for the Class II situation and decide to reduce its size. However, if we look at the NSar angle and find a value of 119.3 degrees, for example, which together with SNA

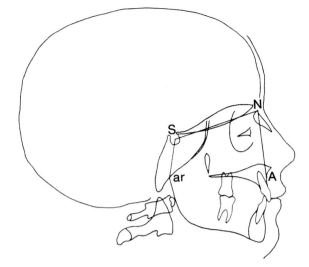

Figure 22–1. Cephalometric landmarks. *Ar,* Articulare; *S,* sella turcica; *N,* nasion; *A,* Downs' point A.[4]

gives a CV of 204.3 degrees, we may question whether there is truly a maxillary protrusion. Maybe for the given saddle angle (smaller than the average value) the large SNA angle is well adjusted and an SNB angle of 80 degrees is smaller than needed, in which case a larger mandible would be more appropriate.[4]

Once this relationship is viewed in a new light, it becomes more important than ever that we as professionals have the ability to reposition the mandible forward (Luzi's "larger mandible"). Let us examine the causes behind the retruded mandible to determine if they shed further light on the subject.

MANDIBULAR RETRUSION

There are two primary causes of mandibular retrusion. These are forward head position as a result of an impaired airway and insufficient posterior alveolar bone growth indirectly caused by one of the three universal responses to stress. Let us investigate the situation that arises as the head travels forward first.

Rocabado, a Chilean physical therapist, clearly states that the position of the hyoid bone is directly related to the cranial, mandibular, or cervical spine regions.[7]

The hyoid bone, the only one in the body not directly attached to another bone, plays a key role in the body's skeletal structure through its unique relationship with these other regions.

Until the age of 3 years, any number of common airway problems, including large tonsils and adenoids, abnormal anatomical variations in nasal passages, and allergies, can influence this key bone's future position and the individual's overall posture (Fig. 22–2).

In compensating for a diminished airway, the patient brings the head forward, thus increasing air flow through the mouth rather than breathing through the nose. This single development, the forward positioning of the head, has a profound effect upon the patient's mandible.

It has long been accepted that lowered tongue position, which occurs spontaneously with nonnasal breathing, causes maxillary constriction and

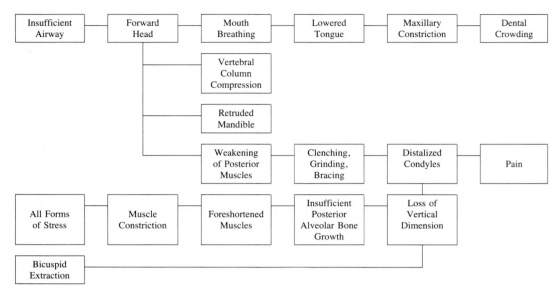

Figure 22–2.

long face syndrome.[8] What is a relatively new concept, however, is the belief that the tongue's new lowered position and the resultant maxillary constriction are both direct results of forward head position.

The mandible and face are further stressed by the effect that the forward head has on the rest of the body. As the head travels forward, the mandible, which is attached to the chest through the hyoid region, retrudes in direct relation to the head position; the farther forward the head is, the more retruded the mandible becomes.

In his same article, Rocabado illustrates what occurs when the head is positioned correctly:

"The functioning of the suprahyoid as it induces tension to the mandible can be observed during normal orthostatic posture (a well-balanced head directly on top of the spinal column),* when the head relies on equal anterior and posterior muscle tension. The craniovertebral joints will remain equally balanced toward the cranium through tensile forces produced by normal function of the supra- and infrahyoid muscles.[7]

Unfortunately, this harmonious balance is not found when the head is positioned forward. Because of the increased relative weight of the head, the posterior muscles begin to weaken. In time, the anterior muscles are also affected. Additionally, two other phenomena occur as the net effect of forward head. The condyles are displaced more distally into the fossa and spinal column compression results in spinal nerve entrapment. The more forward the head, the farther distal the condyles move and the greater the spinal column compression that results.

Thirty-five years ago, Dr. Victor Stoll recognized this cause-and-effect relationship, highlighting it in his report.[9] He noted, "When a part of the body, e.g., the mandible, assumes an abnormal position in relation to the rest of the body, it upsets the correct postural maintenance of the body against gravity. And in order to maintain equilibrium and balance, it calls upon one set of muscles to function at the expense of another.[9]

---

*Rocabado's definition of normal orthostatic posture.

Once the posterior muscles begin to weaken as a result of forward head, the elevator and masticatory muscles come into play, assuming the responsibility for maintaining the body's balance. This action is seen as clenching, constriction, or even mild bracing. The results prevent the patient from achieving normal rest position of the mandible, one of the primary goals of successful facial pain treatment.

THE ROLE STRESS PLAYS IN MANDIBULAR RETRUSION

In his classic text, Dr. Hans Selye describes three universal responses to stress: muscle constriction, lessened resistance to disease, and shutdown somewhere in the gastrointestinal system.[10] Close study of the Funt Symptom Index (an evolutionary, progressive, and cumulative clinical pattern based on symptoms documented in craniomandibular pain patients) leads to the plausible explanation that muscle constriction, one of these three responses, leads to decreased vertical dimension, resulting in teeth being unable to erupt fully into the mouth. In turn, this long-term overclosure and lack of posterior alveolar bone growth result in additional shortening of muscles and distally displaced condyles. This harsh change in maxillary-mandibular relationship ultimately induces many of the signs and symptoms associated with TMJ dysfunction.[11]

According to Eversaul, the catalyst for this action can be any one of a variety of stressful situations. In using the term "stress," he refers to situations that encompass more than the usual definition of stress, which is too commonly perceived as only emotional duress. Eversaul's definition of stress refers to the total body. Diet, environment, physical structure, and dental work can all play key roles in the development of stressful situations.[12]

The muscle constriction and the ensuing decreased length of muscles conspire once again to prevent the patient from achieving normal rest position—the rest position needed for a healthy oral environment.

MANDIBULAR RETRUSION—BREEDING GROUND FOR PROBLEMS

When the oral environment degenerates to this point, the patient becomes a prime candidate for any one of a variety of facial pain–related problems. These include "muscle spasm, emotional stress, dental malocclusion, facial neuralgias, the arthritides, trauma, infection, neoplasm, ear and sinus disorders, salivary gland disease, congenital deformitiés, vascular disorders, and postural discrepancies," according to Shaber.[13] He concludes that out of all these symptoms, "*the single most prevalent common denominator of facial pain (myofacial pain–dysfunction syndrome): muscle spasm* [italics added].[13]

FALL OF THE RATIONAL MODEL

Because of the direct connection between forward head and decreased vertical dimension as a result of stress—both of which lead to mandibular retrusion—the practitioner can no longer treat patients as in the past. Peters and Waterman describe this phenomenon as follows:

What exactly do we mean by the fall of the rational model? Scientists in any field and in any time possess a set of shared beliefs about the world, and for that time the set constitutes the dominant paradigm. Experiments are carried out strictly within the boundaries of those beliefs and small steps towards progress are made. An old but excellent example is the Ptolemic view of the universe (which held until the sixteenth century) that the earth was at the center of the universe. After a paradigm shift begins, progress is fast though fraught with tension. People get angry. New discoveries pour in to support the new belief system. The important point in each instance is that the old "rationality" is eventually replaced with a new, different, and more useful one.[14] [Figure 22–3]

Even if the technology to replace the past is not yet fully developed, it would be impossible to go on as before. That is what we are beginning to see in our profession today.

> rational model = bicuspid extraction
> paradigm shift = move from traditional orthodontics to supplementing traditional
> methods with newer appliances

Figure 22–3.

THE END OF BICUSPID EXTRACTION

It is of extreme importance in orthodontics that nothing is done in treatment to move the mandible or condyle distally. Of equal importance, nothing should be done to the patient to cause loss of vertical dimension. This could move the condyle into a displaced position off the articular disc and onto the weaker fibrous tissue, reducing in size the necessary critical 3 mm. space required for proper tissue function posterior to the condyle (Fig. 22–4). This fibrous tissue contains the nerves and blood vessels supplying the nutrition to the TMJ.

Pressure on the fibrous tissue not only will cause pain but also will lead to disturbances of the circulation (Fig. 22–5). This in turn leads to degeneration of the disc and the fibrous covering of the articulating bones. Pressure can come only from the condylar head.

Because of these reasons, the following three causes of a pathological position of the condyle in the TMJ must be avoided in orthodontic treatment:

1. *Retracted upper anterior teeth after bicuspid extraction.* Retraction can move the condyle into a pathological position and cause loss of vertical dimension by the bicuspid extractions.

2. *Deep overbite* (loss of vertical dimension). A severe loss of vertical dimension occurs with bicuspid extractions and contraction of the dental arches. The loss of vertical dimension should be avoided for normal, healthy TMJ.

3. *Class II, division II malocclusion improperly treated.* As these patients always have deep overbites, it is essential that bicuspids are not removed, which would cause further loss of vertical dimension.

With this realization, the removal of biscupids becomes a thing of the past, since their extraction is no longer advisable. New doors of treatment options are opened once the problem is correctly identified as one of total

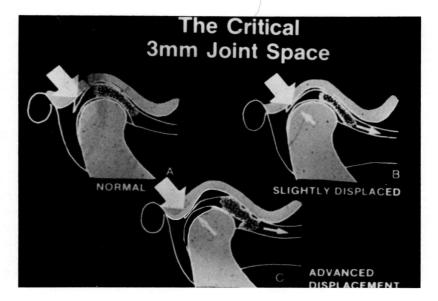

Figure 22–4.

oral environment as opposed to incorrect tooth placement. Too many patients have been left with TMJ pathology, circulation problems, headaches, and facial changes.

If there is a need for removal of tooth structure, there is a reasonable alternative to bicuspid extraction, namely, second molar replacement. The advantages of second molar replacement are readily apparent. Not only will such replacement actually preserve vertical dimension, but in addition it will actually increase it. (This does not apply to younger patients being treated with a Frankel appliance, in whom the goal of 32 teeth is not an unreasonable one.) Long-term results of second molar replacement are a healthy TMJ, finest facial esthetics, a beautiful, full smile, and excellent stability. By utilizing second molar replacement the patient has the potential of having 28 teeth as opposed to 24. How often have we seen third molars removed years after the completion of bicuspid therapy?

Figure 22–5.

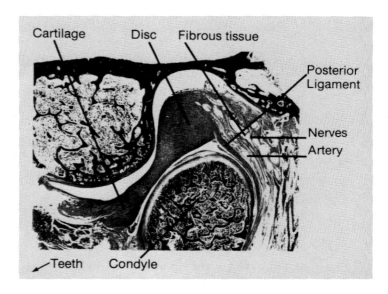

FUNCTIONAL JAW ORTHOPEDICS—A REASONABLE ALTERNATIVE

Mechanically, the solution of the problem is obvious. When necessary, especially in cases of deep overbite, the mandible should be established in a more forward position to meet the upper teeth correctly and permit proper use of the adjacent soft tissues in addition to other benefits.[9]

This correct assumption was made more than 35 years ago by Dr. Stoll. However, at the time his article was published, it was impossible to facilitate the changes he was discussing.

The advent of functional appliances has made it possible to effect changes in the mouth now that were not thought possible even 10 years ago. The bulk of the success that removable appliances have achieved, however, must be attributed to the body's own unique capabilities. In their studies, Carlson and McNamara have demonstrated that muscles stretched beyond their normal length will reattach closer to their optimal length.[15] This makes it possible to reposition the retruded mandible by "retraining" muscles that have been shortened in response to stress or affected by the position of the head.

Through the use of functional appliances, all of the goals of orthodontic treatment may be achieved: (1) pleasing face, (2) attractive, full smile, (3) no TMJ problems, and (4) no relapse later.

THE RELATIONSHIP OF FUNCTIONAL APPLIANCES TO OTHER TREATMENT TECHNIQUES IN THE FUTURE

In order to achieve the best results, functional appliances must be used in conjunction with some traditional orthodontic techniques. In some patients, for instance, teeth will still be uneven after treatment with the newer appliances and need brackets to reposition them.

But even combining these two disciplines may not be enough, nor should it be. Because of the intimate and direct relationship between head position, posture, and the mandible, oral problems cannot be treated effectively without taking these factors into account. Posture not only is a leading factor in the creation of TMJ problems, it must also be a factor in their solution. This can best be facilitated through the use of physical therapy and nonforce chiropractic techniques to retrain the body in posture.

Some of the leading factors of stress, such as diet, must also be investigated when treating a patient. Perhaps behavior modification or changes in diet may be necessary as well.

It is to be hoped, however, that we will continue to search for new answers to provide even more effective treatment.

WHAT IT MEANS TO YOU

The future of functional jaw orthopedics was best stated by King:

The phenomenon of functional jaw orthopedics will not disappear. There are vast cultural and clinical and competitive pressures already in motion which give an importance to what's happening that cannot be denied. You need not choose to participate, but you cannot avoid being touched.[20]

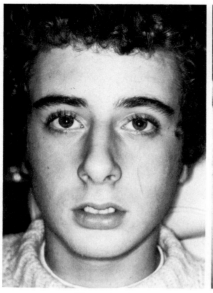

Figure 22–6.

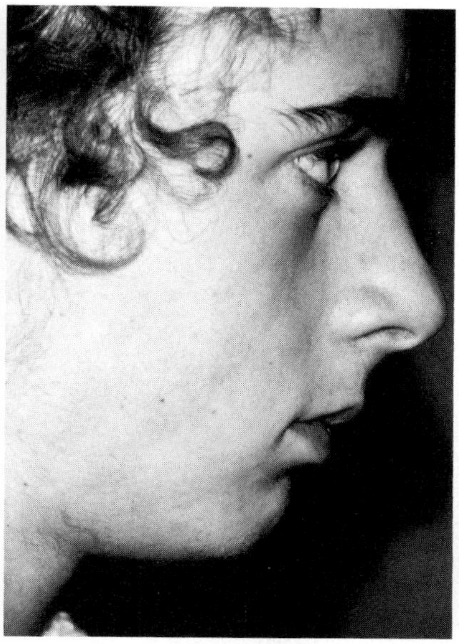

Figure 22–7.

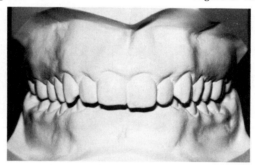

Figure 22–8.

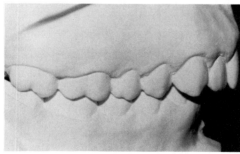

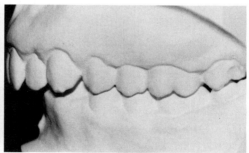

Figure 22–9.

Figure 22–10.

Case 1 (Figs. 22–6 to 22–10)

>*Before treatment*: Age 15 years, 10 months
>*Treatment*: 1. Second molar replacement (upper only)
>2. 6 months upper sagittal appliance
>3. 20 months bionator appliance
>4. NO RETENTION

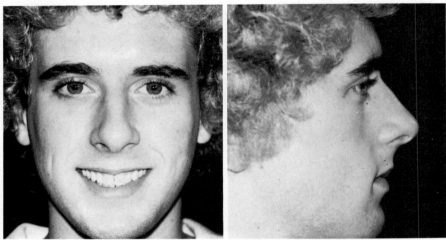

Figure 22–11.   Figure 22–12.

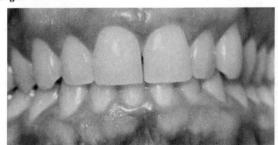

Figure 22–13.

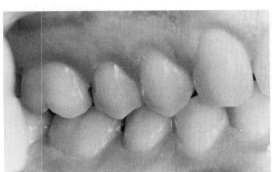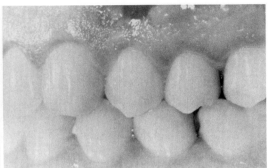

Figure 22–14.

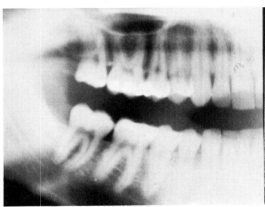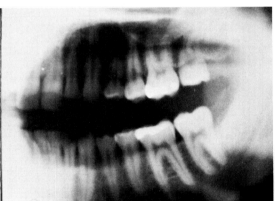

Figure 22–15.   **Figure 22–16.**

Case 1 (Figs. 22–11 to 22–16)

After photography: One year no appliances
Panorex x-ray one year after treatment showing upper third molars replacing upper second molars.

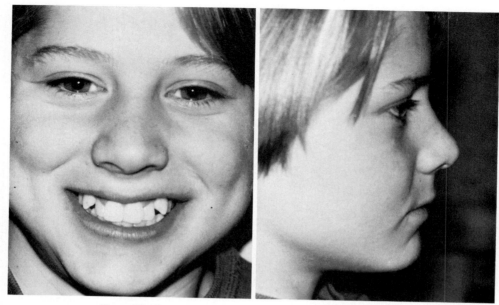

Figure 22–17.   **Figure 22–18.**

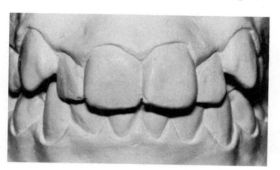

Figure 22–19.

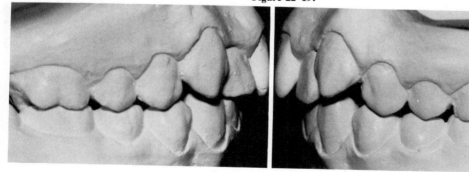

Figure 22–20.   **Figure 22–21.**

Case 2 (Figs. 22–17 to 22–21)

Before treatment: Age 14 years, 5 months

Crowding, blocked out cuspids, skeletal class II

Treatment: 1. Second molar replacement
2. 6 months upper sagittal appliance
3. 5 months upper bonded brackets
4. NO RETENTION

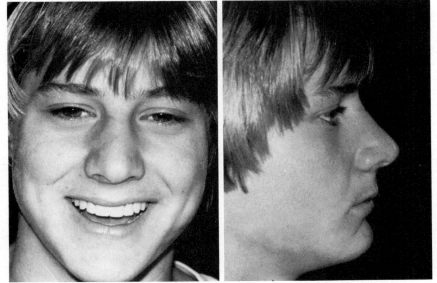

Figure 22–22.   Figure 22–23.

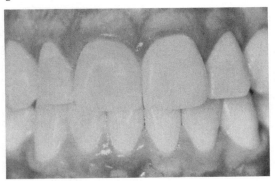

Figure 22–24.

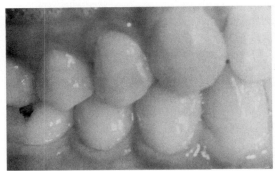   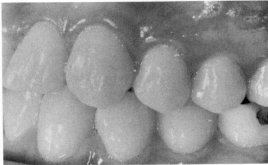

Figure 22–25.   Figure 22–26.

Case 2 (Figs. 22–22 to 22–26)

Photography: One year after all appliances removed

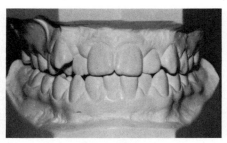

Figure 22–27.

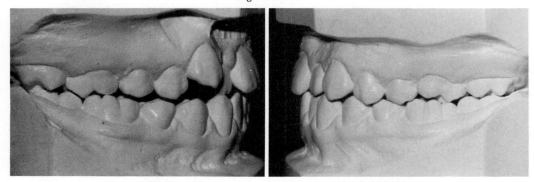

Figure 22–28.   **Figure 22–29.**

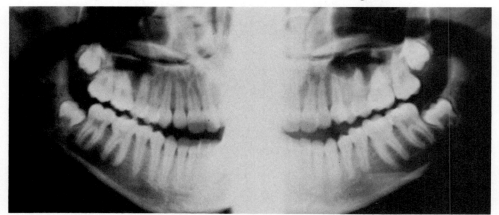

Figure 22–30.

Case 3 (Figs. 22–27 to 22–30)

Preorthodontic treatment by *another* orthodontic office

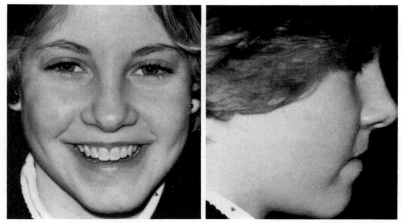

Figure 22–31.

Figure 22–32.

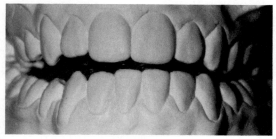

Figure 22–33.

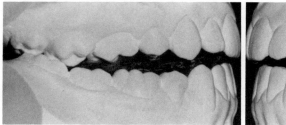

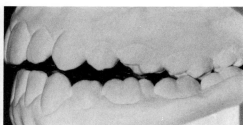

Figure 22–34.

Figure 22–35.

Case 3 (Figs. 22–31 to 22–37)

First appointment with Dr. Witzig for TMJ pain and headaches.

History: Age 16 years, 3 months
    4 bicuspids extracted
    2 years fixed appliances
    Class III elastics
    Vertical elastics—upper and lower anterior teeth
    1½ years positioner

Complaint: 1. TMJ pain
     2. Headaches
     3. Difficulty chewing
     4. Open bite
     5. Clicking and locking of both temporomandibular joints

Arthrogram x-ray: Left TMJ—internal derangement, late stages

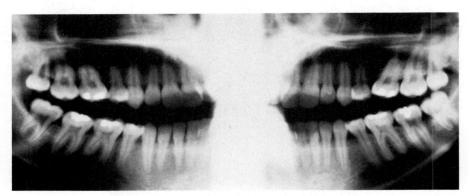

Figure 22–36.

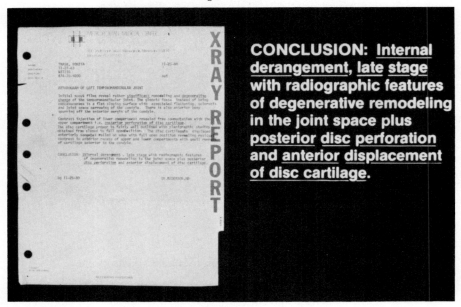

Figure 22–37.

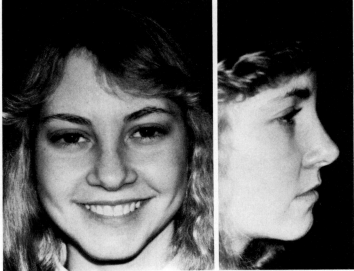

Figure 22–38.   **Figure 22–39.**

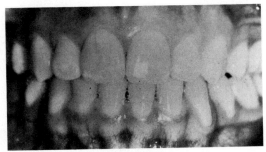

Figure 22–40.

Case 3 (Figs. 22–38 to 22–40)

Completion of Dr. Witzig's TMJ treatment.

After Retreatment: 1. Upper second molar replacement
                2. Lower third molars removed
                3. Crossbite correction
                4. Upper anteriors moved labially to relieve incisal interference and retruded mandible
                5. Surgery to reduce the mandible and incisal interference and to allow the condyle to move forward in the joint
                6. Final tooth positioning with straight wire appliance

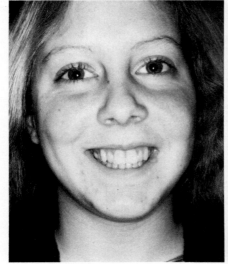

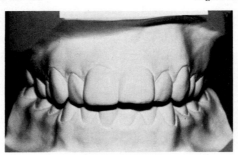

Figure 22–41.   Figure 22–42.

Figure 22–43.

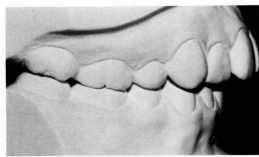

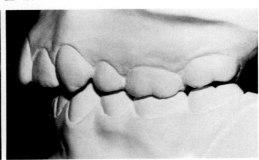

Figure 22–44.   Figure 22–45.

Case 4 (Figs. 22–41 to 22–45)

After conventional orthodontic treatment
First appointment for retreatment by Dr. Witzig
History: Age 16 years, 7 months
        4 years fixed bands, headgear, elastics
        4 bicuspids extracted
        4 third molars extracted
        9 months retainers
Complaint: 1. Overjet returning
        2. Upper anterior crowding
        3. TMJ problems
Retreatment: 1. 5 months upper sagittal appliance
        2. 13 months upper sagittal daytime appliance, bionator home appliance
        3. NO RETENTION

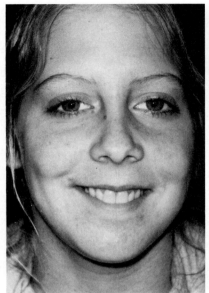
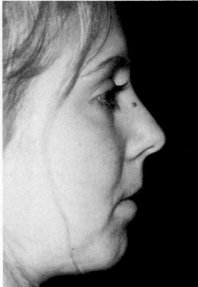

Figure 22–46.   **Figure 22–47.**

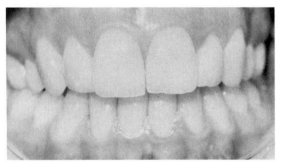

Figure 22–48.

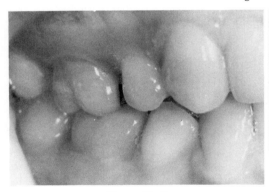

Figure 22–49.   **Figure 22–50.**

Case 4 (Figs. 22–46 to 22–50)

After Photography: 3 years out of all appliances
                    TMJ pain and headache symptoms eliminated
                    Overjet corrected

References

1. Watson, L.: Lifetide. New York, Bantam Books, 1980.
2. King, A.: Nexus, Book IX, Chapter 10. Cave Creek, Arizona, The Nexus Group, Inc., 1983.
3. Graber, T., and Neumann, B.: Removable Orthodontic Appliances. Philadelphia, W. B. Saunders Co., 1977.
4. Luzi, V.: CV value in analysis of sagittal malocclusions. Am. J. Orthod., *81*:478, 1982.
5. Jarvinen, S.: Relation of the SNA angle to the saddle angle. Am. J. Orthod., 78:670, 1980.
6. Enlow, D.: Handbook of Facial Growth. Philadelphia, W. B. Saunders Co., 1978.
7. Rocabado, M.: Biomechanical relationship of the cranial, cervical and hyoid regions. Cranio-Mandibular Pract., *1*:61, 1983.
8. McNamara, J.: Naso-respiratory function and craniofacial growth. Craniofacial Growth Series, Monograph Number 9. Ann Arbor, The University of Michigan, 1979.
9. Stoll, V.: Abstract Lecture delivered before the New Organization Alumni Association, April 22, 1948.
10. Selye, H.: The Stress of Life. New York, McGraw-Hill Book Company, 1978.
11. Gelb, H., and Tarte, J.: A two year clinical dental evaluation of 200 cases of chronic headache: The craniocervical-mandibular syndrome. JADA, *91*:1230, 1975.
12. Eversaul, G.: Dental Kinesiology Text. Los Vegas, Nevada, 1977 (privately published).
13. Shaber, E.: Considerations in the Treatment of Muscle Spasm. Diseases of the Temporomandibular Apparatus. St. Louis, C. V. Mosby Co., 1982.
14. Peters, T., and Waterman, R.: In Search of Excellence. New York, Harper and Row, 1982.
15. Carlson, D., and McNamara, J.: Muscle Adaptation in the Craniofacial Region. Craniofacial Growth Series, Monograph Number 8. Ann Arbor, The University of Michigan, 1978.
16. King, A.: Economic and Behavioral Aspects of Functional Appliances. Cassette Series. Cave Creek, Arizona, The Nexus Group, Inc., 1983.

23

Conclusion

HAROLD GELB, D.M.D

This book was written primarily to bring to the attention of the health professions new information and a better understanding of the multidisciplinary approach to pain and dysfunction of the head, neck, and jaws.

The space age has made us aware that nature itself recognizes no boundaries, and that to continue isolating the various branches of science is a serious obstacle to scientific progress. It is particularly true in both medicine and dentistry that the limited view through the eyes of one discipline is no longer enough. The solution then, is not further fragmentation into increasingly isolated specialties, disciplines, and departments, but the integration of science and scientific knowledge for the enrichment of all branches. Then and only then will those patients, estimated at 30 per cent of the population, suffering from craniomandibular disorders be properly diagnosed and treated.

Since this problem is so complex and the solution relatively obscure to the untrained dental and medical practitioners, it is strongly recommended that we avail ourselves of the teaching and experience already accumulated in this area of practice. Various clinics and their experienced staffs have devoted untold hours in searching for and achieving the alleviation of pain and discomfort for this and other surprisingly common pain disorders. They are ready to offer their knowledge and services to all of us, just for the asking. One of the first and most successful has been that at the University of Washington School of Medicine, headed by Dr. John J. Bonica. Dr. Bonica, who has lectured before many professional groups and at various pain symposia, has superbly outlined the reasons for deficiencies in the management of chronic pain. Although this information was first presented over seven years ago, many of the problems still exist today. His outline is presented below:

1. Insufficient knowledge of chronic pain states
   A. New information acquired from studies of acute pain not very useful for chronic pain patients
      1. Basic scientists not concerned with clinical pain
      2. Experimental animal and human studies led to hypotheses not valid to chronic pain

  B. Inadequate studies of chronic pain states
  1. Difficulties in studying human pathologic pain
  2. Lack of animal models for chronic pain states
  3. Lack of multidisciplinary (team) approach essential to productive research
  C. Inadequate interest in and support for pain research
  1. Only few scientists and clinicians interested in pain research
  2. Insufficient funds for pain research
  3. Only few pain research training programs
  4. Above factors ⟶ insufficient research
  Manpower ⟶ insufficient applications
  ⟶ insufficient funds appropriated
  ⟶ vicious circle
  D. All aforementioned factors ⟶ meager information about chronic pain mechanisms ⟶ inadequate or incorrect therapy
 II. Improper application of knowledge
  A. Little or no teaching of medical and dental students or practitioners
  1. Taught to use pain as diagnostic tool only
  2. Little knowledge of principles of diagnosis and therapy of chronic pain states
  B. Areas managed by patient's physician
  1. Unable to devote sufficient time for comprehensive workup
  a. Frequently incorrect or no diagnosis
  b. Prescription of drugs and other empirical therapy
  2. Inadequate use of consultants
  C. Specialization conducive to "tubular" vision
  1. Chronic pain viewed from perspective of each specialty
  D. Inadequate communication/integration of patient's data
  E. Above factors ⟶ iatrogenic complications
III. Inadequate communications systems
  A. Little or no communication among basic scientists
  1. New information published in highly specialized journals limited to one discipline
  2. Little or no cross-fertilization in the dissemination of information
  B. Little or no communication between scientists and clinicians
  1. Inadequate appreciation between scientists and clinicians
  2. Lag in applying new knowledge to patient care
  C. Lack of universally accepted definition and classification of pain syndromes
  D. Lack of uniform records and retrieval systems; no accurate data on incidence, efficacy of therapy, etc.
  E. Above factors preclude exchange of scientific and clinical data

In all fairness, it must be stated that many new pain centers and clinics have become operational since the first edition of this book was published. Many medical and dental schools have created pain clinics within their health centers. Unfortunately, not enough of the information collected clinically or as a result of basic science research has filtered down to the undergraduate and graduate students.

It is our hope and prayer that the time will soon be at hand when well-trained and experienced medical, dental, osteopathic, and other related health professionals will be integrated staff members of a comprehensive chronic pain center (head, neck, jaw, and low back).

The analyses, conclusions and hypotheses that have been advanced in this book are not the last word on the subject of pain and dysfunction of the head, neck, and jaws. Let us just say they are but a modest positive beginning.

An excellent jumping-off point for further clinical observation and research would be the analysis of the evolution of craniomandibular disorders shown on the following page.

THE F-S INDEX*
OF THE
CRANIOMANDIBULAR PAIN SYNDROME

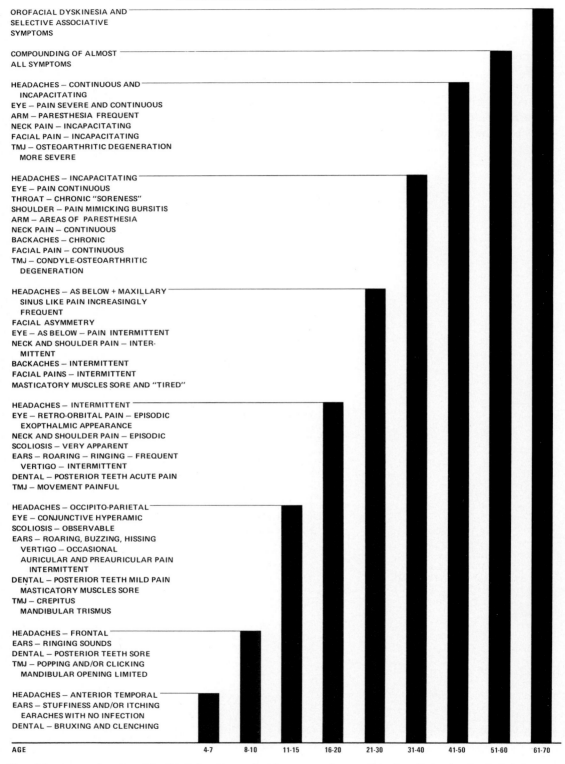

OROFACIAL DYSKINESIA AND
SELECTIVE ASSOCIATIVE
SYMPTOMS

COMPOUNDING OF ALMOST
ALL SYMPTOMS

HEADACHES — CONTINUOUS AND
   INCAPACITATING
EYE — PAIN SEVERE AND CONTINUOUS
ARM — PARESTHESIA FREQUENT
NECK PAIN — INCAPACITATING
FACIAL PAIN — INCAPACITATING
TMJ — OSTEOARTHRITIC DEGENERATION
   MORE SEVERE

HEADACHES — INCAPACITATING
EYE — PAIN CONTINUOUS
THROAT — CHRONIC "SORENESS"
SHOULDER — PAIN MIMICKING BURSITIS
ARM — AREAS OF PARESTHESIA
NECK PAIN — CONTINUOUS
BACKACHES — CHRONIC
FACIAL PAIN — CONTINUOUS
TMJ — CONDYLE-OSTEOARTHRITIC
   DEGENERATION

HEADACHES — AS BELOW + MAXILLARY
   SINUS LIKE PAIN INCREASINGLY
   FREQUENT
FACIAL ASYMMETRY
EYE — AS BELOW — PAIN INTERMITTENT
NECK AND SHOULDER PAIN — INTER-
   MITTENT
BACKACHES — INTERMITTENT
FACIAL PAINS — INTERMITTENT
MASTICATORY MUSCLES SORE AND "TIRED"

HEADACHES — INTERMITTENT
EYE — RETRO-ORBITAL PAIN — EPISODIC
   EXOPTHALMIC APPEARANCE
NECK AND SHOULDER PAIN — EPISODIC
SCOLIOSIS — VERY APPARENT
EARS — ROARING — RINGING — FREQUENT
   VERTIGO — INTERMITTENT
DENTAL — POSTERIOR TEETH ACUTE PAIN
TMJ — MOVEMENT PAINFUL

HEADACHES — OCCIPITO-PARIETAL
EYE — CONJUNCTIVE HYPERAMIC
SCOLIOSIS — OBSERVABLE
EARS — ROARING, BUZZING, HISSING
   VERTIGO — OCCASIONAL
   AURICULAR AND PREAURICULAR PAIN
   INTERMITTENT
DENTAL — POSTERIOR TEETH MILD PAIN
   MASTICATORY MUSCLES SORE
TMJ — CREPITUS
   MANDIBULAR TRISMUS

HEADACHES — FRONTAL
EARS — RINGING SOUNDS
DENTAL — POSTERIOR TEETH SORE
TMJ — POPPING AND/OR CLICKING
   MANDIBULAR OPENING LIMITED

HEADACHES — ANTERIOR TEMPORAL
EARS — STUFFINESS AND/OR ITCHING
   EARACHES WITH NO INFECTION
DENTAL — BRUXING AND CLENCHING

AGE   4-7   8-10   11-15   16-20   21-30   31-40   41-50   51-60   61-70

*An evolutionary, progressive and cumulative clinical index pattern correlated from symptoms documented in craniomandibular pain patients by Dr. Lawrence A. Funt (Bethesda, Maryland) and Dr. Brendan C. Stack (Falls Church, Virginia) — Directors of the National Capital Center for Craniofacial Pain.

INDEX

Note: Page numbers in *italics* refer to illustrations; those followed by t indicate tables.